Public Health Law and Ethics

CALIFORNIA/MILBANK BOOKS ON HEALTH AND THE PUBLIC

Public Health Law and Ethics

A Reader
Revised and Updated Second Edition

Edited by Lawrence O. Gostin

UNIVERSITY OF CALIFORNIA PRESS
Berkeley · *Los Angeles* · *London*

THE MILBANK MEMORIAL FUND
New York

University of California Press, one of the most
distinguished university presses in the United States,
enriches lives around the world by advancing
scholarship in the humanities, social sciences,
and natural sciences. Its activities are supported
by the UC Press Foundation and by philanthropic
contributions from individuals and institutions.
For more information, visit www.ucpress.edu.

The Milbank Memorial Fund is an endowed
operating foundation that engages in nonpartisan
analysis, study, research, and communication on
significant issues in health policy. In the Fund's own
publications, in reports or books it publishes with
other organizations, and in articles it commissions
for publication by other organizations, the Fund
endeavors to maintain the highest standards for
accuracy and fairness. Statements by individual
authors, however, do not necessarily reflect opinions
or factual determinations of the Fund. For more
information, visit www.milbank.org.

University of California Press
Berkeley and Los Angeles, California

University of California Press, Ltd.
London, England

Library of Congress Cataloging-in-Publication Data

Public health law and ethics : a reader / edited by
    Lawrence O. Gostin. — Rev. and updated 2nd ed.
      p.   cm. — (California/Milbank books on health
and the public ; v. 4)
    Includes bibliographical references and index.
    ISBN 978-0-520-26192-1 (alk. paper)
    1. Public health laws—United States. 2. Public
health—Moral and ethical aspects. I. Gostin,
Lawrence O. (Lawrence Ogalthorpe) II. Milbank
Memorial Fund.
    KF3775.P83   2010
    344.73'04—dc22   2010007682

Manufactured in the United States of America

19 18 17 16 15 14 13 12 11 10
10 9 8 7 6 5 4 3 2 1

This book is printed on Cascades Enviro 100, a 100%
post consumer waste, recycled, de-inked fiber. FSC
recycled certified and processed chlorine free. It is
acid free, Ecologo certified, and manufactured by
BioGas energy.

Contents

Illustrations

PHOTOGRAPHS

FIGURES

Tables

Boxes

Foreword

The Milbank Memorial Fund is an endowed operating foundation that works to improve health by helping decision makers in the public and private sectors acquire and use the best available evidence to inform policy for health care and population health. The Fund has engaged in nonpartisan analysis, study, research, and communication about significant issues in health policy since its inception in 1905.

Public Health Law and Ethics: A Reader was the fourth of what are now twenty California/Milbank Books on Health and the Public. The publishing partnership between the Fund and the University of California Press encourages the synthesis and communication of findings from research and experience that could contribute to more effective health policy.

Now in its second edition, *Public Health Law and Ethics: A Reader* is intended as a stand-alone text for those in the interrelated fields of public health, law, and ethics, including scholars, students, practitioners, and the informed public; the *Reader* can also be used as a companion to *Public Health Law: Power, Duty, Restraint*, another book in the California/Milbank series. Containing mostly new material on timely and relevant issues that have been public health staples for years, each chapter offers a detailed commentary that defines a public health problem, frames the relevant questions, and introduces the selected readings, which are certain to provoke debate and informed discussion.

Larry Gostin has carefully chosen selections that explore issues such as emergency preparedness, chronic disease prevention, and the control of infectious disease. Together the selections provide a framework for rigorous analysis of the intersecting philosophical, political, economic, and jurisprudential dimensions of government intervention to ensure and improve population health.

Carmen Hooker Odom
President

Samuel L. Milbank
Chairman

Preface

The field of public health is typically regarded as a positivistic pursuit, and without doubt our understanding of the etiology and response to disease is heavily influenced by scientific inquiry. Public health policies, however, are shaped not only by science but also by ethical values, legal norms, and political oversight. *Public Health Law and Ethics: A Reader* probes and seeks to illuminate this complex interplay through a careful selection of government reports, scholarly articles, and court cases together with discussion and analysis of critical problems at the interface of law, ethics, and public health. This short preface explains the various ways to use the resources in the *Reader,* describes its organization, and acknowledges my colleagues who have supported this scholarly project.

AN ANTHOLOGY

Public Health Law and Ethics: A Reader, now in its second edition, is intended as an independent resource for scholars, students, practitioners, and the informed public. Each chapter offers a detailed commentary that defines a public health problem and frames the relevant questions. The commentary then introduces the selected reading and provides additional resources for readers interested in further pursuing the chapter's subject.

The *Reader* can also be used as a companion to *Public Health Law: Power, Duty, Restraint* (Berkeley: University of California Press; New York: Milbank Memorial Fund, 2d ed., 2008). That treatise offers a theory and definition of public health law, an explanation of its principal analytical methodologies, and an analysis of the major conflicts in public health theory and practice. The books are designed to be used together: the treatise provides a careful description and analysis of public health law, while the *Reader* offers cases and materials that provoke debate and informed discussion. Each provides resources for research, teaching academic courses and seminars, professional practice, and thinking about fascinating problems in public health theory and daily practice.

TEACHING PUBLIC HEALTH LAW: USING THE *READER* AND TREATISE

The purposes of the main treatise and the *Reader* are to aid scholarship, inform the public, and support teaching. Faculty in schools of law, public health, medicine, nursing, and public administration in the United States and abroad have adopted these books for courses and seminars on public health law and/or ethics and on related subjects. Some professors prefer to use the *Reader* alone in their classes. Others use both books, as I do at Georgetown University: the main text offers a scholarly but accessible description and analysis of the field, while the *Reader* provides supplemental materials and an introduction to public health ethics. Each chapter in the second edition of the *Reader* provides resources and reflections on the corresponding chapter in the treatise, enabling readers to easily transition back and forth between the books.

ORGANIZATION OF THE *READER*

The introductory chapter of the *Reader* explores the scope and content of the three fields that intersect in the theory and practice of public health—namely, public health, public health law, and public health ethics. The remainder of the volume is divided into four parts, complementing the organization of the accompanying treatise.

Part 1, "Foundations of Public Health Law and Ethics," contains two chapters—one on the public's health and the second on ethical values and risk regulation. These chapters cover the major concepts in the field of public health (e.g., prevention and the population perspective), ethics (e.g., paternalism and the harm principle), socioeconomic disparities, and the regulation of dangerous activities. Because Part 1 introduces readers to the central issues in the areas of public health law and ethics, these chapters diverge slightly in scope and organization from the corresponding treatise chapters.

Part 2, "The Law and the Public's Health," examines important doctrines and controversies in public health law. The powers and duties of the state in the area of public health and the limitations that our constitutional system places on the exercise of public health powers are addressed in chapters 3 and 4, respectively. The ensuing chapters in Part 2 focus on three areas that are key to the practice of public health law: administrative law, which delineates when an agency is allowed to directly regulate for the public's health (chapter 5); tort law, which indirectly regulates behavior through civil liability (chapter 6); and transnational law, which facilitates a globalized approach to public health (chapter 7). Chapter 7—covering international public health law, world trade law, and human rights—is new to the second edition.

Part 3, "Public Health and Civil Liberties in Conflict," addresses some of the major controversies and trade-offs involved in contemporary public health theory and practice. Chapter 8 discusses surveillance, public health research, and the right to privacy. The interplay between speech and behavior is explored in chapter 9, which looks at health communications and commercial speech against the backdrop of free expression. Chapters 10 and 11 discuss medical countermeasures (immunization, screening, and treatment) and public health strategies (isolation, quarantine, and community containment) for preventing and mitigating the spread of epidemic disease, and the effects of those measures and strategies on bodily integrity and liberty. Chapter 12 is a new chapter, which examines the regulation of businesses and the value of economic liberty.

Concluding reflections on the field of public health law are offered in Part 4, "The Future of the Public's Health." This part consists of chapter 13, which presents case studies on three of the most complex and important of today's public health challenges: bioterrorism and biosecurity, public health genomics, and obesity. The chapter highlights the various themes developed in the *Reader*—public health ethics, the interconnectedness between domestic and global health, and the effects of socioeconomic disparities on public health.

The second edition of this *Reader* contains mostly new materials;

they reflect the contemporary political significance of public health preparedness for emergencies, of the need to prevent chronic diseases that are exacerbated by poor diets and sedentary lifestyles, and of the inexorable spread of infectious and chronic diseases across national borders and regions.

THE *READER*'S OBJECTIVES

The *Reader* probes the interrelated fields of law and ethics and their application to problems affecting the public's health and safety. Its goal is to raise the most important and enduring issues in public health theory and practice. In so doing, it should provoke discussion and debate among students, scholars, practitioners, and policy makers. More importantly, the *Reader* provides a framework for rigorous analysis of the philosophical, political, economic, and jurisprudential dimensions of government intervention to ensure the health of the populace. Nothing is so important to the security and vibrancy of a nation as the well-being of its people.

A RENAISSANCE FOR PUBLIC HEALTH: ACKNOWLEDGING LEADERS

Historians may look at the early twenty-first century as a period of renaissance for public health law and ethics. The field of public health, now expressing its own identity and importance, is reemerging from the shadows of high-technology medicine. Government and the private sector are engaged in a broad set of initiatives to reinvigorate the field. The following list describes many of the important people and organizations that have made my work in national and global health possible, and endlessly fascinating.

The Milbank Memorial Fund and University of California Press jointly publish the treatise and the *Reader*. Daniel M. Fox, then president and now president emeritus of the Fund, and Lynne Withey, director of the Press, above all, have supported and nurtured my scholarship, for which I will always be grateful. I also want to thank the Fund's energetic and talented new president, Carmen Hooker Odom.

Since the publication of the previous edition, remarkable changes have taken place at my home institution. Georgetown University established the O'Neill Institute for National and Global Health Law with the mission of finding innovative solutions to the most complex and enduring problems, thereby enabling people in the United States and throughout the world to lead healthier and longer lives.

I had exceptional editorial and research assistance at the O'Neill Institute. Among the stellar students participating in the research team over several years were Ilina Chaudhuri, Brian A. Fox, Kristen Henderson, Meir Katz, Faiza Mathon-Mathieu, Victoria Ochanda, Morgan Rog, Alia Udhiri, Meagan Winters, and Stelios Xenakis. I want to especially thank a few talented students who played particularly valuable roles in researching and editing the book: Lauren Dunning, Nancy Fullmann, Aimee Kelley, Meredith Larson, Una Lee, and Kate Stewart. The book is much richer for their contributions. Also making valuable contributions to the research and editing effort were the current O'Neill Institute deputy director, Oscar Cabrera; the former deputy director, Ben Berkman; and several O'Neill Institute law fellows: Elenora Connors, John Kraemer, and Paula O'Brien. I want to express my particular gratitude to Susan Kim, who coordinated the final edits, updates, and revisions of the manuscript.

When I began work on the second edition, we had recently hired Katrina Pagonis as a fellow at the O'Neill Institute. Katrina, one of the most talented students I have ever had at Georgetown Law, had just finished her LL.M. at the Yale Law School and a federal District Court clerkship. It would be impossible to overstate the crucial role that she played, brilliantly working with me as a full partner in conceptualizing and writing this book. It is sad to have Katrina leave Georgetown, but she is going on to a bright academic future at Hamline University's Health Law Institute.

Finally, and most important, I express my love and devotion to my family: Jean, Bryn, and Kieran.

Lawrence O. Gostin
Linda D. and Timothy J. O'Neill Professor of Global Health Law
Faculty Director, O'Neill Institute for National and Global Health Law
Georgetown University Law Center
Washington, D.C.
January 2010

Conventions Used
in This Book

The excerpted materials in the *Reader* have been edited for clarity and length. These edits have been made carefully so as not to compromise the meaning or substance of the readings. My intent is to communicate the substance of the case or article, in the words of the author(s), without interfering with its readability. The following editing and other conventions have been used consistently throughout the volume.

Citations follow *The Chicago Manual of Style* (15th ed.). All original references or notes in the excerpts have been deleted, except where they support quotations. In those instances, the references have been added to the bibliography and are indicated within the text of the reading. Citations to and within court cases follow *Bluebook* style (18th ed.), as is usual for legal documents. The styling of headings and subheadings within articles or cases has been standardized, regardless of how they appear in the original text. The indications of deletions and insertions (ellipses and square brackets) follow standard editorial practice.

Abbreviations are spelled out in full at their first appearance in each chapter (e.g., Institute of Medicine [IOM]), unless the abbreviation is more common than the full form (e.g., AIDS); thereafter, the abbreviation is always used. A list of abbreviated terms is included in the front matter.

I welcome comments from readers about the comprehensiveness, readability, and clarity of the *Reader*. I would appreciate being informed if I have omitted major articles or cases important to public health law or ethics.

Abbreviations

ABATE	A Brotherhood against Totalitarian Enactments
ACET	Advisory Council for the Elimination of Tuberculosis
ACIP	Advisory Committee on Immunization Policy
ADA	American Dental Association
AMA	American Medical Association
AVIP	Anthrax Vaccine Immunization Program
BST	bovine somatotropin
CDC	Centers for Disease Control and Prevention
CEA	cost-effectiveness analysis
CLPH	Center for Law and the Public's Health
CSA	Controlled Substances Act
D&E	dilation and evacuation
DES	diethylstilbestrol
DG	director general
DHATs	dental health aide therapists
DHFS	Department of Health and Family Services
DHMH	Department of Health and Mental Hygiene
DoD	Department of Defense

DOT	directly observed therapy
EC	European Communities
EPA	Environmental Protection Agency
EPT	expedited partner therapy
EtO	ethylene oxide
FAAAA	Federal Aviation Administration Authorization Act of 1994
FCGH	Framework Convention on Global Health
FCTC	Framework Convention on Tobacco Control
FDA	Food and Drug Administration
FDCA	Food, Drug, and Cosmetic Act
FTC	Federal Trade Commission
GATT	Global Agreement on Trade in Services
GDP	gross domestic product
GDPpc	per capita gross domestic product
GOARN	Global Outbreak Alert and Response Network
HHS	[Department of] Health and Human Services
HIPAA	Health Insurance Portability and Accountability Act
HPV	human papillomavirus
ICCPR	International Covenant on Civil and Political Rights
ICESCR	International Covenant on Economic, Social, and Cultural Rights
IHR	International Health Regulations
IOM	Institute of Medicine
IRB	institutional review board
IRPOP	investment refinement combined with the public-order principle
KKI	Kennedy Krieger Institute
MDA	Medical Device Amendments
MDR	multidrug resistant
MDR-TB	multidrug-resistant tuberculosis
MMR	measles, mumps, and rubella
MSA	Master Settlement Agreement

MSEHPA	Model State Emergency Health Powers Act
MUSC	Medical University of South Carolina
NCDs	non-communicable diseases
NGO	nongovernmental organization
NLDC	New London Development Corporation
NVAC	National Vaccine Advisory Committee
NVICP	National Vaccine Injury Compensation Program
NYRSA	New York State Restaurant Association
ODWDA	Oregon Death with Dignity Act
OECD	Organisation for Economic Co-operation and Development
OSHA	Occupational Safety and Health Administration
PEPFAR	President's Emergency Plan for AIDS Relief
PHC	Public Health Council
PHI	Protected Health Information
PI	principal investigator
PLCAA	Protection of Lawful Commerce in Arms Act
rBST	recombinant bovine somatotropin
RICO	Racketeer Influenced and Corrupt Organizations
RWJF	Robert Wood Johnson Foundation
SARS	severe acute respiratory syndrome
SES	socioeconomic status
SPS	Agreement on Sanitary and Phytosanitary Measures
STD	sexually transmitted disease
STI	sexually transmitted infection
TB	tuberculosis
TRIPS	Trade-Related Aspects of Intellectual Property Rights
UDHR	Universal Declaration of Human Rights
WHO	World Health Organization
WTO	World Trade Organization
XDR-TB	extensively drug-resistant tuberculosis

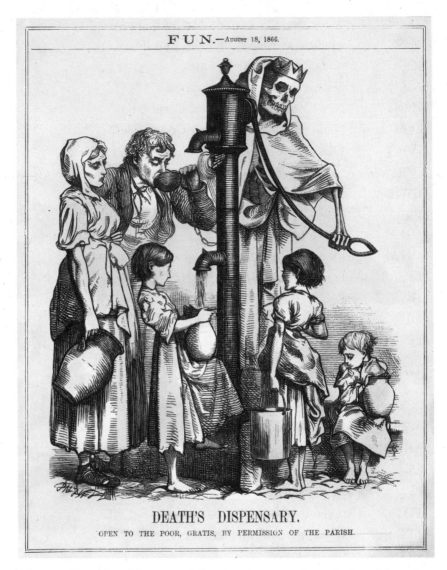

Photo 1. Here "Death" pumps cholera-bearing water from the Broad Street pump in London. John Snow famously proved that its water was the source of a cholera outbreak by removing the pump's handle. Snow went door-to-door in different areas of London to find people suffering from the disease and to pin down its source, a practice described as "shoe-leather epidemiology." Reproduced by permission, © Mary Evans Picture Library/The Image Works.

Mapping the Issues

Public Health, Law, and Ethics

The issues and questions presented in the theory and practice of public health are not resolved solely through scientific inquiry; rather, law and ethics also guide our efforts. Yet despite the closeness of the interplay between public health, law, and ethics, each of these three fields has its separate identity, and cross-fertilization is rare. For the most part, each field has adopted distinct terminologies and forms of reasoning. To the extent that scholars and practitioners in the fields of law and ethics have engaged in sustained examinations of issues in health, they have focused principally on medical care. This introductory chapter maps the important features of, and issues in, law and ethics as they pertain to the theory and practice of public health.

I. PUBLIC HEALTH

In thinking about the application of ethics or law to problems in public health, it is important first to understand what we mean by public health. How is the field defined and what is its content—its mission, functions, and services? Who engages in the practice of public health— government, the private sector, charities, or community-based organizations? What are the principal methods or techniques of public health practitioners (Novak 1996; Turnock 2001)? In truth, finding answers to these fundamental questions is not easy, because the field of public health is highly eclectic and conflicted (Beaglehole and Bonita 1997).

TABLE I. Public health

Definition	Society's obligation to ensure the conditions for people's health
Mission	Promote physical and mental health; prevent disease, injury, and disability
Functions	Assessment—assemble and analyze community health needs Policy development—advance plans informed by scientific knowledge Assurance—provide services necessary for community health
Jurisdiction/Domain	Narrow focus—immediate risk factors (e.g., infectious disease control) Broad focus—fundamental social structures (e.g., discrimination, homelessness, socioeconomic status)
Expertise/Skills	Epidemiology and biostatistics, education and communication, leadership and politics

For a summary of the definition, mission, functions, and jurisdiction of public health, see table 1.

Definitions of public health vary widely, ranging from the World Health Organization's (1946) utopian conception of an ideal state of physical and mental health to a more concrete listing of public health practices. Charles-Edward A. Winslow (1920, 30), for example, defined public health as "the science and the art of preventing disease, prolonging life, and promoting physical health and efficiency through organized community efforts for the sanitation of the environment, the control of community infections, the education of the individual in principles of personal hygiene, and the organization of medical and nursing service for the early diagnosis and preventive treatment of disease." More recent definitions focus on "positive health," emphasizing a person's complete well-being. Definitions of positive health include at least four constructs: a healthy body, high-quality personal relationships, a sense of purpose in life, and self-regard and resilience.

The Institute of Medicine (IOM) (1988, 19), in its landmark report *The Future of Public Health,* proposed one of the most influential contemporary definitions: "Public health is what we, as a society, do collectively to assure the conditions for people to be healthy." The IOM's definition can be appreciated by examining its constituent parts. The emphasis on cooperative and mutually shared obligation ("we, as a society") reinforces the notion that collective entities (e.g., governments and communities) take responsibility for healthy populations. Individuals can do a great deal to safeguard their health, particularly if they have the economic means to do so. They can purchase housing, clothing, food, and medical care. Each person can also behave in ways that promote health and safety by eating healthy foods, exercising, using safety equipment (e.g., seat belts, motorcycle helmets, and smoke detectors), and refraining from smoking, using illicit drugs, or drinking alcoholic beverages to excess. Yet there is a great deal that individuals cannot do to secure their health, and therefore these individuals need to organize and collaborate on building infrastructure and developing shared resources. Acting alone, people cannot achieve environmental protection, hygiene and sanitation, clean air and surface water, uncontaminated food and drinking water, safe roads and products, or control of infectious disease. All these collective goods, and many more, are achievable only through organized and sustained community activities.

The IOM definition also makes clear that even the most organized and socially conscious society cannot guarantee complete physical and mental well-being. There will always be a certain amount of injury and disease in the population that is beyond the reach of individuals or government. The role of public health, therefore, is to ensure the conditions for people to be healthy. These conditions include a variety of educational, economic, social, and environmental factors that are necessary for good health.

Most definitions share the premise that the subject of public health is the health of populations—rather than the health of individuals—and that this goal is reached by a generally high level of health throughout society, rather than the best possible health for a few. The field of public health is concerned with health promotion and disease prevention throughout society. Consequently, public health is interested in devising broad strategies to prevent or ameliorate injury and disease, and to promote longevity and well-being.

Scholars and practitioners are conflicted about the "reach," or domain, of public health. Some prefer a narrow focus on the immediate risk factors for injury and disease (Epstein 2003). The role of public health agencies, according to this perspective, is to identify risks or harms and then intervene to prevent or reduce them. This has been the traditional role of public health—exercising discrete powers such as surveillance (e.g., screening and reporting), injury prevention (e.g., ensuring the safety of consumer products), and infectious disease control (e.g., vaccination, partner notification, and quarantine).

Others prefer a broad focus on the socioeconomic foundations of health (Gostin and Bloche 2003). Those favoring this position see public health as an all-embracing enterprise united by the common value of societal well-being. They claim that the jurisdiction of public health reaches "social ills rooted in distal social structures" (Meyer and Schwartz 2000, 1189). Ultimately, the field is interested in the equitable distribution of social and economic resources because social status, race, and wealth are important influences on the health of populations (Marmot and Wilkinson 1999). Similarly, the field is interested in "social capital" because social networks of family and friends, as well as associations with religious and civic organizations, are important factors in individual well-being and community functioning.

This inclusive view of public health is gaining popularity. Figure 1 illustrates the determinants of health according to the U.S. Department of Health and Human Services: physical environment, behavior and biology, and social environment. In accord with this vision, public health researchers and practitioners have ventured into areas of general social policy, ranging from city planning, safe housing, and diet and exercise to violence, war, and discrimination.

The expansive view of public health may well be justified by the importance of culture, poverty, and powerlessness to the health of populations. Social epidemiologists have found an association between these factors and increased morbidity and premature mortality. Yet to many, this all-embracing notion is troublesome. The first problem is its excessive breadth. Almost every activity in which human beings are engaged affects the population's health, but this fact does not justify an overly inclusive definition of public health. The field of public health appears less credible if it overreaches.

The second problem is lack of expertise. Admittedly, the public health professions incorporate a wide variety of disciplines (e.g., occupational health, health education, epidemiology, laboratory technology, and nursing), with different skills and functions. But public health professionals do not possess the competence in behavioral and social sciences, economics, engineering, and other skills necessary to intervene on behavioral, social, physical, and environmental levels.

The final problem is insufficient political and public support (Burris

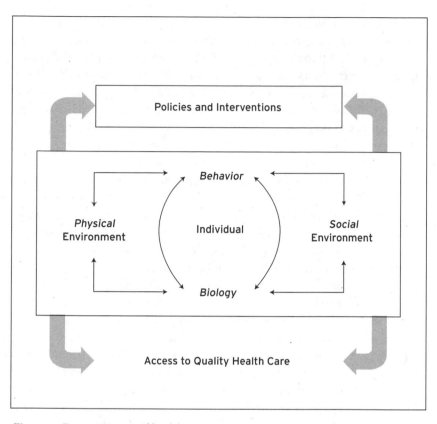

Figure 1. Determinants of health. *Source:* U.S. Department of Health and Human Services [2000a].

1997). By espousing controversial issues of economic redistribution and social restructuring, the field risks losing its legitimacy. Public health gains credibility from its adherence to science, and if the field strays too far into political advocacy, it may lose the appearance of objectivity.

If public health has such a broad meaning, then who engages in the work of public health? The IOM's sequel to its first report, *The Future of the Public's Health in the 21st Century* (2002), stressed the importance of a public health "system" comprising a wide array of public and private entities—government, industry, academia, charities, and community-based organizations. At the governmental level, public health has a significant jurisdictional problem. Even the most powerful public health agency cannot exercise direct authority over the full range of activities that affect health. Many of the determinants of health are normally the province of other agencies (e.g., agencies concerned with education, agriculture, transportation, housing, child welfare, and criminal justice). Furthermore, much of the behavior that public health agencies try to change (e.g., exercise and diet) is not subject to direct legal regulation at all. At the same time, many of the institutions that affect the public's health are outside government, such as managed care organizations, business and labor, community-based groups, and academic institutions. It is for these reasons that government and its partners should pursue a strategy of "health in all policies."

The breadth and variety of public health actors are a relevant practical and theoretical consideration. It matters a great deal in law and ethics to understand who is acting, with what authority, and with what resources. For example, society is prepared to allow government to wield powers to coerce (e.g., to tax, inspect, license, and quarantine) that would be unacceptable in the private sector.

What are the principal methodologies of public health practitioners? Because of the field's broad sweep, the techniques of public health are highly diverse. For example, public health practitioners monitor health status, which calls for skills in epidemiology and biostatistics; inform and educate the public, which calls for skills in education and communication; and create health policy and enforce laws, which call for legal, political, and leadership skills. This description does not account for the many subjects in the field of public health requiring expertise in domains such as infectious diseases (e.g., virology and bacteriology), the environment (e.g., toxicology), and injuries (e.g., behavioral and social sciences). As the IOM (1988, 40) has observed, "Public health's subject matter . . . necessitate[s] the involvement of a broad spectrum of professional disciplines. In fact, . . . public health is a coalition of professions united by their shared mission."

As illustrated in figure 2, the field of public health is caught in a dilemma. If it conceives itself too narrowly, then public health will be accused of lacking vision. It will fail to tackle the root causes of ill health and be unable to employ the broad range of social, economic, and behavioral tools necessary to achieve healthier populations. At the same time, if it conceives itself too expansively, then public health will be accused of overreaching and invading a sphere reserved for politics, not science. It will lose the ability to explain coherently its mission and functions and, consequently, to sell public health in the marketplace of national priorities.

There may be a deeper level of tension here. Public health is an arm

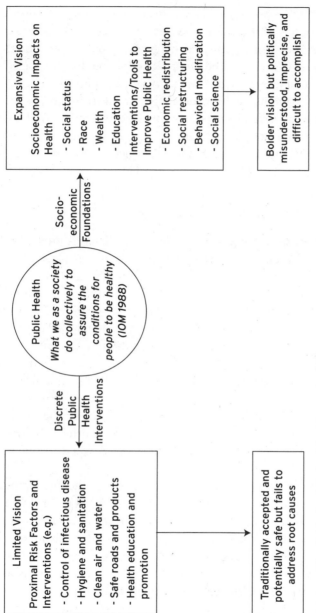

Figure 2. The field of public health: Alternative visions.

of the state and a profession involving public service. It must work within the bounds of the law and respect the judgments of elected officials. At the same time, public health professionals often function as voices of social conscience and champions for the disadvantaged who disproportionately suffer from injury, disability, and disease. It is not always easy for public health officials to "speak truth to power." Yet balance can be achieved by those who understand the myriad political and economic considerations that underlie public policy judgments and the numerous openings in the democratic process for drawing attention to relevant scientific evidence and public health values.

II. PUBLIC HEALTH LAW

As we have just seen, answering the question "What is public health?" is much more difficult than it first appears. Despite this lack of conceptual clarity, it is important to carefully study the legal foundations of public health, as well as its ethical dimensions. Public health law has long taken a backseat to health care law, which primarily examines the financing, organization, and delivery of personal medical services. But important scholarly studies of public health law are gaining prominence both in the United States (Goodman et al. 2007; Grad 2004; Wing 2003) and internationally (Bailey, Caulfield, and Ries 2005; Reynolds 2004; Martin and Johnson 2001). The emergence of the field is underscored by a public health law program at the Centers for Disease Control and Prevention (CDC), a public health law association, and numerous academic centers and institutes devoted to this subject (Goodman et al. 2007).

The preservation of the public's health is among the most important goals of government. The enactment and enforcement of law, moreover, are a primary means by which government creates the conditions for people to lead healthier and safer lives. Laws establish a mission for public health officials, assign their functions, and specify the manner in which they may exercise their power. The law is a tool that is used to influence norms for healthy behavior, to identify and respond to health threats, and to set and enforce health and safety standards. The most important social debates about public health take place in legal fora—legislatures, courts, and administrative agencies—and in the law's language of rights, duties, and justice. It is no exaggeration to say that "the field of public health . . . could not long exist in the manner in which we know it today except for its sound legal basis" (Grad 2004, 4).

In this volume's companion text, I define public health law as "the study of the legal powers and duties of the state, in collaboration with its partners (e.g., health care, business, the community, the media, and academe), to ensure the conditions for people to be healthy and of the limitations on the power of the state to constrain the autonomy, privacy, liberty, proprietary, or other legally protected interests of individuals." Public health law scholars are therefore interested in government authority to prevent injury and disease and to promote the public's health, as well as in the constraints on state action to protect individual freedom. The U.S. government has ample authority to act for the common good, employing "police powers" to safeguard the health, safety, and morals of the population. But the state must exercise that power within the constraints of the Constitution.

Law can be an effective tool to achieve the goal of improved health for the population. Law, regulation, and litigation, like other public health prevention strategies, intervene at a variety of levels, each designed to secure safer and healthier populations. First, government interventions are aimed at individual behavior through education (e.g., health communication campaigns), incentives and disincentives (e.g., taxing and spending powers), and deterrents (e.g., civil and criminal penalties for risk behaviors). Second, the law uses regulations to change behavior by requiring safer product design (e.g., safety standards and indirect regulation through the tort system). Finally, the law alters environments—informational (e.g., through advertising restraints), physical (e.g., through city planning and housing codes), and business (e.g., through inspections and licenses).

Government engages in the work of public health in its three separate branches—legislative, executive, and judicial—with their distinct, albeit overlapping, constitutional authorities: (1) legislatures create health policy and allocate the resources necessary to effect it; (2) executive agencies implement health policy, promulgate health regulations, and enforce regulatory standards; and (3) courts interpret laws and resolve legal disputes. As a society, we forgo the possibility of bold public health governance by any single branch in exchange for constitutional checks and balances that prevent government from overreaching and ensure political accountability.

In practice, public health agencies in the modern state go beyond traditional executive branch functions of implementation and enforcement. Certainly, the legislature assigns the responsibilities and activities of public health agencies. But public health agencies can, in a sense, go beyond that legislation to create law through administrative regulations and interpret law through the regulatory process and their own practices. They can also adjudicate disputes, making such determinations as when a business has violated a safety standard or when a professional is eligible for a license.

Public health law is concerned with the trade-offs that the exercise of government power entails. Under what circumstances should government be permitted to act to achieve a public good when the consequence of that act is to invade a sphere of personal or economic liberty? This is the kind of question that intrigues scholars interested in law and the public's health. Rather than using ethical discourse to resolve these conflicts, the law uses the language of duties, powers, and rights.

It is clear from the above description that public health law is a vast field that incorporates thinking from a variety of legal subspecialties—constitutional, administrative, and tort law. Constitutional law deals with the powers that the Constitution affords the federal government and with limits on the authority of governments at every level in order to protect a sphere of freedom. Administrative law is concerned with the body of statutes and regulations that set health and safety standards, together with the powers of agencies to interpret and enforce those standards. Tort law provides a method of indirect regulation through the courts. By levying damages for certain kinds of harm, tort law can provide powerful disincentives to engage in risk behaviors (e.g., litigation against cigarette and firearm manufacturers). A fourth body of law—international law—is becoming increasingly relevant as infectious and even chronic diseases spill over national borders. International law includes a wide array of treaties involving health, trade, human rights, arms control, and the environment. These legal dimensions will be explored further as the *Reader* unfolds, particularly in Part 2, "The Law and the Public's Health."

III. PUBLIC HEALTH ETHICS

The fields of bioethics and medical ethics have richly informed the development and use of biotechnologies, the practice of medicine, and the allocation of health care resources. Ethicists have not devoted the same sustained attention to problems in public health, but that situation is beginning to change with the appearance of interesting and important scholarship in public health ethics. The Association of Schools of Public Health, for example, has developed a model curriculum for courses

TABLE 2. Public health ethics

Branches of Public Health Ethics	Principal Concerns
Ethics of Public Health (i.e., professional ethics)	Ethical dimensions of professionalism Moral trust society bestows on professionals to act for the common good
Ethics in Public Health (i.e., applied ethics: situation or case oriented)	Ethical dimensions of public health enterprise Moral standing of population's health Trade-offs between collective goods and individual interests Social justice: equitable allocation of benefits and burdens
Advocacy Ethics (i.e., goal-oriented, populist ethics)	Overriding value of healthy communities The interests of populations, particularly the powerless and oppressed

SOURCE: Hastings Center Project on Ethics and Public Health.

in public health ethics that includes materials on the traditions and values of public health, as well as on the ethical issues raised by infectious disease control, environmental health, and health care reform.

Public health ethics seek to understand and clarify principles and values that guide public health actions, offering a framework for making decisions and a means of justifying them. Because public health actions are directed toward populations, the principles and values of the field can differ from those that guide actions in biology and clinical medicine (bioethics and medical ethics), which tend to center on individuals and specific patients.

This discussion raises a critical unanswered question: What are the features that distinguish public health ethics from conventional medical ethics or bioethics? Are ethical principles and values, or the methods of ethical analysis, materially different when applied to populations rather than to individuals? In thinking about this question it will be helpful to consider public health ethics from at least two perspectives: the ethics of public health professionals (professional ethics) and ethics in public health theory and practice (applied ethics and advocacy ethics). See table 2.

The ethics of public health are concerned with the ethical dimensions of professionalism and the moral trust that society bestows on public health professionals to act for the common welfare. This form of ethical discourse stresses the professionalism among public health students and practitioners. It instills in professionals a sense of public duty and trust. Professional ethics are role oriented, helping practitioners to act in virtuous ways as they undertake their functions.

Many professional groups, such as physicians, nurses, and attorneys, hold themselves accountable through a set of ethical guidelines, but public health professionals have no official code of ethics—perhaps because there is no single public health profession. Indeed, some of the different public health disciplines that make up the profession have their own ethical codes—for example, epidemiologists, health educators, and health services researchers.

A code of ethics, or at least a well-articulated values statement, could be helpful to the field. A code could give the profession a moral compass, providing concrete guidelines to help clarify the ethical dilemmas that frequently arise. Public health professionals work in a field of considerable moral ambiguity where guidance could be instructive. A code could also give the field both moral credibility and a higher professional status. After a systematic consultative process, the Public Health Leadership Society developed an unofficial code of ethics, which is reproduced in table 3.

One salient issue in the ethics of public health professionals is that of fiduciary duty. To whom do public health professionals owe a duty of loyalty, and how can these professionals know what actions are morally acceptable? Physicians, attorneys, and accountants have a fiduciary duty to their clients that informs their moral world. For example, client-centered professions usually adhere to the principle that the professional serves the client, advises the client fully and honestly, takes instructions from the client, and avoids acting against the client's best interests.

In the context of public health, the community might be regarded as the "client," but the notion of a "community" is often vague and fragmented. In any given situation, different groups may claim to represent community interests. If the community's wants and needs are not easily ascertained, should public health professionals make their own judgments about communal interests? Public health professionals may, at times, coerce some members of the community to take actions that are in the best interests of others but not necessarily themselves. In

TABLE 3. Principles of the ethical practice of public health

1. Public health should address principally the fundamental causes of disease and requirements for health, aiming to prevent adverse health outcomes.

2. Public health should achieve community health in a way that respects the rights of individuals in the community.

3. Public health policies, programs, and priorities should be developed and evaluated through processes that ensure an opportunity for input from community members.

4. Public health should advocate and work for the empowerment of disenfranchised community members, aiming to ensure that the basic resources and conditions necessary for health are accessible to all.

5. Public health should seek the information needed to implement effective policies and programs that protect and promote health.

6. Public health institutions should provide communities with the information they have that is needed for decisions on policies or programs and should obtain the community's consent for their implementation.

7. Public health institutions should act in a timely manner on the information they have within the resources and mandate given to them by the public.

8. Public health programs and policies should incorporate a variety of approaches that anticipate and respect diverse values, beliefs, and cultures in the community.

9. Public health programs and policies should be implemented in a manner that most enhances the physical and social environment.

10. Public health institutions should protect the confidentiality of information that can bring harm to an individual or community if made public. Exceptions must be justified on the basis of the high likelihood of significant harm to the individual or others.

11. Public health institutions should ensure the professional competence of their employees.

12. Public health institutions and their employees should engage in collaborations and affiliations in ways that build the public's trust and the institutions' effectiveness.

SOURCE: Public Health Leadership Society, http://phls.org/CMSuploads/PHLSposter-68526.pdf.

thinking about public health's complex relationship to populations, is the concept of fiduciary duty helpful as an ethical value?

Do public health professionals have a duty to tell the full truth and, if so, by what standard should they be judged? Public health professionals may earnestly believe that their mission requires vigorous interventions to prevent risk behaviors (e.g., smoking and illicit drug use) or encourage health-promoting behaviors (e.g., exercise and a healthy diet). To achieve these beneficent objectives, public health professionals may exaggerate risks or benefits, or may make claims that are insufficiently grounded in science. Suppose public health professionals know that the risk of sexual transmission of HIV in a middle-class, rural neighborhood is relatively low. Are they obliged to disclose this fact when advising men to wear condoms? How would an ethical code address the nuanced question of "truth telling" by public health professionals?

Another area of public health ethics might be called ethics in public health theory and practice. Ethics in public health are concerned not so much with the character of professionals as with the ethical dimensions of the public health enterprise itself. Here, scholars undertake a philosophical analysis of the kind of reasoning necessary for careful thinking and decision making in creating and implementing public health policy. This type of "applied" ethics is situation or case oriented, seeking to understand morally appropriate decisions in concrete cases. Scholars can make significant contributions to this area by applying general ethical theory and disinterested reasoning to the societal debates common in public health. In each case, public health ethicists could identify and clarify the ethical dilemma posed, describe the benefits and burdens, specify the alternative courses of action, and offer guidance about an ethically appropriate intervention.

The application of ethical principles and values to public health decisions can be complex and controversial. Problems in public health often involve numerous risk factors, multiple stakeholders, and diverse perspectives on matters of individual liberty and the population's well-being. Since a principal aim of public health is to achieve the greatest health benefits for the greatest number of people, it draws from the traditions of consequentialism, which judges the rightness of an action by the consequences, effects, or outcomes that it produces. Utilitarianism, one of the most influential forms of consequentialist ethical theory, holds that actions are justified insofar as they promote the greatest happiness of the greatest number of people.

The "public health model" of ethical reasoning, argue Allen Buchanan and colleagues (2000), uncritically assumes that the appropriate mode of evaluating options is some form of cost-benefit (or cost-effectiveness) calculation—the aggregation of goods and bads (benefits and costs) across individuals. Public health, according to this view, appears to permit, or even require, that the most fundamental interests of individuals be sacrificed in order to produce the best overall outcome.

This characterization is based on an erroneous or, at best, oversimplified understanding of the public health approach. The field of public health is certainly interested in securing the greatest benefits for the most people. And public health officials, as part of government, must concern themselves with efficiencies, benefits, and costs. But public health does not simply aggregate benefits and burdens, choosing the policy that produces the most good and the least harm. Rather, the overwhelming majority of public health interventions are intended to benefit the whole population without knowingly harming individuals or groups. Public health authorities working in the areas of tobacco control, the environment, and occupational safety, for example, believe that everyone will benefit from smoking cessation, clean air, and safe workplaces.

Certainly, public health focuses almost exclusively on one vision of the "common good" (health, not wealth or prosperity). And public health actions can diminish personal and economic freedoms such as privacy or free enterprise. But such individual losses are not the salient characteristics of public health ethics. The field rarely sacrifices fundamental interests to produce the best overall outcome, except perhaps when an individual's behavior threatens the equally fundamental interests of others to live in health and safety—for example, persons with multidrug-resistant tuberculosis are sometimes forced into isolation. At the very least, when a public health action pits one fundamental interest against another, public health ethics should facilitate vigorous debate, and the action should be subject to legal oversight.

Of course, the public health approach does follow a version of the harm principle. Thus, public health authorities regulate individuals or businesses that endanger the community. The objective is to prevent unreasonable risks that jeopardize the public's health and safety—for example, by polluting a stream, exposing others to infectious disease, or selling dangerous toys for children. When public health officials regulate to curtail activities that harm others, they are acting squarely within a widely accepted Western liberal tradition.

More controversially, public health officials at times recommend and undertake paternalistic interventions, such as mandating the wearing of motorcycle helmets or banning trans fat in foods. Public health officials reason that the sacrifice asked of individuals is relatively small and the communal benefits are substantial. Few public health experts advocate that truly fundamental individual liberties be taken away in the name of paternalism. In the public health model, individual interests in autonomy, privacy, liberty, and property are taken seriously, but they do not invariably trump community health benefits.

The public health approach thus differs from modern liberalism primarily in how it balances interests: public health places greater weight on community benefits, whereas liberalism favors individual liberty. Characterizing public health as a utilitarian sacrifice of fundamental personal interests is as unfair as characterizing liberalism as an individualistic sacrifice of vital communal interests. Both traditions would protest this kind of oversimplification.

Scholars in medical ethics and bioethics have convincingly demonstrated the power and importance of individual freedom. However, until recently they have paid insufficient attention to the equally strong values of partnership, citizenship, and community (Beauchamp 1988). As members of a society in which we have a common bond, we also have an obligation to protect and defend the community against threats to health, safety, and security. Members of society owe one another a duty to promote the common good. A new public health ethic should advance the idea that individuals benefit from being part of a well-regulated society that reduces the risks that all members share.

There remains much work to do in public health ethics. What is the moral standing that should be attached to the collective good? Does the health of a community have a moral standing that is independent of the health of individuals within that population? Under what circumstances should individual interests yield in favor of an aggregate benefit for the population? And, at a more fundamental level, what counts as a "harm" or "benefit"? Must the person's behavior pose a risk to others for it to become a matter of concern, or can public health officials justifiably restrict self-regarding behavior?

Social justice is one of the most basic and widely understood aspects of public health ethics. Justice requires fairness or reasonableness, especially in the way people are treated or decisions are made. Social justice stresses the importance of fair distribution of common advantages and the sharing of common burdens. Does an otherwise effective policy become unfair if it disproportionately disadvantages a particular racial, ethnic, or religious group? For example, public health professionals often advocate primary enforcement of seat belt laws so that police can stop a driver simply for failure to comply with the law. But what if the primary enforcement of such laws falls disproportionately on African Americans, as now appears to be the case?

Social justice, of course, not only encompasses fair distribution of resources but also requires the preservation of human dignity and the showing of equal respect for the interests of all members of the community. As Hurricane Katrina taught us, "[a] failure to act expeditiously and with equal concern for all citizens, including the poor and less powerful, . . . erod[es] public trust and undermin[es] social cohesion. It signals to the disadvantaged and to everyone else that the basic human needs of some matter less than those of others, and it thereby fails to show the respect due to all members of the community" (Gostin and Powers 2006, 1058–59).

In addition to "professional" and "applied" ethics, it is possible to think of an "advocacy" ethic informed by the single overriding value of a healthy community. According to this rationale, public health authorities perceive of themselves as knowing what is ethically appropriate and understand their function as advocating for that social goal. This populist ethic serves the interests of populations, especially the powerless and oppressed, and its methods are mainly pragmatic and political. Public health professionals strive to convince the public and its representative political bodies that healthy populations and reduced inequalities are the preferred social goals.

The language and concepts of human rights are often invoked by those advancing an advocacy ethic, and with good reason. Human rights, as part of the body of international law, afford individuals rights against state interference. These include civil and political rights, such as autonomy, bodily integrity, privacy, and nondiscrimination. Human rights, moreover, impose affirmative duties on states to act for the welfare of society. Economic, social, and cultural rights include the rights to social security, education, work, and enjoyment of the benefits of scientific advances.

Most importantly, human rights require governments to recognize "the right of everyone to the highest attainable standard of physical and mental health" (International Covenant on Economic, Social, and Cultural Rights, art. 12). Critics of this approach point to the vagaries of the right to health, such as its lack of definable standards and enforcement mechanisms. Although this critique has force, the United Nation's Committee on Economic, Social and Cultural Rights and a UN special reporter have offered more detailed guidance on the meaning and implementation of the right to health. Public health advocates often invoke this right when seeking improvement in health conditions, reduction of socioeconomic disparities, and universal access to health care.

Public health ethics, therefore, can illuminate the field of public health in several ways. Ethics can offer guidance on (1) the meaning of public health professionalism and the ethical practice of the profession, (2) the moral weight and value of the community's health and well-being, (3) the recurring themes of the field and the dilemmas faced in everyday public health practice, and (4) the role of advocacy to achieve the goal of safer and healthier populations, highlighting the importance of the human right to health.

There needs to be a much more sustained, sophisticated discussion of ethics among students, practitioners, and scholars in public health. Today, ethics instruction in schools of public health is scarce and targeted primarily at biomedical or medical ethics, but this too may be changing, as the Association of Schools of Public Health's model curriculum illustrates (available at www.asph.org/document.cfm?page=782). Further, few public health employers in the public and private sectors offer continuing education that includes ethical issues. Government and academic institutions should consider the value of including ethics in their accreditation of schools, credentialing of professionals, and promotion of public health research.

IV. CONCLUSION

Ensuring and improving population health requires the consideration of broad and divergent issues, from the philosophical to the economic and jurisprudential. Traditionally, these dimensions of public health theory and practice have been analyzed independently by public health practitioners, lawyers, and ethicists, who each apply the distinctive terminology and analytical methods of their respective fields. That these approaches differ is not inherently problematic: members of each field bring their own richly diverse expertise to the theory and practice of public health. But the key to analyzing and practicing public health in a coherent way is the integration of these methodologies into a unified framework. In pursuit of this goal, the *Reader* seeks to integrate and foster dialogue among the fields of public health, law, and ethics.

RECOMMENDED READINGS

Beaglehole, Robert, and Ruth Bonita. 1997. *Public Health at the Crossroads: Achievements and Prospects.* New York: Cambridge Univ. Press. (Considers the global and interdisciplinary aspects of public health and describes the need to integrate rigorous epidemiological research with broad-minded policy making)

Burris, Scott. 1997. The invisibility of public health: Population-level measures in a politics of market individualism. *American Journal of Public Health* 87: 1607–10. (Examines the methods and flaws of the prevailing political attack on public health regulation)

Epstein, Richard A. 2003. Let the shoemaker stick to his last: A defense of the "old" public health. *Perspectives in Biology and Medicine* 46: 138–59. (Argues for a traditional definition of public health that limits its scope to communicable diseases and pollution)

Gostin, Lawrence O., and M. Gregg Bloche. 2003. The politics of public health: A response to Epstein. *Perspectives in Biology and Medicine* 46: 160–75. (Contends that public health must be understood to have a wider scope that encompasses non-communicable diseases and social determinants of health)

Marmot, Michael, and Richard G. Wilkinson, eds. 1999. *Social Determinants of Health.* Oxford: Oxford Univ. Press. (Sets forth the idea that population health is largely determined by social factors—the social determinants of health)

Powers, Madison, and Ruth Faden. 2006. *Social Justice: The Moral Foundations of Public Health and Health Policy.* New York: Oxford Univ. Press. (Confronts foundational issues about health and justice, such as how much inequality in health a just society can tolerate and which inequalities matter most and are the most morally urgent to address)

Turnock, Bernard J. 2001. *Public Health: What It Is and How It Works.* Gaithersburg, MD: Aspen. (Provides a guide to the scope of public health systems, research, and policy development)

PART ONE

Foundations of Public Health Law and Ethics

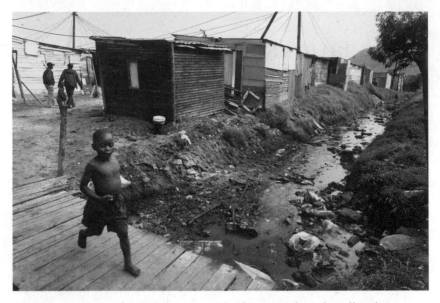

Photo 2. A South African boy crosses a bridge over a heavily polluted river running through Cape Town's densely populated Masiphumelele slum. Left to rely on contaminated water supplies, children in Masiphumelele are at high risk for waterborne diseases, particularly diarrheal diseases. Diarrheal diseases—easily preventable and treatable in the developed world—are often deadly in the developing world, claiming millions of lives each year. Reprinted by permission, © Nic Bothma/epa/Corbis, April 6, 2008.

ONE

The Public's Health

Health is among the most important conditions of human
life and a critically significant constituent of human
capabilities which we have reason to value. Any conception
of social justice that accepts the need for a fair distribution
as well as efficient formation of human capabilities cannot
ignore the role of health in human life and the opportunities
that persons, respectively, have to achieve good health—free
from escapable illness, avoidable afflictions and premature
mortality. Equity in the achievement and distribution of
health gets, thus, incorporated and embedded in a larger
understanding of justice.

Amartya Sen, 2002

The readings in this chapter and the next examine the fields of public
health and public health ethics. The first chapter contains classic readings that illuminate the core values of public health: prevention and
the population-based perspective, the role of community and civic participation, the significance of social justice, and modern perspectives
on the "public health system." Chapter 2 then turns to contemporary
explanations of public health ethics, examining how ethical principles
and values can inform society about the justifiability of actions taken
to safeguard the public's health and safety. The readings on public
health ethics analyze the inevitable trade-offs between personal liberty
and public health, and discuss the ethics of risk regulation.

I. PREVENTION AND THE POPULATION-BASED PERSPECTIVE

Public health interventions are designed to prevent or ameliorate injury,
disease, and premature death among populations. This section offers

two foundational articles explaining the population-based focus of the field of public health. The article by Ali H. Mokdad and colleagues from the Centers for Disease Control and Prevention (CDC) is based on the groundbreaking work of J. Michael McGinnis and William H. Foege (1993), who described the major preventable causes of death in the United States. Mokdad and colleagues introduce readers to differences in the way causes of mortality are framed in medicine and public health.

Medical explanations of death, often in the form of code numbers from the International Classification of Disease (ICD) on death certificates, point to discrete pathophysiological conditions, such as cancer, heart disease, cerebrovascular disease, and pulmonary disease. The biomedical model of record keeping and the societal need to explain a cause of death with a discrete medical condition can distract the public from real contributors to mortality. In contrast, public health explanations examine the root causes of disease. Seen in this way, the leading causes of death are environmental, social, and behavioral factors. The statistics cited by Mokdad and colleagues demonstrate the magnitude of the mortality associated with preventable causes of death and the potential impacts of successful public health campaigns.

ACTUAL CAUSES OF DEATH IN THE UNITED STATES, 2000*

Ali H. Mokdad, James S. Marks, Donna F. Stroup, and Julie L. Gerberding

In a seminal 1993 article, McGinnis and Foege described the major external (nongenetic) modifiable factors that contributed to death in the United States and labeled them the "actual causes of death." During the 1990s, substantial lifestyle pattern changes may have led to variations in actual causes of death. Mortality rates from heart disease, stroke, and cancer have declined. At the same time, behavioral changes have led to an increased prevalence of obesity and diabetes.

Most diseases and injuries have multiple potential causes and several factors and conditions may contribute to a single death. Therefore, it is a challenge to estimate the contribution of each factor to mortality. In this article, we used published causes of death reported to the [CDC] for 2000, relative risks (RRs), and prevalence estimates from published literature and governmental reports to update actual causes of death in the United States—a method similar to that used by McGinnis and Foege. . . .

RESULTS

The number of deaths in the United States in 2000 was 2.4 million, which is an increase of more than 250,000 deaths in comparison with the 1990 total, due largely

*Reprinted from *JAMA* 291 (2004): 1238–45. Copyright © 2004 American Medical Association. All rights reserved.

TABLE 4. Actual causes of death in the United States
in 1990 and 2000

Actual Cause	No. (%) in 1990*		No. (%) in 2000	
Tobacco	400,000	(19)	435,000	(18.1)
Poor Diet and Physical Inactivity	300,000	(14)	400,000	(16.6)
Alcohol Consumption	100,000	(5)	85,000	(3.5)
Microbial Agents	90,000	(4)	75,000	(3.1)
Toxic Agents	60,000	(3)	55,000	(2.3)
Motor Vehicles	25,000	(1)	43,000	(1.8)
Firearms	35,000	(2)	29,000	(1.2)
Sexual Behavior	30,000	(1)	20,000	(0.8)
Illicit Drug Use	20,000	(<1)	17,000	(0.7)
Total	1,060,000	(50)	1,159,000	(48.2)

SOURCE: Mokdad et al. 2004, 1240, table 2.
*Data are from McGinnis and Foege 1993. The percentages are for all deaths.

to population growth and increasing age. Leading causes of death were diseases of the heart, malignant neoplasms, and cerebrovascular diseases. . . .

Tobacco

. . . A slight decline in smoking was observed from 1995–1999 to 2000. The prevalence of smoking in 1995–1999 was 22.8% for current smokers, 24.1% for former smokers, and 53.1% for never-smokers. In 2000, these estimates were 22.2% for current smokers, 24.4% for former smokers, and 53.4% for never-smokers. [Men were consistently more likely than women to be current or former smokers.]

We estimate that approximately 435,000 deaths were attributable to smoking in 2000, which is an increase of 35,000 deaths from 1990 [see table 4]. This increase is due to the inclusion of 35,000 deaths due to secondhand smoking and 1,000 infant deaths due to maternal smoking, which were not included in the article by McGinnis and Foege.

Poor Diet and Physical Inactivity

To assess the impact of poor diet and physical inactivity on mortality, we computed annual deaths due to overweight. [Increases in overweight and obesity have been reported frequently in recent years, and National Health and Nutrition Examination Surveys from 1999 and 2000 indicate that nearly 30% of Americans are overweight or obese.] . . .

. . . In 2000, the mean estimate of the total number of overweight-attributable deaths among nonsmokers or never-smokers was 543,797. [The estimate of overweight-attributable deaths increased 76.6% from 1991.]

The prevalence of overweight used in this study is based on data from 1999–2000. Because the effects of overweight on mortality may not appear until some years after a person becomes overweight, it is likely that the increase in prevalence of overweight in the 1990s overestimates the current actual number of deaths. However, the total number of deaths from the 1999–2000 data may well be the expected number of deaths in the next few years. Thus, we believe a more accurate and conservative estimate for overweight mortality in 2000 [would be] 385,000, which is the rounded average of 2000 and 1991 estimates. . . .

[In addition to overweight-attributable deaths,] we estimate that poor diet and physical inactivity will cause an additional 15,000 deaths a year, although this too may be conservative.

We estimate that 400,000 deaths were attributable to poor diet and physical inactivity, an increase of one third from 300,000 deaths estimated by McGinnis and Foege, and the largest increase among all actual causes of death. However, poor diet and physical inactivity could account for even more deaths (>500,000) when the 1999–2000 prevalence estimates of overweight have their full effect. . . .

Alcohol Consumption

. . . In 2000, 18,539 deaths were reported . . . as alcohol induced. In addition, 16,653 persons were killed in alcohol-related crashes. We estimate another 34,797 deaths in 2000 using . . . alcohol consumption data and [relative risks for a number of alcohol-associated diseases]. This totals to 69,989 deaths in 2000 from these factors alone. . . .

Total alcohol-attributable deaths would reach about 140,000 if mortality among previous alcohol drinkers were included. It is unclear whether excess mortality among former alcohol drinkers is due to damage or illness from past alcohol consumption.

Taking these various numbers into account, our best estimate for total alcohol-attributable deaths in 2000 is approximately 85,000, based on the conservative estimate from cause-specific deaths and the high estimate using all-cause mortality. This is a reduction of 15,000 deaths from the 1990 estimates. . . .

Microbial Agents

. . . In the past, infectious agents were the leading cause of mortality. These agents still present a major threat to the nation's health and are associated with high morbidity. Several improvements in the health system have led to a decline in mortality from infectious diseases. The increase in US immunization rates led to a decline in mortality from many vaccine-preventable diseases. . . . There also have been substantial improvements in sanitation and hygiene, antibiotics and other antimicrobial medicines, and hospital-infection control.

In 2000, influenza and pneumonia accounted for 65,313 deaths, septicemia for 31,224, and tuberculosis for 776. In general, mortality from infectious and parasitic diseases has declined since 1990. Because pneumonia and septicemia occur at higher rates among patients with cancer, heart disease, lung disease, or liver disease, some of these deaths really are attributable to smoking, poor diet, and alcohol consumption. We estimate that approximately 75,000 deaths were attributable to microbial agents in 2000. . . . This contrasts with 90,000 deaths attributed to microbial agents in 1990 estimates. [These deaths caused by microbial agents do not include those from HIV/AIDS, which are included under "Sexual Behavior."]

Toxic Agents

. . . In the 1990s, many improvements were made in controlling and monitoring pollutants. There is more systematic monitoring of pollutants at state and county levels, and exposure to asbestos, benzene, and lead have declined. In fact, the US Environmental Protection Agency reported a decline of 25% from 1970 to 2001 in 6 principal air pollutants: carbon monoxide, lead, ozone, nitrogen dioxide, sulfur dioxide, and particulate matter.

Toxic agents are associated with increased mortality from cancer, respiratory, and cardiovascular diseases. [We estimate] 24,000 deaths per year from air pollution alone.

The National Institute for Occupational Safety and Health (NIOSH) estimates that about 113,000 deaths are due to occupational exposure from 1968 to 1996 [with deaths declining during this period]. Although particulate air pollution accounts for the majority (about 60%) of mortality related to toxic agents, indoor air pollution, environmental tobacco smoke, radon, lead in drinking water, and food contamination are associated with increased mortality. We estimate that toxic agents (excluding environmental tobacco exposure) were associated with 2% to 3.5% of total mortality in 2000. We estimate approximately 55,000 deaths attributable to toxic agents in 2000. . . .

Motor Vehicles

Motor-vehicle crashes involving passengers and pedestrians resulted in 43,354 deaths in 2000. This decline from 47,000 deaths in 1990 represents successful public health efforts in motor-vehicle safety. Deaths from alcohol-related crashes declined from 22,084 in 1990 to 16,653 in 2000. Major contributing factors include the use of child safety seats and safety belts, decreases in alcohol-impaired driving, changes in vehicle and highway design, and national goals to reduce motor-vehicle-related mortality and injury. . . . Efforts to educate the public and enforce laws against driving while intoxicated have accounted for most of the decline in deaths related to motor-vehicle crashes.

Firearms

Firearm-related incidents resulted in 28,663 deaths among individuals in the United States in 2000. This is a decline from approximately 36,000 deaths in 1990. The largest declines were in deaths from homicides and unintentional discharge of firearms. In 2000, 16,586 deaths were due to intentional self-harm (suicide) by discharge of firearms. Assault (homicide) by discharge of firearms resulted in 10,801 deaths. Unintentional discharge of firearms resulted in 776 deaths, while discharge of firearms, undetermined intent, resulted in 230 deaths. The remaining 270 deaths were due to legal intervention. . . .

Sexual Behavior

Sexual behavior is associated with an increased risk of preventable disease and disability. An estimated 20 million persons are newly infected with sexually transmitted diseases each year in the United States. Mortality from sexually transmitted diseases is declining due to the availability of earlier and better treatment, especially for HIV. In 2000, HIV disease resulted in 14,578 deaths [a 48% decline from the 27,695 HIV deaths in 1990. In total,] we estimate that 20,000 deaths in 2000 were due to sexual behavior, [including deaths from HIV, hepatitis B and C, and cervical cancer].

Illicit Use of Drugs

Illicit drug use is associated with suicide, homicide, motor-vehicle injury, HIV infection, pneumonia, violence, mental illness, and hepatitis. An estimated 3 million individuals in the United States have serious drug problems. . . . In keeping with the report by McGinnis and Foege, we included deaths caused indirectly by illicit drug use in this category. . . . Overall, we estimate that illicit drug use resulted in approximately 17,000 deaths in 2000, a reduction of 3,000 deaths from the 1990 report.

Other Factors

Several other factors contribute to an increased rate of death. There are factors that we do not know of such as unknown pollutants or perhaps exposures that may cause a considerable number of deaths. Poverty and low education levels are associated with increased mortality from many causes, partly due to differential exposure to the risks described above. However, controlling for differential exposure to risk factors is unlikely to explain the entire impact on mortality. Lack of access to proper medical care or preventive services is associated with increased mortality. Biological characteristics and genetic factors also greatly affect risk of death. In most studies we reviewed, low education levels and income were associated with increased risk of cardiovascular disease, cancer, diabetes, and injury. The Healthy People 2010 initiative has made the elimination of health disparities, especially racial and ethnic disparities, a primary goal.

COMMENT

We found that about half of all deaths that occurred in the United States in 2000 could be attributed to a limited number of largely preventable behaviors and exposures. Overall, we found relatively minor changes from 1990 to 2000 in the estimated number of deaths due to actual causes. Our findings indicate that interventions to prevent and increase cessation of smoking, improve diet, and increase physical activity must become much higher priorities in the public health and health care systems.

The most striking finding was the substantial increase in the number of estimated deaths attributable to poor diet and physical inactivity[—which now stand at roughly 400,000 a year]. The gap between deaths due to poor diet and physical inactivity and those due to smoking has narrowed substantially. Because rates of overweight increased rapidly during the 1990s, we used a conservative approach to make our estimates, accounting for the delayed effects of overweight on mortality. . . . It is clear that if the increasing trend of overweight is not reversed over the next few years, poor diet and physical inactivity will likely overtake tobacco as the leading preventable cause of mortality.

The most disappointing finding may be the slow progress in reducing tobacco-related mortality. A few states, notably California, have had major success in programs that led to reducing deaths from heart disease and cancer. However, efforts in most other states are too recent or short-term to have a similar effect. . . .

Despite the call to action on these risk factors a decade ago, there has been little progress in reducing the total number of deaths from these causes. The progress that has occurred primarily involves actual causes of death that are less prominent. With the shift in the age distribution of the population, more adults now are in the age group at highest risk because of the cumulative effects of their behavior. The net effect is that both total deaths and total burden due to the actual causes have increased. . . .

In summary, smoking and the deaths attributed to the constellation of poor diet and physical inactivity currently account for about one third of all deaths in the United States. . . . In ancient times, Hippocrates stated that "the function of protecting and developing health must rank even above that of restoring it when it is impaired." The findings in this study argue persuasively for the need to establish a more preventive orientation in health care and public health systems in the United States.

. . . . .

Like Mokdad and colleagues, Geoffrey Rose offers a comparison of medicine and public health. In his influential article, Rose compares the scientific methods and objectives of medicine with those of public health. "Why did this patient get this disease at this time?" is a common question in medicine, and it underscores a physician's central concern for sick·individuals and an individual etiology. By contrast, those interested in public health seek knowledge about why ill health occurs in the population and how it can be prevented.

According to Rose's "prevention paradox," measures that have the greatest potential for improving the public's health (e.g., seat belt use) offer little absolute benefit to any individual, whereas measures that heroically save individual lives (e.g., heart transplants) make no significant contribution to the population's health. This tension between the individual and the population can also be seen in how success is quantified for health interventions. The answer to the question "Did this person survive?" indicates success for the physician. For the public health professional, the key question is "How many person-years of life were saved?" Although Rose acknowledges that medical interventions appear more heroic and are more likely to be welcomed by patients, he favors the broad and powerful impact of successful population-based campaigns.

SICK INDIVIDUALS AND SICK POPULATIONS*
Geoffrey Rose

THE DETERMINANT OF INDIVIDUAL CASES

In teaching epidemiology to medical students, I have often encouraged them to consider a question which I first heard enunciated by Roy Acheson: "Why did this patient

*Reprinted from *International Journal of Epidemiology* 14 (March 1985): 32–38 by permission of Oxford University Press.

get *this* disease at *this* time?" It is an excellent starting-point, because students and doctors feel a natural concern for the problems of the individual. Indeed, the central ethos of medicine is seen as an acceptance of responsibility for sick individuals.

It is an integral part of good doctoring to ask not only, "What is the diagnosis, and what is the treatment?" but also, "Why did this happen, and could it have been prevented?" Such thinking shapes the approach to nearly all clinical and laboratory research into the causes and mechanisms of illness. Hypertension research, for example, is almost wholly preoccupied with the characteristics which distinguish individuals at the hypertensive and normotensive ends of the blood pressure distribution. . . . The constant aim in such work is to answer Acheson's question: "Why did *this* patient get this disease at this time?"

The same concern has continued to shape the thinking of all of us who came to epidemiology from a background in clinical practice. The whole basis of the case-control method is to discover how sick and healthy individuals differ. Equally the basis of many cohort studies is the search for "risk factors," which identify certain individuals as being more susceptible to disease; and from this we proceed to test whether these risk factors are also causes, capable of explaining why some individuals get sick while others remain healthy, and applicable as a guide to prevention. . . .

Applied to aetiology, the individual-centered approach leads to the use of relative risk as the basic representation of aetiological force: that is, "the risk in exposed individuals relative to risk in non-exposed individuals." . . . It may generally be the best measure of aetiological force, but it is no measure at all of aetiological outcome or of public health importance. . . .

THE DETERMINANTS OF POPULATION INCIDENCE RATE

I find it increasingly helpful to distinguish two kinds of aetiological questions. The first seeks the causes of cases, and the second seeks the causes of incidence. "Why do some individuals have hypertension?" is a quite different question from "Why do some populations have much hypertension, whilst in others it is rare?" The questions require different kinds of study, and they have different answers. . . .

To find the determinants of prevalence and incidence rates, we need to study characteristics of populations, not characteristics of individuals. . . . Within populations it has proved almost impossible to demonstrate any relation between an individual's diet and his serum cholesterol level; and the same applies to the relation of individual diet to blood pressure and to overweight. But at the level of populations it is a different story: it has proved easy to show strong associations between population mean values for saturated fat intake *versus* serum cholesterol level and coronary heart disease incidence, sodium intake *versus* blood pressure, or energy intake *versus* overweight. The determinants of incidence are not necessarily the same as the causes of cases.

HOW DO THE CAUSES OF CASES RELATE TO THE CAUSES OF INCIDENCE?

This is largely a matter of whether exposure varies similarly within a population and between populations (or over a period of time within the same population). Softness of water supply may be a determinant of cardiovascular mortality, but it is unlikely to be identifiable as a risk factor for individuals, because exposure tends to be locally uniform. Dietary fat is, I believe, the main determinant of a population's incidence rate for coronary heart disease; but it quite fails to identify high-risk individuals.

In the case of cigarettes and lung cancer it so happened that the study populations contained about equal numbers of smokers and non-smokers, and in such a
situation case-control and cohort studies were able to identify what was also the
main determinant of population differences amid time trends.

There is a broad tendency for genetic factors to dominate individual susceptibility, but to explain rather little of population differences in incidence. Genetic
heterogeneity, it seems, is mostly much greater within than between populations.
This is the contrary situation to that seen for environmental factors. Thus migrants,
whatever the colour of their skin, tend to acquire the disease rates of their country
of adoption.

Most non-infectious diseases are still of largely unknown cause. . . . We know
quite a lot about the personal characteristics of individuals who are susceptible to
them, but for a remarkably large number of our major non-infectious diseases we
still do not know the determinants of the incidence rate. . . .

There is hardly a disease whose incidence rate does not vary widely, either over
time or between populations at the same time. This means that these causes of
incidence rate, unknown though they are, are not inevitable. It is possible to live
without them, and if we knew what they were it might be possible to control them.
[Identifying them, however, requires a difference of exposure within the population;
if such variation does not exist,] the clues must be sought from differences between
populations or from changes within populations over time.

PREVENTION

These two approaches to aetiology—the individual and the population-based—have
their counterparts in prevention. In the first, preventive strategy seeks to identify
high-risk susceptible individuals and to offer them some individual protection. In
contrast, the "population strategy" seeks to control the determinants of incidence
in the population as a whole.

The "High-Risk" Strategy

This is the traditional and natural medical approach to prevention. If a doctor
accepts that he is responsible for an individual who is sick today, then it is a short
step to accept responsibility also for the individual who may well be sick tomorrow.
Thus, screening is used to detect certain individuals who hitherto thought they were
well but who must now understand that they are in effect patients. . . .

What the "high-risk" strategy seeks to achieve is something like a truncation of
the risk distribution. This general concept applies to all special preventive action in
high-risk individuals—in at-risk pregnancies, in small babies, or in any other particularly susceptible group. It is a strategy with some clear and important advantages.

Its first advantage is that it leads to intervention which is appropriate to the
individual. A smoker who has a cough or who is found to have impaired ventilatory
function has a special reason for stopping smoking. . . . The intervention makes
sense because that individual already has a problem which that particular measure
may possibly ameliorate. . . .

For rather similar reasons the "high-risk" approach also motivates physicians.
Doctors, quite rightly, are uncomfortable about intervening in a situation where
their help was not asked for. Before imposing advice on somebody who was getting

on all right without them, they like to feel that there is a proper and special justification in that particular case.

The "high-risk" approach offers a more cost-effective use of limited resources. . . . [I]t is more effective to concentrate limited medical services and time where the need—and therefore also the benefit—is likely to be greatest.

A final advantage of the "high-risk" approach is that it offers a more favourable ratio of benefits to risks. If intervention must carry some adverse effects or costs, and if the risk and cost are much the same for everybody, then the ratio of the costs to the benefits will be more favourable where the benefits are larger.

Unfortunately the "high-risk" strategy of prevention also has some serious disadvantages and limitations. The first centers around the difficulties and costs of screening. [Consider screening for high cholesterol.] The disease process we are trying to prevent (atherosclerosis and its complications) begins early in life, so we should have to initiate screening perhaps at the age of ten. However, the abnormality we seek to detect is not a stable lifetime characteristic, so we must advocate repeated screening at suitable intervals.

In all screening one meets problems with uptake, and the tendency for the response to be greater amongst those sections of the population who are often least at risk of the disease. Often there is an even greater problem: screening detects certain individuals who will receive special advice, but at the same time it cannot help also discovering much larger numbers of "borderliners," that is, people whose results mark them as at increased risk but for whom we do not have an appropriate treatment to reduce their risk. . . .

The second disadvantage of the "high-risk" strategy is that it is palliative and temporary, not radical. It does not seek to alter the underlying causes of the disease but to identify individuals who are particularly susceptible to those causes. Presumably in every generation there will be such susceptibles, and if prevention and control efforts were confined to these high-risk individuals, then that approach would need to be sustained year after year and generation after generation. It does not deal with the root of the problem, but seeks to protect those who are vulnerable to it; and they will always be around.

The potential for this approach is limited—sometimes more than we could have expected—both for the individual and for the population. There are two reasons for this. The first is that our power to predict future disease is usually very weak. Most individuals with risk factors will remain well, at least for some years; contrariwise, unexpected illness may happen to someone who has just received an "all clear" report from a screening examination. One of the limitations of the relative risk statistic is that it gives no idea of the absolute level of danger. . . .

This point came home to me only recently. I have long congratulated myself on my low levels of coronary risk factors, and I joked to my friends that if I were to die suddenly, I should be very surprised. I even speculated on what other disease—perhaps colon cancer—would be the commonest cause of death for a man in the lowest group of cardiovascular risk. The painful truth is that for such an individual in a Western population the commonest cause of death—by far—is coronary heart disease! Everyone, in fact, is a high-risk individual for this uniquely mass disease. . . .

A further disadvantage of the "high-risk" strategy is that it is behaviourally inappropriate. Eating, smoking, exercise and all our other lifestyle characteristics are constrained by social norms. If we try to eat differently from our friends, it will not only be inconvenient, but we risk being regarded as cranks or hypochondriacs. If a man's work environment encourages heavy drinking, then advice that he is damaging his liver is unlikely to have any effect. No one who has attempted any sort of health education effort in individuals needs to be told that it is difficult for such people to step out of line with their peers. This is what the "high-risk" preventive strategy requires them to do.

The Population Strategy

This is the attempt to control the determinants of incidence, to lower the mean level of risk factors, to shift the whole distribution of exposure in a favourable direction. In its traditional "public health" form it has involved mass environmental control methods; in its modern form it is attempting (less successfully) to alter some of society's norms of behaviour.

The advantages are powerful. The first is that it is radical. It attempts to remove the underlying causes that make the disease common. It has a large potential—often larger than one would have expected—for the population as a whole....

The approach is behaviourally appropriate. If nonsmoking eventually becomes "normal," then it will be much less necessary to keep on persuading individuals. Once a social norm of behaviour has become accepted and (as in the case of diet) once the supply industries have adapted themselves to the new pattern, then the maintenance of that situation no longer requires effort from individuals. The health education phase aimed at changing individuals is, we hope, a temporary necessity, pending changes in the norms of what is socially acceptable.

Unfortunately the population strategy of prevention has also some weighty drawbacks. It offers only a small benefit to each individual, since most of them were going to be all right anyway, at least for many years. This leads to the Prevention Paradox (Rose 1981): "A preventive measure which brings much benefit to the population offers little to each participating individual." This has been the history of public health—of immunization, the wearing of seat belts and now the attempt to change various lifestyle characteristics. Of enormous potential importance to the population as a whole, these measures offer very little—particularly in the short term—to each individual; and thus there is poor motivation of the subject....

In mass prevention each individual has usually only a small expectation of benefit, and this small benefit can easily be outweighed by a small risk.... This makes it important to distinguish two approaches. The first is the restoration of biological normality by the removal of an abnormal exposure (e.g., stopping smoking, controlling air pollution, moderating some of our recently acquired dietary deviations); here there can be some presumption of safety. This is not true for the other kind of preventive approach, which leaves intact the underlying causes of incidence and seeks instead to interpose some new, supposedly protective intervention (e.g., immunization, drugs, jogging). Here the onus is on the activists to produce adequate evidence of safety.

CONCLUSIONS

Case-centered epidemiology identifies individual susceptibility, but it may fail to identify the underlying causes of incidence. The "high-risk" strategy of prevention is an interim expedient, needed in order to protect susceptible individuals, but only for so long as the underlying causes of disease remain unknown or uncontrollable; if causes can be removed, susceptibility ceases to matter.

Realistically, many diseases will long continue to call for both approaches, and fortunately competition between them is usually unnecessary. Nevertheless, the priority of concern should always be the discovery and control of the causes of incidence.

II. COMMUNITY AND CIVIC PARTICIPATION

A prevention-oriented and population-based approach requires evaluating health risks and intervening to improve health on a community level. The interaction between public health practitioners and communities should not be only in one direction, however. Experience has shown that community involvement and civic participation at every stage of public interventions—from the initial assessment of health needs to the ultimate evaluation of an intervention's impact—promote effective public health activities. Community action itself may also improve the public's health (Putnam 2000, 326): "Social connectedness is one of the most powerful determinants of our well-being. The more integrated we are with our community, the less likely we are to experience colds, heart attacks, strokes, cancer, depression, and premature death of all sorts. [Thus growing social disconnectedness] represents one of the nation's most serious public health challenges."

In emphasizing the value of community, those in public health should not elide the underlying tensions between the community and the individual. It is important to consider the nature of our social and moral obligations to those in our community. Why should society prefer population health over other social values? That disease prevention is possible does not necessarily make it a desirable goal. Why should the government promote the public's health?

As the following discussion suggests, some political theorists see the common good of society as an ethical imperative, even if the benefit to individuals is small. In *Spheres of Justice* (1983, 65), Michael Walzer explains the value and importance of membership in a community as a vehicle for the provision of communal needs. He tells us that "men and women come together because they literally cannot live apart." By providing for those needs on a community basis, individuals reaffirm and strengthen the sense of membership in a political community.

In the following reading, Dan Beauchamp, a pioneer of public health ethics, builds on the work of Walzer. He analyzes a classic conflict between the need for population-based measures to improve the well-being of the entire community and the ethos of American individualism, which, at times, seems to require only restraint from harming others. Beauchamp argues that communal needs often are mistakenly framed as collections of individual needs to prevent harm to other individuals. For example, instead of viewing pollution controls as fulfilling the societal need for clean air, we often perceive regulations as laws that prevent harm to individuals who may be affected by poor-quality air. To advance his argument, he describes the "second language" of republicanism—a language that acknowledges the community roots of the republican tradition, a language that is not drowned out by individualism and paternalism. This second language, he claims, brings the community together to work toward common goals and, in turn, strengthens its desire to achieve public health goals.

COMMUNITY: THE NEGLECTED TRADITION OF PUBLIC HEALTH*
Dan Beauchamp

What are the limits of government in protecting the health and safety of the public? As more and more states regulate personal behavior to protect the public health and safety, this question again becomes central. Can there be good reasons for public health paternalism in a democracy? Are health and safety individual interests, or also common and shared ends?

The growing public awareness of the role of personal behavior in determining the health of the public can be traced to the "limits to medicine" debates of the early seventies. A substantial literature questioned the efficacy of medical care expenditures for improving health. . . . This new perspective was quickly taken up by many Western governments, particularly in the U.S. and Canada, where national budgets were straining under escalating costs of medical care. . . .

[Proposals to influence lifestyle choices] stirred rhetoric but produced little action. To the contrary the lifestyle debate worked to undermine the legitimacy of the idea that the government is responsible for the health and safety of the public. The lifestyle debate reopened an old theme in democratic theory—paternalism and the meaning of the common good.

THE MEANING OF THE COMMON GOOD

In one version of democratic theory, the state has no legitimate role in restricting personal conduct that is substantially voluntary and that has little or no direct consequence for anyone other than the individual. This strong antipaternalist position is associated with John Stuart Mill. In this view the common good consists in maximizing the freedom of each individual to pursue his or her own interests, subject to a like freedom for every other individual. . . .

*Reprinted from *Hastings Center Report* 15, no. 6 (December 1985): 28–36.

In a second version, health and safety remain private interests but some paternalism is accepted, albeit reluctantly.... Common sense makes us reject a thoroughgoing antipaternalism. Many restrictions on liberty are relatively minor and the savings in life and limb extremely great. Further, often voluntary choices are not completely so; many choices are impaired in some sense....

This reluctant acceptance of paternalism leaves many democrats uneasy. Another alternative is to redefine voluntary risks to an individual as risks to others. Indeed, many argue that all such risks have serious consequences for others, and that the state may therefore limit such activities on the basis of the harm principle. Others challenge the category of voluntariness head on, arguing that most such risks, like cigarettes and alcohol use, have powerful social determinants.

The constitutional basis for the protection of the public health and safety has largely been ignored in this debate. This tradition, and particularly the regulatory power (often called the police power), flows from a view of democracy that sees the essential task of government as protecting and promoting both private and group interests. Government is supposed to defend both sets of interests through an evolving set of practices and institutions, and it is left to the legislatures to determine which set of interests predominate when conflicts arise.

In the constitutional tradition, the common good refers to the welfare of individuals considered as a group, the public or the people generally, the "body politic" or the "commonwealth" as it was termed in the early days of the American Republic. The public or the people were presumed to have an interest, held in common, in self-protection or preservation from threats of all kinds to their welfare. The commonwealth idea was widely influential among New England states during the first half of the nineteenth century.

... The central principles underlying the police or regulatory power were the treatment of health and safety as a shared purpose and need of the community and (aside from basic constitutional rights such as due process) the subordination of the market, property, and individual liberty to protect compelling community interests.

This republican image of democracy was a blending of social contract and republican thought, as well as Judeo-Christian notions of covenant. In the republican vision of society, the individual has a dual status. On the one hand, individuals have private interests and private rights; political association serves to protect these rights. On the other hand, individuals are members of a political community—a body politic.

This common citizenship, despite diversity and divergence of interests, presumes an underlying shared set of loyalties and obligations to support the ends of the political community, among which public health and safety are central. In this scheme, public health and safety are not simply the aggregate of each private individual's interest in health and safety, interests which can be pursued more effectively through collective action. Public health and safety are community or group interests (often referred to as "state interests" in the law), interests that can transcend and take priority over private interests if the legislature so chooses.

The idea of democracy as promoting the common or group interest is captured in Joseph Tussman's classic work (1960, 27–28) on political obligation: "[T]he government's concern for the individual is not to be understood as special concern for *this* or *that* individual but rather as concern for all individuals. Government, that is to say, serves the welfare of the community." ...

THE LANGUAGE OF PUBLIC HEALTH

What are we to make of this constitutional tradition surrounding the development of the regulatory power for health and safety? What relevance does it have for the policy disputes of today, particularly those concerning the limitation of lifestyle risks?

The constitutional tradition for public health constitutes one of those "second languages" of republicanism that Robert Bellah and his coauthors speak of in . . . *Habits of the Heart.* In their book, the first language (or tradition of moral discourse) of American politics is political individualism. But there are "second languages" of community rooted in the republican and biblical tradition that limit and qualify the scope and consequences of political individualism.

Public health as a second language reminds us that we are not only individuals, we are also a community and a body politic, and that we have shared commitments to one another and promises to keep. . . .

The danger is that we can come to discuss public health exclusively within the dominant discourse of political individualism, relying either on the harm principle or a narrow paternalism justified on grounds of self-protection alone. By ignoring the communitarian language of public health, we risk shrinking its claims. We also risk undermining the sense in which health and safety are a signal commitment of the common life—a central practice by which the body politic defines itself and affirms its values.

. . . Public health belongs to the realm of the political and the ethical. Public health belongs to the ethical because it is concerned not only with explaining the occurrence of illness and disease in society, but also with ameliorating them. Beyond instrumental goals, public health is concerned with integrative goals—expressing the commitment of the whole people to face the threat of death and disease in solidarity.

Public health is also a practical science. Spanning the world of science and practical action, it seeks reasonable and practical means of altering property arrangements or limiting liberty to promote the health of the public generally.

These two ideas, the ideas of second languages and of social practices, shed light on why paternalism—at least public health paternalism—plays an affirmative role in the republican tradition. In the constitutional categories for protecting the public health, the regulatory power is to protect not individual citizens, but rather citizens considered as a group, the public health. In this tradition, the public, as well as the community itself, has a reality apart from the citizens who comprise it. Fundamental constituents of the community and the common life are its practices and institutions.

Practices are communal in nature, and concerned with the well-being of the community as a whole and not just the well-being of any particular person. Policy, and here public health paternalism, operates at the level of practices and not at the level of individual behavior. . . .

This distinction between practices and behavior should help us see the difference between public health paternalism aimed at the group and the "personal paternalism" of the doctor-patient, lawyer-client relationship. While there are public elements of these professional relationships, and while the state can (rightly or wrongly) structure these relationships in a paternalistic fashion, their essence is based on a personal encounter between a professional and a client. This is not the case with public health paternalism. Public health paternalism should also be kept separate from the legal doctrine of *parens patriae*, where the state assumes the role of parent in instances where parental supervision is absent or deemed deficient.

This suggests that public health paternalism and the language of community on which it is based fit the parent-child analogy very poorly. To Mill (1961, 273), all paternalism was wrong because the individual is best placed to know his own good: "He is the person most interested in his own well-being: the interest which any other person, except in cases of strong personal attachment, can have in it, is trifling. . . ."

But precisely because public health paternalism is aimed at the group and its practices, and not the specific individual, Mill's point is wrong. The good of the particular person is not the aim of health policy in a democracy which defends both the community and the individual. In fact, Mill is wrong twice, because particular individuals are often very poorly placed to judge the effects that market arrangements and practices have on the population as a whole. This is the task for legislatures, for organized groups of citizens, and for other agents of the public, including the citizen as voter.

Mill's dichotomy of either the harm principle or self-protection is too limited; the world of harms is not exhausted by self-imposed and other-imposed injuries. There is a third and very large set of problems that afflicts the community as a whole and that results primarily from inadequate safeguards over the practices of the common life. Economists and others often refer to this class of harms as "summing up problems" or "choice-in-the-small versus choice-in-the-large."

Creating, extending, or strengthening the practices of public health—and the collective goods principle that underlies it—ought to be the primary justification for our health and safety policy. Instead we usually base these regulations on the harm principle. We usually justify regulating the steel or coal industry on the grounds that workers and the general public have the risks of pollution or black lung visited on them, but consumers are not obliged to drink alcohol or smoke cigarettes. While this may be true, in the communitarian language and categories of public health, fixing blame is not the main point. We regulate the steel or coal industry because market competition undervalues collective goods like a clean environment or workers' safety. Using social organization to secure collective goods like public health, not preventing harms to others, is the proper rationale for health and safety regulations imposed on the steel or coal industry, or the alcohol or cigarette industry. . . .

The main lesson to learn from public health paternalism as it has developed in the constitutional tradition may well be that the second language of community and the virtues of cooperation and beneficence still exist, albeit precariously, alongside a tradition of political individualism. Strengthening the public health includes not only the practical task of improving aggregate welfare, it also involves the task of reacquainting the American public with its republican and communitarian heritage, and encouraging citizens to share in reasonable and practical group schemes to promote a wider welfare, of which their own welfare is only a part. In political individualism, seat belt legislation or signs on the beach restricting swimming when a lifeguard is not present restrict the individual's liberty for his or her own good. In this circumstance the appropriate slogan is: "The life you save may be your own." But in the second language of public health these restrictions define a common practice which shapes our life together, for the general or the common good. In the language of public health, the motto for such paternalistic legislation might be: "The lives we save together might include your own."

III. SOCIAL JUSTICE: SOCIOECONOMIC INEQUALITIES

Demography is destiny.
Attributed to Auguste Comte (1798–1857)

Deep and enduring socioeconomic inequalities form the backdrop to any public health policy, and these disparities help explain why social justice is a core value of public health. As Angus Deaton (2002, 13) explains, "Poorer people die younger and are sicker than richer people; indeed, mortality and morbidity rates are inversely related to many correlates of socioeconomic status [SES] such as income, wealth, education, or social class." Scholars often refer to the relationship as a "gradient" to emphasize the correlation between SES and health, with health improving continuously as wealth and social status rise. Various explanatory variables for the gradient have been proposed. The poor and uneducated may not have sufficient access to life's necessities, such as food, clothing, housing, and health care. Or they may engage more frequently in risk behaviors, such as smoking, illicit drug use, and high-fat diets. Alternatively, poor health may impede individuals from making a living and getting an education. Whatever the explanation, inequalities in health appear persistent over time and across cultures.

The British epidemiologist Sir Michael Marmot offers a powerful illustration of the SES gradient (2006). For every mile traveled on the Metro's Red Line in the District of Columbia from the impoverished northeast to the affluent northwest, the population lives one and a half years longer. Marmot, a pioneer of the theory of a "social gradient for health," elsewhere observes that a person's relative social standing appears to be important for a healthy, happy, and long life (2004).

Relying on Marmot's work, the London *Times* offers some intriguing, tongue-in-cheek pointers on how to better one's lot in life in its editorial "Social Climbing Is Good Exercise" (June 7, 2004):

> First, be very intelligent, very well educated and very married. If you are not those things, become them as soon as possible. Being a homeowner is also a key. But don't set up home in places where all the neighbours are likely to be richer than you. So avoid Silicon Valley, Dubai and pockets of Hampshire and West Sussex (though the ambitious should start house-hunting there immediately). You'll also do better in an inclusive society not one where some are excluded from social situations, such as Hollywood or London's Ivy Restaurant on Saturday night. Last, you should not be "hostile." Except, of course, to the maitre d' who forgets just how winning you are.

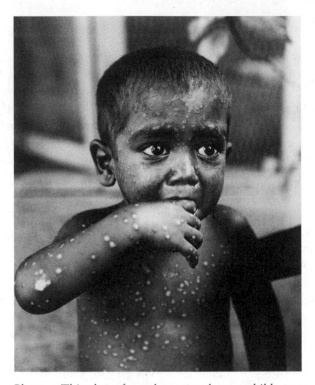

Photo 3. This photo from the 1960s shows a child
suffering from smallpox at the Infectious Diseases
Hospital in Madras. He bears the multiple small
lesions typical of smallpox. International cooperation,
intensive disease surveillance, and targeted vaccination
efforts led to the eradication of smallpox in 1979.
Reproduced by permission, © Bettman/Corbis.

Acknowledging the social gradient for health, public health advocates
often favor redistributive social policies to reduce health disparities.
This "big idea," as the *British Medical Journal* (Editor's Choice 1996,
985) has called it, suggests that "what matters in determining mortality and health in a society is less the overall wealth of that society
and more how evenly wealth is distributed. The more equally wealth is
distributed the better the health of that society." Some ethicists, relying
on these studies, say that "justice is good for our health," as argued by
Norman Daniels and colleagues below.

But before turning to Daniels's claim, it is worth considering whether
there is indeed sufficient evidence for this "big idea." John Lynch and

colleagues (2004, 5) draw the following conclusion after reviewing ninety-eight studies examining the associations between income inequality and health:

> Overall, there seems to be little support for the idea that income inequality is a major, generalizable determinant of population health differences within or between countries. Income inequality may, however, directly influence some health outcomes, such as homicide in the United States, but even that is somewhat mixed. Despite little support for a direct effect of income inequality on health per se, reducing income inequality by raising incomes of the most disadvantaged will improve their health, help reduce health inequalities, and generally improve population health.

Norman Daniels and his colleagues, using a Rawlsian theory, predict the political conditions necessary to achieve health equity. In the excerpt that follows theirs, Madison Powers and I go further, offering a template of what social justice requires for the public's health. In particular, we claim that social justice demands more than fair distribution of resources. Fundamentally, justice requires treating the most disadvantaged in society with dignity and as equal members of the political community. Our commentary explores how social justice sheds light on major ongoing controversies in the field and provides examples of the kinds of policies that public health agencies, guided by a robust conception of justice, would adopt.

JUSTICE IS GOOD FOR OUR HEALTH*
Norman Daniels, Bruce Kennedy, and Ichiro Kawachi

We have long known that the more affluent and better-educated members of a society tend to live longer and healthier lives.... Recent research suggests that the correlations between income and health do not end there. We now know, for example, that countries with a greater degree of socioeconomic inequality show greater inequality in health status; also, that middle-income groups in relatively unequal societies have worse health than comparable, or even poorer, groups in more equal societies. Inequality, in short, seems to be bad for our health.

... Universal access to health care does not necessarily break the link between social status and health. Our health is affected not simply by the ease with which we can see a doctor—though that surely matters—but also by our social position and the underlying inequality of our society. We cannot, of course, infer causation from these correlations, [but] the evidence suggests that there are *social determinants of health*.

*Reprinted from the *Boston Review*, February/March 2000: 6–15.

These social determinants offer a distinctive angle on how to think about justice, public health, and reform of the health care system. If social factors play a large role in determining our health, then efforts to ensure greater justice in health care should not focus simply on the traditional health sector. . . . We should be looking as well to improve social conditions—such as access to basic education, levels of material deprivation, a healthy workplace environment, and equality of political participation—that help to determine the health of societies. . . .

We hope to [explore] some broader issues about health and social justice. To avoid vague generalities about justice, we shall advance a line of argument inspired principally by the theory of "justice as fairness" put forth by the philosopher John Rawls. . . .

Rawls's theory of justice as fairness was not designed to address issues of health care. He assumed a completely healthy population, and argued that a just society must assure people equal basic liberties, guarantee that the right of political participation has roughly equal value for all, provide a robust form of equal opportunity, and limit inequalities to those that benefit the least advantaged. When these requirements of justice are met, Rawls argued, we can have reasonable confidence that others are showing us the respect that is essential to our sense of self-worth.

Recent empirical literature about the social determinants of health suggests that the failure to meet Rawlsian criteria for a just society is closely related to health inequality. The conjecture we propose to explore, then, is that by establishing equal liberties, robustly equal opportunity, a fair distribution of resources, and support for our self-respect—the basics of Rawlsian justice—we would go a long way to eliminating the most important injustices in health outcomes. . . .

SOCIAL DETERMINANTS OF HEALTH

Cross-National Inequalities

A country's prosperity is related to its health. . . . In richer countries people tend to live longer. . . . As a country or region develops economically average health improves. But the evidence suggests that things are more complicated. Figure [3] shows the relationship between the wealth of nations, as measured by per capita gross domestic product (GDPpc), and the health of nations, as measured by life expectancy. Clearly, GDPpc and life expectancy are closely associated, but only up to a point. The relationship levels off when GDPpc reaches $8,000 to $10,000; beyond this threshold, further economic advance buys virtually no further gains in life expectancy. This leveling effect is most apparent among the advanced industrial economies, which largely account for the upper tail of the curve in figure [3]. [Ed.–Figure 3 updates Daniels and colleagues' figure comparing life expectancy and income.]

Relative Income

. . . The health of a population depends not just on the size of the economic pie, but on how the pie is shared. Differences in health outcomes among developed nations cannot be explained simply by the absolute deprivation associated with low economic development. . . . The degree of relative deprivation within a society also matters.

. . . This *relative-income hypothesis* [states that] inequality is strongly associated with population mortality and life expectancy across nations. To be sure, wealthier countries generally have higher average life expectancy. But rich countries, too,

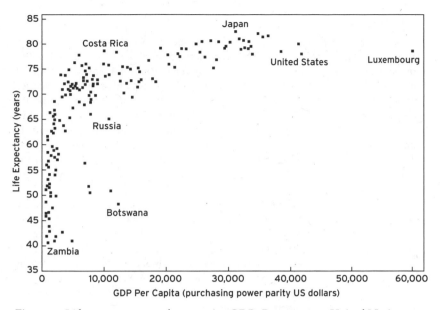

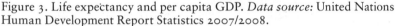

Figure 3. Life expectancy and per capita GDP. *Data source:* United Nations Human Development Report Statistics 2007/2008.

vary in life expectancy (see the tail of figure [3]), and that variation dovetails with income distribution. Wealthy countries with more equal income distributions, such as Sweden and Japan, have higher life expectancies than does the United States, despite their having lower per capita GDP. Likewise, countries with low GDPpc but remarkably high life expectancy, such as Costa Rica, tend to have a more equitable distribution of income. . . .

Individual [Socioeconomic Status (SES)]

Finally, when we move from comparing whole societies to comparing their individual members, we find, once more, that inequality is important. . . . Numerous studies have documented what has come to be known as the *socioeconomic gradient:* at each step along the socioeconomic ladder, we see improved health outcomes over the rung below. This suggests that differences in health outcomes are not confined to the extremes of rich and poor, but are observed across all levels of socioeconomic status.

Moreover, the SES gradient does not appear to be explained by differences in access to health care. Steep gradients have been observed even among groups of individuals, such as British civil servants, who all have adequate access to health care, housing, and transport. . . .

The slope of the gradient [varies substantially across societies and] appears to be fixed by the level of income inequality in a society: the more unequal a society is in economic terms, the more unequal it is in health terms. Moreover, middle income groups in a country with high income inequality typically do worse in terms of health than comparable or even poorer groups in a society with less income inequality. . . .

Pathways

... Correlations between inequality and health do not necessarily imply causation. Still, there are plausible and identifiable pathways through which social inequalities appear to produce health inequalities. In the United States, the states with the most unequal income distributions invest less in public education, have larger uninsured populations, and spend less on social safety nets. ... Educational opportunities for children in high-income-inequality states are quite different from those in states with more egalitarian distributions. These effects on education have an immediate impact on health. [Similarly, between countries, differential investment in human capital is a strong predictor of health. For example, adult literacy (particularly the disparity between male and female adult literacy) is one of the strongest predictors of life expectancy.]

These societal mechanisms—for example, income inequality leading to educational inequality leading to health inequality—are tightly linked to the political processes that influence government policy. For example, income inequality ... erodes social cohesion [leading] to lower participation in political activity, [which], in turn, undermines the responsiveness of government institutions in addressing the needs of the worst off. States with the highest income inequality, and thus lowest levels of social capital and political participation, are less likely to invest in human capital and provide far less generous social safety nets.

In short, the case for social determinants of health is strong. What are the implications of this fact for ideas of justice?

INEQUALITIES AND INEQUITIES

When is a health inequality between two groups "inequitable"? Margaret Whitehead and Goran Dahlgren [Dahlgren and Whitehead 1991] have suggested a useful and influential answer: health inequalities count as inequities when they are avoidable, unnecessary, and unfair.

... The analysis of inequity is only as good as our understanding of what is avoidable or unnecessary. [Biological differences might be unavoidable, but what about behavioral differences between cultural groups and social classes?] Whitehead and Dahlgren's term leaves us with an unresolved complexity of judgments about responsibility, ... fairness and avoidability.

The poor in many countries lack access to clean water, sanitation, adequate shelter, basic education, vaccinations, and prenatal and maternal care. As a result of some, or all, of these factors, infant mortality rates for the poor exceed those of the rich. Since social policies could supply the missing determinants of infant health, these inequalities are avoidable.

Are these inequalities also unfair? Most of us would think they are, perhaps because we believe that policies that create and sustain poverty are unjust, and perhaps also because we object to social policies that compound economic poverty with lack of access to the determinants of health. [But] we cannot eliminate health inequalities simply by eliminating poverty. Health inequalities persist even in societies that provide the poor with access to [social services, including health and education], and they persist as a gradient of health throughout the social hierarchy, not just between the very poorest groups and those above them.

[Does justice require then that all socioeconomic inequalities be eliminated to eliminate health inequalities? Or are some socioeconomic inequalities not unjust?] On issues of this kind, we should take guidance from a well-articulated account of social justice—the one put forth by John Rawls.

JUSTICE AS FAIRNESS

In *A Theory of Justice,* Rawls sought to show that a social contract designed to be fair to free and equal people would lead to equal basic liberties and equal opportunity, and would permit inequalities only when they work to make the worst-off groups fare as well as possible. Though Rawls's account was devised for the most general questions of social justice [and did not deal with health or disease, it nonetheless] provides a set of principles for the just distribution of the social determinants of health. . . .

Let us start by considering what a just society would require with regard to the distribution of the social determinants of health. In such an ideal society, everyone is guaranteed equal basic liberties, including the right to participate in politics. . . . Since, as we argued above, there is evidence that political participation is a social determinant of health, the Rawlsian ideal assures institutional protections that counter the usual effects of socioeconomic inequalities on participation—and thus on health.

Moreover, according to Rawls, justice requires fair equality of opportunity. This principle condemns discriminatory barriers and requires robust measures aimed at mitigating the effects of socioeconomic inequalities and other contingencies on opportunity. [Such measures would include equitable public education, appropriate day care, and accessible graduate and professional education.]

The equal opportunity principle also requires extensive public health, medical, and social support services aimed at promoting normal functioning for all. . . . Obviously, this focus requires provision of universal access to comprehensive health care, including public health, primary health care, and medical and social support services. . . .

Finally, a just society restricts allowable inequalities in income and wealth to those that benefit the least advantaged. . . .

In short, Rawlsian justice—though not devised for the case of health—regulates the distribution of the key social determinants of health, including the social bases of self-respect. There is nothing about the theory that should make us focus narrowly on medical services. Properly understood, justice as fairness tells us what justice requires in the distribution of all socially controllable determinants of health. . . .

Suppose we reduce socioeconomic inequalities, and thereby reduce health inequalities—but the result is that the health of all is worsened because productivity is reduced so much that important institutions are undermined. That is not acceptable. Our commitment to reducing health inequality should not require steps that threaten to make health worse off for those with less-than-equal health status. So the theoretical issue reduces to this: would it ever be reasonable to allow some health inequality in order to produce some non-health benefits for those with the worst health prospects? . . .

Rawls gave priority to the principle of protecting equal basic liberties because he believed that once people achieve some threshold level of material well-being, they will not trade away the fundamental importance of liberty for other goods. Making such a trade might deny them the liberty to pursue their most cherished ideals. . . .

Can we make the same argument about trading health for other goods? [Perhaps rational people should refrain from trading health for other goods because, without health, they cannot pursue what they value most. But this priority is not clear-cut where the conditions on choice are fair, particularly if goods gained are highly valued. Refusing to allow trades of health risks in such cases might be unjustifiably paternalistic in a way that refusal to allow trades of basic liberties is not.]

We propose a pragmatic route around this problem. Fair equality of opportunity is only approximated even in an ideally just system. . . . We cannot achieve complete equality in health any more than we can achieve completely equal opportunity. Justice is always rough around the edges.

[Provided that] everyone has a fair chance to participate [in the political process and that participants span the health gradient,] a democratic process that involved deliberation about the trade-off and its effects might be the best we could do to provide a resolution of the unanswered theoretical question.

In contrast, where the fair value of political participation is not adequately assured—and we doubt it is so assured in even our most democratic societies—we have much less confidence in the fairness of a democratic decision about how to trade health against other goods. It is much more likely under actual conditions that those who benefit most from the inequalities—that is, those who are better off—also wield disproportionate political power and will influence decisions about trade-offs to serve their interests. It may still be that the use of a democratic process in non-ideal conditions is the fairest resolution we can practically achieve, but it still falls well short of what an ideally just democratic process involves.

If we were to achieve a just distribution of resources, then, with the least well-off being as well off as possible, there would still be health inequalities. But decisions about whether to reduce those inequalities even more are matters for democratic process. Justice itself does not command their reduction.

WHAT DOES SOCIAL JUSTICE REQUIRE FOR THE PUBLIC'S HEALTH? PUBLIC HEALTH ETHICS AND POLICY IMPERATIVES*

Lawrence O. Gostin and Madison Powers

Justice is viewed as so central to the mission of public health that it has been described as the field's core value: "The historic dream of public health . . . is a dream of social justice" (Beauchamp 1999). This Commentary addresses a single question of extraordinary social and political importance: What does social justice require for the public's health? Our thesis is that justice can be an important organizing principle for public health. . . .

WHAT IS "JUSTICE," AND HOW IMPORTANT IS IT IN PUBLIC HEALTH?

Among the most basic and commonly understood meanings of justice is fairness or reasonableness, especially in the way people are treated or decisions are made. Our account of justice stresses the fair disbursement of common advantages and the

*Reprinted from *Health Affairs* 25 (July/August 2006): 1053–60.

sharing of common burdens. It captures the twin moral impulses that animate public health: to advance human well-being by improving health and to do so by focusing on the needs of the most disadvantaged. . . .

A core insight of social justice is that there are multiple causal pathways to numerous dimensions of disadvantage. These include poverty, substandard housing, poor education, unhygienic and polluted environments, and social disintegration. These and many other causal agents lead to systematic disadvantage not only in health, but also in nearly every aspect of social, economic, and political life. Inequalities beget other inequalities, and existing inequalities compound, sustain, and reproduce a multitude of deprivations. . . .

THE JUSTICE PERSPECTIVE IN PUBLIC HEALTH

. . . Some believe that government's purpose should not be to redress economic and social disadvantage, and this may be doubly so for administrative agencies dedicated to public health and the pursuit of science. We believe that it is time to rethink this view, and the justice perspective offers an alternative. Values of socioeconomic fairness are just as important to health as the prevailing values of personal license and free enterprise. The justice perspective offers a different way of seeing problems that have long plagued the field of public health.

Legitimate Scope of the Public Health Enterprise

Perhaps the deepest, most persistent critique of public health is that the field has strayed beyond its natural boundaries. Instead of focusing solely on narrow interventions for discrete injuries and diseases, the field has turned its attention to broader health determinants. It is when public health strays into the social/political sphere in matters of war, violence, poverty, and racism that critics become most upset.

The justice perspective does not provide a definitive defense against claims of overreaching. But social justice does provide a counterweight to the prevailing political view of health as primarily a private matter. The justice perspective shows why health is a matter of public concern, with the state having a role not only in the traditional areas of infectious diseases and sanitation, but also in emerging areas such as chronic diseases caused by diet, lifestyle, and the environment. Public health agencies have an obligation to address the root causes of ill health, even while they recognize that socioeconomic determinants have many causes, and solutions, that are beyond public health's exclusive expertise.

Balancing Individual and Collective Interests

The exercise of the state's coercive power has been highly contentious throughout U.S. history. When public health officials act, they face troubling conflicts between the collective benefits of population health on the one hand, and personal and economic interests on the other. Public health powers encroach on fundamental civil liberties such as privacy, bodily integrity, and freedom of movement and association [as well as economic liberties]. Justice demands that government take actions to safeguard the public's health, but that it do so with respect for individuals and sensitivity to the needs of the underprivileged.

In the realm of public health and civil liberties, then, both sides claim the mantle of justice. . . . What is most important to justice is abiding by the rule of law, which requires modern public health statutes that designate clear authority to act and provide fair processes. Policymakers, therefore, should modernize antiquated public health laws to provide adequate power to reduce major risks to the population but ensure that government power is exercised proportionately and fairly. Fairness requires just distributions of burdens and benefits to all, but also procedural due process for people subjected to compulsory interventions.

Certainly, the justice perspective cannot answer many of the most perplexing problems at the intersection of public health and civil liberties such as paternalistic interventions (for example, seat belt laws) or the exercise of powers in health emergencies (for example, avian flu or bioterrorism). However, a more serious failure of public policy would be a failure to recognize and give great weight to the demands of social justice when faced with such challenges. . . .

THE POLICY IMPERATIVES OF THE JUSTICE PERSPECTIVE

The public health community has not been successful in gaining attention to or resources for its core mission and essential services. [Public health efforts directed at prevention and population-based services are chronically underfunded, and resources are frequently allocated only in response to a disaster or threat, rather than in response to long-term needs.] This leads not to core, stable funding and attention but, rather, to a "disease du jour" mentality. This type of response creates silos, disproportionately funds biomedical solutions, and poses a "no-win" situation for public health agencies, which must respond to the latest fashion but seldom gain the kind of ongoing political attention and economic resources they need to improve the public's health.

The justice perspective offers an opportunity to change this dynamic, and the remainder of this Commentary offers concrete proposals based on the imperatives of population improvement and just distribution of benefits.

The Public Health System

Justice, with its concern for human well-being, requires a serious commitment to the public's health. It is for that reason that justice demands a tangible, long-term pledge to the public's health and the needs of the least well-off. Such a commitment, as countless reports have made clear, is lacking. Funding for prevention and population-based services is inordinately low, and categorical funding for special programs such as bioterrorism and avian flu is limited to a single issue and is time restricted. . . . There must be a substantial and stable commitment to the public's health at the federal, state, and local levels. . . . Congress and the executive branch should create a Trust Fund for Public Health to provide generous and stable resources to rebuild the eroded public health infrastructure and implement core public health functions.

Addressing Health Determinants

If justice is outcome oriented, then inevitably public health must deal with the underlying causes of poor and good health. The key health determinants include the built environment (e.g., transportation and buildings); the natural environment (e.g., clean air and water); the informational environment (e.g., health information and advertising restrictions); the social environment (e.g., social networks and support); and the economic environment (e.g., socioeconomic status). These are all public health problems, but they are not solvable solely by public health agencies. Public health researchers and agencies can provide the intellectual tools for understanding the factual basis of the problems policymakers face. They can act directly and as conveners that mobilize and coordinate government agencies, health care institutions, businesses, the media, academia, and the community.

Fair Treatment of the Disadvantaged

Fair distribution of burdens and benefits, as discussed, is a core attribute of justice. Allocations based on the market or political influence favor the rich, powerful, and socially connected. Even neutral or random allocations can be unjust because they do not benefit those with greatest need. For example, health officials who direct a population to evacuate or shelter in place should foresee that the poor will not have private transportation or the means to stock up on food or supplies. For that reason, justice requires public health officials to devise plans and programs with particular attention to the disadvantaged. . . .

. . . Social justice thus demands more than fair distribution of resources in extreme health emergencies. A failure to act expeditiously and with equal concern for all citizens, including the poor and less powerful, predictably harms the whole community by eroding public trust and undermining social cohesion. It signals to those affected and to everyone else that the basic human needs of some matter less than those of others, and it thereby fails to show the respect due to all members of the community. Social justice thus encompasses not only a core commitment to a fair distribution of resources, but it also calls for policies of action that are consistent with the preservation of human dignity and the showing of equal respect for the interests of all members of the community. . . .

A POLICY LANDSCAPE INFORMED BY SOCIAL JUSTICE

What would the policy landscape look like if it were informed by a robust conception of social justice? The political community would embrace, rather than condemn, a wide scope for the public health enterprise; value the public good as much as personal and economic liberty; [and] view the public good as involving a commitment to the health and equal worth of all members of the community. . . .

The central claim of this Commentary is that a commitment to social justice lies at the heart of public health. This commitment is to the advancement of human well-being. It aims to lift up the systematically disadvantaged and in so doing further advance the common good by showing equal respect to all individuals and groups who make up the community. Justice in public health is purposeful, positivistic, and humanistic. The aims of public health deserve a great deal more societal attention and resources than the political community has allowed.

IV. THE PUBLIC HEALTH SYSTEM

Our modern understanding of public health entails a more nuanced and coherent understanding of the causes of ill health that encompasses socioeconomic factors as well as the environmental, behavioral, and microbial causes of disease. The evolution from a focus on infectious diseases to today's more expansive approach to public health has occurred largely over the past few decades. In 1988, the Institute of Medicine (IOM) released its groundbreaking report, the *Future of Public Health,* which defined public health as the obligation of organized society to assure people of the conditions to be healthy. In the sequel published in 2003, *The Future of the Public's Health,* the IOM expounded on this understanding and proposed bold and innovative strategies for health promotion and prevention.

The public health vision articulated by the IOM involves (1) strengthening the governmental public health infrastructure, (2) encouraging major private-sector actors to promote the health of their members and surrounding communities, and (3) improving the broad determinants of population health. This vision pits those advocating on behalf of an expansive public health philosophy grounded in fundamental socioeconomic and cultural transformation against critics in and outside of the public health community who charge that such an ethos moves far beyond public health's conventionally understood purview. In the following paper, Jo Ivey Boufford, Rose Marie Martinez, and I defend the IOM committee of which we were a part, while proposing strategies for achieving an expansive construct of the public health enterprise.

THE FUTURE OF THE PUBLIC'S HEALTH: VISION, VALUES, AND STRATEGIES*

Lawrence O. Gostin, Jo Ivey Boufford, and Rose Marie Martinez

The health of the U.S. public continuously improved throughout the twentieth century. By every measure, Americans are now healthier, live longer, and enjoy lives that are less likely to be marked by injury, ill health, or premature death. During the past century, for example, infant mortality decreased, and the average life span rose from forty-five years to nearly eighty. Public health achievements include safer foods, fluoridation of drinking water, control of infectious diseases, fewer deaths from heart disease and stroke, motor vehicle safety, and safer workplaces.

The public's health still has room to improve. Although the United States has one of the highest levels of per capita gross domestic product (GDP) in the world, Americans' health status is poor compared with the health status of populations that have similar levels of economic development. [Among the thirty member countries of the Organisation for Economic Co-operation and Development (OECD), the United States has the third-highest GDP, but] it ranks twenty-third in infant mortal-

*Reprinted from *Health Affairs* 23 (July/August 2004): 96–107.

ity (7.1 deaths per 1,000 live births) and eighteenth in life expectancy at birth (76.7 years for both sexes). The World Health Organization (WHO) ranks the United States thirty-seventh among global health systems, reflecting concerns about access to and cost of health care, relatively poor health indicators, and sizable racial and socioeconomic disparities.

The relatively poor U.S. health status is even more noteworthy because of high U.S. health spending—$4,373 per capita—which is the highest in the world and more than double the OECD median of $2,000....

... More than 95 percent of U.S. federal and state health spending is directed toward personal health care and biomedical research; only 1-2 percent is directed toward prevention. These governmental funding priorities, consistent for decades, do not reflect scientific understandings of population health. There is strong evidence that access to medical care is a less important determinant of health than behavior and environment, which are responsible for more than 70 percent of avoidable deaths. This history of investment skewed toward personal health care offers a political strategy that is unlikely to achieve a maximum impact on the public's health.

STRATEGIES FOR IMPROVING THE PUBLIC'S HEALTH

If current policies do not ensure the highest attainable health for the U.S. population, then what strategies would be more effective? . . .

Strengthen the Governmental Public Health Infrastructure

Government has primary authority and responsibility for assuring the conditions in which people can be healthy. Yet public health agencies are structurally weak in each of their core components, which led the IOM to conclude that the agencies are largely in disarray. [The CDC similarly concluded that the public health infrastructure is "structurally weak in nearly every area." Structural deficiencies include outdated statutes, a poorly prepared workforce, and inadequate facilities (e.g., information and communications systems and laboratory capacity).]

To address these weaknesses, we offer the following recommendations.

Recommendation 1: Congress should establish a national Public Health Council (PHC). The PHC, comprising the secretary of the Department of Health and Human Services (HHS) and state health commissioners, with representative local health officials and outside experts, would (1) collaborate on action to achieve national health goals as articulated in *Healthy People 2010;* (2) advise the HHS secretary on financing, policy, and regulations affecting the public's health; (3) develop a funding system to sustain the public health infrastructure; and (4) evaluate the impact of domestic policies on national health outcomes and reductions of health disparities. It would improve collaboration among levels of government, provide a forum for strategic planning and monitoring progress, and elevate the status of public health within government.

Recommendation 2: HHS should report annually to Congress on the state of the nation's health.... The assessment should include a systematic evaluation of progress in meeting national health goals (for example, leading health indicators); funding and technical assistance for public health agencies to ensure sustainability; and identification of strengths and gaps In system capacity. Such assessments are needed to keep Congress and the public informed and would play an important role in policy development.

Recommendation 3: Congress should establish a stable funding mechanism, such as a "trust fund" to support state and local public health agencies. Agencies suffer from two interrelated problems: lack of adequate funding to support ongoing services, and inflexible sources of funds. . . . "Silo" or "stovepipe" funding [which is earmarked for particular purposes or constituencies] cannot sustain a permanent infrastructure and discourages evidence-based planning, policies, and programs. . . .

Recommendation 4: Congress should set conditions for receipt of funds based on states' progress toward and adherence to quality standards. HHS, through the PHC, should establish national standards of quality and hold states accountable for meeting them. . . . If agencies are charged with improving the public's health and receive adequate funding, they should be held accountable under these quality standards.

Engage Nongovernmental Actors in Partnerships for Public Health

Although the duty to safeguard the public's health has been assigned historically to government, through the work of national, state, tribal, and local health agencies, no single agency can assure all of the conditions for the public's health. Public health agencies can act as a catalyst for action by other government departments and nongovernmental actors. . . .

[On this point,] we propose the following governmental programs and incentives.

Recommendation 5: The federal government should lead a national effort to achieve stable health care coverage for every person residing in the United States. This coverage should include age-appropriate preventive services and oral health, mental health, and substance abuse treatment. The uninsured have difficulty getting care, and the services they receive may not be timely, appropriate, or well coordinated. Insurance coverage is associated with better health outcomes for children and adults.

Recommendation 6: Federal and state governments should support community-led public health efforts. Community organizations are close to the populations they serve and therefore are a crucial part of the public health system. Public health agencies should provide adequate funding and technical assistance to, and engage in partnerships with, communities. . . .

Recommendation 7: Public health agencies should create incentives for (and, if necessary, regulate) businesses to strengthen health promotion and disease and injury prevention for their employees and communities. Government should provide incentives through the tax code and conditional spending to encourage the private sector to engage in health-promoting activities. [Furthermore,] the state must strengthen regulations relating to occupational health and safety, sanitary food and living conditions, and the environment, among other areas.

Recommendation 8: The media should increase the time devoted to public service announcements and contribute to a well-informed public on matters of health. An ongoing dialogue and collaborative efforts between public health agencies and the media would benefit the public's health. . . .

Recommendation 9: Academic institutions should increase interdisciplinary learning opportunities for public health students, strengthen and expand their training of the current public health workforce, and reward faculty for both basic and applied public health research. Academe is critically important in the education and training of the public health workforce and in providing a science base for public health policy. . . .

Improve the Multiple Conditions for the Public's Health

. . . To achieve population health, it is necessary to transform national health policy, with its traditional dominant investments in personal health care and biomedical research to treat disease after it happens, to a more balanced policy that invests in the multiple determinants of societal health. . . .

Perhaps the two farthest-reaching, and therefore most controversial, determinants of health relate to the "built" and socioeconomic environments. Public health has a long history of designing the built environment to reduce injury (workplace safety, traffic calming, and fire codes), infectious diseases (sanitation, zoning, and housing codes), and environmentally associated harms (lead paint, asbestos, and toxic emissions). The United States is facing an epidemiological transition from infectious to chronic diseases such as cardiovascular disease, cancer, diabetes, asthma, and depression. The challenge is to enable communities to facilitate physical and mental well-being. . . .

A strong and consistent finding of epidemiological research is that socioeconomic status (SES) is correlated with morbidity, mortality, and functioning. SES is a complex phenomenon based on income, education, and occupation. The relationship between SES and health often is referred to as a "gradient" because of the graded and continuous nature of the association. . . .

Some researchers go further, suggesting that the overall level of socioeconomic inequality in a society affects health. That is, societies with large disparities between the rich and poor tend to have inferior health status. The validity of these studies has been challenged recently. However, some claim that from an ethical perspective, "social justice is good for our health." Government can take active steps to improve the built and socioeconomic environments in several ways.

Recommendation 10: State and local governments should engage in land-use planning to encourage healthier lifestyles and habitats. [Strategies include] economic incentives to encourage green spaces and recreational facilities; building and housing codes to reduce toxic exposures; zoning to increase availability of wholesome foods and products; and school requirements to serve healthy foods and promote exercise among students. . . .

Recommendation 11: The federal government and the states should adopt more comprehensive strategies to reduce health disparities. Health policymakers have documented major health disparities within the population and have set a goal of reducing them. . . . Disparities can be reduced through targeted public health interventions to serve . . . populations [with the greatest need, including the poor and racial minorities, and through] general improvements in access to essential services such as income support, education, and health care.

JUSTIFICATIONS FOR AN EXPANDED VISION OF PUBLIC HEALTH

Critics have argued powerfully against the foregoing proposals for achieving a healthier population. In this section we respond to these challenges, recognizing that the questions posed are incisive and deserve careful scrutiny.

Why should health be a primary social undertaking? [Although other priorities, such as transportation, energy, education and national security, compete with health] there are good reasons to give special attention to health. . . .

. . . If individuals have physical and mental health, they are better able to social-ize, work, and engage in the activities of family and social life that bring meaning and happiness. . . . Health is also essential for the functioning of populations. Without minimum levels of health, people cannot fully engage in social interactions, partici-pate in the political process, exercise rights of citizenship, generate wealth, create art, and provide for the common security. Notably, evidence is emerging that direct investments in health can have positive effects on the economy. A safe and healthy population builds strong roots for a country—its governmental structures, social organizations, cultural endowment, economic prosperity, and national defense. Understood in this way, then, population health becomes a transcendent value.

Are fundamental changes in physical [and social] conditions warranted? Critics argue that public health agencies overreach and lose their legitimacy when they address the broad determinants of health. There are . . . political dangers in straying too far from what many consider public health's traditional mandate [but] address-ing the broad determinants of health leads to more effective social policy. . . . As the main proponent of population health in society, the public health community must call attention to the "upstream" causes of morbidity and premature death and must propose a broad range of social, economic, and behavioral tools needed to make populations healthier.

[Though critics may challenge evidence of an SES gradient, the fact that the causal pathways between low SES and poor health are not fully understood should not doom public health to waiting for definitive research before helping the poor. Critics also challenge the appropriateness of efforts to modify the built environment in healthful ways, characterizing efforts as "coercive" and "moralistic." But the gov-ernment has been and is actively involved in land-use planning; therefore, it has an] obligation to carefully consider the population's health in its land-use policies.

ASSURING THE PUBLIC'S HEALTH: FUTURE CHALLENGES

We are acutely aware that key obstacles await the strategies we have enumerated. Achieving a highly functioning governmental public health system is difficult; the necessary tasks are technically within our reach but require political will. There are many reasons to question the political commitment to population health—a history of underinvestment, silo funding, and a culture of individualism. In matters of fund-ing, standard setting, and accountability, federalism poses another problem. Which government—federal, tribal, state, or local—holds the power and duty to devote resources and create policy?

The challenges to achieving effective partnerships in public health are equally apparent. The private and voluntary sectors possess no duty to act for the public good, and there is little political consensus about creating incentives and require-ments to do so. The government's role vis-à-vis the private sector has always been controversial. Those who support limited government and a broad sphere of eco-nomic freedom may oppose partnerships that go beyond the purely voluntary, but the potential value of closer cooperation is becoming more clear.

Finally, and self-evidently, there are deep challenges in creating policy to improve the socioeconomic conditions of health. Socioeconomic determinants evoke images of redistribution of wealth and status, which are unpopular in many circles. However, this is not merely a question of ideology but one of science. The task will be to demonstrate an evidence-based way to reduce socioeconomic disparities and to show that this improves health outcomes.

Given these challenges, we understand that our aspirations for "healthy people in healthy communities" need to compete in the marketplace of ideas. Yet we think that population health does deserve a special place in national debates and priorities, and it has taken a backseat to other political interests for too long.

V. CONCLUSION

The field of public health, as we have seen, is deeply complex, riddled with contradictions, and influenced by politics, culture, and economics, and it has undergone profound developments over the past few decades. Practitioners and scholars have cultivated a common understanding of core concepts in public health, the contours of which are being delineated through experience and scholarly debate. Likewise, the practice of public health has improved; workers in this field are beginning to develop a sense of professionalism, expertise, and competency comparable to that of practitioners of older disciplines such as medicine.

The field of public health has struggled through the years to gain attention, respect, and adequate resources. In the aftermath of recent natural and human-caused tragedies, however, public health has become more visible. The terrorist attacks of 9/11 and subsequent anthrax letters have driven momentous changes in public health policy. The United States and the rest of the world have witnessed the devastation wrought by natural disasters, such as the South Asian tsunami and the Gulf Coast hurricanes. Global society also faces the threat of the catastrophic health consequences of an emerging infectious disease, such as smallpox, severe acute respiratory syndrome (SARS), or pandemic influenza—whether naturally occurring or intentionally inflicted.

Consequently, policy makers have been preoccupied by the perceived need for preparedness for public health emergencies, including stockpiles of vaccines and pharmaceuticals and "surge" capacity for hospital beds and equipment. Emergency public health preparedness funding purportedly allows for "dual use," meaning that funds can also go toward strengthening the public health infrastructure and basic public health activities (e.g., routine surveillance and prevention activities).

Improved visibility and funding constitute only one edge of the double-edged sword of public health preparedness, however. Preparedness activities have also created special programs and "silos" that divert attention from traditional public health services.

But when one steps back from the day-to-day struggles for funding and attention, it is apparent that the field of public health holds great promise for the future. No endeavor is more important than promoting health and preventing injury and disease among the population. As the field improves its scientific methods for measuring effectiveness and as it demonstrates its importance, public health will gain the political attention and resources it deserves.

RECOMMENDED READINGS

Community and Civic Participation

Beauchamp, Dan. 1988. *The Health of the Republic: Epidemics, Medicine, and Moralism as Challenges to Democracy.* Philadelphia: Temple Univ. Press. (Provides an expanded vision of republican equality and further develops his community-oriented perspective on health)

Pearce, Neil, and George Davey Smith. 2003. Is social capital the key to inequalities in health? *American Journal of Public Health* 93: 122–29. (Questions some of Putnam's conclusions, arguing that social capital has a marginal impact on health as compared to macro-level economic and social policies and that overemphasizing the role of social capital produces ineffective or potentially harmful policies)

Putnam, Robert D. 2000. Health and happiness. In *Bowling Alone: The Collapse and Revival of American Community,* 326–35. New York: Simon & Schuster. (Asserts that social connectedness is itself a determinant of health)

Social Justice: Socioeconomic Inequalities

Daniels, Norman. 2006. Equity and population health: Toward a broader bioethics agenda. *Hastings Center Report* 36 (4): 22–35. (Argues that bioethics' traditionally narrow focus on clinical relationships and new technologies should be broadened to address population health, health disparities, and issues of justice)

Deaton, Angus. 2002. Policy implications of the gradient of health and wealth. *Health Affairs* 21 (2): 13–30. (Explains the deep, persistent, and cross-cultural relationship between socioeconomic status and health outcomes, which he terms the gradient of health and wealth)

Lynch, John, George Davey Smith, Sam Harper, Marianne Hillemeier, Nancy Ross, George A. Kaplan, and Michael Wolfson. 2004. Is income inequality a determinant of population health? Part 1: A systematic review. *Milbank*

Quarterly 82: 5–95. (Casts doubt on the assertion that societies where income is distributed on a more equal basis are necessarily healthier)

Powers, Madison, and Ruth Faden. 2006. *Social Justice: The Moral Foundations of Public Health and Health Policy.* New York: Oxford Univ. Press. (Outlines a theory of social justice focused on the nondistributive aspects of well-being and applies it to public health)

The Public Health System

Institute of Medicine. 2003. *The Future of the Public's Health in the 21st Century.* Washington, DC: National Academies Press. (Articulates a broad and ambitious vision for public health that is centered on strengthening government public health infrastructure, coordinating the activities of various state and nonstate actors, and addressing the multiple determinants of health)

Rothstein, Mark A. 2002. Rethinking the meaning of public health. *Journal of Law, Medicine & Ethics* 30: 144–49. (Argues for a narrower understanding of public health's scope that is focused on government officials providing traditional public health services)

Weeks, Elizabeth. 2006. After the catastrophe: Disaster relief for hospitals. *North Carolina Law Review* 85: 223–300. (Provides an evaluation of the public health infrastructure supplied by hospitals in times of disaster, with a specific focus on the Gulf Coast hurricanes)

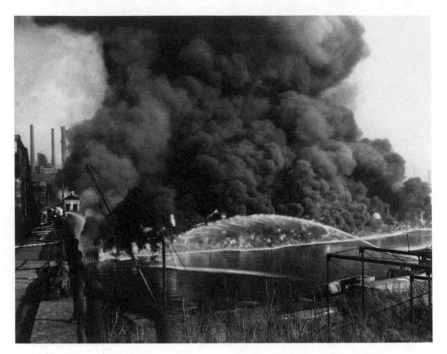

Photo 4. The Cuyahoga River in flames on November 3, 1952. The Cleveland, Ohio, river caught fire several times during the twentieth century when oil and other contaminants on the water's surface ignited. The 1969 river fire prompted outrage nationwide and galvanized the environmental movement. Today, the Environmental Protection Agency regulates the risks posed by environmental contaminants like those responsible for the Cuyahoga fires. Photograph courtesy of James Thomas.

Public Health Ethics

The field of public health ethics applies principles and values to evaluate the justifiability of public health actions. A central question posed is, "What are the appropriate limits on the state's power when its exercise to safeguard the public's health and safety interferes with individual interests?" In answering this question, ethicists take account of the personal and economic interests of individuals, as well as the collective benefits to the population of improved health and safety. This ethical analysis of public health interventions does not dictate policy choices; rather, it enables public health ethicists to identify a range of ethically appropriate actions to promote health and prevent diseases. It is then up to democratically elected officials to choose among ethically viable alternatives for public health action.

The field should not be understood as providing the "right" answer, because public health practice is far too complex to be amenable to simple solutions. The principles and values that ethicists use, moreover, are often in tension. It is not unusual for ethicists to arrive at differing conclusions on the same question, at least in part because ethicists may differ in the values they emphasize. Consequently, public health ethics should be understood more as a helpful methodology for examining difficult problems in public health than as a means of finding ideal solutions.

The companion text to this volume discusses three general ethical justifications for coercive public health interventions: risk to others, protection of incompetent persons, and risk to self. The first justification—the "harm principle"—holds that the state may prevent harm to others or punish individuals for inflicting such harm. The second justification—the "best interests" of the individual—holds that the state may protect the health and safety of those individuals, such as children or persons with mental disabilities, who are incapable of safeguarding their own interests. These two justifications are widely accepted by ethicists. However, the third justification—paternalism—is deeply controversial. Paternalism is "the interference with a person's liberty of action justified by reasons referring exclusively to the welfare, good, happiness, needs, interests, or values of the person being coerced" (Dworkin 2008, 281). Paternalistic interventions are those designed solely or primarily to protect a competent person's own health and safety, irrespective of her wishes. They typically regulate "self-regarding" behaviors—those behaviors that only, or primarily, endanger the health of the actor (e.g., not wearing a seat belt).

The extent to which the government should compel a competent person to refrain from self-regarding behaviors is far from settled. On the one hand, self-destructive behaviors (e.g., high-fat diets, sedentary lifestyles, and smoking) pose a heavy burden of disease and early death in the population. Should public health officials intervene to prevent individuals from engaging in such behaviors even when there is no harm posed to others? If doing so is off-limits, then public health officials miss an important opportunity to prevent injuries and diseases, especially among the vulnerable populations that disproportionately bear the burden of such injuries and diseases. Further, by intruding a little on a person's autonomy now, a health-promoting intervention may provide much greater autonomy later by enabling that person to avoid the constraints on choice that diseases cause (Gostin and Gostin 2009). On the other hand, individuals are supposed to have the freedom to make their own choices. If they make an unhealthy choice, whose responsibility is it—theirs or the state's?

The companion text to this reader discusses five ethical criteria for systematically evaluating government regulation. The first step is determining whether the risk is sufficiently significant to warrant state action. To do so, one must assess the nature of the risk (the hazard faced), the duration of the risk (when the risk will diminish or end), the probability of harm (the likelihood of the event), and the severity of the harm (the degree of injury to individuals and populations). The second step focuses on whether the proposed regulation is likely to be effective in preventing or ameliorating the harm. If the intervention is unlikely to succeed, it is usually not worth undertaking.

Third, the cost of the intervention should be evaluated. Public health regulations impose economic costs—resources of agencies to devise and implement policies, costs to individuals and businesses subject to regulation, and lost opportunities to intervene with a different measure that might be more effective. Fourth, it is important to consider the burden that the regulation will place on individuals. State interventions can infringe on a variety of individual interests, including bodily integrity, privacy, freedom of expression, freedom of association, freedom of religion, and liberty of person. The final step is to determine whether the policy is fair. That is, does the policy demonstrate equal respect for all persons and fairly allocate benefits, burdens, and costs? These five ethical criteria for evaluating public health regulations are not a means of "correctly" determining whether a particular regulation should be implemented, but they do provide a structured method for assessing the appropriateness of coercive state action.

This chapter provides an overview of public health ethics, in three parts. It begins with the evolution from bioethics to public health ethics, moves to the most controversial aspect of public health ethics (paternalism), and concludes with the subject of risk regulation.

I. FROM BIOETHICS TO PUBLIC HEALTH ETHICS

When thinking about the most appropriate principles and values for evaluating public health actions, it is useful to start with perhaps the most famous articulation of bioethical principles, the 1978 "Belmont Report" of the National Commission for the Protection of Human Subjects of Biomedical and Behavioral Research. Although this report is geared principally to the ethics of human subjects research, its explanation of three basic principles—respect for persons, beneficence, and justice—has been highly influential in the broader field of bioethics.

THE BELMONT REPORT: ETHICAL PRINCIPLES AND GUIDELINES FOR THE PROTECTION OF HUMAN SUBJECTS OF RESEARCH*
The National Commission for the Protection of Human Subjects of Biomedical and Behavioral Research

Three basic [ethical] principles, among those generally accepted in our cultural tradition, are particularly relevant to the ethics of research involving human subjects: the principles of respect of persons, beneficence, and justice.

Federal Register 44 (April 18, 1979): 23192–97.

1. RESPECT FOR PERSONS

Respect for persons incorporates at least two ethical convictions: first, that individuals should be treated as autonomous agents, and second, that persons with diminished autonomy are entitled to protection. The principle of respect for persons thus divides into two separate moral requirements: the requirement to acknowledge autonomy and the requirement to protect those with diminished autonomy.

An autonomous person is an individual capable of deliberation about personal goals and of acting under the direction of such deliberation. To respect autonomy is to give weight to autonomous persons' considered opinions and choices while refraining from obstructing their actions unless they are clearly detrimental to others. To show lack of respect for an autonomous agent is to repudiate that person's considered judgments, to deny an individual the freedom to act on those considered judgments, or to withhold information necessary to make a considered judgment, when there are no compelling reasons to do so.

However, not every human being is capable of self-determination. The capacity for self-determination matures during an individual's life, and some individuals lose this capacity wholly or in part because of illness, mental disability, or circumstances that severely restrict liberty. Respect for the immature and the incapacitated may require protecting them as they mature or while they are incapacitated.

. . . The extent of protection afforded should depend upon the risk of harm and the likelihood of benefit. The judgment that any individual lacks autonomy should be periodically reevaluated and will vary in different situations.

In most cases of research involving human subjects, respect for persons demands that subjects enter into the research voluntarily and with adequate information. In some situations, however, application of the principle is not obvious. The involvement of prisoners as subjects of research provides an instructive example. On the one hand, it would seem that the principle of respect for persons requires that prisoners not be deprived of the opportunity to volunteer for research. On the other hand, under prison conditions they may be subtly coerced or unduly influenced to engage in research activities for which they would not otherwise volunteer. . . . Whether to allow prisoners to "volunteer" or to "protect" them presents a dilemma. Respecting persons, in most hard cases, is often a matter of balancing competing claims urged by the principle of respect itself.

2. BENEFICENCE

Persons are [also] treated in an ethical manner . . . by making efforts to secure their well-being. . . . The term "beneficence" is often understood to cover acts of kindness or charity, [but here] beneficence is understood in a stronger sense, as an obligation. Two general rules have been formulated as complementary expressions of beneficent actions in this sense: (1) do not harm and (2) maximize possible benefits and minimize possible harms.

. . . Claude Bernard extended [the Hippocratic maxim "do no harm"] to the realm of research, saying that one should not injure one person regardless of the benefits that might come to others. However, even avoiding harm requires learning what is harmful; and . . . learning what will in fact benefit may require exposing persons to risk. The problem posed by these imperatives is to decide when it is justifiable to seek certain benefits despite the risks involved, and when the benefits should be forgone because of the risks. . . .

The principle of beneficence often occupies a well-defined justifying role in many areas of research involving human subjects. An example is found in research involving children. Effective ways of treating childhood diseases and fostering healthy development are benefits that serve to justify research involving children—even when individual research subjects are not direct beneficiaries. . . . But the role of the principle of beneficence is not always so unambiguous. A difficult ethical problem remains, for example, about research that presents more than minimal risk without immediate prospect of direct benefit to the children involved. . . . Here again, as with all hard cases, the different claims covered by the principle of beneficence may come into conflict and force difficult choices.

3. JUSTICE

Who ought to receive the benefits of research and bear its burdens? . . . An injustice occurs when some benefit to which a person is entitled is denied without good reason or when some burden is imposed unduly. Another way of conceiving the principle of justice is that equals ought to be treated equally. However, this statement requires explication. . . . Almost all commentators allow that distinctions based on experience, age, deprivation, competence, merit, and position do sometimes constitute criteria justifying differential treatment for certain purposes. It is necessary, then, to explain in what respects people should be treated equally. There are several widely accepted formulations of just ways to distribute burdens and benefits. Each formulation mentions some relevant property on the basis of which burdens and benefits should be distributed. These formulations are (1) to each person an equal share, (2) to each person according to individual need, (3) to each person according to individual effort, (4) to each person according to societal contribution, and (5) to each person according to merit.

. . . During the 19th and early 20th centuries the burdens of serving as research subjects fell largely upon poor ward patients, while the benefits of improved medical care flowed primarily to private patients. Subsequently, the exploitation of unwilling prisoners as research subjects in Nazi concentration camps was condemned as a particularly flagrant injustice. In this country, in the 1940's, the Tuskegee syphilis study used disadvantaged, rural black men to study the untreated course of a disease that is by no means confined to that population. These subjects were deprived of demonstrably effective treatment in order not to interrupt the project, long after such treatment became generally available. [See box 1.]

Against this historical background, it can be seen how conceptions of justice are relevant to research involving human subjects. For example, the selection of research subjects needs to be scrutinized in order to determine whether some classes . . . are being systematically selected simply because of their easy availability, their compromised position, or their manipulability, rather than for reasons directly related to the problem being studied. Finally, whenever research supported by public funds leads to the development of therapeutic devices and procedures, justice demands both that these not provide advantages only to those who can afford them and that

BOX 1

TUSKEGEE: RACE, RESEARCH, AND BIOETHICS

The Belmont Report was published seven years after accounts of the infamous Tuskegee syphilis study appeared on the front pages of national newspapers in July 1972. The study, which was begun in 1932, was framed as a "study in nature" that focused on observing the course of untreated syphilis. The test subjects (all African American men living in Macon, Alabama) were denied standard medical treatments throughout the study—even after penicillin became widely available in the 1940s. In fact, as Allan M. Brandt, a professor of the history of medicine, details, the doctors devising and directing the study recruited subjects under the guise of providing care. They provided ineffectual ointments and characterized diagnostic tests (including painful and risky spinal taps) as treatment. In order to ensure that accepted medical therapies would not interfere with the study, the doctors prevented test subjects from receiving treatment from other sources—including local doctors, the Alabama Health Department, and the U.S. Army. Brandt (1978, 23) describes the "essentially racist nature" of the study: "The premise that blacks, promiscuous and lustful, would not seek or continue treatment, shaped the study. A test of untreated syphilis seemed 'natural' because the [U.S. Public Health Service] presumed the men would never be treated; the Tuskegee Study made that a self-fulfilling prophecy."

such research should not unduly involve persons from groups unlikely to be among the beneficiaries of subsequent applications of the research.

.   .   .   .   .

One of the central debates in the field of public health ethics is whether the bioethical principles enunciated in the Belmont Report are sufficient for assessing population-based interventions. It may be that these principles can be adapted to the needs of public health interventions by focusing on public—instead of individual—well-being. Alternatively, bioethical principles may overly constrain public health activities because they stress individual autonomy at the expense of a more communitarian view of the public good. As the bioethicist and prominent political philosopher Onora O'Neill (2004, 1135) notes, "road safety, food safety, water safety, safe medicines and measures that protect against infection cannot be tailored to individual choice," making an individualistic, autonomy-centered ethic less applicable in public health. Other ethical traditions that focus on values of community, solidarity, and the needs of the collective provide a useful counterbalance to the more individualistic bioethical principles.

Many notable scholars are now writing on the subject of public health ethics (e.g., Bayer, Gostin, et al. 2007; Dawson and Verweij 2007; Kass 2001, 2004; Bradley and Burls 2000; Coughlin and Beauchamp 1996), but I have chosen three contributions. First, Ronald Bayer and Amy L. Fairchild offer a historical account of public health ethics' origins and evolution. They start with the autonomy-centered values of bioethics ("in the beginning there was bioethics") and then trace more modern efforts to articulate an ethics of public health.

In the second excerpt, James F. Childress and colleagues provide an overview of the basic principles of and tensions in public health ethics, identifying and weighing general moral considerations in public health: benefits, harms, utility, justice, autonomy, privacy, honesty, transparency, and trust. Like Bayer and Fairchild, Childress and colleagues struggle with how and to what extent individual autonomy should be integrated into public health ethics. They, too, are also interested in teasing out a rubric for determining whether paternalistic interventions are ethically justified in particular cases.

In the last excerpt of this section, Daniel Callahan and Bruce Jennings helpfully examine the scope of public health ethics, which they claim is as broad as public health itself—covering activities ranging from health promotion and disease prevention to the amelioration of socioeconomic disparities. In the process, they draw attention to the correspondingly wide-ranging methods of ethical analysis that are applicable to the practice of public health. Public health ethics continue today to rapidly evolve and develop. Greater engagement of public health practitioners, scholars, and students in ethical discourse will enrich the field and the ongoing political, academic, popular, and professional debates concerning the proper scope of public health and the appropriateness of government interventions to protect communal well-being.

THE GENESIS OF PUBLIC HEALTH ETHICS*
Ronald Bayer and Amy L. Fairchild

In the beginning there was bioethics. The 1960s and 1970s witnessed extraordinary challenges to the broadly understood authority of medicine. Perhaps most strik-

*Reprinted from *Bioethics* 18, no. 6 (2004): 473–92.

ingly, the paternalistic authority of physicians was brought into question by a new medical ethics that gave pride of place to the concept of autonomy. Paralleling the challenges to medical practice were those that involved the research enterprise. Against a backdrop of scandal and abuse, . . . a new ethics of research took hold. . . . The ethics of clinical research and the ethics of medical practice were conjoined by a commitment to autonomy and individual rights.

Remarkably, as bioethics emerged and began to have enormous impacts on the practice of medicine and research . . . little attention was given to the question of the ethics of public health. This was all the more striking since the core values and practices of public health, often entailing the subordination of the individual for the common good, seemed to stand as a rebuke to the ideological impulses of bioethics. . . .

Of what relevance is autonomy-focused bioethics for public health, with its mix of justifications including those that are either implicitly or explicitly paternalistic or that seek to impose strictures on individuals and communities in the name of collective welfare? To examine the deep divide between the central commitments of bioethics and the values that animate the practice of public health, we focus on a series of controversies implicating the concepts of privacy, liberty, and paternalism.

FIRST ENCOUNTERS: EPIDEMIOLOGICAL RESEARCH AND THE LIMITS OF CONSENT

. . . Beginning in the 1970s, a discussion began about whether the emerging rules and regulations for human subjects' research would apply to epidemiological studies. Was informed consent necessary when research involved the use of extant records? Would imposing consent requirements for the examination of data sets involving large numbers of people . . . render epidemiological research virtually impossible? . . . In 1981, . . . regulations for the protection of human subjects explicitly exempt[ed] epidemiological research involving already existing data from informed consent requirements provided the risk to subjects was minimal, the research did not record data in a way that was individually identifiable, and the research could not otherwise be conducted. The concession represented a relaxation of the fundamental principle that individuals could not be conscripted into research without their consent. . . .

AIDS, PUBLIC HEALTH, AND ETHICS

. . . It is not surprising that when those schooled in bioethics first sought to address the ethical challenges posed by AIDS, they did so guided by the principles and values that had shaped the confrontation with medicine and the research enterprise. Their efforts were informed by the intense concern of gay men about threats to privacy and civil liberties advocates fearful that AIDS would provide the occasion for the erosion of a set of substantive and procedural constitutional rights forged by the US Supreme Court. . . .

. . . In lieu of the compulsory tradition [for controlling epidemics] that often involved mandatory case reporting by name, contact investigation, and where necessary the use of isolation, an "exceptionalist" perspective took hold. Focused on the centrality of education for mass behavioural change, the protection of the rights and privacy of people infected with HIV, and a rejection of coercive measures, the approach to AIDS was voluntarist at its core. A simple dictum emerged: no public health policy that violated the rights of individuals could be effective in controlling the spread of HIV. There was, therefore, no tension between public health and civil liberties. Indeed, the protection of civil liberties was critical to the public health. . . .

SURVEILLANCE AND THE LIMITS OF PRIVACY

Since the end of the nineteenth century, surveillance has served as a critical element in the practice of public health. Central to the effort to monitor and intervene in the face of threats to the public health, surveillance has imposed on healthcare institutions and especially physicians the duty to report cases to confidential registries. Almost always such reports have included the names of the afflicted. . . .

[Soon after the first cases of AIDS were identified, state health departments began to require that physicians report by name each newly diagnosed case. Once a test for the HIV antibody became available, it was only a matter of time until reporting requirements were extended to HIV.] The rationale for such reporting drew upon the history of public health: reporting would alert public health officials to the presence of individuals infected with a lethal infection; would allow them to counsel infected individuals about what they needed to do to prevent further transmission; would permit the authorities to monitor the incidence and prevalence of infection. Alert to concerns about privacy and confidentiality, health officials underscored the existence of administrative, regulatory, and statutory protections for reported names. . . .

To these propositions, gay community-based antagonists to name-based reporting and civil liberties advocates retorted that AIDS was different: social hostility and AIDS-related hysteria could lead to changes in policy, legislatively imposed, that would permit breaches that would never occur with other conditions. And then those in registries would lose their jobs, their housing, and perhaps their liberty. . . . Many health officials in states with relatively large AIDS caseloads [came to believe that reporting] would be counterproductive; it would drive people away from testing and counseling. . . . It did not matter that public health departments had an exemplary record in protecting name-based reports. If those most at risk for HIV had fears about what would happen to them, then that was all that mattered. . . .

The debates that occurred over name-based reporting in the context of the AIDS epidemic would inevitably raise questions about the practice of surveillance itself as advocates of privacy, to the astonishment of public health practitioners, suggested that the warrant for the violation of privacy in the early twentieth century no longer deserved unquestioned obeisance.

CONFINEMENT AND THE LIMITS OF LIBERTY

Isolation and quarantine represent the most plenary exercise of the state's authority in the name of public health. Historically, the imposition of isolation and quarantines to control infectious threats was bounded by few procedural protections. The rights of the individual were viewed as subservient to the judgements of those with public health authority. As the pattern of morbidity and mortality underwent an epidemiological transformation in the twentieth century, as chronic conditions replaced infectious diseases as the pre-eminent threat, the role of quarantine and isolation became marginal to the practice of public health in the United States. . . .

[During the 2002 outbreak of severe acute respiratory syndrome (SARS), however, countries relied on these ancient public health tools—isolation and quarantine—to contain the epidemic.] Confinement of individuals with disease and those exposed raised questions about the level of risk that justified loss of liberty. . . . Uncertainty about how wide to cast the net of quarantine for exposed, asymptomatic individuals was framed by the absence of a diagnostic assay that could rapidly distinguish between the infected and merely exposed with high specificity. But very broad quarantines were viewed as justifiable because of the uncertainties of risk. . . .

In the fall of 2003, as the international community braced for the possibility of a resurgence of SARS, it became clear that the isolation procedures used during the initial outbreak had been far too stringent. . . . The [Centers for Disease Control and Prevention (CDC) responded by elaborating] a finer range of surveillance and quarantine recommendations. . . .

PATERNALISM AND THE LIMITS OF AUTONOMY

For government to impose restrictions on those who represent a risk to others falls clearly within the broadly accepted exercise of state power in liberal societies and in principle entails no fundamental problem for the autonomy-focused perspective of bioethics. Problems emerge where the risk to others is uncertain. It is here that an important divide emerges between the judgements of those committed to autonomy and those whose first priority is the public health. It is a divide characterised by complex questions of what moral weight to give to the likelihood and severity of harm. However these matters are resolved, they raise issues that are fundamentally different from those posed by behaviours that represent primarily a threat to individuals themselves. It is here that the spectre of paternalism emerges, and that the tension between public health perspectives and autonomy-focused bioethics is positioned in its boldest relief.

Tobacco consumption . . . serves as an object lesson in the ways in which the antagonism towards paternalism has both shaped and limited public health policy.

Three broad sets of policies were adopted to confront the challenge posed by tobacco [from the 1960s through the turn of the century]: restrictions on advertising; the imposition of taxes; and limits on public smoking. In each case, a public warrant for the measures adopted sought to demonstrate that it was third parties, innocent victims, or children that were the object of protective measures. Only insofar as warnings about tobacco, weak as they were, were posted on cigarette packages, did public health efforts direct themselves to those who bore the full burden of cigarette-related suffering, disease, and death. . . .

. . . By the end of the twentieth century, the willingness to embrace explicitly paternalistic justifications for antismoking policy was becoming more evident, no doubt facilitated by the emergence of a sharp social gradient in cigarette consumption—those who are educated smoke less and less, those at the bottom of the social ladder continue to smoke.

The most dramatic reflection of the willingness to embrace paternalism was to be found in measures seeking to "denormalise" smoking. We typically do not think of health promotion campaigns as paternalistic. But when they go beyond the provision of information and systematically seek to transform the very desires and preferences of those to whom they are directed, they assume a fundamentally different character. Indeed, the use of social marketing techniques to undercut smoking behaviour must be viewed as paternalistic in impulse as well as practice. . . .

TOWARD AN ETHICS OF PUBLIC HEALTH

What the foregoing discussion has demonstrated is that those involved in the practice of public health embrace a set of values that are often, if not always, in conflict with the autonomy-centred values of those who take an individualistic and antipaternalistic stance. But ethos is not ethics. . . . In the context of public health, the question that needs to be addressed is whether paternalism and subordination of the individual for the good of the commonwealth should serve as the foundation for an ethics of public health or whether the perspective derived from the dominant autonomy-focused and antipaternalistic currents in bioethics should serve as a point of departure for a thoroughgoing challenge to the fundamental values and practices of public health.

We begin with the conviction that at the core of public health practice is the charge to protect the common good, to intervene for such ends even in the face of uncertainty. This stance may, we believe, necessitate limits on the choices of individuals on grounds of communal protection against both hazard and paternalism. . . .

[During the twentieth century, public health interventions were often justified by invoking the harm principle. While the harm principle finds support in legal tradition and ethics, there are nonetheless limits to its application.] In recent decades, efforts to bind the harm principle have focused on employing the least restrictive or intrusive alternative that could protect the public health against significant risk. But what constitutes a least restrictive/intrusive alternative and how the significance of risk is to be judged are only in part empirical matters. . . . The tension between autonomy and public health perspectives is reflected in all such judgements. We believe that the standard appropriate to public health cannot be derived from the basic assumptions of a bioethics dominated by individualism.

The case of tuberculosis makes this clear. When individuals fail to complete the course of treatment they run the risk of reactivation and of developing multi-drug resistant strains of mycobacterium tuberculosis. . . . When noncompliance characterises large numbers of individuals . . . there is no question but that the threat to public health attains significance. It is therefore the collective hazard that provides the warrant for intervention even when the threat posed by any individual may not attain the standard of significance. This is, of course, a point suggested by Geoffrey Rose in his now famous formulation of the ways in which small benefits to individuals from public health interventions may produce quite significant collective goods. . . .

In the end, a focus on population-based health requires a population-based analysis and a willingness to recognise that the ethics of collective health may require far more extensive limitations on privacy, as in the case of public health surveillance, and on liberty, as in the case of isolation and quarantine, than would be justified from the perspective of the autonomy-focused orientation of the dominant current in bioethics. Compulsion and, indeed, coercion—so anathema to this tradition of bioethics—are central to public health. Nevertheless, it is important to recognise that while mandatory measures and recourse to coercion may be necessary, efforts designed to elicit the voluntary co-operation of those at risk for acquiring or transmitting infectious diseases are preferable [from an ethical perspective] and, [as a practical matter], may be more effective. . . . Thus, while a public health perspective will not privilege liberty and privacy, it does not follow that it should be insensitive to the importance of protecting individual rights.

More challenging is the question of the role of paternalism in public health. . . . Antipaternalism has struck a powerful cord in American political culture. . . . Animated by a broad utilitarianism that seeks to maximise communal well-being, public health has embraced measures that go far beyond the very limited recognition of justifiable paternalism in conventional bioethical accounts.

. . . [Some defend paternalism by focusing on the protection of those whose choices are limited by a lack of knowledge or understanding, but the] central commitment to collective well-being requires a much more robust embrace of paternalism. . . . We ought, for example, to protect motorcyclists from the hazards of unhelmeted riding not because they may impose costs on the community in the event of accidents or because they are too young to appreciate the hazards entailed, but because we are morally bound to prevent avoidable suffering and death.

. . . Robert Goodin (1989, 30–31), a utilitarian, [offers a forthright defense of public health paternalism]: "We do not leave it to the discretion of consumers, however well informed, whether or not to drink grossly polluted water, ingest grossly contaminated foods, or inject grossly dangerous drugs. We simply prohibit such things. . . . The justification of public health measures, in general, must be baldly paternalistic. Their fundamental point is to promote the wellbeing of people who might otherwise be inclined cavalierly to court certain sorts of diseases." The challenge, we believe, for public health ethics is to define those moments when public health paternalism is justified and to articulate a set of principles that would preserve a commitment to the realm of free choice.

The effort to shape public health policy in liberal societies will require a forthright acknowledgement of the tensions and trade-offs that will inevitably arise when the claims of public welfare and well-being intrude on privacy, individual choice, and liberty. Recognising the role of moral values in decision-making was one of the signal contributions of bioethics in its formative period. . . . [But] bioethics cannot serve as a basis for thinking about the balances required in the defence of the public's health. As we commence the process of shaping an ethics of public health, it is clear that bioethics is the wrong place to start.

PUBLIC HEALTH ETHICS: MAPPING THE TERRAIN*

James F. Childress, Ruth R. Faden, Ruth D. Gaare, Lawrence O. Gostin, Jeffrey Kahn, Richard J. Bonnie, Nancy E. Kass, Anna C. Mastroianni, Jonathan D. Moreno, and Phillip Nieburg

Public health ethics, like the field of public health it addresses, traditionally has focused more on practice and particular cases than on theory, with the result that

*Reprinted from *Journal of Law, Medicine, & Ethics* 30 (2002): 170–78. (Blackwell Publishing)

some concepts, methods, and boundaries remain largely undefined. This paper attempts to provide a rough conceptual map of the terrain of public health ethics. . . .

GENERAL MORAL CONSIDERATIONS

. . . The terrain of public health ethics includes a loose set of general moral considerations—clusters of moral concepts and norms that are variously called values, principles, or rules—that are arguably relevant to public health. . . .

. . . We can establish the relevance of a set of these considerations in part by looking at the kinds of moral appeals that public health agents make in deliberating about and justifying their actions as well as at debates about moral issues in public health. The relevant general moral considerations include:

- producing benefits;
- avoiding, preventing, and removing harms;
- producing the maximal balance of benefits over harms and other costs (often called utility);
- distributing benefits and burdens fairly (distributive justice) and ensuring public participation, including the participation of affected parties (procedural justice);
- respecting autonomous choices and actions, including liberty of action;
- protecting privacy and confidentiality;
- keeping promises and commitments;
- disclosing information as well as speaking honestly and truthfully (often grouped under transparency); and
- building and maintaining trust.

Several of these general moral considerations—especially benefiting others, preventing and removing harms, and utility—provide a *prima facie* warrant for many activities in pursuit of the goal of public health. It is sufficient for our purposes to note that public health activities have their grounding in general moral considerations, and that public health identifies one major broad benefit that societies and governments ought to pursue. The relation of public health to the whole set of general moral considerations is complex. Some general moral considerations support [the pursuit of improved population health]; institutionalizing several others may be a condition for or means to public health; . . . and . . . some of the same general moral considerations may limit or constrain what may be done in pursuit of public health. Hence, conflicts may occur among these general moral considerations.

. . . Whatever theory one embraces, the whole set of general moral considerations roughly captures the moral content of public health ethics. It then becomes necessary to address several practical questions. First, how can we make these general moral considerations more specific and concrete in order to guide action? Second, how can we resolve conflicts among them? Some of the conflicts will concern how much weight and significance to assign to the ends and effects of protecting and promoting public health relative to the other considerations that limit and constrain ways to pursue such outcomes. While each general moral consideration may limit and constrain public health activities in some circumstances[,] . . . justice or fairness, respect for autonomy and liberty, and privacy and confidentiality are particularly noteworthy. . . .

Specifying and Weighting General Moral Considerations

General moral considerations have two major dimensions. One is their meaning and range or scope; the other is their weight or strength. The first determines the extent of conflict among them—if their range or scope is interpreted in certain ways, conflicts may be increased or reduced. The second dimension determines when different considerations yield to others in cases of conflict. . . .

Resolving Conflicts among General Moral Considerations

[The various general moral considerations are not absolute. Each may conflict with another and each may have to yield in some circumstances. In such cases, it is necessary to determine which has priority based on their relative weighting in the particular context at issue. Five "justificatory conditions" can be used to assess the relative weight of general moral considerations:] effectiveness, proportionality, necessity, least infringement, and public justification. These conditions are intended to help determine whether promoting public health warrants overriding such values as individual liberty or justice in particular cases.

Effectiveness: It is essential to show that infringing one or more general moral considerations will probably protect public health. For instance, a policy that infringes one or more general moral considerations in the name of public health but has little chance of realizing its goal is ethically unjustified.

Proportionality: It is essential to show that the probable public health benefits outweigh the infringed general moral considerations. . . . For instance, the policy may breach autonomy or privacy and have undesirable consequences. All of the positive features and benefits must be balanced against the negative features and effects.

Necessity: Not all effective and proportionate policies are necessary to realize the public health goal that is sought. The fact that a policy will infringe a general moral consideration provides a strong moral reason to seek an alternative strategy that is less morally troubling. . . .

Least infringement: Even when a proposed policy satisfies the first three justificatory conditions . . . public health agents should seek to minimize the infringement of general moral considerations. For instance, when a policy infringes autonomy, public health agents should seek the least restrictive alternative; when it infringes privacy, they should seek the least intrusive alternative; and when it infringes confidentiality, they should disclose only the amount and kind of information needed, and only to those necessary, to realize the goal. . . .

Public justification: When public health agents believe that one of their actions, practices, or policies infringes one or more general moral considerations, they also have a responsibility . . . to explain and justify that infringement . . . to the relevant parties, including those affected by the infringement. . . . This transparency stems in part from the requirement to treat citizens as equals and with respect by offering moral reasons, which in principle they could find acceptable, for policies that infringe general moral considerations. Transparency is also essential to creating and maintaining public trust; and it is crucial to establishing accountability. . . .

PROCESS OF PUBLIC ACCOUNTABILITY

[The fifth justificatory condition—public justification—is particularly applicable] in the political context. While public accountability includes public justification, it is broader—it is prospective as well as retrospective. It involves soliciting input from the relevant publics (the numerical, political, and communal publics) in the process of formulating public health policies, practices, and actions, as well as justifying to the relevant publics what is being undertaken. . . . At a minimum, public accountability involves transparency in openly seeking information from those affected and in honestly disclosing relevant information to the public; it is indispensable for engendering and sustaining public trust, as well as for expressing justice. [Procedural fairness is particularly important to public accountability, because "in a pluralistic society we are likely to find disagreement about which principles should govern." As Norman Daniels (2000, 1301) further explains, "Since we may not be able to construct principles that yield fair decisions ahead of time, we need a process that allows us to develop those reasons over time as we face real cases."]

PUBLIC HEALTH INTERVENTIONS VS. PATERNALISTIC INTERVENTIONS

An important empirical, conceptual, and normative issue in public health ethics is the relationship between protecting and promoting the health of individuals and protecting and promoting public health. Although public health is directed to the health of populations, the indices of population health, of course, include an aggregation of the health of individuals. [And individual health may be influenced by substantially voluntary, self-regarding behavior.] The ethical question then is, when can paternalistic interventions . . . be ethically justified if they infringe general moral considerations such as respect for autonomy, including liberty of action? . . .

Whether an agent's other-regarding conduct is voluntary or non-voluntary, the society may justifiably intervene in various ways, including the use of coercion, to reduce or prevent the imposition of serious risk on others. Societal intervention in non-voluntary self-regarding conduct is considered weak (or soft) paternalism, if it is paternalistic at all, and it is easily justified. By contrast, societal interference in voluntary self-regarding conduct would be strong (or hard) paternalism. Coercive intervention in the name of strong paternalism would be insulting and disrespectful to individuals because it would override their voluntary actions for their own benefit, even though their actions do not harm others. Such interventions are thus very difficult to justify in a liberal, pluralistic democracy.

Because of this difficulty, proponents of public health sometimes contend that [there are only a small class of cases in which an individual's actions are both self-regarding and voluntary;] individuals' risky actions are, in most cases, other-regarding or non-voluntary, or both. Thus, they insist, even if we assume that strong or hard paternalism cannot be ethically justified, the real question is whether most public health interventions in personal life plans and risk budgets are paternalistic at all, at least in the morally problematic sense.

To a great extent, the question is where we draw the boundaries of the self and its actions; that is, whether various influences on agents so determine their actions that they are not voluntary, and whether the adverse effects of those actions extend beyond the agents themselves. . . . On the one hand, it is not sufficient to show that social-cultural factors influence an individual's actions; it is necessary to show that those influences render that individual's actions substantially non-voluntary and warrant societal interventions to protect him or her. Controversies about the strong influence of food marketing on diet and weight (and, as a result, on the risk of disease and death) illustrate the debates about this condition.

On the other hand, it is not sufficient to show that an individual's actions have some adverse effects on others; it is necessary to show that those adverse effects on others are significant enough to warrant overriding the individual's liberty. [For example, even if the societal costs of an activity] are morally relevant as a matter of social utility, it [is] still necessary to show that they are significant enough to justify the intervention.

Either kind of attempt to reduce the sphere of autonomous, self-regarding actions, in order to warrant interventions in the name of public health, or, more broadly, social utility, can sometimes be justified, but either attempt must be subjected to careful scrutiny. Sometimes both may represent rationalization and bad faith as public health agents seek to evade the stringent demands of the general moral consideration of respect for autonomy. Requiring consistency across an array of cases may provide a safeguard against rationalization and bad faith, particularly when motives for intervention may be mixed.

Much of this debate reflects different views about whether and when strong paternalistic interventions can be ethically justified. In view of the justificatory conditions identified earlier, relevant factors will include the nature of the intervention, the degree to which it infringes an individual's fundamental values, the magnitude of the risk to the individual apart from the intervention (either in terms of harm or lost benefit), and so forth. . . .

SOCIAL JUSTICE, HUMAN RIGHTS, AND HEALTH

We have noted potential and actual conflicts between promoting the good of public health and other general moral considerations. But it is important not to exaggerate these conflicts. . . . Social injustices expressed in poverty, racism, and sexism have long been implicated in conditions of poor health. In recent years, some evidence suggests that societies that embody more egalitarian conceptions of socioeconomic justice have higher levels of health than ones that do not. Public health activity has traditionally encompassed much more than medicine and health care. Indeed, historically much of the focus of public health has been on the poor and on the impact of squalor and sanitation on health. The focus today on the social determinants of health is in keeping with this tradition. The data about social determinants . . . warrant close attention to the ways conditions of social justice contribute to the public's health.

. . . Some in public health argue that embodying several other general moral considerations, especially as articulated in human rights, is consistent with and may even contribute to public health. . . . Sometimes public health programs burden human rights, but human rights violations "have adverse effects on physical, mental, and social well-being" and "promoting and protecting human rights is inextricably linked with promoting and protecting health" (Mann 1997, 11–12). [Often, the most effective ways to protect public health respect general moral considerations rather than violate them.]

While more often than not public health and human rights—or general moral considerations not expressed in human rights—do not conflict and may even be synergistic, conflicts do sometimes arise and require resolution.... We have tried to provide elements of a framework for thinking through and resolving such conflicts. This process needs to be transparent in order to engender and sustain public trust.

ETHICS AND PUBLIC HEALTH: FORGING A STRONG RELATIONSHIP*

Daniel Callahan and Bruce Jennings

[Bioethics emerged as a discipline separate from medical ethics in the 1960s and 1970s. Today, public health ethics have begun to emerge as a discipline distinct from, but still connected to, bioethics and its principles. In part, this emergence is due to "the unwelcome reminder that infectious disease has not, in fact, been conquered" and "the recognition that the health of populations is a function more of good public health measures and socioeconomic conditions than of biomedical advances."]

[Incorporating bioethics principles and public health principles is not always easy. While bioethics emphasizes an individualistic orientation, public health maintains a focus on populations and societies. There is an additional] tension produced by the predominant orientation in favor of civil liberties and individual autonomy that one finds in bioethics, as opposed to the utilitarian, paternalistic, and communitarian orientations that have marked the field of public health throughout its history. The ethical and policy issues concerning, for example, HIV and multidrug-resistant tuberculosis already have thrust public health ethics into the thick of this clash of values. And, if the issue of paternalism (limiting the freedom of the individual for the sake of his or her own greater good or best interests) were not enough, the cognate clash between individualistic civil liberties and a communitarian orientation (limiting the freedom of the individual for the sake of the common good or public interest) will also provoke lively discussion....

THE SCOPE OF PUBLIC HEALTH ETHICS

Just as public health is broad in its scope, the range of ethical issues in the field is uncommonly wide, encompassing ethics in public health as well as the ethics of public health. If ethics is understood to be a search for those values, virtues, and principles necessary for people to live together in peace, mutual respect, and justice, then there are few issues in public health that do not admit of an ethical perspective. To begin to map the scope of this broad terrain, general categories of such issues should be noted: health promotion and disease prevention, risk reduction, epidemiological and other forms of public health research, and structural and socioeconomic disparities in health status.

Health Promotion and Disease Prevention

Programs designed to promote health and prevent disease and injury raise questions about the responsibility of individuals to live healthy lives; about the govern-

*Reprinted from *American Journal of Public Health* 92 (2002): 169–76.

ment's role in creating an environment in which individuals are able to exercise their health-related responsibility; about the role of government in coercing or influencing health-related behavior or in developing educational programs; about the use of incentives, economic or otherwise, to promote good health; and about the relative importance for society of pursuing good health, particularly in a culture that prizes autonomy and does not always look fondly on government intervention.

Risk Reduction

Risks to the health of the public are many, and many methods are used to reduce or eliminate them. Almost all can pose one or more ethical problems. The concept of risk itself is seemingly impossible to define in value-neutral terms and is inherently controversial. Even more ethically charged is the question of what level or degree of risk is socially acceptable to individuals and communities. Who should decide about that, and how should exposure to risk be distributed across the affected population? . . .

Epidemiological and Other Public Health Research

. . . Is the biomedical model—focused on individual informed consent and tightly regulated research with those at risk of exploitation—an appropriate model for public health, one that may either pose no medical or other risks to individuals or make consent impractical to gain in research encompassing large communities? And should the research standards used in the United States be exactly the same for research in other countries, particularly developing countries?

Structural and Socioeconomic Disparities

It has been known for many years that socioeconomic disparities have a major impact on health status. Equitable access to decent health care and reductions in health status disparities have been long-sought goals in American society but have not always been dealt with in the context of socioeconomic disparities. What is the appropriate role for the public health community in seeking greater justice in health care, and how should it balance its fact-finding and educational role with its historically strong advocacy mission? . . . Finally, to what extent, if any, should the field adopt a politically partisan posture, taking a public stand on important policy issues and legislative initiatives?

TYPES OF ETHICAL ANALYSIS

While the preceding classification of broad issues by no means exhausts the possible categories of topics, it is sufficient to make evident that no single method of ethical analysis can be used for all of them. . . . Ethical analysis can be usefully divided into a number of different types, depending on the point of view and needs from which it originates. One or more of them might be appropriate for any specific ethical problem.

Professional Ethics

The study of professional ethics tends to seek out the values and standards that have been developed by the practitioners and leaders of a given profession over a long period of time and to identify those values that seem most salient and inherent in the profession itself. Applied to public health, this perspective entails identifying the central mission of the profession (e.g., protection and promotion of the health of all members of society) and building up a body of ethical principles and standards that would protect the trust and legitimacy the profession should maintain.

Applied Ethics

... The applied ethics perspective differs from the professional ethics perspective principally in that it adopts a point of view from outside the history and values of the profession. From this more general moral and social point of view, applied ethics seeks to devise general principles that can then be applied to real-world examples of professional conduct or decision making. These principles and their application are designed to give professionals guidance and to provide those individuals affected by professional behavior, as well as the general public, with standards to use in assessing the professions. Thus, in applied ethics, there is a tendency to reason abstractly and to draw from general ethical theories rather than from the folkways and knowledge base of the professions. ...

Advocacy Ethics

... While on occasion it can pose difficulties for civil servants, the ethical persuasion most lively in the field is a stance of advocacy for those social goals and reforms that public health professionals believe will enhance general health and well-being, especially among those least well off in society. Such advocacy is in keeping with the natural priorities of those who devote their careers to public health. It has a strong orientation toward equality and social justice. Much of the research and expertise in public health throughout its history has shown how social deprivation, inequality, poverty, and powerlessness are directly linked to poor health and the burden of disease. ...

Critical Ethics

... For want of a better term, we label [this final perspective] "critical ethics." In many ways, it attempts to combine the strengths of the other perspectives mentioned. Like professional ethics, it is historically informed and practically oriented toward the specific real-world and real-time problems of public health, but, like applied ethics, it brings larger social values and historical trends to bear in its understanding of the current situation of public health and the moral problems faced. These problems are not only the result of the behavior of certain disease organisms or particular individuals. They are also the result of institutional arrangements and prevailing structures of cultural attitudes and social power.

... One possible advantage of critical ethics is its call for discussions of ethics and public health policy to be genuinely public or civic endeavors: not the advocacy of a well-intentioned elite on behalf of needy clients, but a search for forums and programs of meaningful participation, open deliberation, and civic problem solving and capacity building. ...

AN ETHICAL CODE?

The work of the Public Health Leadership Society in initiating a process to establish a code of ethics for public health is important. Where does a code of ethics fit into a broader confrontation with ethical issues? Most professions have a code, and of course many professionals in public health belong to one or another of such professions. Considering this, is there any need for an additional code for public health? There are at least 3 reasons to have a code. One ... is to respond to scandals in a field, aiming to ensure better future conduct.... Another is to help establish the moral credibility of a field and its professional status and to provide principles to deal with common dilemmas.... Still another purpose is to provide a profession with a moral compass and to set forth its ideals....

... [But codifying ethical norms in a field is not without difficulties.] The greatest challenge in writing a code is to specify clearly the ideals of the field and then to specify some general guidelines that will be illuminating for the wide array of problems practitioners can encounter. Historically, many if not most professional codes have been written because of structural changes in a profession that have generated new ethical problems and made it necessary to shore up public confidence in the profession's integrity.

We believe that the integrity of the profession of public health is sound, but the changing situation of public health practice may be a good reason to more precisely specify the ethical obligations that those in the field take on when they become practitioners. Code developments and revisions, it might be noted, have often been most successful when they are accompanied by lengthy and strenuous debate engaging the entire professional community and not simply those with a special interest in ethics.

LAW AND ETHICS

Public health is one of the few professions that has, in many matters, legal power—in particular, the police power of the state—behind it. It can, through use of the law, coerce citizens into behaving in some approved, healthy way.... Public health also has the distinction ... of being a profession in which many practitioners are government employees and officials. It thus has an obligation both toward government, which controls it, and toward the public that it serves.

Because of its public and governmental roles, public health has ethical problems unlike those of most other professions. The relationship between ethics and law is a long and tangled one, but it is safe to say that most public health laws and regulations have behind them an explicitly moral purpose: that of promoting and protecting the lives of citizens. Because the police power of the state is involved, however, a number of moral conflicts are generated. The tension between individual health and rights, on the one hand, and government obligations and population health, on the other, is an obvious instance of this kind of conflict. The economic and social impact on communities of public health measures, requiring some form of cost-benefit analysis, is another.

Health is an important human need, and good health is highly valued. But health is not the only need or good health the only value. Laws must always find ways of balancing various goods, and the centrality of laws for the work of public health brings uncommon visibility to its actions and an uncommon need for public accountability.

POLITICS AND PUBLIC HEALTH

As public arguments over fluoridation or HIV disease amply demonstrate, public health measures can quickly become politicized. Political controversy is often

treated as some kind of disaster for calm reflection and measured rationality...
[but] politics is unavoidable and necessary. It is unavoidable because there is no
way to stop the public from turning to legislatures or the courts to express their
values and needs; nor should there be. Politics is a necessary component of public
health, moreover, precisely in order to achieve public health policies and practices
consistent with American traditions and values. Politics is the messy arena in which
ultimate questions of the public good are worked out....

Yet, there can be responsible and irresponsible politics. Public health can best
serve the cause of responsible politics, even when it has a self-interested stake in
the outcome, when it makes available good data, when it is sensitive to community
sentiments, and when it makes clear by all of its actions that it is not (as the stereotype would have it) just one more self-serving, distant government bureaucracy....

THE TEACHING OF PUBLIC HEALTH ETHICS

[A crucial question, then, is how to promote greater awareness and a more sustained, sophisticated discussion of ethical issues among public health practitioners
and researchers themselves, as well as among the broader public. An important
step is to promote the teaching of ethics in all schools of public health and among
practitioners through continuing education programs. This may be controversial,
intellectually difficult, institutionally challenging, and expensive, but it needs to be
done if there is going to be serious study and discussion of the myriad ethical issues
arising in public health.]

II. PUBLIC HEALTH PATERNALISM: A CASE STUDY ON MOTORCYCLE HELMET LAWS

As mentioned, paternalism remains the most politically controversial
justification for public health action. Classic liberalism rejects paternalism, holding that the only justification for interference with liberty is to
prevent harm to others. There are many examples of paternalistic policies, including seat belt laws, water fluoridation, and prohibitions on
gambling and illicit drugs. In the treatise accompanying this volume,
I use motorcycle helmet laws as an illustration. Here, I present two
readings offering starkly different justifications for motorcycle helmet
laws. In *Benning v. State,* the Vermont Supreme Court upholds a state
law mandating that motorcycle riders wear helmets, stressing the socioeconomic harms that motorcycle crashes cause to families and society.
The public health ethicists Marian Moser Jones and Ronald Bayer also
support these laws, but they rely primarily on paternalistic arguments.

In both pieces, it is clear that antipaternalistic rhetoric—often
couched in terms of liberty and free choice—has been central to motorcyclists' efforts to repeal helmet laws. Recent data, however, confirm
the danger of a strict antipaternalistic stance: repeals of motorcycle

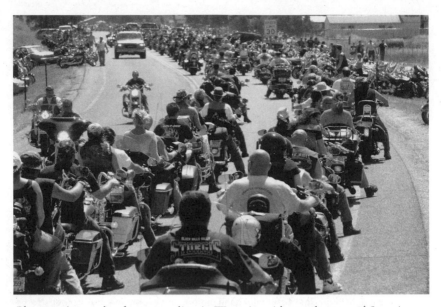

Photo 5. A parade of motorcyclists in Wyoming rides to the annual Sturgis
motorcycle rally in South Dakota. The riders are largely helmetless, reflecting
the absence of motorcycle helmet laws in both Wyoming and South Dakota.
Avid motorcyclists frequently oppose motorcycle helmet laws, claiming that
motorcyclists themselves should be responsible for making personal safety
decisions. Reproduced by permission, © Peter Turnley/Corbis, August 8,
2007.

helmet laws increase motorcyclist fatality rates by more than 12 percent on average (Houston and Richardson 2007). At times, choice has
disastrous consequences. Those states that adhere to a classic liberal
tradition eschewing paternalism may face an increased social and economic burden of injury and disease.

BENNING V. STATE*
Supreme Court of Vermont
Decided January 28, 1994

Justice DOOLEY delivered the opinion of the court.

[Plaintiffs bring a state constitutional challenge against Vermont's motorcycle
law, Vermont Statutes Annotated, Title 23, §1256, which requires motorcyclists to
wear reflective helmets with neck or chin straps when on highways. The challenge is
based on the language in the first amendment of the Vermont Constitution guaran-

*641 A.2d 757 (Vt. 1994).

teeing citizens the right of "enjoying and defending ... liberty" and "pursuing and obtaining ... safety."]

At the center of plaintiffs' argument is the assertion that Vermont values personal liberty interests so highly that the analysis under the federal constitution or the constitutions of other states is simply inapplicable here. In support of this contention, plaintiffs rely on political theorists, sociological materials, and incidents in Vermont's history. Without detailing this argument, we find it unpersuasive not because it overvalues Vermont's devotion to personal liberty and autonomy, but because it undervalues the commitment of other governments to those values. ... Certainly, if there was a heightened concern for personal liberty, there is no evidence of it in the text of the Constitution. ...

As a result, we reject the notion that this case can be resolved on the basis of a broad right to be let alone without government interference. We accept the federal analysis of such a claim in the context of a public safety restriction applicable to motorists using public roads. We agree with Justice Powell, recently sitting by designation with the Court of Appeals for the Eleventh Circuit, who stated:

> There is no broad legal or constitutional "right to be let alone" by government. In the complex society in which we live, the action and notation of citizens are subject to countless local, state, and federal laws and regulations. Bare invocation of a right to be let alone is an appealing rhetorical device, but it seldom advances legal inquiry, as the "right"—to the extent it exists—has no meaning outside its application to specific activities. ... (*Picou v. Gillum,* 874 F.2d 1519, 1521 [11th Cir. 1989])

... We are left then with the familiar standard for evaluating police power regulations—essentially, that expressed in *State v. Solomon,* 260 A.2d 377, 379 (Vt. 1969) [holding that §1256 did not exceed the state's police power or violate due process of law and was "directly related to highway safety" because without a helmet, a motorcyclist could be affected by highway hazards, lose control, and injure other motorists]. Plaintiffs urge us to overrule *Solomon* because it was based on an analysis of the safety risk to other users of the roadway that is incredible. In support of their position, they offered evidence from motorcycle operators that the possibility of an operator losing control of a motorcycle and becoming a menace to others is remote. On the other hand, these operators assert that helmets make a motorcycle operator dangerous. Plaintiffs also emphasize that even supporters of helmet laws agree that their purpose is to protect the motorcycle operator, not other highway users.

We are not willing to abandon the primary rationale of *Solomon* because of plaintiffs' evidence. The statute is entitled to a presumption of constitutionality. Plaintiffs are not entitled to have the courts act as a super-legislature and retry legislative judgments based on evidence presented to the court. Thus, the question before us is whether the link between safety for highway users and the helmet law is rational, not whether we agree that the statute actually leads to safer highways. The *Solomon* reasoning has been widely adopted in the many courts that have considered the constitutionality of motorcycle helmet laws. We still believe it supports the constitutionality of §1256.

There are at least two additional reasons why we conclude §1256 is constitutional. ... Although plaintiffs argue that the only person affected by the failure to wear a helmet is the operator of the motorcycle, the impact of that decision would be felt well beyond that individual. Such a decision imposes great costs on the public. As Professor Laurence Tribe (1988, 1372) has commented, ours is "a society unwilling to abandon bleeding bodies on the highway, [and] the motorcyclist or driver who endangers himself plainly imposes costs on others." This concern has been echoed in a number of opinions upholding motorcycle helmet laws.... Whether in taxes or insurance rates, our costs are linked to the actions of others and are driven up when others fail to take preventive steps that would minimize health care consumption. We see no constitutional barrier to legislation that requires preventive measures to minimize health care costs that are inevitably imposed on society.

A second rationale supports this type of a safety requirement on a public highway. Our decisions show that in numerous circumstances the liability for injuries that occur on our public roads may be imposed on the state, or other governmental units, and their employees. It is rational for the state to act to minimize the extent of the injuries for which it or other governmental units may be financially responsible. The burden placed on plaintiffs who receive the benefit of the liability system is reasonable....

As a result, we reiterate our conclusion that §1256 "in no way violates any of the provisions of our state and federal constitutions." *Solomon,* 260 A.2d at 380.

PATERNALISM AND ITS DISCONTENTS: MOTORCYCLE HELMET LAWS, LIBERTARIAN VALUES, AND PUBLIC HEALTH*
Marian Moser Jones and Ronald Bayer

In the face of overwhelming epidemiological evidence that motorcycle helmets reduce accident deaths and injuries, state legislatures in the United States have rolled back motorcycle helmet regulations during the past 30 years.... There are many ways to account for the historical arc; we focus here on the enduring impact libertarian and antipaternalistic values may have on US public health policy....

THE ORIGIN OF MOTORCYCLE HELMET LAWS

... The 1966 National Highway Safety Act introduced drastic and unwelcome changes to US motorcycle culture. The law ... included a provision that withheld federal funding for highway safety programs to states that did not enact mandatory motorcycle helmet laws within a specified time frame. This provision was added after a study showed that helmet laws would significantly decrease the rate of fatal accidents.... Adoption of this measure drew upon a broader movement within public health to expand its purview beyond infectious disease to "prevention of disability and postponement of untimely death." Several years later, this shift sparked debate on the role of both individual and collective behaviors in contemporary patterns of morbidity and mortality....

As of 1966, only 3 states ... had passed motorcycle helmet laws, but between 1967 and 1975, nearly every state passed statutes to avoid penalties under the National Highway Safety Act....

*Reprinted from the *American Journal of Public Health* 97 (2007): 208–17.

THE BIKER LOBBY ROARS INTO ACTION

Motorcyclists had long been organized . . . and the passage of motorcycle helmet laws galvanized the groups to become political. [During the 1970s, state-level and nationwide groups committed to advocating the repeal of helmet laws—so-called motorcyclists' rights organizations—began to form around the country. Soon, motorcyclists evolved into an organized and powerful national lobby. Group representatives were invited to hearings in July 1975 to discuss revisions to the National Highway Safety Act.]

Recognizing that proponents of motorcycle helmet laws, in the tradition of public health, had used statistical evidence of injury and death to make their case, the first motorcyclist to speak at these hearings, Bruce Davey of ABATE [A Brotherhood against Totalitarian Enactments] opened with a frontal attack on such data. . . . Davey then advanced a series of constitutional claims that were rooted in an antipaternalistic ethic, which enshrined a concept of personal liberty. . . . Not surprisingly, the issue of choice emerged as the central theme in the arguments of those opposed to helmet laws. . . . ABATE chapter literature stated "ABATE does not advocate that you ride without a helmet when the law is repealed, only that you have the right to decide." . . .

[The tide had turned against proponents of mandatory helmet laws.] On December 13, 1975, the Senate voted 52 to 37 to approve a bill that revised the National Highway Safely Act. The House passed a similar measure. . . . The bill was signed by President Gerald Ford on May 5, 1976.

HELMETLESS RIDERS: AN UNPLANNED PUBLIC HEALTH EXPERIMENT

During the next 4 years, 28 states repealed their mandatory helmet laws. . . . Overall, deaths from motorcycle accidents increased 20%, from 3,312 in 1976 to 4,062 in 1977. . . .

For those concerned about public health, the unfolding events were viewed with alarm. In the June 1980 issue of the *American Journal of Public Health*, Susan Baker . . . compared the situation to one where "scientists, having found a successful treatment for a disease, were impelled to further prove its efficacy by stopping the treatment and allowing the disease to recur." Invoking the 1905 US Supreme Court decision in *Jacobson v. Massachusetts* that upheld compulsory immunization statutes, Baker asserted that the state had the authority to limit individual liberty to protect the public's health and the rights of others. . . . Baker emphasized the social burden created by motorcycle accidents and fatalities.

In 1981, the *American Journal of Public Health* published a counterpoint to Baker's editorial. . . . Richard Perkins . . . attacked the argument that the motorcyclist was reducing the freedom of others by not wearing a helmet as "so ridiculous as to be ammunition for the anti-helmet law forces." . . . He argued that laws should consider not only safety but also "such intangible consequences as potential loss of opportunity for individual fulfillment and loss of social vitality."

Baker and Stephen Teret [1981] offered a rebuttal to Perkins and stated that his argument "implies that if policy is not applied at the outer limits of a continuum of circumstances, it would be unreasonable to apply that policy at any point along the continuum." They defended their reliance on *Jacobson v. Massachusetts* by pointing out that the decision has been used as a precedent for decisions that cover "manifold" restraints on liberty for the common good beyond the scope of contagious disease.

During the next decade, evidence of the human and social costs of repeal continued to mount. Medical costs among helmetless riders increased 200% compared with helmeted riders, and in some states, helmetless riders were more likely to be uninsured. . . . Posing a challenge to the antipaternalism that had inspired the repeal of laws, [an editorial in *Texas Medicine*] contended, "[a] civilized society makes laws not only to protect a person from his fellowman, but also sometimes from himself as well" (Narayan 1987, 5–6). . . .

HELMET LAWS IN THE CONGRESS ONCE AGAIN

In May 1989, [Senator John Chaffee introduced] a bill—the National Highway Fatality and Injury Reduction Act of 1989—that would empower the US Department of Transportation to withhold up to 10% of federal highway aid from any state that did not require motorcyclists to wear helmets and front-seat automobile passengers to wear seat belts. . . .

. . . [Robert Ford, representing an antihelmet lobbying group, spoke at a hearing on the bill.] Ford did not quibble with statistics that showed seat belts make people safer. Instead, he argued that the issue was about fundamental individual liberty.

> We do not want to be told how to behave in matters of personal safety. We do not want to be forced to wear seat belts or helmets because others think that it is good for us. We do not want to be forced to eat certain diets because some think that it too may be good for us, reduce deaths and medical costs, and make us more productive citizens. We do not want to be forced to give up certain pastimes simply because some may feel they entail any amount of unnecessary risk.

Instead of confronting the moral arguments made by opponents of helmet laws, proponents of such measures sought once again to marshal the compelling force of evidence. In 1991 . . . the General Accounting Office issued a comprehensive report that documented the toll. The report reviewed 46 studies and found that they overwhelmingly showed helmet use rose and fatalities and serious injuries plummeted after enactment of mandatory universal helmet laws.

[Despite the fierce opposition of motorcycle groups, a motorcycle helmet provision was enacted as part of a major highway funding bill in 1991. Under the law states that failed to pass helmet laws would have 3% of their highway funds withheld. This public health success was short-lived, however.] In 1995, after the "Gingrich Revolution," in which conservative Republicans took control of Congress, the national motorcycle lobby succeeded in getting the federal 3% highway safety fund penalties repealed.

CONCLUSIONS

Over the past 30 years, helmet law advocates have gathered a mountain of evidence to support their claims that helmet laws reduce motorcycle accident fatalities and severe injuries. Thanks to the rounds of helmet law repeals, advocates have been able to conclusively prove the converse as well: helmet law repeals increase fatalities and the severity of injuries. But the antihelmet law activists . . . have learned a lesson about how persuasive unadorned appeals to libertarian values can be.

This history of motorcycle helmet laws in the United States illustrates the profound impact of individualism on American culture and the manner in which this ideological perspective can have a crippling impact on the practice of public health. . . . Abundant evidence makes it clear . . . that in the absence of mandatory motorcycle helmet laws, preventable deaths and great suffering will continue to occur. The NHTSA [National Highway Traffic Safety Administration] estimated that 10,838 additional lives could have been saved between 1984 and 2004 had all riders and passengers worn helmets. The success of those who oppose such statutes shows the limits of evidence in shaping policy when strongly held ideological commitments are at stake.

Early on in the battles over helmet laws, advocates for mandatory measures placed great stress on the social costs of riding helmetless. . . . Such a perspective . . . mask[s] the extent to which concerns for the welfare of cyclists themselves were the central motivation for helmet laws. The inability to successfully and consistently defend these measures for what they were—acts of public health paternalism—was an all but fatal limitation. . . .

The challenge for public health is to expand on this base of justified paternalism and to forthrightly argue in the legislative arena that adults and adolescents need to be protected from their poor judgments about motorcycle helmet use. . . . Paternalistic protective legislation is part of the warp and woof of public health practice in America. . . .

With the latest round of helmet law repeals, motorcycle helmet use has dropped precipitately to 58% nationwide, and fatalities have risen. Need anything more be said to show that motorcyclists have not been able to make sound safety decisions on their own and that mandatory helmet laws are needed to ensure their own safety?

III. ETHICAL REASONING IN RISK REGULATION

Scholars have lamented the sharp differences in the way that "experts" and laypersons assess risk. Risk is a highly complex concept, and a great deal of literature exists about its analysis, perception, characterization, communication, and management. Scientists understand risk according to probabilistic assessments focusing on the chance that a dangerous event will occur and, if it does, on the severity of its effects. Such an inquiry is said to be objective. The lay public's understanding of risk, in contrast, takes account of more subjective matters, including personal, social, and cultural values. People seem interested in whether the risk is fairly distributed among the population, voluntarily assumed or externally imposed, and naturally occurring or introduced by novel technologies.

Given this apparent rift between scientific and popular risk assessments, how are policy makers in a democratic government to decide which risks should be regulated and how heavily? Frank B. Cross (1994, 888), a business law scholar, explains the problem:

Should the government concern itself with public opinion when addressing public health risks, such as cancer? What if the public opinion is at odds with all the best scientific evidence? Suppose the public demands extensive government regulation or even prohibition of a valuable substance or activity, when scientific studies indicate that the substance or activity presents little or no risk. The result is a conflict between the goals of a democratically responsive government and an effective public heath protection program. Because it is impossible to reduce all human health risks, as publicly perceived or as scientifically identified, a trade-off is unavoidable. This problem is complicated because the general populace and scientists do not even agree on the meaning of the term "risk."

The current regulatory system purports to use scientific methods to measure risk, but policy in the real world is complicated by scientific uncertainties, human values, and political compromises. The result is a combination of "overregulated risk," such as the removal of apples treated with the pesticide Alar from supermarkets, and "underregulated risk," such as the failure to regulate personal handguns.

Justice Stephen Breyer's book *Breaking the Vicious Circle* sharply criticizes existing public health regulation, particularly in the environmental area. In the excerpt below, Breyer discusses one of the most important factors contributing to what he sees as inefficient risk regulation: public risk perception. He outlines the cognitive attributions and schemata the public uses to inaccurately assess risk. Faulty public perception of risk, together with politics and the technical uncertainties of the regulatory process, creates what he terms the "vicious circle" of risk regulation. The vicious circle, argues Breyer, leads agencies to overregulate tiny health risks while ignoring larger, more pressing health concerns.

· · · · ·

BREAKING THE VICIOUS CIRCLE: TOWARD EFFECTIVE RISK REGULATION*
Stephen Breyer

Study after study shows that the public's evaluation of risk problems differs radically from any consensus of experts in the field. Risks associated with toxic waste dumps and nuclear power appear near the bottom of most expert lists; they appear near the top of the public's list of concerns, which more directly influences regula-

*Reprinted from *Breaking the Vicious Circle: Toward Effective Risk Regulation* by Stephen Breyer (Cambridge, Mass.: Harvard University Press) by permission of the publisher. Copyright © 1993 by the President and Fellows of Harvard College.

tory agendas. To some extent, these differences may reflect that the public fears certain risks more than others with the same probability of harm. . . . Of two equal risks, one could rationally dislike or fear more the risk that is involuntarily suffered, new, unobservable, uncontrollable, catastrophic, delayed, a threat to future generations, or likely accompanied by pain or dread.

Still, these differences in the source, quality, or nature of a risk may not account for the different ranking by the public and the experts. A typical member of the public would like to minimize risks of death to himself, to his family, to his neighbors; he would normally prefer that regulation buy more safety for a given expenditure or the same amount of safety for less. Not many of us would like to shift resources to increase overall risks of death significantly in order to increase the likelihood that death will occur on a bicycle or in a fire, rather than through disease. There is a far simpler explanation for the public's aversion to toxic waste dumps than an enormous desire for supersafety, or a strong aversion to the tiniest risk of harm—namely, the public does not *believe* that the risks are tiny. The public's "nonexpert" reactions reflect not different values but different understandings about the underlying risk-related facts.

My assumption that the public assigns "rational" values to risks, however, does not entail rational public reactions to risk. Psychologists have found several examples of thinking that impede rational understanding, but may have helped us survive as we lived throughout much of prehistory, in small groups of hunter-gatherers, depending upon grain, honey, and animals for sustenance. The following, rather well-documented aspects of risk perception are probably familiar.

Rules of Thumb

In daily life most of us do not weigh all the pros and cons of feasible alternatives. We use rules of thumb, more formally called "heuristic devices." We simplify radically; we reason with the help of a few readily understandable examples; we categorize (events and other people) in simple ways that tend to create binary choices—yes/no, friend/foe, eat/abstain, safe/dangerous, act/don't act—and may reflect deeply rooted aversions, such as fear of poisons. The resulting categorizations do not always accurately describe another person or circumstance, but they help us make quick decisions, most of which prove helpful. This kind of quick decision-making may help cut a swath through the modern information jungle, but it oversimplifies dramatically and thereby inhibits an understanding of risks, particularly small risks.

Prominence

People react more strongly, and give greater importance, to events that stand out from the background. Unusual events are striking. We more likely notice the (low-risk) nuclear waste disposal truck driving past the school than the (much higher-risk) gasoline delivery trucks on their way to local service stations. Journalists, whose job is to write interesting stories, know this psychological fact well. The American Medical Association examined how the press treated two similar stories, one finding increased leukemia rates among nuclear workers, the other finding no increased cancer rates among those living near nuclear plants. More than half of the newspapers in the study mentioned the first story but not the second; and more than half of those that mentioned both emphasized the first.

Ethics

The strength of our feelings of ethical obligation seems to diminish with distance. That is to say, feelings of obligation are stronger (or we have different, more time-consuming obligations) toward family, neighbors, friends, community, and those with whom we have direct contact, those whom we see, than toward those who live in distant places, whom we do not see but only read or hear about.

Trust in Experts

People cannot easily judge between experts when those experts disagree with each other. The public, since the mid-1960s, has shown increasing distrust of experts and the institutions, private, academic, or governmental, that employ them.

Fixed Decisions

A person who has made up his or her mind about something is very reluctant to change it.

Mathematics

Most people have considerable difficulty understanding the mathematical probabilities involved in assessing risk. People consistently overestimate small probabilities. What is the likelihood of death by botulism? (One in two million.) They underestimate large ones. What is the likelihood of death by diabetes? (One in fifty thousand.) People cannot detect inconsistencies in their own risk-related choices. . . .

These few, near-commonsense propositions, with strong statistical support in the technical literature, verify Oliver Wendell Holmes's own observation that "most people think dramatically, not quantitatively." They also have important consequences. Consider the public reaction to toxic waste dumps. Start with the mathematical facts about the probability of various occurrences: In 1985 a New Jersey woman won the state lottery twice. What are the odds against this, billions to one? Given the vast number of lotteries in the world, the odds come close to favoring someone somewhere winning a lottery twice. Given the population of the world, and the number of dreams each night, the odds favor someone somewhere dreaming he marries a girl who looks very much like the girl he meets the next day and marries. Given the number of toxic waste dumps in the United States (26,000) and the number of places with above-average cancer rates (half of all places), obviously many cities, towns, and rural areas near toxic waste dumps must also have seriously elevated cancer rates ("mathematics").

Add what sells newspapers—interesting stories—and you can be fairly certain the press will write about the double lottery-winner, perhaps the dreamer, and, if the mathematical evidence is somewhat less crude than my example, the toxic waste dump ("prominence"). Will it be easy to convince the cancer victim that the waste dump (water that is "pure" or "not pure") had nothing to do with the disease ("rules of thumb")? And how will the public react to the image of the angry family member on nightly television ("ethics"), particularly if experts disagree ("trust in experts") as they might, for the relation between the disease and the toxic site may not be strictly chance (the lottery, too, might be fixed). If further study exonerates the dump, will the viewing public change its mind ("fixed decision")?

When we think about nuclear power controversies, we should take account of the fact that hearing about an accident is what psychologists tell us is a heuristic "tip-off" of danger, whether or not anyone is hurt. We have "seen" Chernobyl and Three Mile Island, and we may therefore doubt nuclear power's safety, whether or not experts tell us that the reactor at Chernobyl was not properly designed, that the accident at Three Mile Island hurt no one, that military weapons, not electric power generators, are responsible for 99 percent of all nuclear waste, that nuclear power's risks are minuscule compared to the risks of coal-generated power. Add a few disagreements among experts and the fact that most members of the public made up their minds long ago, and one can understand nuclear power's position on the public perception risk charts.

These few propositions suggest that better "risk communications," such as efforts to explain risks to the public at open meetings, may not suffice to alleviate risk regulation problems. It is not surprising that, after the EPA [Environmental Protection Agency] Administrator William Ruckelshaus spent days at such meetings in Tacoma, Washington, explaining why an ASARCO chemical plant that was leaking small amounts of arsenic could remain open, he was misunderstood, criticized, and accused of trying to drive a wedge between environmentalists and blue collar workers. The plant eventually closed, although perhaps for other reasons. Nor is it surprising that after special public discussions of nuclear power plants were held in Sweden, surveys of the eighty thousand Swedes who participated showed no consensus, but increased confusion.

There is little reason to hope for better risk communication over time. To the contrary, as science improves, scientists may more easily detect and identify ever tinier risks—the risks associated, for example, with the migration of a single molecule of plastic from a container into a soft drink; they may more easily identify geographical areas near toxic waste dumps with higher than average cancer rates. As international communications improve, the press will have an ever larger pool of unusual, and therefore more interesting, accident stories to write about. Why should we not expect an outcry from a public that reads about Love Canal, Times Beach, Alar, Chilean grapes laced with cyanide, and the leaflet of Villejuif, whether or not such examples reflect meaningful danger? (At the same time, how can one expect public reaction to potentially greater but more mundane problems, of which it is unaware?)

It is hard to make the normal human mind grapple with this inhuman type of problem. To change public reaction, one would either have to institute widespread public education in risk analysis or generate greater public trust in some particular group of experts or the institutions that employ them. The first alternative seems unlikely. The second, over the past thirty years, has not occurred. Ordinary, human, public perception, then, forms one element of the vicious circle.

.   .   .   .   .

The courts appear to apply a scientific understanding of risk. In *School Board of Nassau County, Florida v. Arline*, 480 U.S. 273 (1987), Justice William Brennan reasons that risks should be weighed based on their nature, the probability of their occurrence, and the severity of the harm should the risk materialize. Although Brennan's arguments are presented in the context of disability discrimination law, they say something important about how the courts should weigh risk. In actual cases, the courts confront real and complex problems in digesting expressions of risks and determining acceptable levels of risks.

A few years before *Breaking the Vicious Circle* was published, Justice Breyer, then a judge on the United States Court of Appeals for the First Circuit, delivered the court's opinion in *United States v. Ottati & Goss*, 900 F.2d 429 (1st Cir. 1990), a famous case involving the "Superfund" toxic cleanup law. The court rejected the claim of the Environmental Protection Agency (EPA) that the International Minerals and Chemical Corporation did not clean up a toxic waste site sufficiently. Breyer expressed frustration at the cost and complexity of adjudicating a case involving a nearly 50,000-page record:

> Why . . . has this case taken ten years to litigate? The issues are complex, but not unfathomable. Why has the government not found a way to express its technical problems in English (e.g., "small children will eat tiny amounts of dirt when they play in a yard"), instead of relying upon maze-like patterns of cross-references among regulations, statutes, and "expert jargon"? . . . Has the government, in fact, spent enormous administrative (and judicial) resources in an effort to force improvement from "quite clean" . . . to "extremely clean," at three to four times the "quite clean" costs?

Determining appropriate levels of toxicity in *Ottati* turned on seemingly trivial questions, such as "Will a child playing in the dirt consume contaminated soil on 70 or 245 days out of the year?"

Breyer's thinking on risk regulation was also influenced by the Supreme Court's decision in *Industrial Union Department, AFL-CIO v. American Petroleum Institute*, 448 U.S. 607 (1980). The "benzene case," as it is often called, illustrates an equally challenging problem in risk regulation: determining how much exposure to a harmful chemical is "safe." If exposure to benzene at a certain level is associated with an increased rate of leukemia, does any exposure increase the risk of leukemia? Alternatively, is there a "safe" level at which benzene exposure will have no physical effects? The Occupational Safety and Health Administration (OSHA) decided that in the absence of scientific data, there is no "safe" level of benzene exposure. The Supreme Court disagreed, holding that OSHA had the burden of proving, on the basis of substantial evidence, that long-term exposure to benzene at low levels presents a "significant risk of material health impairment."

Inconsistencies in risk regulation not only are the result of conflicting scientific and popular understandings of risks, but are also the
product of inherent variance in how scientists understand, prioritize,
compare, and express risks. Experts believe that scientific risk assessments lead to more cost-effective interventions because they encourage
policy makers to concentrate resources on preventing hazards that are
highly probable and would cause significant harm. But there are tensions between probability and magnitude of harm. Should policy makers devote resources to events of high likelihood and low consequence,
or vice versa? For example, the common cold is highly likely but of
small consequence, while bioterrorism or avian influenza (H_5N_1) is
unlikely but of major consequence. So, should policy makers devote
more resources to preventing routine events or catastrophic ones?
Alternatively, should policy makers concentrate on preventing endemic
health threats (both likely and harmful), such as seasonal influenza,
obesity, and smoking? In the following excerpt, the physicists Richard
Wilson and E. A. C. Crouch describe how risks—of varying certainties
and magnitudes—are assessed, compared, and expressed.

RISK ASSESSMENT AND COMPARISONS: AN INTRODUCTION*
Richard Wilson and E. A. C. Crouch

Every day we take risks and avoid others....
    Most of us act semi-automatically to minimize our risks. We also expect society to
minimize the risks suffered by its members, subject to overriding moral, economic,
or other constraints. In some cases these constraints will dominate, in others there
will be trade-offs between the values assigned to risks and the constraints. Risk
assessments, except in the simplest of circumstances, are not designed for making
judgments, but to illuminate them. To effectively illuminate, and then to minimize,
risks requires knowing what they are and how big they are. This knowledge usually
is gained through experience, and the essence of risk assessment is the application
of this knowledge of past mistakes (and deliberate actions) in an attempt to prevent
new mistakes in new situations.
    The results of risk assessments will necessarily be in the form of an estimate
of probabilities for various events, usually injurious. The goal in performing a risk
assessment is to obtain such estimates, although we consider the major value in performing a risk assessment is the exercise itself, in which (ideally) all aspects of some
action are explored.... Cultural values will presumably be factors influencing societal decisions and may differ even for risk estimates that are identical in probability.

*Excerpted from *Science* 236 (1987): 267–70. Reprinted with permission from the
American Association for the Advancement of Science.

RISK AND UNCERTAINTY

The concept of risk and the notion of uncertainty are closely related. We may say that the lifetime risk of cancer is 25%, meaning that approximately 25% of all people develop cancer in their lifetimes. Once an individual develops cancer, we can no longer talk about the risk of cancer, for it is a certainty. Similarly if a man lies dying after a car accident, the risk of his dying of cancer drops to near zero. Thus estimates of risks, insofar as they are expressions of uncertainty, will change as knowledge improves.

Different uncertainties appear in risk estimation in different ways. There is clearly a risk that an individual will be killed by a car if that person walks blindfolded across a crowded street. One part of this risk is stochastic; it depends on whether the individual steps off the curb at the precise moment that a car arrives. Another part of the risk might be systematic; it will depend on the nature of the fenders and other features of the car. . . .

Some estimates of uncertainties are subjective, with differences of opinion arising because there is a disagreement among those assessing the risks. Suppose one wishes to assess the risk (to humans) of some new chemical being introduced into the environment, or of a new technology. Without any further information, all we can say about any measure of the risk is that it lies between zero and unity. [Extreme opinions might be voiced in response, with some assuming a risk of unity because safety has not been demonstrated, and others assuming a risk of zero because nothing has been proven dangerous.] We argue that it is the task of the risk assessor to use whatever information is available to obtain a number between zero and one for a risk estimate, with as much precision as possible, together with an estimate of the imprecision. . . .

. . . The assumption of zero risk can arise because people and government agencies have a propensity to ignore anything that is not a proven hazard. We argue that this attitude is inconsistent if the objective is to improve the public health, may also lead to economic inefficiencies, and often leads to unnecessary contention between experts who disagree strongly. . . .

RISK VALUE VERSUS CERTAINTY OF INFORMATION

After risks of a number of situations have been assessed, we often want to order them in order to decide which should command our attention. [The risk value and the certainty of information may both influence the ordering.]

Vinyl chloride gas has been found to cause angiosarcomas both in people and in rats. Since an angiosarcoma is a rare tumor, the risk ratio (the ratio of the observed number of cancers in those exposed to the number expected by chance) is of order 100 or more in some cases. If an angiosarcoma is seen in a vinyl chloride worker, the attribution to vinyl chloride exposure is almost certain. On the other hand, the number of persons who have been heavily exposed to vinyl chloride is small. . . . Now that exposures in the workplace have been greatly reduced, . . . no more than one cancer is expected in several years.

We can compare this with the possible cancer incidence that was predicted by the Food and Drug Administration (FDA) in 1977 from use of saccharin. This was based on experiments with rats leading to an additional uncertainty. More people ate saccharin than were exposed to vinyl chloride, and nearly 500 cancers per year were estimated for the United States alone. For vinyl chloride . . . the individual risk is now low, yet there is considerable certainty that there is a risk. For saccharin the risk is higher, but there is more uncertainty about the value of the risk. Some . . . may demand that more attention be given to the risk from vinyl chloride than to the risk from saccharin; for other persons or situations the reverse may be the case.

COMPARISON OF RISKS

The purpose of risk assessment is to be useful in making decisions about the hazards causing risks, and so it is important to gain some perspective about the meaning of the magnitude of the risk. Comparisons can be useful. . . . It is particularly helpful to compare risks that are calculated in a similar way. For example, the risk of traveling by automobile can be compared to that of traveling by horse with the use of historical data. . . .

CONTRASTING RISKS

Objections have been raised to risk comparisons on the ground that they are misleading. This would be true if all risks of the same numerical magnitude were treated in the same way. But they are not. In some cases it is useful to contrast risks to indicate the different ways in which they are treated in society. . . .

[For example, the] small risk of a large accident in a nuclear power plant can . . . be contrasted with the more numerous small accidents or events that occur every day in the mining, transport, and burning of coal. One feature that is brought out clearly here is that we do not always compare the risk averaged over time, but worry more about risks that are sharply peaked in time.

EXPRESSION OF RISKS

Just as a comparison of risks is an aid in understanding them, so is a careful selection of the methods of expression. It is hard to comprehend the statistical (stochastic) nature of risk. . . . When we talk about the expectation of life being 79 years (for a nonsmoking male in the United States) we all know that some die young and that many live to be over 80. Thus the expression of a risk as the reduction of life expectancy caused by the risky action conveys some of the statistical concept essential to its understanding. . . .

It is important to realize that risks appear to be very different when expressed in different ways. One example of this can be seen if we consider the cancer risk to those persons exposed to radionuclides after the Chernobyl disaster. [Across the lifetimes of those 24,000 persons living between 3 and 15 kilometers from the plant, we can expect 131 cancers; in comparison, 31 people within the plant itself died within 60 days of acute radiation sickness and burns.] Dividing the 131 again by the approximately 5,000 cancer deaths expected from other causes, the accident caused "only" a 2.6% increase in cancer. This seems small compared to the 30% of cancers attributable to cigarette smoking. [In the total population of Ukraine and Byelorussia, the 3,500 "extra" cancers caused by Chernobyl will result in an] "insignificant" increase of 0.0047%. Of course, none of the methods of expressing the risk can be considered "right" in an absolute sense. Indeed, it is our belief that a full understanding of the risk involves expressing it in as many different ways as possible.

COST OF REDUCING A RISK

Another interesting and instructive way of comparing risks is by comparing the amount people have paid in the past to reduce them. . . . Society is willing to spend more on environmental protection to prevent cancer (over $1 million per life) than on cures (about $50,000 per life with the high value of $200,000 for kidney dialysis raising some objections). This ratio is in rough accord with the maxim "an ounce of protection is better than a pound of cure." People are willing to spend still more on radiation protection at nuclear power plants and on waste disposal. Economists and others often argue that efficiency depends on adjusting society until the amounts spent to save lives in different situations are equalized. It seems to us that society does not work that way. People are aware of the order of magnitude of these differences, and approve of them. Nonetheless, we believe that providing this information to a decision-maker is essential for an informed decision.

.   .   .   .   .

As Wilson and Crouch note, the varying prices that society is willing to pay to mitigate various risks might be seen as a reflection of underlying societal values or as an indication of troubling economic inefficiencies. Economists generally take the latter view. Using quantitative reasoning, they evaluate public health regulations and seek to understand both the costs of an intervention and its effects. Economic costs include the resources of agencies that must devise and implement the regulation (transaction costs), added expenses to individuals and businesses subject to the regulation (direct costs), and lost opportunities to intervene with different, potentially more effective techniques (opportunity costs). Similarly, economists seek to understand the effects of regulation—the effectiveness of the intervention in the real world and its societal benefits. Using this "cost-effectiveness" analysis (CEA), health economists can compare the estimated costs and benefits of various proposed interventions. According to standard economic theory, government should favor regulatory responses that maximize health benefits (e.g., saving the most years of life or quality-adjusted years of life) at the least cost.

Much of the CEA scholarship relies on a classic empirical study by John F. Morrall III (1986) purporting to show that government often spends exorbitant sums to avert very small risks. However, Lisa Heinzerling offers a powerful critique of Morrall's methods and thereby calls into question some of the risk scholarship that relies on his findings (Heinzerling 1998b; Ackerman and Heinzerling 2004). Heinzerling points out that the work by Morrall and others systematically downgrades the importance of regulation aimed at preventing long-latency diseases and long-term ecological harm. She also suggests that Morrall's estimates are inflated because they reflect only one regulatory benefit (cancer sickness and death) without taking into account other regulatory benefits, such as preventing respiratory illness and ecological harms: "Given all the benefits, some quantifiable, some not, most of the regulatory programs that have been portrayed as clunkers are not just barely cost-justified. They are bargains" (Heinzerling 1998a, 42).

Methodological debates aside, not everyone believes that sterile estimates of costs and benefits represent a fair way of evaluating policies. Many argue that market exchanges should not be the principal measure of the value of human lives. In particular, critics argue that public health policies cannot be compressed, through ever more complex economic methods, into a single aggregate number, such as costs per quality-adjusted life saved. Before spending five years working to pursue "smarter regulation" as a top official with the Bush administration's Office of Management and Budget, John D. Graham reminded those advocating greater reliance on CEA that noneconomic factors are nonetheless relevant to regulatory decisions. He emphasized "what is obvious but sometime forgotten: Cost-effectiveness is only one of the considerations that should inform allocations of limited resources. Other important factors include: notions of justice, equity, personal freedom, political feasibility, and the constraints of current law. It is important for advocates of CEA to recognize that what they have to offer should inform rather than dictate allocation of resources within the health sector of the economy" (Graham et al. 1998, 149).

RECOMMENDED READINGS

From Bioethics to Public Health Ethics

Buchanan, David R. 2008. Autonomy, paternalism, and justice: Ethical priorities in public health. *American Journal of Public Health* 98: 15–20. (Examines the underlying currents of paternalism in public health and incorporates a discussion of justice principles)

Kass, Nancy. 2001. An ethics framework for public health. *American Journal of Public Health* 91: 1776–82. (Introduces public health ethics primarily in reference to public health programs and provides a set of six framing questions for analyzing the ethics of a particular program)

Thomas, James C., Michael Sage, Jack Dillenberg, and V. James Guillory. 2002. A code of ethics for public health. *American Journal of Public Health*

92: 1057–59. (Reviews efforts to create an ethical code for public health and the necessary components found in one such code)

Public Health Paternalism: A Case Study on Motorcycle Helmet Laws

Dworkin, Gerald. 2008. Paternalism. In *Philosophy of Law,* ed. Joel Feinberg and Jules Coleman, 281–91. 8th ed. Belmont, CA: Wadsworth Publishing. (Provides the best-known scholarly examination of paternalism)

Ethical Reasoning in Risk Regulation

Arrow, Kenneth J., Maureen L. Cropper, George C. Eads, Robert W. Hahn, Lester B. Lave, Roger G. Noll, Paul R. Portney, et al. 1996. Is there a role for benefit-cost analysis in environmental, health, and safety regulation? *Science* 272: 221–22. (Explains the applications of cost-benefit analysis to health and environmental regulatory policy and gives eight guiding principles for the use of cost-benefit analysis)

Rodricks, Joseph V. 1994. Risk assessment, the environment, and public health. *Environmental Health Perspectives* 102: 258–64. (Provides an introduction to the science of risk assessment and argues for broader use of risk assessment principles and methods in public health)

Sunstein, Cass R. 1996. Health-health tradeoffs. *University of Chicago Law Review* 63: 1533–71. (Explores the problem that arises when averting a given health risk exacerbates another)

PART TWO

The Law and the Public's Health

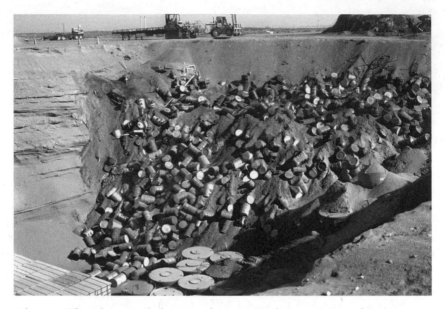

Photo 6. This photograph depicts a dump in Washington State, where at one time the nation sent much of its nuclear waste. In the 1980s, the federal government attempted to facilitate cooperative agreements between states for nuclear waste disposal. But the Supreme Court held in *New York v. United States,* 505 U.S. 144 (1992), that Congress had exceeded its authority in penalizing states for failure to participate in the program. Reproduced by permission, © Roger Ressmeyer/Corbis, October 18, 1988.

THREE

Public Health Duties
and Powers

The United States Constitution provides the framework for the distribution of governmental power. It divides power between the federal government and the states, separates power among the three branches of government, and limits governmental power over individuals to protect a sphere of liberty (see figure 4). Federal and state public health agencies carry out public health functions within these constitutional boundaries. Governmental actors must use their power to protect and promote the public's health according to this constitutional design and within the scope of legislative mandates. When disputes regarding governmental powers arise, courts often determine the lawfulness of particular public health interventions.

In thinking about government intervention to promote the common good, we should ask at least three important questions: (1) Does government have a *duty* to protect the public's health and safety? (2) What *power* does government have to regulate in the name of public health? (3) What *limits* exist in the exercise of public health powers? These three issues—governmental duties, powers, and limits—are central to understanding the role of public health authorities in the constitutional design. In the next chapter, I evaluate the third issue—constitutional restraints on the exercise of public health power. The readings in this chapter examine government's duty and power and also explore a corollary question: Which government—federal or state—may act to avert a health threat? The first portion discusses American federalism—the allocation of powers between federal and state governments—and examines

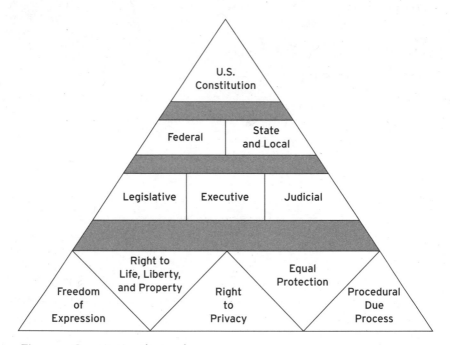

Figure 4. Constitutional triangle.

the pivotal role played by federal preemption of state regulation, which can virtually foreclose effective public health governance. In the second section, the readings offer historical and modern-day perspectives on the duties of government to safeguard the public's health and safety. And the next two sections explore state and federal public health powers.

The chapter concludes by returning to the contentious issue of public health federalism and the Supreme Court's resuscitation of the "reserved powers" doctrine to block federal public health regulation. The Court's rulings have placed significant obstacles in the way of public health governance: preemption impedes state regulation, while reserved powers impede federal regulation. Yet though the current judicial environment is unfavorable toward regulation, public health governance is not impossible.

I. AMERICAN FEDERALISM: THE ANTIREGULATORY EFFECTS OF FEDERAL PREEMPTION

One of the Constitution's primary functions is to divide governmental powers between the federal and state governments. Under the

Constitution, the federal government is a government of limited powers: that is, for the government to act, the basis of its power must be enumerated in the Constitution. The Constitution grants the federal government a number of powers, perhaps the most expansive being the power to regulate interstate and foreign commerce (see Article I, section 8, clause 3). Many federal public health statutes were passed under Congress's power to regulate interstate commerce, including laws governing food and drugs, occupational health and safety, and the environment. States, however, retain those powers inherent in sovereign governments but not delegated to the federal government by the Constitution. Two powers retained by the states are particularly relevant in public health law: the police power (protecting the health, safety, and morals of the community) and the *parens patriae* power (protecting the interests of minors and incompetent persons). The police powers are vast and enable states to regulate broadly to protect the health, safety, and morals of the population.

Federalism acts as a sorting device, helping to determine when a matter is exclusively or primarily a federal or state concern. Sometimes the boundary lines are uncertain, and in such circumstances decisive action can be thwarted. One of the principal questions in times of a public health emergency is, "Who is in charge?" During the Gulf Coast hurricanes, for example, lines of authority between the federal government, the state, and the city were blurred, which hampered the emergency response.

Conflicts between national and state regulation are resolved in favor of the federal government because federal law is supreme. The Constitution's Supremacy Clause declares that the "Constitution, and the Laws of the United States . . . and all Treaties made . . . shall be the supreme law of the Land" (Article VI). Consequently, Congress can enact legislation with the express or implied intent to supersede state law.

The doctrine of preemption holds that if Congress has enacted legislation on a particular subject, it is controlling over state or local laws. At times such federal action advances effective public health governance. For example, federal law sometimes sets a floor of minimum protection and allows states to go further. As a result, there are myriad examples of vigorous state regulation addressing health, safety, and the environment, even in the same sphere as federal legislation. But in recent years the courts have interpreted some federal statutes to virtually preclude state regulation. The recurrent debate on the interplay of federal and state regulation has "radically shifted from regulatory compliance to federal preemption" (Sharkey 2007, 1018).

Preemption has had antiregulatory effects in fields ranging from tobacco, occupational hazards, and motor vehicle safety to unsafe foods, pharmaceuticals, and medical devices. Indeed, from 2001 to 2006, Congress enacted twenty-seven statutes that preempted state health, safety, and environmental regulations or other social policy (U.S. Congress 2006). The effects of federal preemption are not simply to block direct state regulation but also to thwart common law tort actions to redress harms from unsafe products (see chapter 6).

In several cases in the past decade, the Supreme Court has held that federal laws preempt state tobacco control laws, stymieing state public health efforts. In *Lorillard Tobacco Co. v. Reilly*, 533 U.S. 525 (2001), the Court ruled that the Federal Cigarette Labeling and Advertising Act preempts Massachusetts regulations governing outdoor and point-of-sale cigarette advertising that were intended to prevent youth exposure to tobacco ads. (For a discussion of the commercial speech aspects of *Lorillard*, see chapter 9.) In 2008, the Supreme Court returned to the issue of federal preemption of state tobacco regulation in *Rowe v. New Hampshire Motor Transport Association*, 128 S. Ct. 989 (2008). At issue was whether the Federal Aviation Administration Authorization Act of 1994 (FAAAA) preempts Maine's Tobacco Delivery Law, which was designed to prevent Internet sales to minors. Maine's law required Internet tobacco retailers to use a delivery service that verifies the buyer's age. The Court held that Maine's law was preempted, rejecting the state's argument that it helps prevent minors from obtaining cigarettes, and thereby protects its citizens' health. Justice Stephen Breyer stressed that the FAAAA does not create a public health exception.

The Supreme Court has also held that some tort actions, based on state common law, are preempted by federal laws and regulations. In these cases, manufacturers have won by arguing that compliance with federal regulations for a product provides not only a compliance defense but also a preemptive shield against liability. In *Geier v. American Honda Motor Co., Inc.*, 529 U.S. 861 (2000), Alexis Geier sought damages under District of Columbia tort law for injuries he incurred in a crash while driving a 1987 Honda Accord that did not have an air bag. At the time, federal regulations required automobile manufacturers to equip some, but not all, of their vehicles with passive restraints. The Supreme Court held that the suit was preempted, reasoning that the imposition of liability would conflict with the objectives of the federal law. Two years later, however, in *Sprietsma v. Mercury Marine*, 537 U.S. 51 (2002), the Court held that a preemption provision in the Federal Boat Safety Act did not bar a husband from suing the manufacturer of a ski boat for the death of his wife. The boat's propeller blades had not been equipped with a guard, and Jeanne Sprietsma died after she fell overboard and was struck by the propeller.

Similarly, the Supreme Court has turned its attention to preemption in the field of drug and medical device safety. In *Buckman Co. v. Plaintiffs' Legal Committee*, 531 U.S. 341 (2001), the Court held that state tort law claims asserting that a medical device manufacturer is liable to injured consumers for having committed fraud on the FDA conflicts with the FDA's statutory responsibility to police fraud itself. The Medical Device Amendments (MDA) to the Federal Food, Drug, and Cosmetic Act (FDCA) therefore implicitly preempted the tort action. The Court recently revisited implied preemption of "fraud-on-the-FDA" in *Warner-Lambert Co. v. Kent*, 128 S. Ct. 1168 (2008). In *Warner-Lambert*, a group of Michigan residents sued for injuries caused by the diabetes drug Rezulin. At issue was a Michigan statute that shields pharmaceutical manufacturers from liability for harms caused by FDA-approved drugs, but removes that shield if there is evidence that the FDA approval was fraudulently secured. The Second Circuit Court of Appeals distinguished the case from *Buckman,* finding that the tort action did not conflict with the FDA's ability to police fraud. Because the eight Supreme Court justices hearing the case were evenly divided, the circuit decision was affirmed. While the suit will now be allowed to move forward, the split decision creates no precedent; thus the underlying legal issues have not been resolved by the Court.

The MDA, in addition to creating the federal scheme for policing compliance that implicitly preempts fraud-on-the-FDA claims under *Buckman,* also expressly preempts state regulation of medical devices. Recently, the Court has grappled with the question of whether state tort claims are preempted by state regulations that address medical devices. In *Medtronic v. Lohr,* 518 U.S. 470 (1996), the Court held that FDA approval of a pacemaker does not preempt claims of defective design under state tort law when the device had not been approved under the FDA's premarket approval process for new devices, but had instead been grandfathered in as a device "substantially equivalent" to devices on the market when the MDA was enacted. In 2008, the Supreme Court reconsidered the scope of preemption for medical devices, this time in a products liability case involving a device that had undergone the premarket approval process. The plaintiff in that case, Charles Riegel, brought suit after a balloon catheter burst during his angioplasty. Justice Antonin Scalia, writing for the Court in

Riegel v. Medtronic, Inc., 128 S. Ct. 999 (2008), said that the plaintiff's tort action could not proceed, because the MDA bars common law claims challenging the safety or effectiveness of a medical device marketed in a form that received premarket approval from the FDA. Justice Ruth Bader Ginsburg, the sole dissenter in the case, favored an approach based on sound regulation for the public's health and safety and argued, "Preemption analysis starts with the assumption that the historic police powers of the States are not to be superseded . . . unless that was the clear and manifest purpose of Congress." She referred to a "series of high-profile medical device failures that caused extensive injuries and loss of life," most notably the deaths and injuries from the Dalkon Shield intrauterine device (128 S. Ct. at 1013).

Lohr and *Riegel* both deal with the reach of the express preemption provision for medical devices. But the recent wave of preemption decisions has raised the question of whether and when FDA approval of pharmaceuticals similarly preempts state court action. In March 2009, the Court heard *Wyeth v. Levine*, 129 S. Ct. 1187 (2009). Diana Levine claimed that Wyeth was liable for the injury she sustained when she inadvertently received an intra-arterial injection of an antinausea drug while a health care provider was attempting to give the drug intravenously. After the injection, Levine developed gangrene and her arm had to be amputated. The Court considered whether the FDA's approval of the drug and its label preempted Levine's failure-to-warn claim. Wyeth argued that it could not have more adequately warned of the risk of administering its drug in the use that led to Diana Levine's injury. The company asserted that it could not alter a drug label that had been approved by the FDA without rendering the drug mislabeled under the federal FDCA. Further, it argued that compliance with heightened state law requirements would obstruct the purposes of the FDCA by substituting a jury's perceptions of drug safety for FDA expert assessment. The Court disagreed, and instead ruled that Wyeth could have altered the label under a regulation that allows drug safety information to be added while FDA approval is pending. The Court also found no evidence that Congress intended to preempt state law products liability. Justice Stevens wrote for the majority, "If Congress thought state-law suits posed an obstacle to its objectives, it surely would have enacted an express pre-emption provision at some point during the FDCA's 70-year history," as it did for medical devices (128 S. Ct. at 1200).

The Supreme Court's preemption jurisprudence, as it has developed over the past decade, demonstrates the potentially broad sweep of federal supremacy that enables Congress to override state regulation to promote the public's health.

II. THE NEGATIVE CONSTITUTION: GOVERNMENT'S DUTY TO PROTECT HEALTH AND SAFETY

Conventional wisdom holds that the Constitution places no affirmative duty on the government to protect individuals from harm or to promote the common good. Under this view, the Constitution is purely "negative" or "defensive" in character, protecting individuals against government's overreaching; it places no positive obligation on government to act. But influential scholars question this conventional position, arguing that states historically have had responsibilities to protect the populace. Professor Wendy Parmet (1992), for example, suggests that protection from infectious diseases was so important to our ancestors that government's duty to prevent epidemics was in effect assumed. The *DeShaney* and *Castle Rock* cases, excerpted below, make clear that the modern Supreme Court has a very different understanding of the extent to which such obligations are imposed under the Constitution.

The tragic case of Joshua DeShaney, a victim of child abuse, sets the backdrop for a landmark Supreme Court decision that limits the responsibility of government to protect the health of citizens. Professors Louis M. Seidman and Mark V. Tushnet (1996, 52) describe the facts of *DeShaney:*

> In Joshua DeShaney's first year of life, his parents divorced, and a court granted custody of the infant to his father, Randy DeShaney. For the next four years, the child lived through a nightmare of pain and violence. Randy DeShaney beat his son repeatedly and with increasing savagery. Eventually, the toddler fell into a life-threatening coma, and emergency brain surgery revealed injuries, inflicted over an extended period, that left Joshua permanently and severely retarded.
>
> As these tragic events unfolded, many of them came to the attention of county officials in the Wisconsin community where the DeShaneys lived. A battery of judges, lawyers, pediatricians, psychologists, police officers, and social workers became involved in Joshua's case. With Kafkaesque efficiency, these functionaries performed their particular assigned task within the social welfare bureaucracy. They held hearings, filed reports, completed forms. Yet despite all the purposeful bustling and the show of activity and concern, no one actually intervened to stop the violence until it was too late.
>
> After the damage had already been done, Joshua and his mother filed an action against [Winnebago County] in United States District Court. They argued that county officials had deprived Joshua of his liberty with-

out due process of law, thereby violating his rights under the Fourteenth Amendment.

If government officials had beaten Joshua themselves, his suit—even against their employers—might well have succeeded. Supreme Court decisions have made it clear that government agents who unjustifiably inflict physical injury violate the Due Process Clause. But because Joshua and his mother could not claim that the injury was directly inflicted by state officials, the suit foundered on the so-called "state action" requirement.

The Supreme Court's decision expresses a vision of a "negative" constitution according to which the judiciary is reluctant to impose on government an affirmative duty to safeguard the well-being of its citizens. The dissenting opinion of Justice Harry A. Blackmun conveys an alternative view of the constitutional obligation to protect vulnerable citizens. This dissent also expresses a sense of moral outrage at the notion that government cannot be held accountable for a failure to act in the interest of a citizen's health. As Justice Blackmun said, simply, "Poor Joshua."

The Supreme Court returned to the issue of government's duties to protect citizens in *Castle Rock v. Gonzales.* The case poses a set of heart-wrenching facts, with important public health and constitutional implications. Simon Gonzales, who had a history of erratic and suicidal behavior, violated a restraining order by abducting his three young daughters. His estranged wife, Jessica Gonzales, made repeated pleas to the police to enforce the restraining order, but to no avail. Nearly eight hours after she had first contacted police, her husband opened fire on the police station with a semiautomatic handgun he purchased after abducting his daughters. He was fatally shot, and police found the bodies of the three young girls, murdered by their father, in the cab of his truck.

The Supreme Court held that state law did not create an "entitlement" to enforce restraining orders issued in response to domestic abuse. Justice Scalia, writing for the majority, said that the arrest of a person who violates a protective order is purely discretionary. However, the Colorado statute declares that a peace officer "shall" arrest a person who violates a restraining order. If the state had promised its eligible citizens a service (e.g., education) or a benefit (e.g., Medicaid), there certainly would be an "entitlement." Police protection against violence is just as valuable as any other government service or benefit. Unfortunately, the Court made it clear that the Constitution does not offer vulnerable people a remedy, even in the face of the direst need.

When reading *DeShaney* and *Castle Rock,* consider whether the history and text genuinely support the view that the Constitution rarely imposes a responsibility on government to protect individuals and

populations. Even if the Constitution imposes no affirmative obligations, is there a reason, based on principle, for the distinction between
government's acts and omissions? Suppose a public health department,
knowing there is a high risk of an infectious disease outbreak, does
nothing to inform the public or intervene. Should the agency's failure to
prevent the outbreak be actionable under the due process clause of the
Fourteenth Amendment? Finally, if government does act to establish a
protective agency (e.g., child welfare or public health), should citizens
have a reasonable expectation that they can rely on that agency to safeguard their health and safety?

DESHANEY V. WINNEBAGO COUNTY DEPARTMENT OF SOCIAL SERVICES*

Supreme Court of the United States
Decided February 22, 1989

Chief Justice REHNQUIST delivered the opinion of the Court.

Petitioner [Joshua DeShaney] sued respondents [Winnebago County social workers and other officials] claiming that their failure to act deprived him of his liberty
in violation of the Due Process Clause of the Fourteenth Amendment to the United
States Constitution. We hold that it did not. . . .

The Due Process Clause of the Fourteenth Amendment provides that "[n]o State
shall . . . deprive any person of life, liberty, or property, without due process of
law." Petitioners contend that the State deprived Joshua of his liberty interest in
"free[dom from . . . unjustified intrusions on personal security," by failing to provide
him with adequate protection against his father's violence. The claim is one invoking
the substantive rather than the procedural component of the Due Process Clause;
petitioners do not claim that the State denied Joshua protection without according
him appropriate procedural safeguards, but that it was categorically obligated to
protect him in these circumstances. . . .

. . . Nothing in the language of the Due Process Clause itself requires the State
to protect the life, liberty, and property of its citizens against invasion by private
actors. The Clause is phrased as a limitation on the State's power to act, not as a
guarantee of certain minimal levels of safety and security. It forbids the State itself
to deprive individuals of life, liberty, or property without "due process of law," but
its language cannot fairly be extended to impose an affirmative obligation on the
State to ensure that those interests do not come to harm through other means.
Nor does history support such an expansive reading of the constitutional text. Like
its counterpart in the Fifth Amendment, the Due Process Clause of the Fourteenth
Amendment was intended to prevent government "from abusing [its] power, or
employing it as an instrument of oppression." . . . Its purpose was to protect the
people from the State, not to ensure that the State protected them from each other.

*489 U.S. 189 (1989).

The Framers were content to leave the extent of governmental obligation in the latter area to the democratic political processes.

Consistent with these principles, our cases have recognized that the Due Process Clause generally confers no affirmative right to governmental aid, even where such aid may be necessary to secure life, liberty, or property interests of which the government itself may not deprive the individual. . . . As we said in *Harris v. McRae:* "Although the liberty protected by the Due Process Clause affords protection against unwarranted government interference . . . , it does not confer an entitlement to such [governmental aid] as may be necessary to realize all the advantages of that freedom." 448 U.S. 297, 317–18 (1980). If the Due Process Clause does not require the State to provide its citizens with particular protective services, it follows that the State cannot be held liable under the Clause for injuries that could have been averted had it chosen to provide them. As a general matter, then, we conclude that a State's failure to protect an individual against private violence simply does not constitute a violation of the Due Process Clause.

Petitioners contend, however, that even if the Due Process Clause imposes no affirmative obligation on the State to provide the general public with adequate protective services, such a duty may arise out of certain "special relationships" created or assumed by the State with respect to particular individuals. Petitioners argue that such a "special relationship" existed here because the State knew that Joshua faced a special danger of abuse at his father's hands, and specifically proclaimed, by word and by deed, its intention to protect him against that danger. Having actually undertaken to protect Joshua from this danger—which petitioners concede the State played no part in creating—the State acquired an affirmative "duty," enforceable through the Due Process Clause, to do so in a reasonably competent fashion. Its failure to discharge that duty, so the argument goes, was an abuse of governmental power that so "shocks the conscience," as to constitute a substantive due process violation.

We reject this argument. It is true that in certain limited circumstances the Constitution imposes upon the State affirmative duties of care and protection with respect to particular individuals. In *Estelle v. Gamble,* 429 U.S. 97 (1976), we recognized that the Eighth Amendment's prohibition against cruel and unusual punishment, made applicable to the States through the Fourteenth Amendment's Due Process Clause, requires the State to provide adequate medical care to incarcerated prisoners. We reasoned that because the prisoner is unable "by reason of the deprivation of his liberty [to] care for himself," it is only "just" that the State be required to care for him. 429 U.S. at 103–04.

In *Youngberg v. Romeo,* 457 U.S. 307 (1982), we extended this analysis beyond the Eighth Amendment setting, holding that the substantive component of the Fourteenth Amendment's Due Process Clause requires the State to provide involuntarily committed mental patients with such services as are necessary to ensure their "reasonable safety" from themselves and others. . . .

Taken together, [these cases] stand only for the proposition that when the State takes a person into its custody and holds him there against his will, the Constitution imposes upon it a corresponding duty to assume some responsibility for his safety and general well-being. . . . The affirmative duty to protect arises . . . from the limitation which it has imposed on his freedom to act on his own behalf. In the substantive due process analysis, it is the State's affirmative act of restraining the individual's freedom to act on his own behalf—through incarceration, institutionalization, or other similar restraint of personal liberty—which is the "deprivation of liberty" triggering the protections of the Due Process Clause, not its failure to act to protect his liberty interests against harms inflicted by other means. . . .

[This] analysis simply has no applicability in the present case. Petitioners concede that the harms Joshua suffered occurred . . . while he was in the custody of his natural father, who was in no sense a state actor. While the State may have been aware of the dangers that Joshua faced in the free world, it played no part in their creation, nor did it do anything to render him any more vulnerable to them. That the State once took temporary custody of Joshua does not alter the analysis, for when it returned him to his father's custody, it placed him in no worse position than that in which he would have been had it not acted at all; the State does not become the permanent guarantor of an individual's safety by having once offered him shelter. Under these circumstances, the State had no constitutional duty to protect Joshua . . . [and] its failure to do so—though calamitous in hindsight—simply does not constitute a violation of the Due Process Clause.

Judges and lawyers, like other humans, are moved by natural sympathy in a case like this to find a way for Joshua and his mother to receive adequate compensation for the grievous harm inflicted upon them. But before yielding to that impulse, it is well to remember once again that the harm was inflicted not by the State of Wisconsin, but by Joshua's father. The most that can be said of the state functionaries in this case is that they stood by and did nothing when suspicious circumstances dictated a more active role for them. In defense of them it must also be said that had they moved too soon to take custody of the son away from the father, they would likely have been met with charges of improperly intruding into the parent-child relationship, charges based on the same Due Process Clause that forms the basis for the present charge of failure to provide adequate protection.

The people of Wisconsin may well prefer a system of liability which would place upon the State and its officials the responsibility for failure to act in situations such as the present one. They may create such a system, if they do not have it already, by changing the tort law of the State in accordance with the regular lawmaking process. But they should not have it thrust upon them by this Court's expansion of the Due Process Clause of the Fourteenth Amendment.

Affirmed.

Justice BLACKMUN, dissenting.

Today, the Court purports to be the dispassionate oracle of the law, unmoved by "natural sympathy." But, in this pretense, the Court itself retreats into a sterile formalism which prevents it from recognizing either the facts of the case before it or the legal norms that should apply to those facts. . . . The facts here involve not mere passivity, but active state intervention in the life of Joshua DeShaney—intervention that triggered a fundamental duty to aid the boy once the State learned of the severe danger to which he was exposed.

The Court fails to recognize this duty because it attempts to draw a sharp and rigid line between action and inaction. But such formalistic reasoning has no place in the interpretation of the broad and stirring Clauses of the Fourteenth Amendment. Indeed, I submit that these Clauses were designed, at least in part, to undo the formalistic legal reasoning that infected antebellum jurisprudence.

Like the antebellum judges who denied relief to fugitive slaves, the Court today claims that its decision, however harsh, is compelled by existing legal doctrine. On the contrary, the question presented by this case is an open one, and our Fourteenth Amendment precedents may be read more broadly or narrowly depending upon how one chooses to read them. Faced with the choice, I would adopt a "sympathetic" reading, one which comports with dictates of fundamental justice and recognizes that compassion need not be exiled from the province of judging.

Poor Joshua! Victim of repeated attacks by an irresponsible, bullying, cowardly, and intemperate father, and abandoned by respondents who placed him in a dangerous predicament and who knew or learned what was going on, and yet did essentially nothing except, as the Court revealingly observes, "dutifully recorded these incidents in [their] files." It is a sad commentary upon American life, and constitutional principles—so full of late of patriotic fervor and proud proclamations about "liberty and justice for all"—that this child, Joshua DeShaney, now is assigned to live out the remainder of his life profoundly retarded. Joshua and his mother, as petitioners here, deserve—but now are denied by this Court—the opportunity to have the facts of their case considered in the light of . . . constitutional protection.

CASTLE ROCK V. GONZALES*
Supreme Court of the United States
Decided June 27, 2005

Justice SCALIA delivered the opinion of the Court.

The horrible facts of this case are contained in the complaint that respondent Jessica Gonzales filed in Federal District Court. [She] alleges that petitioner, the town of Castle Rock, Colorado, violated the Due Process Clause of the Fourteenth Amendment to the United States Constitution when its police officers, acting pursuant to official policy or custom, failed to respond properly to her repeated reports that her estranged husband was violating the terms of a restraining order. . . .

The Fourteenth Amendment . . . provides that a State shall not "deprive any person of life, liberty, or property, without due process of law." . . . Respondent claims . . . that she had a property interest in police enforcement of the restraining order against her husband; and that the town deprived her of this property without due process by having a policy that tolerated nonenforcement of restraining orders. . . .

The procedural component of the Due Process Clause does not protect everything that might be described as a "benefit": To have a property interest in a benefit, a person clearly must have more than an abstract need or desire and more than a unilateral expectation of it. He must, instead, have a legitimate claim of entitlement to it. Such entitlements are not created by the Constitution. Rather, they are created and their dimensions are defined by existing rules or understandings that stem from an independent source such as state law. . . .

. . . The ultimate issue [is] whether what Colorado law has given respondent constitutes a property interest for purposes of the Fourteenth Amendment. [Stated differently, the central question is] whether Colorado law gave respondent a right to police enforcement of the restraining order. . . .

*545 U.S. 748 (2005).

The critical language in the restraining order came not from any part of the order itself . . . but from the preprinted notice to law-enforcement personnel that appeared on the back of the order. That notice effectively restated the statutory provision describing "peace officers' duties" related to the crime of violation of a restraining order. At the time of the conduct at issue in this case, that provision read as follows:

"(a) Whenever a restraining order is issued, the protected person shall be provided with a copy of such order. *A peace officer shall use every reasonable means to enforce a restraining order.*

"(b) *A peace officer shall arrest, or, if an arrest would be impractical under the circumstances, seek a warrant for the arrest of a restrained person* when the peace officer has information amounting to probable cause that:

"(I) The restrained person has violated or attempted to violate any provision of a restraining order; and

"(II) The restrained person has been properly served with a copy of the restraining order or the restrained person has received actual notice of the existence and substance of such order.

"(c) In making the probable cause determination described in paragraph (b) of this subsection (3), a peace officer shall assume that the information received from the registry is accurate. *A peace officer shall enforce a valid restraining order whether or not there is a record of the restraining order in the registry.*" (Colo. Rev. Stat. § 18-6-803.5[3] [emphases added]) . . .

We do not believe that these provisions of Colorado law truly made enforcement of restraining orders *mandatory*. A well established tradition of police discretion has long coexisted with apparently mandatory arrest statutes. . . .

Against that backdrop, a true mandate of police action would require some stronger indication from the Colorado Legislature than "shall use every reasonable means to enforce a restraining order" (or even "shall arrest . . . or . . . seek a warrant"). . . . It is hard to imagine that a Colorado peace officer would not have some discretion to determine that—despite probable cause to believe a restraining order has been violated—the circumstances of the violation or the competing duties of that officer or his agency counsel decisively against enforcement in a particular instance. The practical necessity for discretion is particularly apparent in a case such as this one, where the suspected violator is not actually present and his whereabouts are unknown. . . .

Respondent does not specify the precise means of enforcement that the Colorado restraining-order statute assertedly mandated. . . . Such indeterminacy is not the hallmark of a duty that is mandatory. Nor can someone be safely deemed "entitled" to something when the identity of the alleged entitlement is vague. . . . After the warrant is sought, it remains within the discretion of a judge whether to grant it, and after it is granted, it remains within the discretion of the police whether and when to execute it. Respondent would have been assured nothing but the seeking of a warrant. This is not the sort of "entitlement" out of which a property interest is created. . . .

Even if the statute could be said to have made enforcement of restraining orders "mandatory" because of the domestic-violence context of the underlying statute, that would not necessarily mean that state law gave *respondent* an entitlement to enforcement of the mandate. Making the actions of government employees obligatory can serve various legitimate ends other than the conferral of a benefit on a specific class of people. The serving of public rather than private ends is the normal course of the criminal law. . . .

Respondent's alleged interest stems only from a State's *statutory* scheme—from a restraining order that was authorized by and tracked precisely the statute. . . . She does not assert that she has any common-law or contractual entitlement to enforcement. If she was given a statutory entitlement, we would expect to see some indication of that in the statute itself. Although Colorado's statute spoke of "protected person[s]" such as respondent, it did so in connection with matters other than a right to enforcement. . . . The protected person's express power to "initiate" civil contempt proceedings contrasts tellingly with the mere ability to "request" initiation of criminal contempt proceedings—and even more dramatically with the complete silence about any power to "request" (much less demand) that an arrest be made.

The creation of a personal entitlement to something as vague and novel as enforcement of restraining orders cannot "simply g[o] without saying." We conclude that Colorado has not created such an entitlement.

Even if we were to think otherwise concerning the creation of an entitlement by Colorado, it is by no means clear that an individual entitlement to enforcement of a restraining order could constitute a "property" interest for purposes of the Due Process Clause. Such a right would not, of course, resemble any traditional conception of property. Although that alone does not disqualify it from due process protection, . . . the right to have a restraining order enforced does not "have some ascertainable monetary value," as even our [previous] cases have implicitly required. Perhaps most radically, the alleged property interest here arises *incidentally*, not out of some new species of government benefit or service, but out of a function that government actors have always performed—to wit, arresting people who they have probable cause to believe have committed a criminal offense. . . .

We conclude, therefore, that respondent did not, for purposes of the Due Process Clause, have a property interest in police enforcement of the restraining order against her husband. . . .

In light of today's decision and that in *DeShaney*, the benefit that a third party may receive from having someone else arrested for a crime generally does not trigger protections under the Due Process Clause, neither in its procedural nor in its "substantive" manifestations. . . .

Justice STEVENS, with whom Justice GINSBURG joins, dissenting.

The central question in this case is . . . whether, as a matter of Colorado law, respondent had a right to police assistance comparable to the right she would have possessed to any other service the government or a private firm might have undertaken to provide. . . .

. . . The crucial point is that, under the statute, the police were *required* to provide enforcement; *they lacked the discretion to do nothing.* The Court suggests that the fact that "enforcement" may encompass different acts infects any entitlement to enforcement with "indeterminacy." But this objection is also unfounded. Our cases have never required the object of an entitlement to be some mechanistic, unitary thing. . . . The enforcement of a restraining order is not some amorphous, indeterminate thing. Under the statute, if the police have probable cause that a violation has occurred, enforcement consists of either making an immediate arrest or seeking a warrant and then executing an arrest–traditional, well-defined tasks that law enforcement officers perform every day. . . .

Police enforcement of a restraining order is a government service that is no less concrete and no less valuable than other government services. . . . In this case, Colorado law *guaranteed* the provision of a certain service, in certain defined circumstances, to a certain class of beneficiaries, and respondent reasonably relied on that guarantee. . . .

Because respondent had a property interest in the enforcement of the restraining order, state officials could not deprive her of that interest without observing fair procedures. . . . According to respondent's complaint the process she was afforded by the police constituted nothing more than a "'sham or a pretense.'"

Accordingly, I respectfully dissent.

III. STATE POLICE POWERS: PROTECTING HEALTH, SAFETY, AND MORALS

I define police power in the *Reader*'s companion text as "the inherent authority of the state (and, through delegation, local government) to enact laws and promulgate regulations to protect, preserve, and promote the health, safety, morals, and general welfare of the people. To achieve these communal benefits, the state retains the power to restrict, within federal and state constitutional limits, private interests—personal interests in autonomy, privacy, association, and liberty as well as economic interests in freedom to contract and uses of property."

Chief Justice John Marshall, in *Gibbons v. Ogden*, 22 U.S. 1, 87 (1824), was the first Supreme Court justice to refer to the police powers. Marshall conceived of state police powers as "that immense mass of legislation, which embraces every thing within the territory of a State, not surrendered to the general government: all which can be most advantageously exercised by the States themselves. Inspection laws, quarantine laws, health laws of every description, as well as laws for regulating the internal commerce of a State, and those which respect turnpike roads, ferries, are component parts of this mass." Perhaps the most famous explanation of the police power was the 1905 case of *Jacobson v. Massachusetts,* excerpted in chapter 4.

Santiago Legarre, in a comprehensive article on the history of the police powers (2007), suggests three different meanings of "police power," each favored in turn during different periods of American constitutional history: (1) a broad meaning, conveying the residual sovereignty of the states or the powers inherent in every sovereignty; (2) a narrow meaning, conveying the state's power to protect certain public goods—namely, public health, public safety, and public morals; and (3) a somewhat different broad meaning, encompassing all great public needs, including economic and social interests, such that the state may regulate for the public's health, safety, morals, convenience, and general prosperity.

In the following reading, the University of Chicago historian William J. Novak talks about the rich historical origins of the "police power." More important, he reminds us that early America, far from illustrating laissez-faire philosophy, as is often assumed, was truly a "well-regulated" society, and this regulation principally occurred at the state and local levels.

GOVERNANCE, POLICE, AND AMERICAN LIBERAL MYTHOLOGY*
William J. Novak

She starts old, old, wrinkled and writhing in an old skin.
And there is a gradual sloughing off of the old skin,
towards a new youth. It is the myth of America.

D.H. Lawrence

A distinctive and powerful governmental tradition devoted in theory and practice to the vision of a well-regulated society dominated United States social and economic policymaking from 1787 to 1877. With deep and diverse roots in colonial, English, and continental European customs, laws, and public practices, that tradition matured into a full-fledged science of government by midcentury. At the heart of the well-regulated society was a plethora of bylaws, ordinances, statutes, and common law restrictions regulating nearly every aspect of early American economy and society, from Sunday observance to the carting of offal. These laws—the work of mayors, common councils, state legislators, town and county officers, and powerful state and local judges—comprise a remarkable and previously neglected record of governmental aspiration and practice. Taken together they explode tenacious myths about nineteenth-century government (or its absence) and demonstrate the pervasiveness of regulation in early American versions of the good society: regulations for *public safety* and security (protecting the very existence of the population from catastrophic enemies like fire and invasion); the construction of a *public economy* (determining the rules by which the people would acquire and exchange food and goods); the policing of *public space* (defining common rights in roads, rivers, and public squares); all-important restraints on *public morals* (establishing the social and cultural conditions of public order); and the open-ended regulatory powers granted to public officials to guarantee *public health* (securing the population's well-being, longevity, and productivity). Public regulation—the power of the state to restrict individual liberty and property for the common welfare—colored all facets of early American development. It was the central component of a reigning theory and

*From *The People's Welfare: Law and Regulation in Nineteenth-Century America* by William J. Novak. Copyright © 1996 by the University of North Carolina Press. Used by permission of the publisher.

practice of governance committed to the pursuit of the people's welfare and happiness in a well-ordered society and polity.

These laws [are] what I collectively refer to as "the well-regulated society." . . . To the omnipresent and skeptical social-historical question, Were such laws enforced?, the thousand cases examined here testify simply and unequivocally, yes. A second question is more interesting, more complicated, and more controversial: Why is this governmental regulatory practice so invisible in our traditional accounts of nineteenth-century American history? Why is it at all surprising to discover the pivotal role played by public law, regulation, order, discipline, and governance in early American society? . . .

America's nineteenth-century regulatory past remains something of a trade secret. No comprehensive history of antebellum regulation exists, and the mention of an American regulatory heritage prompts a familiar incredulity if not outright denial. Why? The culprit is a set of four interrelated and surprisingly resilient myths about nineteenth-century America challenged by this [essay]: the myth of statelessness, the myth of liberal individualism, the myth of the great transformation, and the myth of American exceptionalism. . . .

[Ed.—The author discusses these four myths.]

Together these four organizing myths constitute a master narrative of American political development in which liberty *against* government serves as the fulcrum of a constant and distinctively American liberal-constitutional tradition. The reigning paradigms of American politics (self-interested liberalism), law (constitutionalism), and economics (neoclassical market theory) conspire with this mythic historiography to produce a gross overemphasis on individual rights, constitutional limitations, and the invisible hand; and a terminal neglect of the positive activities and public responsibilities of American government over time. . . .

The well-regulated society confronts the myths of statelessness, individualism, transformation, and exceptionalism with four distinguishing principles of positive governance: public spirit, local self-government, civil liberty, and law. While very much at odds with modern conceptions of the sovereign state and the rights-bearing individual, these principles were the heart of the nineteenth-century vision of a well-regulated society.

Public Spirit

Salus populi (the people's welfare) is . . . an abridgment of the influential common law maxim *salus populi suprema lex est* (the welfare of the people is the supreme law) and one of the fundamental ordering principles of the early American polity. Nineteenth-century America was a *public* society in ways hard to imagine after the invention of twentieth-century privacy. Its governance was predicated on the elemental assumption that public interest was superior to private interest. Government and society were not created to protect preexisting private rights, but to further the welfare of the whole people and community. . . .

Local Self-Government

Despite the jilting of the Articles of Confederation and the new supremacy clause in the federal Constitution, nineteenth-century American governance remained decidedly local. Towns, local courts, common councils, and state legislatures were the basic institutions of governance, and they continued to function in ways not unlike their colonial and European forebears. . . . Though its antidespotic thrust is often mistaken for liberal individualism, local self-government conceived of liberty and autonomy as collective attributes—badges of participation, things achieved in common through social and political interaction with others. The independent law-making authority of local communities . . . was to be defended from usurpation by despots, courtly mandarins, or other central powers. But within communities, individuals were expected to conform their behavior to local rules and expectations. No community was deemed free without the power and right of members to govern themselves, *that is,* to determine the rules under which the locality as a whole would be organized and regulated. Such open-ended local regulatory power was simply a necessary attribute of any truly popular sovereignty. . . .

Civil Liberty

Integral to local self-government was a unique conception of civil or regulated liberty. . . . Civil liberty consisted only in those freedoms consistent with the laws of the land. Such liberty was never absolute, it always had to conform to the superior power of self-governing communities to legislate and regulate in the public interest. From time immemorial, as the common law saying went, this liberty was subject to local bylaws for the promotion and maintenance of community order, comfort, safety, health, and well-being. Freedom and regulation in this tradition were not viewed as antithetical but as complementary and mutually reinforcing. . . .

Law

By definition, any history of early American government must also be a legal history. . . . As Thomas Paine (1945, 29) noted, "In America the law is king." John Adams famously added (invoking James Harrington) that this was "a government of laws" (Paine 1945, 29). . . . But the content of the common legal tradition undergirding the well-regulated society runs counter to some classic interpretations of American bench and bar that emphasize solely devotion to private (usually economic) interests and hostility to government. The legal doctrines and practices guaranteeing the rights of municipalities to regulate social and economic life were testaments to the importance of nonconstitutional public law to the American polity. The nineteenth century was not simply an age of private contract and public constitutional limitations. It was an epoch in which strong common law notions of public prerogatives and the duties and obligations of government persisted amid a torrent of private adjudication and constitution writing. The rule of law, a distinctly public and social ideal antedating both Lockean liberalism and Machiavellian civic humanism, dominated most thinking about governance in the nineteenth century. . . .

Public spirit, local self-government, civil liberty, and common law were part of a worldview decidedly different from our own and from the one we have imposed on an unsuspecting past. Their reference point was the relationship of a citizen to a republic rather than an individual subject to a sovereign nation-state. But *salus populi* and well-regulated governance entailed more than a particular legal-political worldview. It was a governmental practice embedded in some of the most important public policies and initiatives of the nineteenth century. In particular, the four principles outlined here found clearest expression in countless nineteenth-century exertions of what is known in legal parlance as *state police power.* . . .

The state police power is one of the most enigmatic phenomena in American legal and political history. To begin with, the phrase "state police power" is triply misleading. First, police power has little to do with our modern notion of a municipal police force. Second, the triumph of this particular legal terminology was part of a late nineteenth-century effort to rein in, constitutionalize, and centralize the disparate powers of states and localities. Using the term to describe earlier developments thus risks importing some anachronistic assumptions. Finally, despite being a "state" power, the police power was usually exercised by local officials.

Generations of judges and scholars have suggested that, in fact, state police power is undefinable. [The definitions proposed by early twentieth-century scholars] cover three essential components of police power: law, regulation, and people's welfare. Police power was the ability of a state or locality to enact and enforce public laws regulating or even destroying private right, interest, liberty, or property for the common good (i.e., for the public safety, comfort, welfare, morals, or health). Such broad compass has led some to conclude that state police power was the essence of governance, the hallmark of sovereignty and statecraft.

The American constitutional basis of state police power was the Tenth Amendment, reserving to the states all power not explicitly delegated or prohibited in the Constitution. But more significant than this formal constitutional sanction were the substantive roots of state regulatory power in early modern notions of police or *Polizei*. . . . Police was a science and mode of governance where the polity assumed control over, and became implicated in, the basic conduct of social life. . . . Police aspirations also included enriching population and state, increasing agricultural yields, minimizing threats to health and safety, promoting communication and commerce, and improving the overall quality of the people's existence.

Such sweeping objectives required the intense regulation and public monitoring of economy and society. Indeed the effect of police was a vast proliferation of regulatory intrusions into the remotest corners of public and private activity [including religion, morals, health, travel, and labor]. No aspect of human intercourse remained outside the purview of police science. . . .

The vast, largely unwritten history of American governance and police regulation suggests that it is time to refocus attention on [a] . . . founding paradox—the myth of American liberty. For . . . the storied history of liberty in the United States, with its vaunted rhetoric of unprecedented rights of property, contract, mobility, privacy, and bodily integrity, was built directly upon a strong and consistent willingness to employ the full, coercive, and regulatory powers of law and government. The public conditions of private freedom remain the great problem of American governmental and legal history.

IV. FEDERAL POWER TO SAFEGUARD THE PUBLIC'S HEALTH

The national government has only those powers expressly enumerated in the Constitution. For public health purposes, the foremost of these are the power to tax and spend for the general welfare and the power to regulate interstate commerce. These powers provide Congress with independent authority to raise revenue for public health services and to regulate, both directly and indirectly, private activities that endanger the public's health. The Constitution also affords Congress other powers important to public health. Congress has the power to enforce the civil rights amendments (the Thirteenth, Fourteenth, and Fifteenth Amendments); and it has the power to "promote the Progress of Science" by securing for inventors the exclusive right to their discoveries through the granting of patents (Article I, section 8, clause 8). The Constitution also grants the president authority to make treaties with the Senate's advice and consent, a power that has significance in global health, as discussed in chapter 7.

The "necessary and proper" clause in Article I, section 8, of the Constitution permits Congress to employ all means reasonably appropriate to achieve the objectives of enumerated national powers. Chief Justice John Marshall's famous remark in *McCulloch v. Maryland*, 17 U.S. 316, 421 (1819), illustrates the potentially expansive powers of Congress: "Let the end be legitimate, let it be within the scope of the constitution, and all means which are appropriate, which are plainly adapted to that end, which are not prohibited, but consistent with the letter and spirit of the constitution, are constitutional." This "implied powers" doctrine has enabled the national government to expand into public health regulation, traditionally a state-level responsibility. Federal regulation now covers broad aspects of public health, such as air and water quality, food and drug safety, pesticide production and sales, consumer product safety, occupational health and safety, and medical care.

A. *The Power to Tax and Spend—the Power to Influence State and Private Behavior*

The power to tax and spend is found in the Constitution's phrase "Congress shall have Power To lay and collect Taxes, Duties, Imposts and Excises, to pay the Debts and provide for the common Defence and general Welfare of the United States" (Article I, section 8, clause 1). The power to tax and spend enables the federal government to raise revenue to provide for the good of the community, making possible such services as health care for the poor, sanitation, and environmental protection. Equally important, the taxing and spending power makes it possible to regulate risk behavior and influence health-promoting activities. Through its taxing powers, government can create incentives to engage in beneficial activities (e.g., employer-sponsored health plans) or disincentives to engage in risk behaviors (e.g., smoking cigarettes). Alternatively, by setting "conditions" on the granting of funds, the United States can induce states to adopt federal regulatory standards.

The spending power has been challenged by states claiming that when it is used inappropriately, the federal government coerces states and violates state sovereignty. This issue came before the Supreme Court in *South Dakota v. Dole*, which addressed the federal government's ability to encourage states to raise the minimum drinking age by setting conditions on the receipt of federal highway funds. *Dole* illustrates the Supreme Court's permissive view that government can allocate resources on the condition that the recipient complies with specified norms. Thus, the conditional spending power can be used to achieve a public health objective.

SOUTH DAKOTA V. DOLE*
Supreme Court of the United States
Decided June 23, 1987

Chief Justice REHNQUIST delivered the opinion of the Court.

[In South Dakota, persons nineteen years of age or older are permitted to purchase beer containing up to 3.2 percent alcohol. Title 23 U.S.C. § 158 directs the secretary of transportation to withhold federal highway funds from states that allow persons under the age of twenty-one years to purchase and possess alcohol. The State of South Dakota argues that § 158 violates the constitutional limitations on congressional spending power under Article I, section 8, clause 1 (tax-and-spend power) of the Constitution and violates the Tenth Amendment (among other constitutional arguments).]

... Incident to [the tax-and-spend power], Congress may attach conditions on the receipt of federal funds, and has repeatedly employed the power "to further broad policy objectives by conditioning receipt of federal moneys upon compliance by the recipient with federal statutory and administrative directives." *Fullilove v. Klutznick*, 448 U.S. 448, 474 (1980)....[Even those] objectives not thought to be within Article I's "enumerated legislative fields" may nevertheless be attained through the use of the spending power and the conditional grant of federal funds.

The spending power is of course not unlimited, but is instead subject to several general restrictions articulated in our cases. The first of these limitations is derived from the language of the Constitution itself: the exercise of the spending power must be in pursuit of "the general welfare." In considering whether a particular expenditure is intended to serve general public purposes, courts should defer substantially to the judgment of Congress. Second, we have required that if Congress desires to condition the States' receipt of federal funds, it "must do so unambiguously...,

*483 U.S. 203 (1987).

enabl[ing] the States to exercise their choice knowingly, cognizant of the consequences of their participation." *Pennhurst State School and Hospital v. Halderman*,
451 U.S. 1, 17 (1981). Third, our cases have suggested (without significant elaboration) that conditions on federal grants might be illegitimate if they are unrelated "to
the federal interest in particular national projects or programs." *Massachusetts v.
United States*, 435 U.S. 444, 461 (1978) (plurality opinion). . . .

South Dakota does not seriously claim that § 158 is inconsistent with any of the
first three restrictions mentioned above. We can readily conclude that the provision is designed to serve the general welfare, especially in light of the fact that
"the concept of welfare or the opposite is shaped by Congress. . . . " *Helvering v.
Davis*, 301 U.S. 619, 645 (1937). Congress found that the differing drinking ages in
the States created particular incentives for young persons to combine their desire to
drink with their ability to drive, and that this interstate problem required a national
solution. The means it chose to address this dangerous situation were reasonably
calculated to advance the general welfare. The conditions upon which States receive
the funds, moreover, could not be more clearly stated by Congress. And the State
itself, rather than challenging the germaneness of the condition to federal purposes,
admits that it "has never contended that the congressional action was . . . unrelated
to a national concern in the absence of the Twenty-first Amendment." Indeed, the
condition imposed by Congress is directly related to one of the main purposes for
which highway funds are expended—safe interstate travel. This goal of the interstate
highway system had been frustrated by varying drinking ages among the States. A
Presidential commission appointed to study alcohol-related accidents and fatalities
on the Nation's highways concluded that the lack of uniformity in the States' drinking
ages created "an incentive to drink and drive" because "young persons commut[e]
to border States where the drinking age is lower." By enacting § 158, Congress conditioned the receipt of federal funds in a way reasonably calculated to address this
particular impediment to a purpose for which the funds are expended. . . .

We have also held that a perceived Tenth Amendment limitation on congressional regulation of state affairs did not concomitantly limit the range of conditions
legitimately placed on federal grants. . . . We think that . . . the [spending] power may
not be used to induce the States to engage in activities that would themselves be
unconstitutional. Thus, for example, a grant of federal funds conditioned on invidi-
ously discriminatory state action or the infliction of cruel and unusual punishment
would be an illegitimate exercise of the Congress's broad spending power. But no
such claim can be or is made here. Were South Dakota to succumb to the blandish-
ments offered by Congress and raise its drinking age to 21, the State's action in so
doing would not violate the constitutional rights of anyone.

Our decisions have recognized that in some circumstances the financial induce-
ment offered by Congress might be so coercive as to pass the point at which "pressure turns into compulsion." *Steward Machine Co. v. Davis*, 301 U.S. 548, 590
(1937). Here, however, Congress has directed only that a State desiring to establish
a minimum drinking age lower than 21 lose a relatively small percentage of certain
federal highway funds. Petitioner contends that the coercive nature of this program
is evident from the degree of success it has achieved. We cannot conclude, however,
that a conditional grant of federal money of this sort is unconstitutional simply by
reason of its success in achieving the congressional objective.

When we consider, for a moment, that all South Dakota would lose if she adheres to her chosen course as to a suitable minimum drinking age is 5% of the funds otherwise obtainable under specified highway grant programs, the argument as to coercion is shown to be more rhetoric than fact. . . . Here Congress has offered relatively mild encouragement to the States to enact higher minimum drinking ages than they would otherwise choose. But the enactment of such laws remains the prerogative of the States not merely in theory but in fact. Even if Congress might lack the power to impose a national minimum drinking age directly, we conclude that encouragement to state action found in § 158 is a valid use of the spending power.

B. Controlling the Stream of Interstate Commerce—the Power to Regulate

The Commerce Clause, more than any other enumerated power, affords Congress potent regulatory authority. Article I, section 8, clause 3, states that "[t]he Congress shall have the power . . . to regulate Commerce with foreign Nations, and among the several states, and with the Indian Tribes." Since Franklin Delano Roosevelt's New Deal era, the Supreme Court has interpreted the Commerce Clause broadly, giving Congress the ability to regulate almost any area of activity as long as that activity has national effects. However, the Supreme Court has begun to rethink the breadth of commerce power, shifting regulatory authority back to the states for activities that are primarily intrastate. In *United States v. Lopez* (excerpted next), the Court was faced with a popular statute in which Congress had restricted gun possession in school zones. Chief Justice William Rehnquist's opinion does not question the importance of firearm control as a legitimate public health function. Rather, he argues that controlling the mere possession of guns in schools is outside the sphere of the federal commerce power.

UNITED STATES V. LOPEZ*
Supreme Court of the United States
Decided April 26, 1995

Chief Justice REHNQUIST delivered the opinion of the Court.

In the Gun-Free School Zones Act of 1990, Congress made it a federal offense "for any individual knowingly to possess a firearm at a place that the individual knows, or has reasonable cause to believe, is a school zone." 18 U.S.C. § 922(q)(1)(A) (1988 ed., Supp. V). The Act neither regulates a commercial activity nor contains a requirement that the possession be connected in any way to interstate commerce.

*514 U.S. 549 (1995).

We hold that the Act exceeds the authority of Congress "[t]o regulate Commerce ... among the several States. ... " U.S. Const., art. I, § 8, cl. 3. ...

... We have identified three broad categories of activity that Congress may regulate under its commerce power. First, Congress may regulate the use of the channels of interstate commerce. Second, Congress is empowered to regulate and protect the instrumentalities of interstate commerce, or persons or things in interstate commerce, even though the threat may come only from intrastate activities. Finally, Congress's commerce authority includes the power to regulate those activities having a substantial relation to interstate commerce, *i.e.*, those activities that substantially affect interstate commerce. ...

Within this final category, admittedly, our case law has not been clear whether an activity must "affect" or "substantially affect" interstate commerce in order to be within Congress's power to regulate it under the Commerce Clause. We conclude, consistent with the great weight of our case law, that the proper test requires an analysis of whether the regulated activity "substantially affects" interstate commerce.

We now turn to consider the power of Congress, in the light of this framework, to enact § 922(q). The first two categories of authority may be quickly disposed of: § 922(q) is not a regulation of the use of the channels of interstate commerce, nor is it an attempt to prohibit the interstate transportation of a commodity through the channels of commerce; nor can § 922(q) be justified as a regulation by which Congress has sought to protect an instrumentality of interstate commerce or a thing in interstate commerce. Thus, if § 922(q) is to be sustained, it must be under the third category as a regulation of an activity that substantially affects interstate commerce. ...

Section 922(q) is a criminal statute that by its terms has nothing to do with "commerce" or any sort of economic enterprise, however broadly one might define those terms. Section 922(q) is not an essential part of a larger regulation of economic activity, in which the regulatory scheme could be undercut unless the intrastate activity were regulated. It cannot, therefore, be sustained under our cases upholding regulations of activities that arise out of or are connected with a commercial transaction, which viewed in the aggregate, substantially affect interstate commerce.

Second, § 922(q) contains no jurisdictional element which would ensure, through case-by-case inquiry, that the firearm possession in question affects interstate commerce. ...

The Government's essential contention [is] that § 922(q) is valid because possession of a firearm in a local school zone does indeed substantially affect interstate commerce. The Government argues that possession of a firearm in a school zone may result in violent crime and that violent crime can be expected to affect the functioning of the national economy in two ways. First, the costs of violent crime are substantial, and, through the mechanism of insurance, those costs are spread throughout the population. Second, violent crime reduces the willingness of individuals to travel to areas within the country that are perceived to be unsafe. The Government also argues that the presence of guns in schools poses a substantial threat to the educational process by threatening the learning environment. A handicapped educational process, in turn, will result in a less productive citizenry. That, in turn, would have an adverse effect on the Nation's economic well-being. As a result, the Government argues that Congress could rationally have concluded that § 922(q) substantially affects interstate commerce.

... Under the Government's "national productivity" reasoning, Congress could regulate any activity that it found was related to the economic productivity of individual citizens.... It is difficult to perceive any limitation on federal power, even in areas such as criminal law enforcement or education where States historically have been sovereign. Thus, if we were to accept the Government's arguments, we are hard pressed to posit any activity by an individual that Congress is without power to regulate....

The possession of a gun in a local school zone is in no sense an economic activity that might, through repetition elsewhere, substantially affect any sort of interstate commerce. Respondent was a local student at a local school; there is no indication that he had recently moved in interstate commerce, and there is no requirement that his possession of the firearm [has] any concrete tie to interstate commerce.

To uphold the Government's contentions here, we would have to pile inference upon inference in a manner that would bid fair to convert congressional authority under the Commerce Clause to a general police power of the sort retained by the States. Admittedly, some of our prior cases have taken long steps down that road, giving great deference to congressional action. The broad language in these opinions has suggested the possibility of additional expansion, but we decline here to proceed any further. To do so would require us to conclude that the Constitution's enumeration of powers does not presuppose something not enumerated, and that there never will be a distinction between what is truly national and what is truly local. This we are unwilling to do.

.   .   .   .   .

In its 1999–2000 term, the Supreme Court revisited the Commerce Clause in *United States v. Morrison,* 529 U.S. 598 (2000). At issue was the private civil rights remedy created by the Violence against Women Act of 1994, which allowed survivors to bring federal lawsuits against perpetrators of gender-motivated crimes of violence. Congress proclaimed that violence against women impairs women's ability to work, harms businesses, and increases national health care costs. But the Court, reiterating its arguments made in *Lopez,* found no national effects of violence against women and struck down the law for exceeding Congress's authority under the Commerce Clause.

Lopez and *Morrison* suggest that the Supreme Court is fully prepared to narrow the scope of the federal commerce power to protect a sphere of state sovereignty. In those cases, the effect was to strike down progressive federal safety regulation relating to guns in schools and violence against women. In *Gonzales v. Raich,* however, the Court said that *Lopez* and *Morrison* should not be read too broadly. The Court held that federal law enforcement authorities could criminally prosecute patients for possessing marijuana prescribed by a physician in accordance with state law. Justice John Paul Stevens said that Congress's authority to regulate interstate commerce includes the power to prohibit purely local cultivation and use of marijuana. He found "striking similarities" between this case and *Wickard v. Filburn*, 317 U.S. 111 (1942), a case that upheld a federal prohibition on a farmer growing wheat for his own consumption: "Like the farmer in *Wickard*, respondents are cultivating, for home consumption, a fungible commodity for which there is an established, albeit illegal, interstate market." The 6–3 decision in *Raich* revealed a fissure within the coalition on the Court that over the past decade has curtailed federal power and safeguarded state sovereignty.

GONZALES V. RAICH*
Supreme Court of the United States
June 6, 2005

Justice STEVENS delivered the opinion of the Court.
. . . The question presented in this case is whether the power vested in Congress by Article I, § 8, of the Constitution "[t]o make all Laws which shall be necessary and proper for carrying into Execution" its authority to "regulate Commerce with foreign Nations, and among the several States" includes the power to prohibit the local cultivation and use of marijuana in compliance with California law.
. . . In 1996, California voters passed Proposition 215, now codified as the Compassionate Use Act of 1996. The proposition was designed to ensure that "seriously ill" residents of the State have access to marijuana for medical purposes, and to encourage Federal and State Governments to take steps toward ensuring the safe and affordable distribution of the drug to patients in need. The Act creates an exemption from criminal prosecution for physicians, as well as for patients and primary caregivers who possess or cultivate marijuana for medicinal purposes with the recommendation or approval of a physician. . . .
Respondents Angel Raich and Diane Monson are California residents who suffer from a variety of serious medical conditions and have sought to avail themselves of medical marijuana pursuant to the terms of the Compassionate Use Act. . . .
On August 15, 2002, county deputy sheriffs and agents from the federal Drug Enforcement Administration (DEA) came to Monson's home. After a thorough investigation, the county officials concluded that her use of marijuana was entirely lawful as a matter of California law. Nevertheless, after a 3-hour standoff, the federal agents seized and destroyed all six of her cannabis plants. . . .
[Respondents brought an action against the attorney general. After the District Court denied the respondent's motion for a preliminary injunction, the Ninth Circuit Court of Appeals reversed, finding that the federal Controlled Substances Act (CSA)

*545 U.S. 1 (2005).

to be "an unconstitutional exercise of Congress' Commerce Clause Authority."] The Court of Appeals distinguished prior Circuit cases upholding the CSA in the face of Commerce Clause challenges by focusing on what it deemed to be the "*separate and distinct class of activities*" at issue in this case: "the intrastate, noncommercial cultivation and possession of cannabis for personal medical purposes as recommended by a patient's physician pursuant to valid California state law." [The Court of Appeals distinguished this class of activities from the illicit drug market because the marijuana does not enter the stream of commerce.]

The obvious importance of the case prompted our grant of certiorari. The case is made difficult by respondents' strong arguments that they will suffer irreparable harm because, despite a congressional finding to the contrary, marijuana does have valid therapeutic purposes. The question before us, however, is not whether it is wise to enforce the statute in these circumstances; rather, it is whether Congress' power to regulate interstate markets for medicinal substances encompasses the portions of those markets that are supplied with drugs produced and consumed locally. Well-settled law controls our answer. The CSA is a valid exercise of federal power, even as applied to the troubling facts of this case. We accordingly vacate the judgment of the Court of Appeals. . . .

[Under the CSA, marijuana is listed as a Schedule I drug, characterized by a high potential for abuse and a lack of any accepted medical use.] By classifying marijuana as a Schedule I drug, as opposed to listing it on a lesser schedule, the manufacture, distribution, or possession of marijuana became a criminal offense, with the sole exception being use of the drug as part of a Food and Drug Administration preapproved research study. . . .

Respondents in this case do not dispute that passage of the CSA, as part of the Comprehensive Drug Abuse Prevention and Control Act, was well within Congress' commerce power. Nor do they contend that any provision or section of the CSA amounts to an unconstitutional exercise of congressional authority. Rather, respondents' challenge is actually quite limited; they argue that the CSA's categorical prohibition of the manufacture and possession of marijuana as applied to the intrastate manufacture and possession of marijuana for medical purposes pursuant to California law exceeds Congress' authority under the Commerce Clause. . . .

[There are] three general categories of regulation in which Congress is authorized to engage under its commerce power. First, Congress can regulate the channels of interstate commerce. Second, Congress has authority to regulate and protect the instrumentalities of interstate commerce, and persons or things in interstate commerce. Third, Congress has the power to regulate activities that substantially affect interstate commerce. Only the third category is implicated in the case at hand. . . .

[In *Wickard v. Filburn*, 317 U.S. 111 (1942), the Court upheld the Agricultural Adjustment Act of 1938, a Depression-era law that sought to stabilize the grain supply and prices by, among other things, prescribing how much wheat a farmer could grow. The Court found that the act was a valid exercise of the Commerce Clause even where it was applied to a farmer who was growing wheat for his personal use and not for sale in the market:] "That [the farmer's] own contribution to the demand for wheat may be trivial by itself is not enough to remove him from the scope of federal regulation where, as here, his contribution, taken together with that of many others similarly situated, is far from trivial." *Wickard*, 317 U.S., at 127-28. *Wickard* thus establishes that Congress can regulate purely intrastate activity that is not itself "commercial," in that it is not produced for sale, if it concludes that failure to regulate that class of activity would undercut the regulation of the interstate market in that commodity.

The similarities between this case and *Wickard* are striking. Like the farmer in *Wickard,* respondents are cultivating, for home consumption, a fungible commodity for which there is an established, albeit illegal, interstate market. Just as the Agricultural Adjustment Act was designed "to control the volume [of wheat] moving in interstate and foreign commerce in order to avoid surpluses . . . " and consequently control the market price, a primary purpose of the CSA is to control the supply and demand of controlled substances in both lawful and unlawful drug markets. In *Wickard* we had no difficulty concluding that Congress had a rational basis for believing that, when viewed in the aggregate, leaving home-consumed wheat outside the regulatory scheme would have a substantial influence on price and market conditions. Here too, Congress had a rational basis for concluding that leaving home-consumed marijuana outside federal control would similarly affect price and market conditions. . . .

. . . We need not determine whether respondents' activities, taken in the aggregate, substantially affect interstate commerce in fact, but only whether a "rational basis" exists for so concluding. Given the enforcement difficulties that attend distinguishing between marijuana cultivated locally and marijuana grown elsewhere and concerns about diversion into illicit channels, we have no difficulty concluding that Congress had a rational basis for believing that failure to regulate the intrastate manufacture and possession of marijuana would leave a gaping hole in the CSA. Thus, as in *Wickard* when it enacted comprehensive legislation to regulate the interstate market in a fungible commodity, Congress was acting well within its authority to "make all Laws which shall be necessary and proper" to "regulate Commerce . . . among the several States." U.S. Const., Art. I, § 8. That the regulation ensnares some purely intrastate activity is of no moment. As we have done many times before, we refuse to excise individual components of that larger scheme.

To support their contrary submission, respondents rely heavily on two of our more recent Commerce Clause cases. In their myopic focus, they overlook the larger context of modern-era Commerce Clause jurisprudence preserved by those cases. Moreover, even in the narrow prism of respondents' creation, they read those cases far too broadly.

Those two cases, of course, are *Lopez* and *Morrison.* As an initial matter, the statutory challenges at issue in those cases were markedly different from the challenge respondents pursue in the case at hand. Here, respondents ask us to excise individual applications of a concededly valid statutory scheme. In contrast, in both *Lopez* and *Morrison,* the parties asserted that a particular statute or provision fell outside Congress' commerce power in its entirety. This distinction is pivotal for we have often reiterated that "[w]here the class of activities is regulated and that class is within the reach of federal power, the courts have no power 'to excise, as trivial, individual instances' of the class." *Perez* v. *United States,* 402 U.S., 146, 154 (1971) (emphasis deleted) (quoting *Maryland v. Wirtz,* 392 U.S., 183, 193 [1968]).

At issue in *Lopez* was the validity of the Gun-Free School Zones Act of 1990, which was a brief, single-subject statute making it a crime for an individual to possess a gun in a school zone. The Act did not regulate any economic activity and did not contain any requirement that the possession of a gun have any connection to past interstate activity or a predictable impact on future commercial activity. Distinguishing our earlier cases holding that comprehensive regulatory statutes may be validly applied to local conduct that does not, when viewed in isolation, have a significant impact on interstate commerce, we held the statute invalid. . . .

The statutory scheme that the Government is defending in this litigation is at the opposite end of the regulatory spectrum [from *Lopez*]. . . . The CSA . . . was a lengthy and detailed statute creating a comprehensive framework for regulating the production, distribution, and possession of five classes of "controlled substances." [It established this "closed regulatory system" in order to accomplish Congress's main objectives—conquering drug abuse and controlling the legitimate and illegitimate traffic in controlled substances. Congress was particularly concerned with preventing the diversion of drugs from legitimate to illicit channels.]

[Similarly, the Court's holding in *Morrison* does not cast doubt on the validity of such a comprehensive regulatory scheme. There the decision rested on the fact that while gender-motivated crimes have an effect on interstate commerce, the statute did not regulate economic activity.]

Unlike those at issue in *Lopez* and *Morrison,* the activities regulated by the CSA are quintessentially economic. . . . The CSA is a statute that regulates the production, distribution, and consumption of commodities for which there is an established, and lucrative, interstate market. Prohibiting the intrastate possession or manufacture of an article of commerce is a rational (and commonly utilized) means of regulating commerce in that product. . . . Because the CSA is a statute that directly regulates economic, commercial activity, our opinion in *Morrison* casts no doubt on its constitutionality. . . .

Indeed, that the California exemptions will have a significant impact on both the supply and demand sides of the market for marijuana is not just "plausible" as the principal dissent concedes, it is readily apparent. The exemption for physicians provides them with an economic incentive to grant their patients permission to use the drug. . . .

The exemption for cultivation by patients and caregivers can only increase the supply of marijuana in the California market. The likelihood that all such production will promptly terminate when patients recover or will precisely match the patients' medical needs during their convalescence seems remote; whereas the danger that excesses will satisfy some of the admittedly enormous demand for recreational use seems obvious. Moreover, that the national and international narcotics trade has thrived in the face of vigorous criminal enforcement efforts suggests that no small number of unscrupulous people will make use of the California exemptions to serve their commercial ends whenever it is feasible to do so. . . .

So, from the "separate and distinct" class of activities identified by the Court of Appeals (and adopted by the dissenters), we are left with "the intrastate, noncommercial cultivation, possession and use of marijuana." Thus the case for the exemption comes down to the claim that a locally cultivated product that is used domestically rather than sold on the open market is not subject to federal regulation. Given the findings in the CSA and the undisputed magnitude of the commercial market for marijuana, our decisions in *Wickard v. Filburn* and the later cases endorsing its reasoning foreclose that claim. . . .

[The judgment of the Court of Appeals is vacated.]

V. NEW FEDERALISM AND THE PUBLIC'S HEALTH

As explained at the beginning of this chapter, public health functions are carried out at multiple levels of government (federal, state, tribal, and local). Some of the most significant, and politically controversial, disputes occur when governments at each of these levels lay claim to particular public health issues. In divisive areas such as gun control, smoking, and the environment, the federal government may choose to act. It is in this context that the Supreme Court may have to decide whether national public health regulations invade a sphere of state sovereignty.

"New federalism" is a principle of political change, spurred by conservative activism, that limits federal authority and returns power to the states. New federalism has taken on significant political importance in public health in the contentious debates over which level of government should set standards, as well as perform and pay for services. The Supreme Court altered the balance between the supremacy of federal law and the separate sovereignty of the states in *Lopez* and *Morrison,* but its decision in *Raich* may signal a retreat from strong federalism.

This section discusses an additional constitutional issue in American federalism: Congress's power to require state governments to implement federal standards. The Supreme Court's federalism jurisprudence has extended beyond the Commerce Clause. The Court has held that Congress cannot directly coerce states to comply with federal regulatory standards, even when it is acting validly within the commerce power. In *New York v. United States* (excerpted below), a federal program regulating radioactive waste removal was held to be unconstitutional because it "commandeered" state governments to implement federal programs in violation of the Tenth Amendment. The Court held that the federal government cannot coerce state legislatures to act according to federal standards.

Five years after *New York,* in *Printz v. United States,* 521 U.S. 898 (1997), the Supreme Court used the same reasoning to strike down provisions of the Brady Handgun Violence Prevention Act directing state and local law enforcement officers to conduct background checks on prospective handgun purchasers. Justice Scalia referred to the "dual sovereignty" established by the Constitution that is the foundation of federalism. His opinion states that the Framers designed the Constitution to allow federal regulation of the people, not the states.

NEW YORK V. UNITED STATES*
Supreme Court of the United States
Decided June 19, 1992

Justice O'CONNOR delivered the opinion of the Court.

[In 1985, Congress enacted the Low Level Radioactive Waste Policy Amendments Act of 1985 (the "Act") amid fears that the nation would be left without any disposal sites for low-level radioactive waste. The Act was intended to encourage states to establish and operate disposal facilities for low-level radioactive waste over the next several years, acting either by themselves or with other states in regional compacts. The Act obligated states to provide for disposal of waste produced within each state's borders, and it provided three types of incentives to encourage compliance. The first were monetary incentives, the second were access incentives, and the final "incentives" were a take title provision. The take title provision mandates that if a state is not able to provide for the disposal of waste generated within its borders, it is obligated, upon request of the generator of the waste, to take possession of that waste. Should the state fail to take possession, it will be liable for all damages incurred by the waste generator as a result. Petitioner, the State of New York, claimed that the Act is inconsistent with the Tenth Amendment.]

These cases implicate one of our Nation's newest problems of public policy and perhaps our oldest question of constitutional law. The public policy issue involves the disposal of radioactive waste.... The constitutional question is as old as the Constitution: It consists of discerning the proper division of authority between the Federal Government and the States. We conclude that while Congress has substantial power under the Constitution to encourage the States to provide for the disposal of the radioactive waste generated within their borders, the Constitution does not confer upon Congress the ability simply to compel the States to do so. We therefore find that only two of the Act's three provisions at issue are consistent with the Constitution's allocation of power to the Federal Government....

... If a power is delegated to Congress in the Constitution, the Tenth Amendment expressly disclaims any reservation of that power to the States; if a power is an attribute of state sovereignty reserved by the Tenth Amendment, it is necessarily a power the Constitution has not conferred on Congress....

... The Tenth Amendment confirms that the power of the Federal Government is subject to limits that may, in a given instance, reserve power to the States. The Tenth Amendment thus directs us to determine, as in this case, whether an incident of state sovereignty is protected by a limitation on an Article I power....

Petitioners do not contend that Congress lacks the power to regulate the disposal of low level radioactive waste.... Petitioners contend only that the Tenth Amendment limits the power of Congress to regulate in the way it has chosen. Rather than addressing the problem of waste disposal by directly regulating the generators and disposers of waste, petitioners argue, Congress has impermissibly directed the States to regulate in this field....

*505 U.S. 144 (1992).

As an initial matter, Congress may not simply "commandeer the legislative processes of the States by directly compelling them to enact and enforce a federal regulatory program." *Hodel v. Virginia Surface Mining & Reclamation Ass'n, Inc.*, 452 U.S. 264, 288 (1981). . . . While Congress has substantial powers to govern the Nation directly, including in areas of intimate concern to the States, the Constitution has never been understood to confer upon Congress the ability to require the States to govern according to Congress's instructions. . . .

In providing for a stronger central government, the Framers explicitly chose a Constitution that confers upon Congress the power to regulate individuals, not States. As we have seen, the Court has consistently respected this choice. We have always understood that even where Congress has the authority under the Constitution to pass laws requiring or prohibiting certain acts, it lacks the power directly to compel the States to require or prohibit those acts.

This is not to say that Congress lacks the ability to encourage a State to regulate in a particular way, or that Congress may not hold out incentives to the States as a method of influencing a State's policy choices. Our cases have identified a variety of methods, short of outright coercion, by which Congress may urge a State to adopt a legislative program consistent with federal interests. Two of these methods are of particular relevance here.

First, under Congress's spending power, "Congress may attach conditions on the receipt of federal funds." *South Dakota v. Dole*, 483 U.S., 203, 206 (1987). Such conditions must (among other requirements) bear some relationship to the purpose of the federal spending; otherwise, of course, the spending power could render academic the Constitution's other grants and limits of federal authority. Where the recipient of federal funds is a State, as is not unusual today, the conditions attached to the funds by Congress may influence a State's legislative choices. . . .

Second, where Congress has the authority to regulate private activity under the Commerce Clause, we have recognized Congress's power to offer States the choice of regulating that activity according to federal standards or having state law pre-empted by federal regulation. . . .

By either of these methods, as by any other permissible method of encouraging a State to conform to federal policy choices, the residents of the State retain the ultimate decision as to whether or not the State will comply. If a State's citizens view federal policy as sufficiently contrary to local interests, they may elect to decline a federal grant. If state residents would prefer their government to devote its attention and resources to problems other than those deemed important by Congress, they may choose to have the Federal Government rather than the State bear the expense of a federally mandated regulatory program, and they may continue to supplement that program to the extent state law is not pre-empted. Where Congress encourages state regulation rather than compelling it, state governments remain responsive to the local electorate's preferences; state officials remain accountable to the people.

By contrast, where the Federal Government compels States to regulate, the accountability of both state and federal officials is diminished. If the citizens of New York, for example, do not consider that making provision for the disposal of radioactive waste is in their best interest, they may elect state officials who share their view. That view can always be pre-empted under the Supremacy Clause if it is contrary to the national view, but in such a case it is the Federal Government that makes the decision in full view of the public, and it will be federal officials that suffer the consequences if the decision turns out to be detrimental or unpopular. But where the Federal Government directs the States to regulate, it may be state officials who will bear the brunt of public disapproval, while the federal officials who devised the regulatory program may remain insulated from the electoral ramifications of their decision. Accountability is thus diminished when, due to federal coercion, elected state officials cannot regulate in accordance with the views of the local electorate in matters not pre-empted by federal regulation. . . .

[The Court upholds the first two sets of incentives under the commerce and spending powers.] The take title provision is of a different character. This third so-called "incentive" offers States, as an alternative to regulating pursuant to Congress's direction, the option of taking title to and possession of the low level radioactive waste generated within their borders and becoming liable for all damages waste generators suffer as a result of the States' failure to do so promptly. In this provision, Congress has crossed the line distinguishing encouragement from coercion. . . . The take title provision offers state governments a "choice" of either accepting ownership of waste or regulating according to the instructions of Congress. . . .

Because an instruction to state governments to take title to waste, standing alone, would be beyond the authority of Congress, and because a direct order to regulate, standing alone, would also be beyond the authority of Congress, it follows that Congress lacks the power to offer the States a choice between the two. Unlike the first two sets of incentives, the take title incentive does not represent the conditional exercise of any congressional power enumerated in the Constitution. In this provision, Congress has not held out the threat of exercising its spending power or its commerce power; it has instead held out the threat, should the States not regulate according to one federal instruction, of simply forcing the States to submit to another federal instruction. A choice between two unconstitutionally coercive regulatory techniques is no choice at all. Either way, "the Act commandeers the legislative processes of the States by directly compelling them to enact and enforce a federal regulatory program," *Hodel,* 452 U.S. at 288, an outcome that has never been understood to lie within the authority conferred upon Congress by the Constitution. . . .

The take title provision appears to be unique. No other federal statute has been cited which offers a state government no option other than that of implementing legislation enacted by Congress. Whether one views the take title provision as lying outside Congress's enumerated powers, or as infringing upon the core of state sovereignty reserved by the Tenth Amendment, the provision is inconsistent with the federal structure of our Government established by the Constitution. . . .

. . . Respondents . . . observe that public officials representing the State of New York lent their support to the Act's enactment. . . . [and] then pose what appears at first to be a troubling question: How can a federal statute be found an unconstitutional infringement of state sovereignty when state officials consented to the statute's enactment?

The answer follows from an understanding of the fundamental purpose served by our Government's federal structure. The Constitution does not protect the sover-

eignty of States for the benefit of the States or state governments as abstract political entities, or even for the benefit of the public officials governing the States. To the
contrary, the Constitution divides authority between federal and state governments
for the protection of individuals. . . .

State officials thus cannot consent to the enlargement of the powers of Congress
beyond those enumerated in the Constitution. Indeed, the facts of these cases raise
the possibility that powerful incentives might lead both federal and state officials to
view departures from the federal structure to be·in their personal interests. Most
citizens recognize the need for radioactive waste disposal sites, but few want sites
near their homes. As a result, while it would be well within the authority of either
federal or state officials to choose where the disposal sites will be, it is likely to be
in the political interest of each individual official to avoid being held accountable to
the voters for the choice of location. If a federal official is faced with the alternatives of choosing a location or directing the States to do it, the official may well
prefer the latter, as a means of shifting responsibility for the eventual decision. If a
state official is faced with the same set of alternatives—choosing a location or having
Congress direct the choice of a location—the state official may also prefer the latter,
as it may permit the avoidance of personal responsibility. The interests of public
officials thus may not coincide with the Constitution's intergovernmental allocation
of authority. Where state officials purport to submit to the direction of Congress in
this manner, federalism is hardly being advanced.

.   .   .   .   .   .

The readings in this chapter illustrate the complexity of constitutional
law in creating government powers and duties to preserve the public's
health and safety. Generally speaking, the Supreme Court sees few
affirmative obligations, but does permit wide-ranging powers to act
for the common good. The federal government possesses enumerated
powers that enable it to regulate in virtually all areas of public health.
The states retain the police powers that provide inherent authority to
safeguard the health, safety, and morals of the community. Perhaps
the most divisive issues in constitutional law involve matters of federalism. In recent years, the Court has shifted the balance of power,
denying the national government the authority to invade a sphere of
state sovereignty.

As a society, we have to seriously consider the competing claims of
the national and state governments in matters of public health. If the
states refuse to deal effectively with contentious public health issues
such as gun control, violence against women, or tobacco, will the
courts allow the federal government to intervene?

Another matter has preoccupied and divided the country every bit
as much as American federalism: the claim of government to act for the

welfare of the population and the countervailing claim of individuals to be free from government interference. The Constitution, of course, has a great deal to say about the competing interests of communal goods and individual rights. That is the topic of the next chapter.

RECOMMENDED READINGS

American Federalism: The Antiregulatory Effects of Federal Preemption

Parmet, Wendy E. 1992. Health care and the Constitution: Public health and the role of the state in the Framing Era. *Hastings Constitutional Law Quarterly* 20: 267–335. (Discusses the historical view of government's duty to protect the population from epidemics)

Sharkey, Catherine M. 2007. Federalism in action: FDA regulatory preemption in pharmaceutical cases in state versus federal courts. *Brooklyn Journal of Law and Policy* 15: 1013–48. (Discusses the differing approaches of state and federal courts in deciding whether the Federal Food, Drug, and Cosmetic Act [FDCA] preempts state claims against pharmaceutical companies)

The Negative Constitution: Government's Duty to Protect Health and Safety

Seidman, Louis Michael, and Mark V. Tushnet. 1996. *Remnants of Belief: Contemporary Constitutional Issues.* New York: Oxford Univ. Press. (Argues that historically it has been the responsibility of the states to take care of population health)

State Police Powers: Protecting Health, Safety, and Morals

Legarre, Santiago. 2007. The historical background of the police power. *University of Pennsylvania Journal of Constitutional Law* 9: 745–96. (Explains the meanings of the term "police power" and its historical usage as a broad and narrow term)

Federal Power to Safeguard the Public's Health

Hodge, James G., Jr. 1997. Implementing modern public health goals through government: An examination of new federalism and public health law. *Journal of Contemporary Health Law and Policy* 14: 93–126. (Discusses the impact of new federalism and its impact on public health)

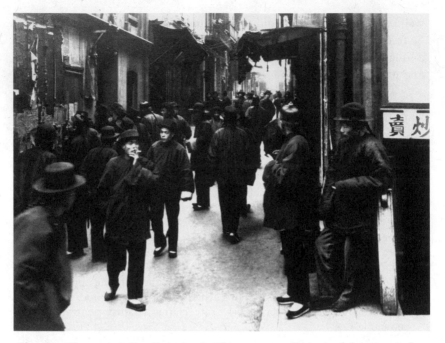

Photo 7. The scene is San Francisco's Chinatown at the turn of the twentieth century. In 1900, the city quarantined a twelve-block area of that neighborhood, targeting Chinese homes and businesses for enforcement. In *Jew Ho v. Williamson*, 103 F. 10 (C.C.N.D. Cal. 1900), the Circuit Court for the Northern District of California held that selective enforcement of a valid quarantine violated the constitutional guarantee of equal protection of the laws. Reproduced by permission, © Corbis, ca. 1900.

FOUR

Public Health and the Protection of Individual Rights

Government has a long tradition of regulating for the community's welfare. Regulations target individuals (e.g., setting forth infectious disease powers), professionals and institutions (e.g., requiring licenses), and businesses (e.g., mandating inspections and safety standards). The previous chapter emphasized the broad *powers and duties* of government to safeguard the public's health. This chapter considers the *restraints* on government power that protect individual interests in autonomy, privacy, liberty, and property.

The cases and commentary in this chapter trace the evolution in judicial thought on the balance between public health power and protection of individual rights. Public health jurisprudence is neither static nor immune from political and social influences. Rather, judicial review of public health interventions has changed over time with the varying composition of the Supreme Court. These changes, moreover, often reflect prevailing social and political thought. The Warren Court's defense of personal freedom and nondiscrimination can be traced to the civil rights movements for African Americans and women during the 1960s. Decisions by the Rehnquist Court favoring federalism were influenced by a predisposition toward states' rights and against large central government. And a pro-business, antiregulatory environment appears to be shaping the Roberts Court.

Several different meanings may be attributed to constitutional

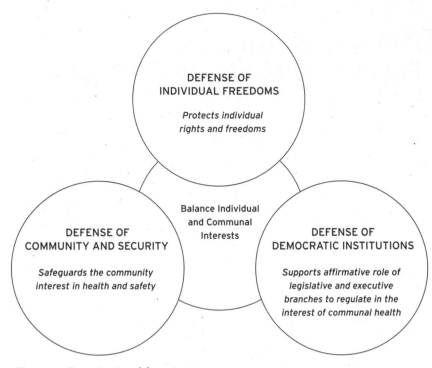

Figure 5. Constitutional functions.

adjudication (see figure 5). The primary role of the Constitution may be seen as defending freedom, defending community and security, or defending democratic institutions. It is possible to perceive the various phases of Supreme Court decision making as in turn vindicating, or repudiating, each of these values. But judges often reject these political explanations, claiming simply that they objectively read the text and history of the Constitution. In the eyes of these jurists, their primary task is to discover the original intent of the Framers or to neutrally construe the language of the Constitution.

The Constitution's primary purpose is often seen as the protection of individual rights against excessive government interference. According to this view, people are born free with inalienable rights to liberty and property that can be impeded by the government only if the justification is highly persuasive. This perspective restrains public health power. It assumes that one value—freedom—ought to prevail over other values, including health and security, except in unusual cases. Courts that adhere to this view scrutinize the exercise of public health powers more closely. Public health officials, knowing that they are subject to intense scrutiny, may be reluctant to use power aggressively. The result may be firm protection of individual rights but diminished protection of the community's health and safety.

Others perceive the Constitution's primary purpose as the defense of common goods. According to this view, the principal purpose of government is to safeguard communal interests in health and security, even at the expense of individual interests. This perspective affords public health officials the most extensive and flexible authority. It assumes that the exercise of public health powers is legitimate unless they further an insubstantial purpose or unjustifiably trample individual rights. Courts that adhere to this view adopt a low level of constitutional scrutiny, encouraging public health officials to employ a broad range of powers.

Finally, some perceive the Constitution's primary purpose as the defense of democratic institutions. According to this view, the formulation and enforcement of policy are left largely to the political branches of government. It assumes that public health powers involve highly complex policy choices that are best made by lawmakers and agency officials. Not only do these branches have greater policy expertise, they are also politically accountable. If the electorate is displeased with the decision of a legislator or public health official, the ballot box can usually provide a remedy. If the public is displeased with a court's decision involving a constitutional principle, the electoral remedy is not as clear. Courts that adhere to this view are deferential to legislatures and executive agencies, giving them wide latitude in formulating and executing public health policy (see box 2).

Whatever view one takes about judicial review, it is helpful to underscore the exceptional power of public health officials. Few actors in the American system of government exercise such broad discretionary powers and enjoy such a high level of respect and deference. This public trust should vest a responsibility in public health officials to exercise their powers wisely and justly.

This chapter contains two sections—one focusing on early limits on the exercise of police powers, and the other on modern limits. Both are important, providing a sense of history and tradition as well as articulating judicial principles on the rightful exercise of public health authority.

BOX 2

The courts have a long tradition of deferring to legislatures and agencies, believing that elected officials have greater policy expertise and are democratically accountable to voters. Such deference is particularly common when officials allocate scarce resources, such as access to experimental medicines. In the highly controversial case of *Abigail Alliance v. Von Eschenbach*, 495 F.3d 695 (D.C. Cir. 2007), *cert. denied*, 128 S. Ct. 1069 (2008), the United States Court of Appeals for the D.C. Circuit examined whether terminally ill patients have a constitutional right to investigational drugs—that is, drugs under study but not yet approved for public use by the FDA—regardless of the drugs' potential lifesaving properties.

The case has been characterized as capturing a "microcosm of contemporary health policy tensions, [raising] challenging issues regarding drug safety at the limits of scientific knowledge, the role of markets vs regulators, medical care of terminally ill patients, individual rights vs protection of public health, and the allocation of scarce resources" (Jacobson and Parmet 2007, 206). Initially, a panel of the circuit court concluded that when no alternative government-approved treatment options exist, a terminally ill, mentally competent adult patient has a substantive due process right of access to potentially lifesaving investigational drugs that have been found, on the basis of Phase 1 trials, to be sufficiently safe for expanded human trials (445 F.3d 470 [D.C. Cir. 2006]). The case was then reheard by the entire circuit court, which vacated the panel's decision, concluding that terminal patients do not have a fundamental right to access such drugs. The court, citing *Jacobson v. Massachusetts*, stressed the prerogatives of the legislature and agency:

> Although in the Alliance's view the FDA has unjustly erred on the side of safety in balancing the risks and benefits of experimental drugs, this is not to say that the FDA's balance can never be changed. The Alliance's arguments about morality, quality of life, and acceptable levels of medical risk are certainly ones that can be aired in the democratic branches, without injecting the courts into unknown questions of science and medicine. Our Nation's history and traditions have consistently demonstrated that the democratic branches are better suited to decide the proper balance between the uncertain risks and benefits of medical technology, and are entitled to deference in doing so. As the Supreme Court [held in *Jacobson*]: "We must assume that, when the statute in question was passed, the legislature . . . was not unaware of these opposing theories, and was compelled, of necessity,

to choose between them. It was not compelled to commit a matter involving the public health and safety to the final decision of a court or jury. It is no part of the function of a court or a jury to determine which one of two modes was likely to be the most effective for the protection of the public health against disease."

Consistent with that precedent, our holding today ensures that this debate among the Alliance, the FDA, the scientific and medical communities, and the public may continue through the democratic process.

I. EARLY TWENTIETH-CENTURY LIMITS ON THE POLICE POWER

This section on historical limits on police powers features two classic public health cases from the early twentieth century, *Jacobson v. Massachusetts* and *Jew Ho v. Williamson*. The story of public health law often begins with the refusal of Henning Jacobson to comply with an early twentieth-century Cambridge, Massachusetts, ordinance compelling smallpox vaccination. The resulting case is perhaps the most important Supreme Court opinion in the history of American public health law. In an article marking the centenary of *Jacobson v. Massachusetts,* the public health lawyers and scholars Wendy Parmet, Richard Goodman, and Amy Farber (2005, 653–54) shed light on its historical background:

By 1902, vaccination was well established in Massachusetts. Nevertheless, smallpox remained a persistent visitor: in 1900, more than 100 cases were reported in the state; in 1901, there were 773 cases and 97 deaths, and in 1902, 2,314 cases and 284 deaths.

In response, local public health officials resorted to a variety of measures, many of which were scientifically sound but not all of which were apt to inspire public trust. For example, on March 15, 1902, Boston public health doctors, accompanied by guards, descended on the railroad yards and forcibly vaccinated "Italians, negroes and other employees." In nearby Cambridge, a heated political battle brewed over the mayor's nominations for the board of health. It was in this contentious climate, in which politicians and public health officials debated and vulnerable groups were targeted, that [Reverend Henning] Jacobson and at least three others . . . refused to be vaccinated and were prosecuted.

At the time, vaccination was highly regarded in the medical community. Nevertheless, opposition to it was widespread and long-standing. "Antivaccinationism" had many roots, including religious beliefs and concern about civil liberties, as well as skepticism about medicine. . . .

. . . Born in Yllestad, Sweden, in 1856, Jacobson immigrated to the United States in 1870. . . . Known as a charismatic preacher and a community leader, Jacobson practiced a form of pietism in which spirituality was infused into everyday life. That pietism probably influenced his resistance to vaccination. His status as an immigrant and as a member of a minority religion may also have widened the gulf between him and the Cambridge Board of Health. . . .

As we consider public health interventions today . . . we would do well to recall *Jacobson*. Although much has changed in the past century, many of the conflicts and tensions involved in the case remain unresolved. We continue to debate the relationship between liberty and public health. Like vaccination laws, isolation or quarantines imposed for communicable diseases and laws about reporting sexually transmitted diseases rely on the state police power affirmed in *Jacobson*. Each such legal measure limits the rights of individuals in the name of public health, and each is widely accepted as an important tool by the public health community.

JACOBSON V. MASSACHUSETTS*
Supreme Court of the United States
Decided February 20, 1905

Justice HARLAN delivered the opinion of the Court.

[The board of health of the City of Cambridge, pursuant to a Massachusetts statute, adopted an ordinance providing for mandatory vaccination for smallpox of all city inhabitants over the age of twenty-one who had not been recently vaccinated. The board passed the ordinance to address the growing prevalence of smallpox in the city. The vaccinations were provided to the citizens free of charge. Under the statute, those who did not comply would be subject to a fine of $5. Jacobson refused to be vaccinated, and as a result, he was criminally charged. He alleged that the statute was unconstitutional, arguing, among other things, that it violated the Due Process, Equal Protection, and Privileges and Immunities clauses of the Fourteenth Amendment.]

This case involves the validity, under the Constitution of the United States, of certain provisions in the statutes of Massachusetts relating to vaccination. . . .

The authority of the state to enact this statute is to be referred to what is commonly called the police power—a power which the state did not surrender when becoming a member of the Union under the Constitution. Although this court has refrained from any attempt to define the limits of that power, yet it has distinctly recognized the authority of a state to enact quarantine laws and "health laws of every description" *Gibbons v. Ogden*, 22 U.S. (9 Wheat.) 1, 87 (1824); indeed, all

*197 U.S. 11 (1905).

laws that relate to matters completely within its territory and which do not by their necessary operation affect the people of other states. According to settled principles, the police power of a state must be held to embrace, at least, such reasonable regulations established directly by legislative enactment as will protect the public health and the public safety.... The mode or manner in which those results are to be accomplished is within the discretion of the state, subject, of course, so far as Federal power is concerned, only to the condition that no rule prescribed by a state, nor any regulation adopted by a local governmental agency acting under the sanction of state legislation, shall contravene the Constitution of the United States, nor infringe any right granted or secured by that instrument. A local enactment or regulation, even if based on the acknowledged police powers of a state, must always yield in case of conflict with the exercise by the general government of any power it possesses under the Constitution, or with any right which that instrument gives or secures.

We come, then, to inquire whether any right given or secured by the Constitution is invaded by the statute as interpreted by the state court. The defendant insists that his liberty is invaded when the state subjects him to fine or imprisonment for neglecting or refusing to submit to vaccination; that a compulsory vaccination law is unreasonable, arbitrary, and oppressive, and, therefore, hostile to the inherent right of every freeman to care for his own body and health in such way as to him seems best; and that the execution of such a law against one who objects to vaccination, no matter for what reason, is nothing short of an assault upon his person. But the liberty secured by the Constitution of the United States to every person within its jurisdiction does not import an absolute right in each person to be, at all times and in all circumstances, wholly freed from restraint. There are manifold restraints to which every person is necessarily subject for the common good.... Real liberty for all could not exist under the operation of a principle which recognizes the right of each individual person to use his own, whether in respect of his person or his property, regardless of the injury that may be done to others. This court has more than once recognized it as a fundamental principle that "persons and property are subjected to all kinds of restraints and burdens in order to secure the general comfort, health, and prosperity of the state; of the perfect right of the legislature to do which no question ever was, or upon acknowledged general principles ever can be, made, so far as natural persons are concerned." *Hannibal & St. J.R. Co. v. Husen,* 95 U.S. 465, 471 (1877). In *Crowley v. Christensen,* 137 U.S. 86, 89 (1890), we said: "The possession and enjoyment of all rights are subject to such reasonable conditions as may be deemed by the governing authority of the country essential to the safety, health, peace, good order, and morals of the community. Even liberty itself, the greatest of all rights, is not unrestricted license to act according to one's own will. It is only freedom from restraint under conditions essential to the equal enjoyment of the same right by others. It is, then, liberty regulated by law." In the Constitution of Massachusetts adopted in 1780 it was laid down as a fundamental principle of the social compact that the whole people covenants with each citizen, and each citizen with the whole people, that all shall be governed by certain laws for "the common good," and that government is instituted "for the common good, for the protection, safety, prosperity, and happiness of the people, and not for the profit, honor, or private interests of any one man, family, or class of men." The good and welfare of the commonwealth, of which the legislature is primarily the judge, is the basis on which the police power rests in Massachusetts.

Applying these principles to the present case, it is to be observed that the legislature of Massachusetts required the inhabitants of a city or town to be vaccinated only when, in the opinion of the board of health, that was necessary for the public health or the public safety. The authority to determine for all what ought to be done in such an emergency must have been lodged somewhere or in some body; and surely it was appropriate for the legislature to refer that question, in the first instance, to a board of health composed of persons residing in the locality affected, and appointed, presumably, because of their fitness to determine such questions. To invest such a body with authority over such matters was not an unusual, nor an unreasonable or arbitrary, requirement. Upon the principle of self-defense, of paramount necessity, a community has the right to protect itself against an epidemic of disease which threatens the safety of its members. It is to be observed that when the regulation in question was adopted smallpox, according to the recitals in the regulation adopted by the board of health, was prevalent to some extent in the city of Cambridge, and the disease was increasing. If such was the situation,—and nothing is asserted or appears in the record to the contrary,—if we are to attach any value whatever to the knowledge which, it is safe to affirm, is common to all civilized peoples touching smallpox and the methods most usually employed to eradicate that disease, it cannot be adjudged that the present regulation of the board of health was not necessary in order to protect the public health and secure the public safety. Smallpox being prevalent and increasing at Cambridge, the court would usurp the functions of another branch of government if it adjudged, as matter of law, that the mode adopted under the sanction of the state, to protect the people at large was arbitrary, and not justified by the necessities of the case. We say necessities of the case, because it might be that an acknowledged power of a local community to protect itself against an epidemic threatening the safety of all might be exercised in particular circumstances and in reference to particular persons in such an arbitrary, unreasonable manner, or might go so far beyond what was reasonably required for the safety of the public, as to authorize or compel the courts to interfere for the protection of such persons. . . . If the mode adopted by the commonwealth of Massachusetts for the protection of its local communities against smallpox proved to be distressing, inconvenient, or objectionable to some,—if nothing more could be reasonably affirmed of the statute in question,—the answer is that it was the duty of the constituted authorities primarily to keep in view the welfare, comfort, and safety of the many, and not permit the interests of the many to be subordinated to the wishes or convenience of the few. There is, of course, a sphere within which the individual may assert the supremacy of his own will, and rightfully dispute the authority of any human government,—especially of any free government existing under a written constitution, to interfere with the exercise of that will. But it is equally true that in every well-ordered society charged with the duty of conserving the safety of its members the rights of the individual in respect of his liberty may at times, under the pressure of great dangers, be subjected to such restraint, to be enforced by reasonable regulations, as the safety of the general public may demand. . . . The liberty secured by the 14th Amendment, this court has said, consists, in part, in the right of a person "to live and work where he will" (*Allgeyer v. Louisiana,* 165 U.S. 578 [1897]);

and yet he may be compelled, by force if need be, against his will and without regard to his personal wishes or his pecuniary interests, or even his religious or political convictions, to take his place in the ranks of the army of his country, and risk the chance of being shot down in its defense. It is not, therefore, true that the power of the public to guard itself against imminent danger depends in every case involving the control of one's body upon his willingness to submit to reasonable regulations established by the constituted authorities, under the sanction of the state, for the purpose of protecting the public collectively against such danger.

It is said, however, that the statute, as interpreted by the state court, although making an exception in favor of children certified by a registered physician to be unfit subjects for vaccination, makes no exception in case of adults in like condition. But this cannot be deemed a denial of the equal protection of the laws to adults; for the statute is applicable equally to all in like condition, and there are obviously reasons why regulations may be appropriate for adults which could not be safely applied to persons of tender years.

Looking at the propositions embodied in the defendant's rejected offers of proof, it is clear that they are more formidable by their number than by their inherent value. Those offers in the main seem to have had no purpose except to state the general theory of those of the medical profession who attach little or no value to vaccination as a means of preventing the spread of smallpox, or who think that vaccination causes other diseases of the body. What everybody knows the court must know, and therefore the state court judicially knew, as this court knows, that an opposite theory accords with the common belief, and is maintained by high medical authority. We must assume that, when the statute in question was passed, the legislature of Massachusetts was not unaware of these opposing theories, and was compelled, of necessity, to choose between them. It was not compelled to commit a matter involving the public health and safety to the final decision of a court or jury. It is no part of the function of a court or a jury to determine which one of two modes was likely to be the most effective for the protection of the public against disease. That was for the legislative department to determine in the light of all the information it had or could obtain. It could not properly abdicate its function to guard the public health and safety. The state legislature proceeded upon the theory which recognized vaccination as at least an effective, if not the best-known, way in which to meet and suppress the evils of a smallpox epidemic that imperiled an entire population. Upon what sound principles as to the relations existing between the different departments of government can the court review this action of the legislature? If there is any such power in the judiciary to review legislative action in respect of a matter affecting the general welfare, it can only be when that which the legislature has done comes within the rule that, "if a statute purporting to have been enacted to protect the public health, the public morals, or the public safety has no real or substantial relation to those objects, or is, beyond all question, a plain, palpable invasion of rights secured by the fundamental law, it is the duty of the courts to so adjudge, and thereby give effect to the Constitution." *Mugler v. Kansas,* 123 U.S. 623 (1887).

Whatever may be thought of the expediency of this statute, it cannot be affirmed to be, beyond question, in palpable conflict with the Constitution. Nor, in view of the methods employed to stamp out the disease of smallpox, can anyone confidently assert that the means prescribed by the state to that end has no real or substantial

relation to the protection of the public health and the public safety. Such an assertion would not be consistent with the experience of this and other countries whose
authorities have dealt with the disease of smallpox. And the principle of vaccination
as a means to prevent the spread of smallpox has been enforced in many states by
statutes making the vaccination of children a condition of their right to enter or
remain in public schools.

The latest case upon the subject of which we are aware is *Viemester v. White*, 72
N.E. 97 (N.Y. Ct. App. 1904), decided very recently by the court of appeals of New
York. That case involved the validity of a statute excluding from the public schools
all children who had not been vaccinated. One contention was that the statute and
the regulation adopted in exercise of its provisions was inconsistent with the rights,
privileges, and liberties of the citizen. The contention was overruled, the court saying, among other things: "Smallpox is known of all to be a dangerous and contagious
disease. If vaccination strongly tends to prevent the transmission or spread of this
disease, it logically follows that children may be refused admission to the public
schools until they have been vaccinated. The appellant claims that vaccination does
not tend to prevent smallpox, but tends to bring about other diseases, and that it
does much harm, with no good. It must be conceded that some laymen, both learned
and unlearned, and some physicians of great skill and repute, do not believe that
vaccination is a preventive of smallpox. The common belief, however, is that it has a
decided tendency to prevent the spread of this fearful disease, and to render it less
dangerous to those who contract it. While not accepted by all, it is accepted by the
mass of the people, as well as by most members of the medical profession. It has
been general in our state, and in most civilized nations for generations. It is generally
accepted in theory, and generally applied in practice, both by the voluntary action of
the people, and in obedience to the command of law. Nearly every state in the Union
has statutes to encourage, or directly or indirectly to require, vaccination; and this
is true of most nations of Europe. . . . A common belief, like common knowledge, does
not require evidence to establish its existence, but may be acted upon without proof
by the legislature and the courts. . . . The fact that the belief is not universal is not
controlling, for there is scarcely any belief that is accepted by everyone. The possibility that the belief may be wrong, and that science may yet show it to be wrong,
is not conclusive; for the legislature has the right to pass laws which, according to
the common belief of the people, are adapted to prevent the spread of contagious
diseases. In a free country, where the government is by the people, through their
chosen representatives, practical legislation admits of no other standard of action,
for what the people believe is for the common welfare must be accepted as tending
to promote the common welfare, whether it does in fact or not. Any other basis would
conflict with the spirit of the Constitution, and would sanction measures opposed to
a Republican form of government. While we do not decide, and cannot decide, that
vaccination is a preventive of smallpox, we take judicial notice of the fact that this is
the common belief of the people of the state, and, with this fact as a foundation, we
hold that the statute in question is a health law, enacted in a reasonable and proper
exercise of the police power." 72 N.E. [at 98–99].

Since, then, vaccination, as a means of protecting a community against smallpox,
finds strong support in the experience of this and other countries, no court, much
less a jury, is justified in disregarding the action of the legislature simply because

in its or their opinion that particular method was—perhaps, or possibly—not the best either for children or adults.

Did the offers of proof made by the defendant present a case which entitled him, while remaining in Cambridge, to claim exemption from the operation of the statute and of the regulation adopted by the board of health? We have already said that his rejected offers, in the main, only set forth the theory of those who had no faith in vaccination as a means of preventing the spread of smallpox, or who thought that vaccination, without benefitting the public, put in peril the health of the person vaccinated. But there were some offers which it is contended embodied distinct facts that might properly have been considered. Let us see how this is.

The defendant offered to prove that vaccination "quite often" caused serious and permanent injury to the health of the person vaccinated; that the operation "occasionally" resulted in death; that it was "impossible" to tell "in any particular case" what the results of vaccination would be, or whether it would injure the health or result in death; that "quite often" one's blood is in a certain condition of impurity when it is not prudent or safe to vaccinate him; that there is no practical test by which to determine "with any degree of certainty" whether one's blood is in such condition of impurity as to render vaccination necessarily unsafe or dangerous; that vaccine matter is "quite often" impure and dangerous to be used, but whether impure or not cannot be ascertained by any known practical test; that the defendant refused to submit to vaccination for the reason that he had, "when a child," been caused great and extreme suffering for a long period by a disease produced by vaccination; and that he had witnessed a similar result of vaccination, not only in the case of his son, but in the cases of others.

These offers, in effect, invited the court and jury to go over the whole ground gone over by the legislature when it enacted the statute in question. The legislature assumed that some children, by reason of their condition at the time, might not be fit subjects of vaccination; and it is suggested—and we will not say without reason—that such is the case with some adults. But the defendant did not offer to prove that, by reason of his then condition, he was in fact not a fit subject of vaccination at the time he was informed of the requirement of the regulation adopted by the board of health. It is entirely consistent with his offer of proof that, after reaching full age, he had become, so far as medical skill could discover, and when informed of the regulation of the board of health was, a fit subject of vaccination, and that the vaccine matter to be used in his case was such as any medical practitioner of good standing would regard as proper to be used. The matured opinions of medical men everywhere, and the experience of mankind, as all must know, negative the suggestion that it is not possible in any case to determine whether vaccination is safe. Was defendant exempted from the operation of the statute simply because of his dread of the same evil results experienced by him when a child, and which he had observed in the cases of his son and other children? Could he reasonably claim such an exemption because "quite often," or "occasionally," injury had resulted from vaccination, or because it was impossible, in the opinion of some, by any practical test, to determine with absolute certainty whether a particular person could be safely vaccinated?

It seems to the court that an affirmative answer to these questions would practically strip the legislative department of its function to care for the public health and the public safety when endangered by epidemics of disease. Such an answer would mean that compulsory vaccination could not, in any conceivable case, be legally enforced in a community, even at the command of the legislature, however widespread the epidemic of smallpox, and however deep and universal was the belief of the community and of its medical advisers that a system of general vaccination was vital to the safety of all.

We are not prepared to hold that a minority, residing or remaining in any city or town where smallpox is prevalent, and enjoying the general protection afforded by an organized local government, may thus defy the will of its constituted authorities, acting in good faith for all, under the legislative sanction of the state. If such be the privilege of a minority, then a like privilege would belong to each individual of the community, and the spectacle would be presented of the welfare and safety of an entire population being subordinated to the notions of a single individual who chooses to remain a part of that population. We are unwilling to hold it to be an element in the liberty secured by the Constitution of the United States that one person, or a minority of persons, residing in any community and enjoying the benefits of its local government, should have the power thus to dominate the majority when supported in their action by the authority of the state. While this court should guard with firmness every right appertaining to life, liberty, or property as secured to the individual by the supreme law of the land, it is of the last importance that it should not invade the domain of local authority except when it is plainly necessary to do so in order to enforce that law. The safety and the health of the people of Massachusetts are, in the first instance, for that commonwealth to guard and protect. They are matters that do not ordinarily concern the national government. So far as they can be reached by any government, they depend, primarily, upon such action as the state, in its wisdom, may take; and we do not perceive that this legislation has invaded any right secured by the Federal Constitution.

Before closing this opinion we deem it appropriate, in order to prevent misapprehension as to our views, to observe—perhaps to repeat a thought already sufficiently expressed, namely—that the police power of a state, whether exercised directly by the legislature, or by a local body acting under its authority, may be exerted in such circumstances, or by regulations so arbitrary and oppressive in particular cases, as to justify the interference of the courts to prevent wrong and oppression. Extreme cases can be readily suggested. Ordinarily such cases are not safe guides in the administration of the law. It is easy, for instance, to suppose the case of an adult who is embraced by the mere words of the act, but yet to subject whom to vaccination in a particular condition of his health or body would be cruel and inhuman in the last degree. We are not to be understood as holding that the statute was intended to be applied to such a case, or, if it was so intended, that the judiciary would not be competent to interfere and protect the health and life of the individual concerned. "All laws," this court has said, "should receive a sensible construction. General terms should be so limited in their application as not to lead to injustice, oppression, or an absurd consequence. It will always, therefore, be presumed that the legislature intended exceptions to its language which would avoid results of this character. The reason of the law in such cases should prevail over its letter." *United States v. Kirby*, 74 U.S. 482 (1868). Until otherwise informed by the highest court of Massachusetts, we are not inclined to hold that the statute establishes the absolute rule that an adult must be vaccinated if it be apparent or can be shown with reasonable certainty that he is not at the time a fit subject of vaccination, or that vaccination, by reason of his then condition, would seriously impair his health, or probably cause his death. No such case is here presented. It is the case of an adult who, for aught that appears, was himself in perfect health and a fit subject of vaccination, and yet, while remaining in the community, refused to obey the statute and the regulation adopted in execution of its provisions for the protection of the public health and the public safety, confessedly endangered by the presence of a dangerous disease.

We now decide only that the statute covers the present case, and that nothing clearly appears that would justify this court in holding it to be unconstitutional and inoperative in its application to the plaintiff in error.

.   .   .   .   .

Justice Harlan's eloquent opinion in *Jacobson* rings with the values of community and the common good. But beyond passively accepting state legislative discretion in matters of public health, the Court makes the first systematic statement of the constitutional limitations imposed on public health officials. In *Jacobson*, the Court establishes four constitutional standards.

- *Public health necessity*—Public health powers can be exercised only when necessary to prevent an avoidable harm. Justice Harlan insisted that police powers must be based on the "necessities of the case" and cannot be exercised in "an arbitrary, unreasonable manner" or go "beyond what was reasonably required for the safety of the public."

- *Reasonable means*—The methods used must be designed to prevent or ameliorate a health threat. Even though the objective of the legislature may be valid and beneficent, the methods adopted must have a "real or substantial relation" to protection of the public health, and cannot be "a plain, palpable invasion of rights."

- *Proportionality*—The public health regulation may be unconstitutional if the burden imposed is wholly disproportionate to the expected benefit. "[T]he police power of a state," said Justice Harlan, "may be exerted in such circumstances, or by regulations so arbitrary and oppressive in particular cases, as to justify the interference of the courts to prevent wrong and oppression."

- *Harm avoidance*—The control measure should not pose an undue health risk to its subject. Justice Harlan emphasized that Henning Jacobson was a "fit subject" for smallpox vaccination, but asserted that requiring a person to be immunized who would be harmed is "cruel and inhuman in the last degree." If there had been evidence that the vaccination would seriously impair Jacobson's health, he might have prevailed in this historic case. The courts have required safe and habitable environments for persons subject to isolation on the theory that public health powers are designed to promote well-being, and not to punish the individual. For example, in *Kirk v. Wyman*, 65 S.E. 387 (S.C. 1909) (excerpted in chapter 11), the South Carolina Supreme Court found isolation in a pest house to be unconstitutional where "even temporary isolation in such a place would be a serious affliction and peril to an elderly lady, enfeebled by disease."

During the same time period as *Jacobson*, the judiciary expressed its displeasure with governmental action motivated by animus against an ethnic group. In *Yick Wo v. Hopkins*, 118 U.S. 356 (1886), the Supreme Court found unlawful discrimination when a San Francisco ordinance prohibiting the washing of clothes in public laundries after 10 P.M. was enforced only against Chinese owners. By 1900 public health authorities were implementing a quarantine in San Francisco within a twelve-block district known as Chinatown that housed a population of 12,000. Police, moreover, closed only businesses owned by nonwhite persons. The quarantine was challenged in *Jew Ho v. Williamson*, and a federal appellate court held it unconstitutional on the grounds that it was unfair: the health authorities had acted with an "evil eye and an unequal hand." *Jew Ho* serves as a reminder that public health measures can be motivated by prejudice and used as an instrument of subjugation.

JEW HO V. WILLIAMSON*
Circuit Court, Northern District of California
. Decided June 15, 1900

Circuit Judge MORROW delivered the opinion of the court (orally).
   [The board of health of San Francisco adopted a resolution authorizing the board to quarantine twelve city blocks after nine people in the area died of bubonic plague.

*103 F. 10 (C.C.N.D. Cal. 1900).

The complainant, who resided within the limits of the quarantined district, alleged, inter alia, that the resolution was enforced only against persons of Chinese race and nationality, and not against persons of other races. Additionally, the complainant alleged that there were not any cases of bubonic plague within the limits of the quarantined district within the thirty days preceding the filing of this complaint.]

It is ... contended that the acts of the defendants in establishing a quarantine district in San Francisco are authorized by the general police power of the state, intrusted to the city of San Francisco. . . .

. . . The question therefore arises as to whether or not the quarantine established by the defendants in this case is reasonable, and whether it is necessary, under the circumstances of this case. . . . This court will, of course, uphold any reasonable regulation that may be imposed for the purpose of protecting the people of the city from the invasion of epidemic disease. In the presence of a great calamity, the court will go to the greatest extent, and give the widest discretion, in construing the regulations that may be adopted by the board of health or the board of supervisors. But is the regulation in this case a reasonable one? Is it a proper regulation, directed to accomplish the purpose that appears to have been in view? That is a question for this court to determine. . . .

The purpose of quarantine and health laws and regulations with respect to contagious and infectious diseases is directed primarily to preventing the spread of such diseases among the inhabitants of localities. In this respect these laws and regulations come under the police power of the state, and may be enforced by quarantine and health officers, in the exercise of a large discretion, as circumstances may require. . . . This is a system of quarantine that is well recognized in all communities, and is provided by the laws of the various states and municipalities: That, when a contagious or infectious disease breaks out in a place, they quarantine the house or houses first; the purpose being to restrict the disease to the smallest number possible, and that it may not spread to other people in the same locality. It must necessarily follow that, if a large section or a large territory is quarantined, intercommunication of the people within that territory will rather tend to spread the disease than to restrict it. . . . The quarantined district comprises 12 blocks. . . . There are, I believe, 7 or 8 blocks in which it is claimed that deaths have occurred on account of what is said to be this disease. In 2 or 3 blocks it has not appeared at all. Yet this quarantine has been thrown around the entire district. The people therein obtain their food and other supplies, and communicate freely with each other in all their affairs. They are permitted to go from a place where it is said that the disease has appeared, freely among the other 10,000 people in that district. It would necessarily follow that, if the disease is there, every facility has been offered by this species of quarantine to enlarge its sphere and increase its danger and its destructive force. . . . The court cannot but see the practical question that is presented to it as to the ineffectiveness of this method of quarantine against such a disease as this. So, upon that ground, the court must hold that this quarantine is not a reasonable regulation to accomplish the purposes sought. It is not in harmony with the declared purpose of the board of health or of the board of supervisors.

But there is still another feature of this case that has been called to the attention of the court, and that is its discriminating character; that is to say, it is said that this

quarantine discriminates against the Chinese population of this city, and in favor of
the people of other races. . . . The evidence here is clear that this is made to operate
against the Chinese population only, and the reason given for it is that the Chinese
may communicate the disease from one to the other. That explanation, in the judgment of the court, is not sufficient. It is, in effect, a discrimination, and it is the
discrimination that has been frequently called to the attention of the federal courts
where matters of this character have arisen with respect to Chinese. . . .

In the case at bar, assuming that the board of supervisors had just grounds
for quarantining the district which has been described, it seems that the board of
health, in executing the ordinance, left out certain persons, members of races other
than Chinese. This is precisely the point noticed by the supreme court of the United
States, namely, the administration of a law "with an evil eye and an unequal hand."
Yick Wo v. Hopkins, 118 U.S. 356, 373-74 (1886). Wherever the courts of the United
States have found such an administration of the law . . . [with] the purpose to enforce
it "with an evil eye and an unequal hand," then it is the duty of the court to interpose,
and to declare the ordinance discriminating in its character, and void under the constitution of the United States. . . .

. . . This quarantine cannot be continued, by reason of the fact that it is unreasonable, unjust, and oppressive, and therefore contrary to the laws limiting the police
powers of the state and municipality in such matters; and, second, that it is discriminating in its character, and is contrary to the provisions of the fourteenth amendment of the constitution of the United States. The counsel for complainant will prepare an injunction, which shall, however, permit the board to maintain a quarantine
around such places as it may have reason to believe are infected by contagious or
infectious diseases, but that the general quarantine of the whole district must not
be continued, and that the people residing in that district, so far as they have been
restricted or limited in their persons and their business, have that limitation and
restraint removed.

II. PUBLIC HEALTH POWERS IN THE MODERN CONSTITUTIONAL ERA

Broadly speaking, it is possible to identify two different kinds of
restraint on police powers. The first restraint is substantive in nature,
requiring government to provide a plausible explanation for its intrusion on individual interests. As the restriction of rights or liberties inten-
sifies, the government must offer an increasingly strong justification.

The second type of restraint on police powers is procedural. Here
the Supreme Court requires government to provide a fair hearing
before depriving individuals of important liberty or property interests.
Police powers that affect important interests—for example, a liberty
interest denied by quarantine or a property interest denied by confiscation of dangerous possessions—may be exercised only with procedural
due process.

A. Substantive Rights: Levels of Scrutiny

The Supreme Court has developed a "tiered" approach to constitutional law, according to which it adopts various levels of scrutiny depending on the importance of the individual interests at stake—strict scrutiny, intermediate scrutiny, or minimum rationality. *City of Cleburne v. Cleburne Living Center* represents one of the Warren Court's clearest articulations of this layered approach to constitutional adjudication.

CITY OF CLEBURNE V. CLEBURNE LIVING CENTER*
Supreme Court of the United States
Decided July 1, 1985

Justice WHITE delivered the opinion of the Court.

A Texas city denied a special use permit for the operation of a group home for the mentally retarded, acting pursuant to a municipal zoning ordinance requiring permits for such homes. The Court of Appeals for the Fifth Circuit held that mental retardation is a "quasi-suspect" classification and that the ordinance violated the Equal Protection Clause because it did not substantially further an important governmental purpose. We hold that a lesser standard of scrutiny is appropriate, but conclude that under that standard the ordinance is invalid as applied in this case. . . .

The Equal Protection Clause of the Fourteenth Amendment commands that no State shall "deny to any person within its jurisdiction the equal protection of the laws," which is essentially a direction that all persons similarly situated should be treated alike. *Plyler v. Doe,* 457 U.S. 202, 216 (1982). Section 5 of the Amendment empowers Congress to enforce this mandate, but absent controlling congressional direction, the courts have themselves devised standards for determining the validity of state legislation or other official action that is challenged as denying equal protection. The general rule is that legislation is presumed to be valid and will be sustained if the classification drawn by the statute is rationally related to a legitimate state interest. When social or economic legislation is at issue, the Equal Protection Clause allows the States wide latitude, and the Constitution presumes that even improvident decisions will eventually be rectified by the democratic processes.

The general rule gives way, however, when a statute classifies by race, alienage, or national origin. These factors are so seldom relevant to the achievement of any legitimate state interest that laws grounded in such considerations are deemed to reflect prejudice and antipathy—a view that those in the burdened class are not as worthy or deserving as others. For these reasons and because such discrimination is unlikely to be soon rectified by legislative means, these laws are subjected to strict scrutiny and will be sustained only if they are suitably tailored to serve a compelling state interest. Similar oversight by the courts is due when state laws impinge on personal rights protected by the Constitution.

*473 U.S. 432 (1985).

Legislative classifications based on gender also call for a heightened standard of review. That factor generally provides no sensible ground for differential treatment.... Rather than resting on meaningful considerations, statutes distributing benefits and burdens between the sexes in different ways very likely reflect outmoded notions of the relative capabilities of men and women. A gender classification fails unless it is substantially related to a sufficiently important governmental interest....

We have declined, however, to extend heightened review to differential treatment based on age:

> While the treatment of the aged in this Nation has not been wholly free of discrimination, such persons, unlike, say, those who have been discriminated against on the basis of race or national origin, have not experienced a "history of purposeful unequal treatment" or been subjected to unique disabilities on the basis of stereotyped characteristics not truly indicative of their abilities. *Massachusetts Board of Retirement v. Murgia*, 427 U.S. 307, 313 (1976)

The lesson of *Murgia* is that where individuals in the group affected by a law have distinguishing characteristics relevant to interests the State has the authority to implement, the courts have been very reluctant, as they should be in our federal system and with our respect for the separation of powers, to closely scrutinize legislative choices as to whether, how, and to what extent those interests should be pursued. In such cases, the Equal Protection Clause requires only a rational means to serve a legitimate end.

Against this background, we conclude for several reasons that the Court of Appeals erred in holding mental retardation a quasi-suspect classification calling for a more exacting standard of judicial review than is normally accorded economic and social legislation. [The Court gives reasons for concluding that mental retardation is not a quasi-suspect classification: Persons with mental retardation are a diverse population, are materially different with less ability to cope, and have a certain level of public and political support.] ...

Doubtless, there have been and there will continue to be instances of discrimination against the retarded that are in fact invidious, and that are properly subject to judicial correction under constitutional norms. But the appropriate method of reaching such instances is not to create a new quasi-suspect classification and subject all governmental action based on that classification to more searching evaluation. Rather, we should look to the likelihood that governmental action premised on a particular classification is valid as a general matter, not merely to the specifics of the case before us. Because mental retardation is a characteristic that the government may legitimately take into account in a wide range of decisions, and because both State and Federal Governments have recently committed themselves to assisting the retarded, we will not presume that any given legislative action, even one that disadvantages retarded individuals, is rooted in considerations that the Constitution will not tolerate.

Our refusal to recognize the retarded as a quasi-suspect class does not leave them entirely unprotected from invidious discrimination. To withstand equal protection review, legislation that distinguishes between the mentally retarded and others must be rationally related to a legitimate governmental purpose. This standard, we believe, affords government the latitude necessary both to pursue policies designed to assist the retarded in realizing their full potential, and to freely and efficiently engage in activities that burden the retarded in what is essentially an incidental manner. The State may not rely on a classification whose relationship to an asserted goal is so attenuated as to render the distinction arbitrary or irrational. Furthermore, some objectives—such as "a bare ... desire to harm a politically unpopular group," *United States Dept. of Agriculture v. Moreno*, 413 U.S. 528, 534 (1973)–are not legitimate state interests. Beyond that, the mentally retarded, like others, have and retain their substantive constitutional rights in addition to the right to be treated equally by the law. [The Court goes on to hold that although mental retardation is not a classification deserving "strict scrutiny," in this case denial of a zoning permit was unreasonable and unconstitutional.]

. . . . . .

Although most justices accept the constitutional standards expressed in *Cleburne*, they are bitterly divided between alternative constitutional visions, particularly in cases that involve privacy interests and sexual and reproductive autonomy. Consider the stridently different judicial perspectives in *Lawrence v. Texas*, 539 U.S. 558 (2003), and *Gonzales v. Carhart*, 550 U.S. 124 (2007)—both cases in which the Supreme Court disregarded established judicial precedent.

   Lawrence expressly overturned *Bowers v. Hardwick*, 478 U.S. 186 (1986), a Burger Court case upholding criminal penalties against two men for having sex. Relying on a series of cases affording constitutional protection to personal decisions relating to marriage, procreation, contraception, family relationships, child rearing, and education, *Lawrence* struck down the penalties. Justice Anthony Kennedy, the swing vote on the Court, said that the Texas statute criminalizing sexual conduct in same-sex couples "furthers no legitimate state interest which can justify its intrusion into the personal and private life of the individual" (539 U.S. at 578). Therefore, he concluded, gay couples have a due process right to engage in consensual sexual activity in their home without government interference. Justice Sandra Day O'Connor, who wrote separately, favored an approach based on the Equal Protection Clause, stating that a "law branding one class of persons as criminal based solely on the State's moral disapproval ... runs contrary to the values of the Constitution and the Equal Protection Clause under any standard of review" (539 U.S. at 585). The majority of the Court, however, focused on the protected conduct instead of the right to equal treatment, reasoning that homosexual couples would continue to be stigmatized as long as consensual sexual acts could be criminalized under *Bowers*. Declining to overturn *Bowers,* Kennedy wrote, would "demean the lives of homosexual persons" (539 U.S. at 575).

Similarly, in *Gonzales v. Carhart* the Supreme Court changed course from its precedent on reproductive freedom. In *Roe v. Wade,* 410 U.S. 113 (1973), and *Planned Parenthood of Southeastern Pennsylvania v. Casey,* 505 U.S. 833 (1992), the Court established three principles governing abortion jurisprudence: (1) prior to viability, the state may not impose an "undue burden" on a woman's right to choose to have an abortion; (2) after viability, the state has the power to restrict abortion if the law contains an exception for pregnancies that endanger a woman's life or health; and (3) the state has legitimate interests from the outset of the pregnancy in protecting the health of the woman and the life of the fetus. Affirming these central holdings numerous times since 1973, the Court stated clearly that the government has an obligation to protect the health of the woman.

In 2000, consistent with these rulings, the Court in *Stenberg v. Carhart,* 530 U.S. 914 (2000), struck down a Nebraska statute criminalizing intact dilation and evacuation (a procedure termed by its critics "partial birth abortion") because it did not contain an exception for the preservation of a woman's health. In unmistakable defiance of the Court's decision, Congress enacted the Partial-Birth Abortion Act of 2003, which banned the same procedure without allowing a health exception. In doing so, Congress found that an intact dilation and evacuation (D&E) is "never" necessary—a statement that sharply contradicts the American College of Obstetricians and Gynecologists' finding that the procedure is necessary and proper in certain cases.

By the time the act was challenged in the Supreme Court in 2007, the Court's membership had significantly changed with the appointment of Chief Justice John Roberts and Associate Justice Samuel Alito. In their confirmation hearings, both justices had pledge to "respect" the precedents of *Roe* and *Casey* under principles of *stare decisis* (literally, "to stand by things decided"). Despite settled precedent, the Supreme Court upheld the act. On one level, *Gonzales v. Carhart* does not broadly restrict the practice of reproductive medicine because only a small proportion of abortions use intact D&E. But on another level, the decision is troubling because it undermines clinical freedom and the physician/patient relationship (Drazen 2007), as well as calling into question the legitimacy of a Court that departs from the principle of *stare decisis.* In a stirring dissent, which she read aloud from the bench, Justice Ruth Bader Ginsburg criticized the majority opinion:

The Act scarcely furthers [the state's interest in preserving and promoting fetal life]: The law saves not a single fetus from destruction, for it targets only a method of performing abortion. . . .

Ultimately, the Court admits that "moral concerns" are at work, concerns that could yield prohibitions on any abortion. Notably, the concerns expressed are untethered to any ground genuinely serving the Government's interest in preserving life. By allowing such concerns to carry the day and case, overriding fundamental rights, the Court dishonors our precedent.

Revealing in this regard, the Court invokes an antiabortion shibboleth for which it concededly has no reliable evidence: Women who have abortions come to regret their choices, and consequently suffer from "[s]evere depression and loss of esteem." Because of women's fragile emotional state and because of the "bond of love the mother has for her child," the Court worries, doctors may withhold information about the nature of the intact D & E procedure. The solution the Court approves, then, is not to require doctors to inform women, accurately and adequately, of the different procedures and their attendant risks. Instead, the Court deprives women of the right to make an autonomous choice, even at the expense of their safety.

In sum, the notion that the Partial-Birth Abortion Ban Act furthers any legitimate governmental interest is, quite simply, irrational. The Court's defense of the statute provides no saving explanation. In candor, the Act, and the Court's defense of it, cannot be understood as anything other than an effort to chip away at a right declared again and again by this Court—and with increasing comprehension of its centrality to women's lives. When "a statute burdens constitutional rights and all that can be said on its behalf is that it is the vehicle that legislators have chosen for expressing their hostility to those rights, the burden is undue." *Stenberg v. Carhart,* 530 U.S. 914, 952 (Ginsburg, J., concurring). (550 U.S. 124, 180–91)

Beyond the equal protection and substantive due process rights contained in the Fifth and Fourteenth Amendments, the Constitution protects a number of other substantive rights and interests. For example, the right of assembly, free speech, and religion (First Amendment); the right to keep and bear arms (Second Amendment); the right to be free from unreasonable searches and seizures (Fourth Amendment); and the right to a speedy trial (Sixth Amendment) are all set forth in the Constitution. At times, these substantive protections are at odds with public health interests (see box 3). But the fact that a regulation encroaches on a protected interest does not necessarily invalidate it. Rather, the courts determine constitutionality by scrutinizing the interests involved under the appropriate standard of review.

In *District of Columbia v. Heller,* 554 U.S. 290 (2008), the Supreme

BOX 3
PARENTAL RIGHTS AND CONTRACEPTIVE ACCESS FOR MINORS

Public health clinics operate in a political environment espousing two values often in tension—ensuring minors' access to reproductive services and respecting parental interests in knowing about, and even approving, such services, including sexually transmitted disease (STD) treatment, contraception, and abortion. Some states have stepped in to expand minors' access—distributing condoms and health information in the schools. Others have contracted access by, for example, requiring health care professionals to notify parents prior to providing reproductive services to minors. Both approaches implicate competing constitutional interests: the minor's right to privacy, on the one hand, and the parents' right to care for and guide their children, on the other.

In *Anspach v. Philadelphia Department of Public Health*, 503 F.3d 256 (3d Cir. 2007), a city-operated health center provided "morning after" contraceptives to a sixteen-year-old minor, Melissa Anspach, at her request. Her parents contended that the state's action infringed on their parental rights. The United States Court of Appeals for the Third Circuit analyzed the nature and extent of parental rights, concluding that the state can provide minors with reproductive health services in a noncoercive manner without infringing on parental rights. Melissa Anspach herself also alleged a constitutional violation, contending that because the state did not tell her that the emergency contraceptives might act in a way that violates her religious beliefs concerning abortion, her right to free exercise of religion was infringed. The court found that the clinic's actions were constitutionally permissible because Anspach was not compelled to act contrary to her beliefs.

Court—again divided along ideological lines—wrestled with the reaches of the Second Amendment right to keep and bear arms. At issue in *Heller* is the constitutionality of the District of Columbia's 1975 handgun law, which was credited with reducing gun homicides by 25 percent and gun suicides by 23 percent (Loftin et al. 1991). The justices were sharply divided on two questions: Does the Second Amendment protect a right of individuals to bear arms for purposes unconnected with militia service? And, if it protects such a right, are the District of Columbia's restrictions on handgun registration and possession reasonable limitations on the right to keep and bear arms? The following excerpt from the *United States Law Week* reviews the Court's opinion in the case.

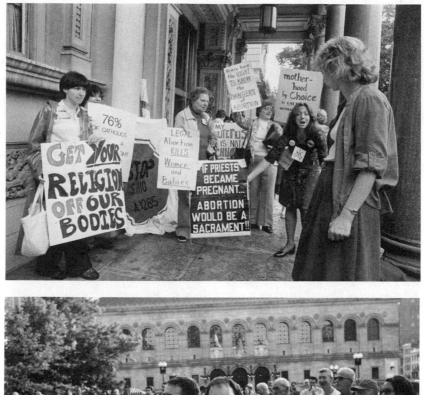

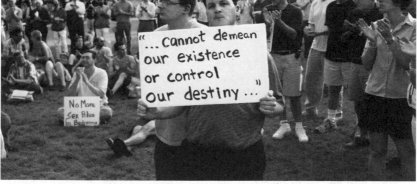

Photo 8. Demonstrators react to two major Supreme Court decisions affecting individual rights. At the top, protesters rally for and against limits on abortion outside the New Jersey statehouse six years after *Roe v. Wade,* 410 U.S. 113 (1973), legalized abortion in the United States. Below, supporters of gay rights gather in Boston's Copley Square to celebrate the Supreme Court ruling in *Lawrence v. Texas,* 539 U.S. 558 (2003), in which the Supreme Court found sodomy laws to be unconstitutional. The sign in the photograph refers to Justice Kennedy's majority opinion, in which he wrote of same-sex couples that "the State cannot demean their existence or control their destiny by making their private sexual conduct a crime." Reproduced by permission. Top: © Bettman/Corbis, June 11, 1979. Bottom: © Rick Friedman/Corbis, July 26, 2003.

SECOND AMENDMENT SHIELDS INDIVIDUAL RIGHTS, IS VIOLATED BY D.C.'S PROHIBITION OF HANDGUNS*
Bureau of National Affairs, Inc.

The Second Amendment protects the individual right to have and use weapons for self-defense, and the District of Columbia's ban on handguns in the home violates that right, the U.S. Supreme Court held . . . by a vote of 5–4.

This was the court's first comprehensive look at the amendment, which states that a "well regulated Militia, being necessary to the security of a free State, the right of the people to keep and bear Arms, shall not be infringed." The court sided with the two appeals courts that have construed it to confer an individual right, rather than a collective right related to militia service as found by most appeals courts.

[Writing for the majority,] Justice Antonin Scalia said that the prefatory clause's reference to the militia reflected concerns that the federal government not eliminate state militias, but does not limit the second, "operative" clause's recognition of a pre-existing individual right to have and carry weapons. The amendment "surely elevates above all other interests the right of law-abiding, responsible citizens to use arms in defense of hearth and home," he said. The D.C. laws are invalid because they frustrate that core right, Scalia said.

A dissent [by Justice Stevens] charged that "not a word in the constitutional text even arguably supports" the latter "overwrought and novel" construction of the amendment. Another dissent [by Justice Breyer] argued that a handgun ban is reasonable in a high-crime urban area, even assuming that the amendment protects individual rights.

At issue were D.C. ordinances that, with certain exceptions, (1) bar registration (and thus possession) of handguns, (2) prohibit carrying a handgun without a license issued by the chief of police, and (3) require that lawfully owned firearms, such as long guns, be kept "unloaded and disassembled or bound by a trigger lock or similar device" unless they are located in a place of business or are being used for lawful recreational activities. The plaintiff, who was denied a registration certificate for a handgun that he wished to keep at home, charged that these ordinances violated the Second Amendment to the extent that they bar use of "functional firearms in the home."

The district court dismissed the suit, ruling that the amendment, at most, protects an individual's right to "*bear* arms for service in the militia." The D.C. Circuit, agreeing with [an earlier ruling by] the Fifth Circuit, reversed. It found that the amendment protects an individual right to possess firearms and that the city's total ban on handguns, and the disassemble-or-lock requirement for lawful firearms, violated that right.

A RIGHT OF THE PEOPLE

Affirming, the Supreme Court said the Second Amendment "is naturally divided into two parts: its prefatory clause and its operative clause. The former does not limit

*Reproduced with permission from the *United States Law Week* 77, no. 1 (July 1, 2008): 1011–13. Copyright 2008 by the Bureau of National Affairs, Inc. (800-372-1033). www.bna.com.

the latter grammatically, but rather announces a purpose." That purpose was "to prevent elimination of the militia," the court said. It explained that the amendment's proponents sought to prevent the federal government's "enabling a select militia or standing army to suppress political opponents" as had occurred in 17th century England via a disarming of the people. The term "militia" refers to "all males physically capable of acting in concert for the common defense," rather than to the "organized" military units of the several states, the court said. And the phrase "security of a free state" meant the "security of a free polity," rather than the security of each of the several states, thus torpedoing the theory of a D.C. Circuit dissenter who reasoned that the amendment did not apply to the District of Columbia because it is not a state.

The amendment's operative clause significantly codifies a "right of the people," the court observed. This language resembles that in the First, Fourth, and Ninth Amendments, which in each case protects individual, not collective, rights, it said. Moreover, "the people" consistently refers "to all members of the political community," rather than to a subset such as the militia, the court said. "Reading the Second Amendment as protecting only the right to 'keep and bear Arms' in an organized militia therefore fits poorly with the operative clause's description of the holder of that right as 'the people,'" it reasoned.

The term "arms" was not limited to military weapons, the court said. "'Keep arms' was simply a common way of referring to possessing arms, for militiamen *and everyone else*," it said. The term "bear" was not limited to military use of weapons, but did signify "confrontation," the court said. It thus concluded that the operative clause's text "guaranteed the individual right to possess and carry weapons in case of confrontation." Being derived from the English Bill of Rights, it "was clearly an individual right, having nothing whatever to do with service in a militia," the court said.

[SUPREME COURT PRECEDENT] HARMONIZED

That interpretation is confirmed by analogous arms-bearing rights in contemporaneous state constitutions, which state courts construed to confer individual rights, the court said. It also invoked post-ratification and 19th century commentary in support.

None of its precedents is to the contrary, the court said. In particular, *United States v. Miller*, 307 U.S. 174 (1939), rejected a Second Amendment challenge by defendants convicted of transporting an unregistered sawed-off shotgun, based on that weapon's lack of a "reasonable relationship to the preservation or efficiency of a well regulated militia." If the *Miller* court "had believed that the Second Amendment protects only those serving in the militia, it would have been odd to examine the character of the weapon rather than simply note that the two crooks were not militiamen," the court here said. It thus read *Miller* "to say only that the Second Amendment does not protect those weapons not typically possessed by law-abiding citizens for lawful purposes, such as short-barreled shotguns."

"Like most rights, the right secured by the Second Amendment is not unlimited," the court cautioned. Thus, restrictions on carrying of concealed weapons, or on possession of weapons by felons or the mentally ill or in sensitive places such as schools or government buildings, are not placed in doubt, it said. Nor are bans on carrying of "dangerous and unusual weapons." But the D.C. handgun ban and disassembly/lock law strike at the "inherent right of self-defense [that] has been central to the Second

Amendment right," and thus are invalid as to possession of those guns in the home, it ruled. But it left the licensing requirement intact.

Dissenting, Justice John Paul Stevens, joined by Justices David H. Souter, Ruth Bader Ginsburg, and Stephen G. Breyer, said that *Miller* recognized that the amendment "protects the right to keep and bear arms for certain military purposes, but that it does not curtail the Legislature's power to regulate the nonmilitary use and ownership of weapons." He found nothing in the amendment's text or history to support an intent of the Framers "to enshrine the common-law right of self-defense in the Constitution." He cited a striking contrast of the Second Amendment's terms with contemporaneous provisions of the Vermont and Pennsylvania Constitutions expressly recognizing individual rights.

Also dissenting, Breyer, joined by Stevens, Souter, and Ginsburg, said that a legislature could reasonably find that an urban handgun ban "will advance goals of great public importance, namely, saving lives, preventing injury, and reducing crime," and thus the D.C. law "falls within the zone that the Second Amendment leaves open to regulation by legislatures."

.   .   .   .   .

The decision has important implications for public health authorities working in violence prevention. The Court did recognize a significant scope for gun control, suggesting that some reasonable limitation on licensing or possession would be permitted. The Court also implied that the right to personal possession did not extend to "dangerous and unusual weapons" not typically used for self-defense or recreation, such as machine guns. But the majority did not articulate the standard of scrutiny that courts should use to evaluate the constitutionality of gun laws. In his dissent, Justice Breyer criticized the majority's failure to set forth a constitutional standard and suggested that an "interest-balancing inquiry" be used. Justice Breyer would have upheld the District of Columbia law because the city had a compelling interest in curbing rampant gun violence, as demonstrated by the striking figures on gun violence:

> From 1993 to 1997, there were 180,533 firearm-related deaths in the United States, an average of over 36,000 per year. Fifty-one percent were suicides, 44% were homicides, 1% were legal interventions, 3% were unintentional accidents, and 1% were of undetermined causes. . . .
>
> The statistics are particularly striking in respect to children and adolescents. In over one in every eight firearm-related deaths in 1997, the victim was someone under the age of 20. . . . More male teenagers die from firearms than from all natural causes combined. . . .
>
> Handguns are involved in a majority of firearm deaths and injuries in the United States. . . . And among children under the age of 20, handguns

account for approximately 70% of all unintentional firearm-related injuries and deaths. In particular, 70% of all firearm-related teenage suicides in 1996 involved a handgun. (128 S. Ct. at 2856)

While many state and municipal firearm laws appear to be permitted under *Heller,* categorical bans on handguns in cities such as Chicago are in serious jeopardy. The National Rifle Association (NRA) has recently filed lawsuits challenging firearm regulations around the country. Gun advocates have even challenged Washington, D.C.'s ban on semiautomatic guns. Shortly after the Court's decision in *Heller,* the *New England Journal of Medicine* published an editorial announcing, "The Supreme Court has launched the country on a risky epidemiologic experiment" (Drazen, Morrissey, and Curfman 2008, 517). The effects of this "experiment" remain to be seen, as the courts continue to define the legal standards for firearm laws and as jurisdictions struggle to write laws that comply with *Heller* but protect the public's health.

B. Procedural Due Process

Hardly any state interest is higher than protecting its citizenry from disease. Hardly any individual interest is higher than the liberty interest of being free from confinement. The consequences of error and abuse are grave for both the state and the individual.

City of Newark v. J.S., 652 A.2d 265
(N.J. Super. Ct. Law Div. 1993)

The due process clause of the Fourteenth Amendment provides that no state shall "deprive any person of life, liberty, or property, without due process of law." Police powers that implicate these important interests in life, liberty, or property may be exercised only with procedural due process. Once the court determines that the government must provide procedural due process, the issue becomes "What process is due?"—that is, how elaborate must the procedures be to satisfy the due process requirement? In *Mathews v. Eldridge,* 424 U.S. 319, 334 (1976), the Court set the modern standard for fair procedures under the due process clause:

> "Due process is flexible and calls for such procedural protections as the particular situation demands." *Morrissey v. Brewer,* 408 U.S. 471, 481 (1972). Accordingly, resolution of the issue whether the administrative procedures provided . . . are constitutionally sufficient requires analysis

of the governmental and private interests that are affected. More precisely, . . . identification of the specific dictates of due process generally requires consideration of three distinct factors: First, the private interest that will be affected by the official action; second, the risk of an erroneous deprivation of such interest through the procedures used, and the probable value, if any, of additional or substitute procedural safeguards; and finally, the Government's interest, including the function involved and the fiscal and administrative burdens that the additional or substitute procedural requirement would entail.

In *Greene v. Edwards* (excerpted next), the West Virginia Supreme Court applied that standard in the public health context of isolation for tuberculosis (TB), enumerating a list of procedural protections that must be accorded to a person involuntarily confined under the state's Tuberculosis Control Act. Since *Greene,* the courts have continued to define what the Constitution requires in terms of procedural protections for those whose liberty is constrained for public health purposes. For example, a unanimous jury verdict and proof beyond a reasonable doubt are not constitutionally required for civil commitment of a TB patient (*Ventura County Public Health Officer v. Adalberto M.,* 67 Cal. Rptr. 3d 277 [Cal. Ct. App. 2007]).

GREENE V. EDWARDS*
Supreme Court of Appeals of West Virginia
Decided March 11, 1980

PER CURIAM:
   William Arthur Greene . . . is involuntarily confined in Pinecrest Hospital under an order of the Circuit Court of McDowell County entered pursuant to the terms of the West Virginia Tuberculosis Control Act. He alleges, among other points, that the Tuberculosis Control Act does not afford procedural due process because: (1) it fails to guarantee the alleged tubercular person the right to counsel; (2) it fails to insure that he may cross-examine, confront and present witnesses; and (3) it fails to require that he be committed only upon clear, cogent and convincing proof. We agree. . . .
   [The West Virginia Tuberculosis Control Act] provides in part:

   If such practicing physician, public health officer, or chief medical officer having under observation or care any person who is suffering from TB in a communicable stage is of the opinion that the environmental conditions of such person are not suitable for proper isolation or control by any type of local quarantine as prescribed by the state health department, and that such person is unable or unwilling to conduct himself and to live in such a manner as not to expose mem-

*263 S.E.2d 661 (W. Va. 1980).

bers of his family or household or other persons with whom he may be associated to danger of infection, he shall report the facts to the department of health which shall forthwith investigate or have investigated the circumstances alleged. If it shall find that any such person's physical condition is a health menace to others, the department of health shall petition the circuit court of the county in which such person resides, or the judge thereof in vacation, alleging that such person is afflicted with communicable TB and that such person's physical condition is a health menace to others, and requesting an order of the court committing such person to one of the state institutions. Upon receiving the petition, the court shall fix a date for hearing thereof and notice of such petition and the time and place for hearing thereof shall be served personally, at least seven days before the hearing, upon the person who is afflicted with TB and alleged to be dangerous to the health of others. If, upon such hearing, it shall appear that the complaint of the department of health is well founded, that such person is afflicted with communicable TB, and that such person is a source of danger to others, the court shall commit the individual to an institution maintained for the care and treatment of persons afflicted with TB. . . . [ellipsis in the original]

It is evident from an examination of this statute that its purpose is to prevent a person suffering from active communicable TB from becoming a danger to others. A like rationale underlies our statute governing the involuntary commitment of a mentally ill person.

In *State ex rel. Hawks v. Lazaro*, 202 S.E.2d 109 (W. Va. 1974), we examined the procedural safeguards which must be extended to persons charged under our statute governing the involuntary hospitalization of the mentally ill. We noted that Article 3, Section 10 of the West Virginia Constitution and the Fifth Amendment to the United States Constitution provide that no person shall be deprived of life, liberty, or property without due process of law. . . .

We concluded that due process required that persons charged under [the West Virginia statute governing involuntary commitment for the mentally ill] must be afforded: (1) an adequate written notice detailing the grounds and underlying facts on which commitment is sought; (2) the right to counsel; (3) the right to be present, cross-examine, confront and present witnesses; (4) the standard of proof to warrant commitment to be by clear, cogent and convincing evidence; and (5) the right to a verbatim transcript of the proceeding for purposes of appeal.

Because the Tuberculosis Control Act and the Act for the Involuntary Hospitalization of the Mentally Ill have like rationales, and because involuntary commitment for having communicable TB impinges upon the right to "liberty, full and complete liberty" no less than involuntary commitment for being mentally ill, we conclude that the procedural safeguards set forth in *State ex rel. Hawks v. Lazaro*, must, and do, extend to persons charged under [the Tuberculosis Control Act]. . . .

We noted in *State ex rel. Hawks v. Lazaro* that where counsel is to be appointed in proceedings for the involuntary hospitalization of the mentally ill, the law contemplates representation of the individual by the appointed guardian in the most zealous, adversary fashion consistent with the Code of Professional Responsibility. Since this decision, we have concluded that appointment of counsel immediately prior to a trial in a criminal case is impermissible since it denies the defendant effective assistance of counsel. It is obvious that timely appointment and reasonable opportunity for adequate preparation are prerequisites for fulfillment of appointed counsel's constitutionally assigned role in representing persons charged ... with having communicable TB.

In the case before us, counsel was not appointed for Mr. Greene until after the commencement of the commitment hearing. Under the circumstances, counsel could not have been properly prepared to defend Mr. Greene. For this reason, he must be accorded a new hearing. . . .

[Mr. Greene's] discharge is hereby delayed for a period of thirty days during which time the State may entertain further proceedings to be conducted in accordance with the principles expressed herein.

· · · · ·

The government has considerable power to safeguard the health and well-being of its citizens. However, this power has limits in a constitutional democracy. The state may regulate in the name of public health, but it may not overreach. It may act on the basis of scientific evidence, but not arbitrarily or with animus. From this point of view, society seeks a reasonable balance between the common goods of public health regulation and individual rights or freedoms. To ensure that we reach a fair balance of interests, the Constitution requires government to have a good reason for public health interventions. And when government does intervene, the Constitution requires that individuals subject to coercion receive a fair hearing.

RECOMMENDED READINGS

Early Twentieth-Century Limits on the Police Power

Albert, Michael, Kristen Ostheimer, and Joel Breman. 2001. The last smallpox epidemic in Boston and the vaccination controversy, 1901–1903. *New England Journal of Medicine* 344: 375–79. (Sets forth the public health history behind *Jacobson*, focusing on Boston's smallpox epidemic and the attendant compulsory vaccination controversy)

Colgrove, James, and Ronald Bayer. 2005. Manifold restraints: Liberty, public health, and the legacy of *Jacobson v. Massachusetts. American Journal of Public Health* 95: 571–76. (Reviews the historical tension between civil rights and public health from *Jacobson* to today)

Gostin, Lawrence O. 2005. *Jacobson v. Massachusetts* at 100 years: Police power and civil liberties in tension. *American Journal of Public Health* 95: 576–81. (Provides a historical perspective on Justice Harlan's opinion in *Jacobson* and its enduring value)

Mariner, Wendy K., George J. Annas, and Leonard H. Glantz. 2005. *Jacobson v. Massachusetts*: It's not your great-great-grandfather's public health law.

American Journal of Public Health 95: 581–90. (Reviews *Jacobson* in light of modern protections for civil liberties and human rights, positing that the vigorous defense of individual rights aids public health by promoting public trust and creating social solidarity)

Public Health Powers in the Modern Constitutional Era

Charo, R. Alta. 2007. The partial death of abortion rights. *New England Journal of Medicine* 356: 2125–28. (Details the Court's decision in *Gonzales v. Carhart* and tracks state laws banning "partial-birth" abortion)

Dresser, Rebecca. 2007. Protecting women from their abortion choices. *Hastings Center Report* 37 (6): 13–14. (Describes the Court's decision in *Carhart* and looks forward toward a case based on South Dakota's mandatory disclosure approach to abortion)

Gostin, Lawrence O. 2007. Abortion politics: Clinical freedom, trust in the judiciary, and the autonomy of women. *JAMA* 298: 1562–64. (Explains the consequences of the Court's departure from precedents in *Carhart*)

———. 2008. The right to bear arms: Constitutional law, politics, and public health. *JAMA* 300: 1575–77. (Examines the *Heller* decision and its connection to public health)

Jacobson, Peter D., and Wendy E. Parmet. 2007. A new era of unapproved drugs: The case of *Abigail Alliance v. Von Eschenbach*. *JAMA* 297: 205–8. (Describes the District of Columbia Circuit Court case holding that terminally ill patients do not have a fundamental right to access investigational drugs found safe for expanded human trials but not approved for public use by the FDA)

Rosenbaum, Sara, and Taylor Burke. 2003. *Lawrence v. Texas:* Implications for public health policy and practice. *Public Health Reports* 118: 559–61. (Provides an examination of the public health implications of the Court's decision in *Lawrence* striking down anti-sodomy laws)

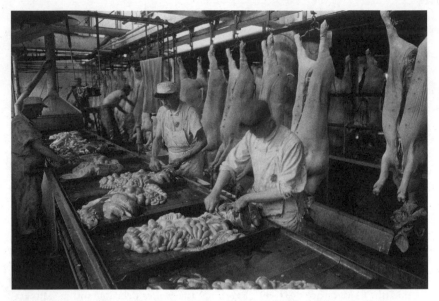

Photo 9. Employees of the Federal Meat Inspection Service inspect the internal organs of pigs in a 1950s meatpacking plant. The Meat Inspection Act, passed in 1906 after Upton Sinclair's *The Jungle* described the unsanitary conditions in such plants in gruesome detail, gives the federal government the authority to perform these inspections. Reproduced by permission, © Hulton-Deutsch Collection/Corbis, ca. 1950s.

FIVE

Public Health Governance

Direct Regulation for the Public's
Health and Safety

The first two chapters in this part of the *Reader* explored the scope and limits of the government's public health powers. In this chapter, we examine how these powers are exercised. To achieve communal health and safety, governments have formed specialized agencies, usually in the executive branch. Local and federal agencies issue and enforce regulations to ensure occupational health and safety; prevent environmental degradation; and protect consumers from unsafe products, impure food and water, and ineffective or dangerous pharmaceuticals and medical devices. They license professionals, businesses, and institutions to ensure adequate qualifications and standards, and inspect premises and commercial establishments to identify unsanitary conditions, unsafe environments, or impure products. (The contours of agencies' licensing and inspection powers will be examined in chapter 12.) Public health advocates see these agency activities—and the regulatory state in general—as necessary to securing the public's health. A well-regulated society generates communal benefits; it promotes health and prevents injury and disease, fulfilling a central purpose of democratic government.

The legal status of the modern public health agency is highly

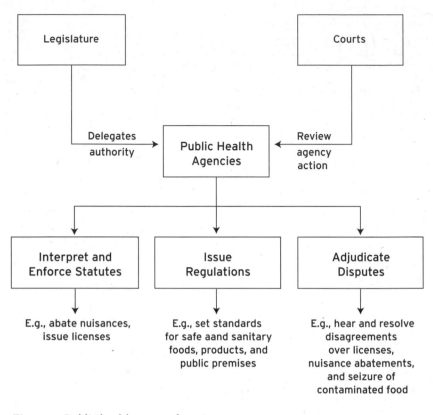

Figure 6. Public health agency functions.

complex, informed by a vast body of administrative law. Administrative
law helps determine when public health agencies are acting openly,
fairly, and within the scope of their legislative mandates. Although the
modern public health agency resides within the executive branch of
government, it not only possesses executive power but may also issue
regulations, interpret statutes, and adjudicate disputes (see figure 6).
The lines between lawmaking, enforcement, and adjudication (inherent
in the doctrine of separation of powers) have become blurred with the
rise of the administrative state.

This chapter begins by exploring two fundamental questions: When
can an agency act? And when *must* an agency act? The first section
explores the former question, examining how courts decide whether
the legislature has granted an agency a specific power. The second

section addresses the latter question, looking at when the courts will compel an agency to regulate a significant health hazard; the hazards in the illustrative cases are ethylene oxide—a dangerous workplace chemical—and greenhouse gas emissions linked to global climate change. The third section undertakes a more fundamental inquiry into the value of the regulatory state in protecting the public's health and safety. The issue in this final section carries particular political significance because the debate over government's role in regulating businesses and individuals is highly charged in contemporary American society.

I. LIMITS OF ADMINISTRATIVE POWER: WHEN CAN AN AGENCY ACT?

Legislatures are the policy-making arm of government and establish public health agencies to carry out legislative policy. Consequently, administrative agencies have only those powers that are delegated by the legislature. In addition, there are limits as to what powers the legislature can lawfully delegate; some policy questions are assigned only to the legislative branch (whose members are directly elected by and accountable to the people) and cannot be handed over to executive agencies. The judiciary reviews statutory grants of power to ensure that agencies act within the scope of their authority and that the legislature has not delegated purely legislative functions. The cases that follow elucidate these two core administrative law doctrines.

A. Scope of Delegated Authority

When courts determine whether an agency action was within the scope of its delegated authority, their central question is whether the legislature intended to grant the power exercised by the public health agency. In examining this question, the judiciary often affords public health agencies deference in decision making. If the agency asserts that it has the delegated authority to act in a certain area, or the agency interprets the authorizing statute in a certain way, the courts tend to defer (see *Chevron U.S.A., Inc. v. Natural Resources Defense Council, Inc.*, 467 U.S. 837 [1984]).

The measure of deference to an agency administering its own statute varies with the circumstances. The courts have looked to the degree of care the agency took in arriving at its interpretations; its consistency, formality of proceedings, and relative expertise; and the persuasiveness of the agency's position (see *United States v. Mead Corp.,* 533 U.S. 218, 227 [2001]).

There are at least three circumstances in which courts will not grant agencies what is known as *Chevron* deference. In the first, the agency has not been granted by Congress the power to interpret the statute; in such cases, the agency's interpretation is entitled to respect only to the extent that it is persuasive (see *Skidmore v. Swift & Co.,* 323 U.S. 134 [1944]). In *Gonzales v. Oregon* (excerpted next), the attorney general interpreted the scope of "legitimate medical purpose" under the Controlled Substances Act so as to effectively criminalize the prescription of potentially lethal drug doses under the Oregon Death with Dignity Act. The Supreme Court, however, declined to give the attorney general any deference.

In the second circumstance, discussed in *Food and Drug Administration v. Brown & Williamson Tobacco Corp.* (excerpted below), Congress has directly spoken to the precise question at issue. Thus, if Congress unambiguously specified its intent, the agency cannot form a different judgment. *Brown & Williamson* dealt with the FDA's effort to regulate tobacco in the 1990s: specifically, its attempt to prevent the direct marketing of cigarettes to minors. The Supreme Court found that Congress clearly intended to exclude tobacco from the FDA's jurisdiction, and thus the FDA's contrary interpretation was not entitled to deference.

In the third circumstance, the agency's action raises significant constitutional questions. In *Solid Waste Agency of Northern Cook County v. United States Army Corps of Engineers,* 531 U.S. 159 (2001), the Supreme Court held that the Army Corps of Engineers exceeded its authority under the Clean Water Act when it regulated waste disposal in intrastate waters. The Court said that when an administrative interpretation of a statute invokes the outer limits of Congress's constitutional power, it is not entitled to *Chevron* deference. Concern that agency action exceeds the limits of power granted by Congress is heightened when the administrative interpretation alters the federal-state framework by permitting federal encroachment on a traditional state power.

GONZALES V. OREGON*

Supreme Court of the United States

Decided January 17, 2006

Justice KENNEDY delivered the opinion of the Court.

In 1994, Oregon became the first State to legalize assisted suicide when voters approved a ballot measure enacting the Oregon Death With Dignity Act (ODWDA). ODWDA . . . exempts from civil or criminal liability state-licensed physicians who . . . dispense or prescribe a lethal dose of drugs upon the request of a terminally ill patient. . . .

A November 9, 2001, Interpretive Rule issued by the [United States] Attorney General . . . determines that using controlled substances to assist suicide is not a legitimate medical practice and that dispensing or prescribing them for this purpose is unlawful under the [Controlled Substances Act]. The Interpretive Rule's validity under the CSA is the issue before us. . . .

. . . A 1971 regulation promulgated by the Attorney General requires that every prescription for a controlled substance "be issued for a legitimate medical purpose by an individual practitioner acting in the usual course of his professional practice." 21 CFR § 1306.04(a) (2005). . . .

. . . To issue lawful prescriptions of [controlled substances], physicians must "obtain from the Attorney General a registration issued in accordance with the rules and regulations promulgated by him." 21 U.S.C. § 822(a)(2). The Attorney General may deny, suspend, or revoke this registration if, as relevant here, the physician's registration would be "inconsistent with the public interest." § 824(a)(4); § 822(a) (2). . . .

Executive actors often must interpret the enactments Congress has charged them with enforcing and implementing. The parties before us are in sharp disagreement both as to the degree of deference we must accord the Interpretive Rule's substantive conclusions and whether the Rule is authorized by the statutory text at all. . . . An administrative rule may receive substantial deference if it interprets the issuing agency's own ambiguous regulation. An interpretation of an ambiguous statute may also receive substantial deference. Deference in accordance with Chevron, however, is warranted only "when it appears that Congress delegated authority to the agency generally to make rules carrying the force of law, and that the agency interpretation claiming deference was promulgated in the exercise of that authority." United States v. Mead Corp., 533 U.S. 218, 226–27 (2001). Otherwise, the interpretation is "entitled to respect" only to the extent it has the "power to persuade." Skidmore v. Swift & Co., 323 U.S. 134, 140 (1944).

The Government first argues that the Interpretive Rule is an elaboration of one of the Attorney General's own regulations, which requires all prescriptions be issued "for a legitimate medical purpose by an individual practitioner acting in the usual course of his professional practice." 21 CFR § 1306.04 (2005). . . .

[The regulation] gives little or no instruction on a central issue in this case: Who

*546 U.S. 243 (2006).

decides whether a particular activity is in "the course of professional practice" or done for a "legitimate medical purpose"? . . . An agency does not acquire special authority to interpret its own words when, instead of using its expertise and experience to formulate a regulation, it has elected merely to paraphrase the statutory language. . . .

. . . If a statute is ambiguous, judicial review of administrative rulemaking often demands *Chevron* deference; and the rule is judged accordingly. All would agree, we should think, that the statutory phrase "legitimate medical purpose" is a generality, susceptible to more precise definition and open to varying constructions, and thus ambiguous in the relevant sense. *Chevron* deference, however, is not accorded merely because the statute is ambiguous and an administrative official is involved. . . .

. . . It is not enough that the terms "public interest," "public health and safety," and "Federal law" are used in the part of the statute over which the Attorney General has authority. The statutory terms "public interest" and "public health" do not call on the Attorney General, or any other Executive official, to make an independent assessment of the meaning of federal law. The Attorney General did not base the Interpretive Rule on an application of . . . the "public health and safety" factor specifically. Even if he had, it is doubtful the Attorney General could cite the "public interest" or "public health" to deregister a physician simply because he deemed a controversial practice permitted by state law to have an illegitimate medical purpose. . . .

. . . Since the Interpretive Rule was not promulgated pursuant to the Attorney General's authority, its interpretation of "legitimate medical purpose" does not receive *Chevron* deference. Instead, it receives deference only [to the extent that it is persuasive]. "The weight of such a judgment in a particular case will depend upon the thoroughness evident in its consideration, the validity of its reasoning, its consistency with earlier and later pronouncements, and all those factors which give it power to persuade, if lacking power to control." *Skidmore*, 323 U.S., at 140. The deference here is tempered by the Attorney General's lack of expertise in this area and the apparent absence of any consultation with anyone outside the Department of Justice who might aid in a reasoned judgment. . . . For the reasons given and for further reasons set out below, we do not find the Attorney General's opinion persuasive. . . .

The judgment of the Court of Appeals is affirmed.

FOOD AND DRUG ADMINISTRATION V. BROWN & WILLIAMSON TOBACCO CORP.*

Supreme Court of the United States
Decided March 21, 2000

Justice O'CONNOR delivered the opinion of the Court.
[The Food and Drug Administration (FDA) has the power to regulate drugs and

*529 U.S. 120 (2000).

medical devices to ensure they are "safe and effective." Pursuant to this power, the FDA claimed jurisdiction to regulate tobacco products as a "nicotine delivery device." The question for the Supreme Court was whether Congress intended to give the agency the power to regulate.]

In 1996, the FDA, after having expressly disavowed any such authority since its inception, asserted jurisdiction to regulate tobacco products. The FDA concluded that nicotine is a "drug" within the meaning of the Food, Drug, and Cosmetic Act (FDCA or Act), 21 U.S.C. § 301 et seq., and that cigarettes and smokeless tobacco are "combination products" that deliver nicotine to the body. Pursuant to this authority, it promulgated regulations intended to reduce tobacco consumption among children and adolescents. The agency believed that, because most tobacco consumers begin their use before reaching the age of 18, curbing tobacco use by minors could substantially reduce the prevalence of addiction in future generations and thus the incidence of tobacco-related death and disease.

Regardless of how serious the problem an administrative agency seeks to address, however, it may not exercise its authority "in a manner that is inconsistent with the administrative structure that Congress enacted into law." ETSI Pipeline Project v. Missouri, 484 U.S. 495, 517 (1998). And although agencies are generally entitled to deference in the interpretation of statutes that they administer, a reviewing "court, as well as the agency, must give effect to the unambiguously expressed intent of Congress." Chevron U.S.A. Inc. v. Natural Resources Defense Council, Inc., 467 U.S. 837, 842–43 (1984). In this case, we believe that Congress has clearly precluded the FDA from asserting jurisdiction to regulate tobacco products. Such authority is inconsistent with the intent that Congress has expressed in the FDCA's overall regulatory scheme and in the tobacco-specific legislation that it has enacted subsequent to the FDCA. . . .

The FDCA grants the FDA . . . the authority to regulate, among other items, "drugs" and "devices." See 21 U.S.C. § 321(g)-(h), 393 (1994 ed. & Supp. III). The Act defines "drug" to include "articles (other than food) intended to affect the structure or any function of the body." Id. at § 321(g)(1)(c). It defines "device," in part, as "an instrument, apparatus, implement, machine, contrivance, . . . or other similar or related article, including any component, part, or accessory, which is . . . intended to affect the structure or any function of the body." Id. at § 321(h). The Act also grants the FDA the authority to regulate so-called "combination products," which "constitute a combination of a drug, device, or biologic product." Id. at § 353(g)(1). The FDA has construed this provision as giving it the discretion to regulate combination products as drugs, as devices, or as both. . . .

The FDA determined that nicotine is a "drug" and that cigarettes and smokeless tobacco are "drug delivery devices," and therefore it had jurisdiction under the FDCA to regulate tobacco products as customarily marketed—that is, without manufacturer claims of therapeutic benefit. First, the FDA found that tobacco products "affect the structure or any function of the body" because nicotine "has significant pharmacological effects." Fed. Reg. 44,418, 44,631 (1996). Specifically, nicotine "exerts psychoactive, or mood-altering, effects on the brain" that cause and sustain addiction, have both tranquilizing and stimulating effects, and control weight. Id. at 44,631–44,632. Second, the FDA determined that these effects were "intended" under the FDCA because they "are so widely known and foreseeable that [they] may be deemed to have been intended by the manufacturers," *id.* at 44,687; consumers use tobacco products "predominantly or nearly exclusively" to obtain these effects, *id.* at 44,807; and the statements, research, and actions of manufacturers revealed that they "have 'designed' cigarettes to provide pharmacologically active doses of nicotine to consumers," *id.* at 44,849. Finally, the agency concluded that cigarettes and smokeless tobacco are "combination products" because, in addition to containing nicotine, they include device components that deliver a controlled amount of nicotine to the body, *id.* at 45,208–45,216.

Having resolved the jurisdictional question, the FDA next explained the policy justifications for its regulations, detailing the deleterious health effects associated with tobacco use. It found that tobacco consumption was "the single leading cause of preventable death in the United States." *Id.* at 44,398. . . . The agency also determined that the only way to reduce the amount of tobacco-related illness and mortality was to reduce the level of addiction, a goal that could be accomplished only by preventing children and adolescents from starting to use tobacco. . . .

Based on these findings, the FDA promulgated regulations concerning tobacco products' promotion, labeling, and accessibility to children and adolescents. . . .

[The Court analyzes the FDA's assertion of authority to regulate tobacco products, specifically the agency's construction of the statute, which is governed by *Chevron*, 467 U.S. 837 (1984). Under *Chevron*, the Court determines whether Congress has directly spoken (the expressed intent of Congress). If Congress has not spoken, the Court must respect the agency's construction of the statute so long as it is permissible. Such deference is justified because the "responsibilities for assessing the wisdom of such policy choices and resolving the struggle between competing views of the public interest are not judicial ones," *id.* at 866, and because of the agency's greater familiarity with the ever-changing facts and circumstances surrounding the subjects regulated.]

. . . We find that Congress has directly spoken to the issue here and precluded the FDA's jurisdiction to regulate tobacco products.

Viewing the FDCA as a whole, it is evident that one of the Act's core objectives is to ensure that any product regulated by the FDA is "safe" and "effective" for its intended use. . . . The Act generally requires the FDA to prevent the marketing of any drug or device where the "potential for inflicting death or physical injury is not offset by the possibility of therapeutic benefit." *United States v. Rutherford*, 442 U.S. 544, 556 (1979).

In its rulemaking proceeding, the FDA quite exhaustively documented that "tobacco products are unsafe," "dangerous," and "cause great pain and suffering from illness." 61 Fed. Reg. 44,412 (1996). . . . These findings logically imply that, if tobacco products were "devices" under the FDCA, the FDA would be required to remove them from the market. . . .

Congress, however, has foreclosed the removal of tobacco products from the market. A provision of the United States Code currently in force states that "[t]he marketing of tobacco constitutes one of the greatest basic industries of the United States with ramifying activities which directly affect interstate and foreign commerce at every point, and stable conditions therein are necessary to the general welfare." 7 U.S.C. § 1311(a). More importantly, Congress has directly addressed the problem of tobacco and health through legislation on six occasions since 1965. . . . Congress has stopped well short of ordering a ban. Instead, it has generally regulated the labeling and advertisement of tobacco products, expressly providing that it is the policy of Congress that "commerce and the national economy may be . . . protected to the maximum extent consistent with [consumers] be[ing] adequately informed about any adverse health effects." 15 U.S.C. § 1331. . . . The collective premise of these statutes is that cigarettes and smokeless tobacco will continue to be sold in the United States. A ban of tobacco products by the FDA would therefore plainly contradict congressional policy. . . .

Nonetheless, . . . the FDA found that, because of the high level of addiction among tobacco users, a ban would likely be "dangerous." 61 Fed. Reg. 44,413 (1996). In particular, current tobacco users could suffer from extreme withdrawal, the health care system and available pharmaceuticals might not be able to meet the treatment demands of those suffering from withdrawal, and a black market offering cigarettes even more dangerous than those currently sold illegally would likely develop. . . .

But the FDA's judgment that leaving tobacco products on the market "is more effective in achieving public health goals than a ban," id. at 44,398, is no substitute for the specific safety determinations required by the FDCA's various operative provisions. . . . In contrast, the FDA's conception of safety would allow the agency, with respect to each provision of the FDCA that requires the agency to determine a product's "safety" or "dangerousness," to compare the aggregate health effects of alternative administrative actions. This is a qualitatively different inquiry. Thus, although the FDA has concluded that a ban would be "dangerous," it has not concluded that tobacco products are "safe" as that term is used throughout the Act. . . .

. . . To accommodate the FDA's conception of safety, however, one must read "any probable benefit to health" to include the benefit to public health stemming from adult consumers' continued use of tobacco products, even though the reduction of tobacco use is the raison d'être of the regulations. In other words, the FDA is forced to contend that the very evil it seeks to combat is a "benefit to health." This is implausible. . . .

. . . What the FDA may not do is conclude that a drug or device cannot be used safely for any therapeutic purpose and yet, at the same time, allow that product to remain on the market. Such regulation is incompatible with the FDCA's core objective of ensuring that every drug or device is safe and effective.

Considering the FDCA as a whole, it is clear that Congress intended to exclude tobacco products from the FDA's jurisdiction. A fundamental precept of the FDCA is that any product regulated by the FDA—but not banned—must be safe for its intended use. . . . Consequently, if tobacco products were within the FDA's jurisdiction, the Act would require the FDA to remove them from the market entirely. But a ban would contradict Congress's clear intent as expressed in its more recent, tobacco-specific legislation. The inescapable conclusion is that there is no room for tobacco products within the FDCA's regulatory scheme. If they cannot be used safely for any therapeutic purpose, and yet they cannot be banned, they simply do not fit.

In determining whether Congress has spoken directly to the FDA's authority to regulate tobacco, we must also consider in greater detail the tobacco-specific legislation that Congress has enacted over the past 35 years. . . .

Congress has enacted six separate pieces of legislation since 1965 addressing
the problem of tobacco use and human health. Those statutes, among other things,
require that health warnings appear on all packages and in all print and outdoor
advertisements....

In adopting each statute, Congress has acted against the backdrop of the FDA's
consistent and repeated statements that it lacked authority under the FDCA to regulate tobacco absent claims of therapeutic benefit by the manufacturer. In fact, on
several occasions over this period, and after the health consequences of tobacco use
and nicotine's pharmacological effect had become well known, Congress considered
and rejected bills that would have granted the FDA such jurisdiction. Under these
circumstances, it is evident that Congress's tobacco-specific statutes have effectively ratified the FDA's long-held position that it lacks jurisdiction under the FDCA
to regulate tobacco products. Congress has created a distinct regulatory scheme
to address the problem of tobacco and health, and that scheme, as presently constructed, precludes any role for the FDA....

Finally, our inquiry into whether Congress has directly spoken to the precise
question at issue is shaped, at least in some measure, by the nature of the question
presented. Deference under *Chevron* to an agency's construction of a statute ... is
premised on the theory that a statute's ambiguity constitutes an implicit delegation
from Congress to the agency to fill in the statutory gaps.... Given this history and
the breadth of the authority that the FDA has asserted, we are obliged to defer not
to the agency's expansive construction of the statute, but to Congress's consistent
judgment to deny the FDA this power....

By no means do we question the seriousness of the problem that the FDA has
sought to address.... Nonetheless, no matter ... how likely the public is to hold the
Executive Branch politically accountable, an administrative agency's power to regulate in the public interest must always be grounded in a valid grant of authority from
Congress.... Reading the FDCA as a whole, as well as in conjunction with Congress's
subsequent tobacco-specific legislation, it is plain that Congress has not given the
FDA the authority that it seeks to exercise here.

.   .   .   .   .   .

To support its claim of jurisdiction, the FDA published voluminous
evidence indicating that the industry manipulated the nicotine content
of tobacco, designed cigarettes to deliver the drug to consumers, and
knew that nicotine was a highly addictive substance. The agency also
cited current statutes making it illegal to market cigarettes to children
and adolescents as it demonstrated that the industry had engaged in
a persistent campaign of advertising to young persons. Should the
Supreme Court have relied on these data to support the FDA's asserted
jurisdiction? And, from a policy perspective, has Congress shirked
its responsibility to safeguard the public's health? The Court made a
pointed reference to the fact that "Congress has persistently acted to

preclude a meaningful role for *any* administrative agency in making policy on the subject of tobacco and health" (529 U.S. at 156). Recently, however, Congress has passed a major bill that expressly grants the FDA jurisdiction to regulate tobacco products. On June 11, 2009, the Family Smoking Prevention and Tobacco Control Act was enacted by Congress, restoring the FDA authority that was invalidated in *Brown & Williamson.*

B. Separation of Powers and Nondelegation

In *Brown & Williamson,* the Supreme Court was concerned only with interpreting the statute granting the FDA regulatory power. The sole issue for the Court was whether Congress intended to grant the FDA jurisdiction to regulate tobacco products. Sometimes, however, even if the legislature does intend to delegate broad authority to administrative agencies, the courts may prohibit such delegation on constitutional grounds.

Conventionally, representative assemblies may not delegate legislative functions to the executive branch. According to the "nondelegation doctrine," policy-making functions should be undertaken by the legislative branch, on the theory that only representative assemblies are politically accountable. Thus, if the legislature does intend to empower an agency to issue rules, it must draw up clear guidelines. If the legislative grant of authority is so vague that the agency has no policy guidance, that delegation may be unconstitutional.

The nondelegation doctrine has rarely been used by the federal courts to limit agency powers. In the 1935 case of *A. L. A. Schechter Poultry Corp. v. United States,* 295 U.S. 495 (1935), the Supreme Court invoked the doctrine to invalidate New Deal–era regulations setting maximum hours and minimum wages under the National Industrial Recovery Act of 1933. However, since that time the Court has not struck down a federal regulatory program on these grounds.

In 2001 the Supreme Court decided a much-anticipated case about the allocation of authority in the modern administrative state. In *Whitman v. American Trucking Associations, Inc.,* 531 U.S. 457 (2001), the Court refused to strike down the Environmental Protection Agency (EPA) rules on air quality standards for ozone and particulate matter (developed pursuant to the Clean Air Act) when they were challenged on the basis of the nondelegation doctrine. Writing for the Court (531 U.S. at 472), Justice Antonin Scalia explained the doctrine as follows:

In a delegation challenge [at the federal level], the constitutional question is whether the statute has delegated legislative power to the agency. Article I § 1 of the Constitution vests "all legislative Powers herein granted . . . in a Congress of the United States." This text permits no delegation of those powers, and so we have repeatedly said that when Congress confers decisionmaking authority upon agencies Congress must "lay down by legislative act an intelligible principle to which the person or body authorized to [act] is directed to conform."

Justice Scalia ruled that the Clean Air Act's delegation of authority to the EPA to set national ambient air quality standards at a level "requisite to protect public health" was not an unconstitutional delegation of power. It contained an "intelligible principle" for setting air quality standards, and it was not necessary for the act to set precise upper limits for pollutants.

Even if the courts do not rigidly apply the nondelegation doctrine, they may use it as an aid to statutory construction, interpreting agency authority narrowly if the grant of rule-making power is vague. Recall the "benzene case" discussed in chapter 2, in which the Supreme Court invalidated a federal agency rule that limited benzene in the workplace to no more than one part per million parts of air. The Court reasoned that the broad congressional delegation of power did not permit the Occupational Safety and Health Administration (OSHA) to impose health standards for exceptionally low risks with inordinately high economic costs.

The nondelegation doctrine has received varying interpretations at the state level; some jurisdictions liberally permit delegation of powers, whereas others are more restrictive. In *Boreali v. Axelrod,* New York's highest court found unconstitutional a health department prohibition on smoking in public places because the legislature, not the health department, should make these "policy" choices.

BOREALI V. AXELROD*
New York Court of Appeals
Decided November 25, 1987

Judge TITONE delivered the opinion of the court.
We hold that the Public Health Council (PHC) overstepped the boundaries of its lawfully delegated authority when it promulgated a comprehensive code to govern

---

*517 N.E.2d 1350 (N.Y. Ct. App. 1987).

tobacco smoking in areas that are open to the public. While the Legislature has given the Council broad authority to promulgate regulations on matters concerning the public health, the scope of the Council's authority under its enabling statute must be deemed limited by its role as an administrative, rather than a legislative, body. In this instance, the Council usurped the latter role and thereby exceeded its legislative mandate, when, following the Legislature's inability to reach an acceptable balance, the Council weighed the concerns of nonsmokers, smokers, affected businesses and the general public and, without any legislative guidance, reached its own conclusions about the proper accommodation among those competing interests. . . .

The growing concern about the deleterious effects of tobacco smoking led our State Legislature to enact a bill in 1975 restricting smoking in certain designated areas, specifically, libraries, museums, theaters and public transportation facilities. Efforts during the same year to adopt more expansive restrictions on smoking in public areas were, however, unsuccessful. . . .

In late 1986, the PHC took action of its own. Purportedly acting pursuant to the broad grant of authority contained in its enabling statute (Public Health Law § 225[5][a]), the PHC published proposed rules, held public hearings and, in February of 1987, promulgated the final set of regulations prohibiting smoking in a wide variety of indoor areas that are open to the public, including schools, hospitals, auditoriums, food markets, stores, banks, taxicabs and limousines. . . .

. . . The only dispute is whether the challenged restrictions were properly adopted by an administrative agency acting under a general grant of authority and in the face of the Legislature's apparent inability to establish its own broad policy on the controversial problem of passive smoking. . . .

Section 225(5)(a) of the Public Health Law authorizes the PHC to "deal with any matters affecting the . . . public health." At the heart of the present case is the question of whether this broad grant of authority contravened the oft-recited principle that the legislative branch of the government cannot cede its fundamental policy-making responsibility to an administrative agency. As a related matter, we must also inquire whether, assuming the propriety of the Legislature's grant of authority, the agency exceeded the permissible scope of its mandate by using it as a basis for engaging in inherently legislative activities. While the separation of powers doctrine gives the Legislature considerable leeway in delegating its regulatory powers, enactments conferring authority on administrative agencies in broad or general terms must be interpreted in light of the limitations that the Constitution imposes.

However facially broad, a legislative grant of authority must be construed, whenever possible, so that it is no broader than that which the separation of powers doctrine permits. Even under the broadest and most open-ended of statutory mandates, an administrative agency may not use its authority as a license to correct whatever societal evils it perceives. Here, we cannot say that the broad enabling statute in issue is itself an unconstitutional delegation of legislative authority. However, we do conclude that the agency stretched that statute beyond its constitutionally valid reach when it used the statute as a basis for drafting a code embodying its own assessment of what public policy ought to be. . . .

A number of coalescing circumstances that are present in this case persuade us that the difficult-to-define line between administrative rulemaking and legislative policy-making has been transgressed. While none of these circumstances, standing alone, is sufficient to warrant the conclusion that the PHC has usurped the Legislature's prerogative, all of these circumstances, when viewed in combination, paint a portrait of an agency that has improperly assumed for itself [a range of actions] which characterizes the elected Legislature's role in our system of government.

First, while generally acting to further the laudable goal of protecting nonsmokers from the harmful effects of "passive smoking," the PHC has, in reality, constructed a regulatory scheme laden with exceptions based solely upon economic and social concerns. . . . They demonstrate the agency's own effort to weigh the goal of promoting health against its social cost and to reach a suitable compromise. . . .

Striking the proper balance among health concerns, cost and privacy interests, however, is a uniquely legislative function. While it is true that many regulatory decisions involve weighing economic and social concerns against the specific values that the regulatory agency is mandated to promote, the agency in this case has not been authorized to structure its decision making in a "cost-benefit" model and, in fact, has not been given any legislative guidelines at all for determining how the competing concerns of public health and economic cost are to be weighed. Thus, [the agency] . . . was "acting solely on [its] own ideas of sound public policy" and was therefore operating outside of its proper sphere of authority. *Picone v. Commissioner of Licenses*, 149 N.E. 336 (N.Y. 1925). This conclusion is particularly compelling here, where the focus is on administratively created exemptions rather than on rules that promote the legislatively expressed goals, since exemptions ordinarily run counter to such goals and, consequently, cannot be justified as simple implementations of legislative values.

The second, and related, consideration is that in adopting the antismoking regulations challenged here the PHC did not merely fill in the details of broad legislation describing the over-all policies to be implemented. Instead, the PHC wrote on a clean slate, creating its own comprehensive set of rules without benefit of legislative guidance. . . .

A third indicator that the PHC exceeded the scope of the authority properly delegated to it by the Legislature is the fact that the agency acted in an area in which the Legislature had repeatedly tried—and failed—to reach agreement in the face of substantial public debate and vigorous lobbying by a variety of interested factions. . . .

In summary, we conclude that while Public Health Law § 225(5)(a) is a valid delegation of regulatory authority, it cannot be construed to encompass the policy-making activity at issue here without running afoul of the constitutional separation of powers doctrine.

.   .   .   .   .

The decision in *Boreali* did not halt efforts to make public spaces in New York State smoke-free. In 1995, the Smoke-Free Air Act came into force in New York City. This local law, which banned smoking in most restaurants, was expanded to cover the city's smaller restaurants and bars in 2003. In that same year, the New York legislature passed the Clean Indoor Act, a comprehensive, statewide law that requires almost all indoor workplaces and public places (e.g., restaurants, bars, and other hospitality venues) to be smoke-free. Because these laws were passed by the legislative branch of the city and state government, they were not subjected to the nondelegation challenges at issue in *Boreali*.

II. OBLIGATIONS OF ADMINISTRATIVE AGENCIES: WHEN REGULATORY ACTION MUST BE TAKEN

Agencies enjoy a relatively wide range of discretion in promulgating and enforcing regulations under their authorizing statutes. Sometimes, however, the legislature clearly instructs an agency to regulate a particular health hazard and, in such cases, the courts may compel the agency to act to ameliorate that threat. Consider, for example, the Occupational Safety and Health Act, which provides that the secretary of labor "shall" issue an emergency occupational health standard when "workers are exposed to grave danger from exposure to substances or agents determined to be toxic or physically harmful or from new hazards," and "such [an] emergency standard is necessary to protect employees from such a danger" (29 U.S.C. § 655[c][1]). Under this provision, once the danger of exposure and the necessity of an emergency standard are established, the secretary is obligated to act regardless of other considerations.

Even when Congress has made an obligation to act clear (by using words like "shall"), agencies, for political or other reasons, sometimes act slowly or not at all. In such cases, litigation may be necessary to enforce the legislature's mandate. At times, this process may span years and may involve numerous court battles. David Vladeck (2006, 192–222), a public interest lawyer and scholar, recounts attempts to use unreasonable delay litigation to force OSHA to set a more stringent regulatory standard for ethylene oxide (EtO), a battle he describes as "the regulatory equivalent of hand-to-hand combat":

> The filing of the petition [to ask OSHA to lower the acceptable occupation exposure level of EtO to a level consistent with new scientific knowledge about the health harms of the chemical—including cancer and spontaneous miscarriage] was the signal event that triggered seven years of proceedings before OSHA, three trips to the federal courts resulting in four published opinions, a contentious congressional hearing, and almost constant behind-the-scenes maneuvering to obstruct the rule-making by the White House's Office of Management and Budget. [The battle was

eventually successful, though the seven years of delay meant that many workers continued to be exposed to unsafe levels of EtO.]

What conclusions can be drawn from the battle to regulate EtO? Perhaps most important, hospital and health care workers are better off with a full EtO standard in place. . . . Regulation can save lives and prevent harm.

Unreasonable delay litigation, a novelty when we first sued, has become a viable option in cases where agencies disregard their statutory duties. . . . Courts understandably remain cautious about granting relief in these cases to avoid upsetting an agency's prerogative to set priorities. But, as the D.C. Circuit said in [*Public Citizen Health Research Group v. Brock*, 823 F.2d 626 (D.C. Cir. 1987)], sometimes an agency's delay is so protracted and so inexplicable that it becomes necessary for a court to say that "enough is enough" and order an agency to take action by a date-certain.

A decade ago, consumer organizations petitioned the EPA to regulate greenhouse gas emissions from motor vehicles. The Clean Air Act (CAA) requires the EPA to set standards for vehicle emissions that contribute to air pollution threatening public health. (See box 4, discussing the impact of climate change on human health, and figure 7.) But the agency denied the petition in 2003, concluding that the act did not grant it authority to regulate greenhouse gas emissions and that such regulation would be unwise besides. In declining to act, the EPA emphasized the Bush administration's efforts to reduce greenhouse gas emissions through voluntary measures. The controversy reached the Supreme Court, and in 2007 the Court decided *Massachusetts v. EPA* (excerpted below). After the Court rejected the EPA's arguments, President George W. Bush promised to issue regulations, but he did not do so before leaving office. In April 2009, the Obama administration began the process that might lead to the regulation of greenhouse gases under the CAA.

MASSACHUSETTS V. EPA*
Supreme Court of the United States
Decided April 2, 2007

Justice STEVENS delivered the opinion of the Court.

On October 20, 1999, a group of 19 private organizations filed a rulemaking petition asking EPA to regulate "greenhouse gas emissions from new motor vehicles

*549 U.S. 497 (2007).

BOX 4
GREENHOUSE GASES AND HEALTH

There is broad scientific agreement that greenhouse gas emissions resulting from human activity are changing the earth's climate. From a public
health perspective, the key questions are, How will climate change affect
human health? And what can be done to minimize climate change's health
effects?

Although the precise impact is uncertain, there is little doubt that climate change will profoundly affect human health. Heat waves and extreme
weather events (e.g., floods and hurricanes) clearly cause excess mortality. Consider, for example, the 15,000 extra deaths in France during a
heat wave in August 2003. Infectious diseases will also take a large toll
in a warming world as the higher temperatures promote the proliferation
of microbes—such as salmonella and cholera—and the insects that carry
vector-borne diseases, such as malaria and dengue fever. Safe drinking
water will become scarcer, as rising sea levels contribute to the salina-
tion of water supplies. Ecosystem changes and water scarcity will in turn
impair crop, livestock, and fisheries yields, leading to food shortages (see
figure 7). These impacts will contribute to larger social, economic, and
political disruptions, further complicating the relationship between climate
change and human health and security. As the epidemiologists Anthony
J. McMichael and Rosalie Woodruff (2004, 1417) note, "Climate change is
not merely another addition to the list of environmental health hazards
each warranting separate epidemiologic study and risk management. It is
a complex global environmental hazard, with knock-on effects.... Hence
the overall risk to health is more than the aggregation of itemized disease
risks due to particular climatic factors."

under . . . the Clean Air Act." Petitioners maintained . . . that greenhouse gas emissions have significantly accelerated climate change. . . . The petition further alleged
that climate change will have serious adverse effects on human health and the
environment. . . .

On September 8, 2003, EPA entered an order denying the rulemaking petition.
The agency gave two reasons for its decision: (1) that contrary to the opinions of its
former general counsels, the Clean Air Act does not authorize EPA to issue mandatory regulations to address global climate change; and (2) that even if the agency
had the authority to set greenhouse gas emission standards, it would be unwise to
do so at this time.

In concluding that it lacked statutory authority over greenhouse gases, EPA
observed that Congress "was well aware of the global climate change issue when
it last comprehensively amended the [Clean Air Act] in 1990," yet it declined to

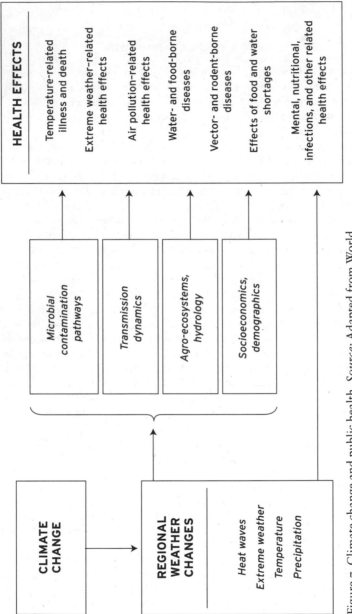

Figure 7. Climate change and public health. *Source:* Adapted from World Health Organization 2003a, 11, figure 3.1.

adopt a proposed amendment establishing binding emissions limitations. 68 Fed. Reg. 52926. Congress instead chose to authorize further investigation into climate change. EPA further reasoned that Congress' "specially tailored solutions to global atmospheric issues," *id.*, at 52926–in particular, its 1990 enactment of a comprehensive scheme to regulate pollutants that depleted the ozone layer–counseled against reading the general authorization of [the Clean Air Act] to confer regulatory authority over greenhouse gases. . . .

Even assuming that it had authority over greenhouse gases, EPA explained in detail why it would refuse to exercise that authority. The agency began by recognizing that the concentration of greenhouse gases has dramatically increased as a result of human activities, and acknowledged the attendant increase in global surface air temperatures. EPA nevertheless gave controlling importance to the NRC [National Research Council] Report's statement that a causal link between the two "cannot be unequivocally established." *Id.*, at 52930. Given that residual uncertainty, EPA concluded that regulating greenhouse gas emissions would be unwise. . . .

. . . As we have repeated time and again, an agency has broad discretion to choose how best to marshal its limited resources and personnel to carry out its delegated responsibilities. That discretion is at its height when the agency decides not to bring an enforcement action. . . . Some debate remains, however, as to the rigor with which we review an agency's denial of a petition for rulemaking. . . .

EPA concluded in its denial of the petition for rulemaking that it lacked authority . . . to regulate new vehicle emissions because carbon dioxide is not an "air pollutant" as that term is defined in [the Clean Air Act]. In the alternative, it concluded that even if it possessed authority, it would decline to do so because regulation would conflict with other administration priorities. As discussed earlier, the Clean Air Act expressly permits review of such an action. We therefore "may reverse any such action found to be . . . arbitrary, capricious, an abuse of discretion, or otherwise not in accordance with law." 42 U.S.C. § 7607(d)(9).

. . . The first question is whether . . . the Clean Air Act authorizes EPA to regulate greenhouse gas emissions from new motor vehicles in the event that it forms a "judgment" that such emissions contribute to climate change. We have little trouble concluding that it does. In relevant part, [the Act] provides that EPA "shall by regulation prescribe . . . standards applicable to the emission of any air pollutant from any class or classes of new motor vehicles or new motor vehicle engines, which in [the Administrator's] judgment cause, or contribute to, air pollution which may reasonably be anticipated to endanger public health or welfare." § 7521(a)(1). Because EPA believes that Congress did not intend it to regulate substances that contribute to climate change, the agency maintains that carbon dioxide is not an "air pollutant" within the meaning of the provision.

The statutory text forecloses EPA's reading. The Clean Air Act's sweeping definition of "air pollutant" includes "*any* air pollution agent or combination of such agents, including *any* physical, chemical . . . substance or matter which is emitted into or otherwise enters the ambient air. . . . " § 7602(g) (emphasis added). On its face, the definition embraces all airborne compounds of whatever stripe, and underscores that intent through the repeated use of the word "any." . . . The statute is unambiguous. . . .

While the Congresses that drafted [the Clean Air Act] might not have appreciated the possibility that burning fossil fuels could lead to global warming, they did
understand that without regulatory flexibility, changing circumstances and scientific developments would soon render the Clean Air Act obsolete. The broad language . . . reflects an intentional effort to confer the flexibility necessary to forestall
such obsolescence. Because greenhouse gases fit well within the Clean Air Act's
capacious definition of "air pollutant," we hold that EPA has the statutory authority
to regulate the emission of such gases from new motor vehicles.

The alternative basis for EPA's decision—that even if it does have statutory
authority to regulate greenhouse gases, it would be unwise to do so at this time—
rests on reasoning divorced from the statutory text. . . .

If EPA makes a finding of endangerment, the Clean Air Act requires the agency to
regulate emissions of the deleterious pollutant from new motor vehicles. . . . Under
the clear terms of the Clean Air Act, EPA can avoid taking further action only if
it determines that greenhouse gases do not contribute to climate change or if it
provides some reasonable explanation as to why it cannot or will not exercise its
discretion to determine whether they do. . . .

EPA has refused to comply with this clear statutory command. Instead, it has
offered a laundry list of reasons not to regulate. . . .

Although we have neither the expertise nor the authority to evaluate these policy
judgments, it is evident they have nothing to do with whether greenhouse gas emissions contribute to climate change. Still less do they amount to a reasoned justification for declining to form a scientific judgment. . . .

Nor can EPA avoid its statutory obligation by noting the uncertainty surrounding various features of climate change and concluding that it would therefore be
better not to regulate at this time. If the scientific uncertainty is so profound that it
precludes EPA from making a reasoned judgment as to whether greenhouse gases
contribute to global warming, EPA must say so. That EPA would prefer not to regulate greenhouse gases because of some residual uncertainty . . . is irrelevant. The
statutory question is whether sufficient information exists to make an endangerment finding.

In short, EPA has offered no reasoned explanation for its refusal to decide
whether greenhouse gases cause or contribute to climate change. Its action was
therefore "arbitrary, capricious . . . or otherwise not in accordance with law." . . .

The judgment of the Court of Appeals is reversed, and the case is remanded for
further proceedings consistent with this opinion.

It is so ordered.

III. DEREGULATION AND NEW GOVERNANCE THEORY

Questions concerning what agencies are legally able or obligated to
regulate are different from the underlying policy questions: What areas
of life should be regulated? How much regulation is desirable? And
how vigorously should regulations be enforced? Public health advocates see community-wide benefits to living in a well-regulated society;

from a public health perspective, the regulatory state is a key element in securing basic health and safety standards. But the free market and laissez-faire economics are powerful values in American culture and politics. Citizens sometimes see government regulation as creating costly bureaucracies that tie up tax dollars and constrain economic liberty. (Of course, when administrative agencies fail to fulfill their mandate—and when that inaction leads to highly visible food-borne disease outbreaks, mining disasters, and unacceptably dangerous pharmaceuticals—these objections typically lose their force.)

Market economists believe that regulation, if desirable at all, should redress market failures rather than restrain free enterprise. They often maintain that historical precedent supports the notion of minimal governmental intervention in the economy, asserting that the free enterprise system was the prevailing value in early America. The historian William J. Novak (1993, 1–2) disputes this claim:

> The relationship of law, state, and economy in America has been the center of legal-historical research for almost 50 years now. But basic assumptions about state regulation and economics have remained surprisingly static. First, regulation and the economy are seen as diametrical opposites. Regulation is a contrived and public interference in a field of invisible economic relations otherwise natural and private. Second, American regulation is understood as a relatively recent invention. . . .
>
> Through a historical reconstruction of 19th century notions of "public economy" and the "well-ordered market," I hope to establish the predominance in theory and practice of an approach to economic life in early America antithetical to the classical separation of market and state. [Numerous] cases, statutes, and ordinances suggest that early Americans understood the economy as simply another part of their "well-regulated society," intertwined with public safety, health, morals, and welfare and subject to the same kinds of legal controls. Far from viewing the state and the economy as adversarial, the notion of "public economy" was part of a worldview slow to separate public and private, government and society. It understood commerce, trade, and economics, like health and morals, as fundamentally public in nature, created, shaped, and regulated by the polity via public law.

Novak argues that economic regulation was deeply rooted in American life and law throughout the pre–Civil War era. The pervasiveness of regulation and the accompanying rationales steeped in a vision of a "well-regulated society" call into question later descriptions of this period as the golden age of market capitalism and individualism. (See chapter 3, which excerpts Novak's historical discussion of the police power and the regulatory state.)

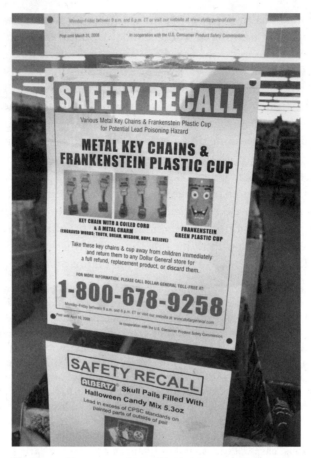

Photo 10. Signs posted in a Virginia store window
in 2007 announce safety recalls of children's toys by
the Consumer Product Safety Commission, which is
responsible for regulating such products. The toys were
potentially contaminated with lead paint. Lead is a
potent neurotoxin that is especially dangerous for children. The series of recalls led Congress to pass legislation in July 2008 banning lead and other toxins in
children's toys. Reproduced by permission, © Sonda
Dawes/The Image Works, December 2007.

In modern America, however, the regulatory state remains the subject of contention; a strong antigovernment movement favors deregulation, devolution, and privatization to dismantle the administrative state. Others have advocated in favor of a hybrid system that falls somewhere in the middle of the spectrum. They draw on the concept of "new governance," which recognizes the importance of nongovernmental stakeholders and their impact on society. The newer forms of governance advocated under this theory tend to favor market- or incentive-based regulation, negotiated rule making, self-regulation, public disclosure, and other methods that aid the agency in coordinating decisions by affected parties rather than merely selecting the regulatory scheme that it prefers. Some new governance strategies might be beneficial, achieving improved health and safety at a lower social and economic cost than pure regulation, but it is unlikely that new governance can or should replace traditional regulation for the public's health. Instead, policy makers and regulators should apply the new or traditional governance tools that are best suited to the task at hand.

While new governance and traditional regulation might complement one another, many new governance strategies have been implemented to the exclusion of effective traditional regulation. In the article excerpted below, I describe the emerging "Deregulatory State" that has come to prominence through preemption and privatization.

THE DEREGULATORY STATE*
Lawrence O. Gostin

Public health can be achieved only through collective action. Individuals acting alone cannot protect themselves from work hazards, unsafe or ineffective vaccines and pharmaceuticals, impure food and water, a polluted environment, or epidemics. Only a well-regulated society can secure the essential conditions for health. Yet in this country, successive administrations have eroded health and safety protections. The consequences include deaths in the mining industry, lead in toys, industrial solvents in toothpaste, harmful bacteria in peanut butter and spinach, and unsafe and ineffective pharmaceuticals.

The "Deregulatory State" is a result of a conservative campaign that has created and reinforced deep-seated concerns about overbearing government. The political dialogue used to describe agency action is pejorative and effective: "big government," "centralized," "top-down," and "bureaucratic." This anti-government narra-

*Reprinted from *Hastings Center Report* 38, no. 2 (March–April 2008): 10–11.

tive has set the terms of the debate about the role of government in protecting the public from market excesses and failures.

The Deregulatory State takes many subtle forms, including self-policing, so that industry discloses and corrects its own safety violations; incapacitating, so that agencies are starved of expertise and resources; devolving, so that residual regulation is focused at the local level; preempting, so that the federal government denies states the authority to protect their citizens; and privatizing, so that government functions are conducted by "for-profit" or voluntary entities.

REGULATORY VACUUMS THROUGH PREEMPTION

Congress has the power to preempt public health regulation at the state level, even if the state is acting squarely within its police powers. Federal preemption may seem like an arcane doctrine, but it has powerful consequences for the public's health and safety. The Supreme Court's preemption decisions can effectively foreclose meaningful state regulation and prevent people from turning to the courts for legal redress.... From 2001 to 2006, Congress enacted twenty-seven statutes that preempt state health, safety, and environmental policies, demonstrating the potential breadth of federal power to override state public health safeguards.

The Bush administration has vigorously advocated preemption to invalidate state public health efforts in both amicus curiae briefs and preambles to agency rules. On February 20, 2008, the Roberts Court handed the administration a victory in two major preemption cases. In *Rowe v. New Hampshire Motor Transport Association*, the Court held that a federal transportation statute preempted Maine's laws designed to prevent minors from buying cigarettes on the Internet. In *Riegel v. Medtronic, Inc.*, the Court ruled that manufacturers are immune from tort liability for medical devices . . . that received pre-market approval and meet Food and Drug Administration specifications.... In effect, the executive and judicial branches are dismantling a long-standing civil justice safety net for consumers and patients who suffer from industry misconduct left unchecked by federal and state regulations.

Outside the courtroom, multiple agencies charged with protecting public health, safety, and the environment have systematically pushed for preemption through administrative rulemaking. Federal agencies have inserted preemptory language in preambles to rules governing everything from seatbelt placement and mattress flammability to drug labeling and railroad safety. This troubling trend is made all the more worrisome by the administration's failure to provide an opportunity for public comment on the preemption language in rule preambles.

This sweeping preemption of state regulation and tort actions has created regulatory vacuums. Instead of advocating devolution or otherwise supporting state authority to protect the public's health, the federal government has consistently derailed state regulation. At the same time, it has dismantled federal safety standards, leaving a large regulatory abyss....

Thus, the public remains unprotected prospectively because the federal government both declines to regulate and suppresses state efforts to do so. And the public is unprotected retrospectively because of the Court's invalidation of state tort law. In short, the public is left to fend for itself.

TRUSTING THE PRIVATE SECTOR

Privatization, understood broadly, is the government's abdication of responsibility for health governance by assigning public functions to the private sector. It can happen directly, when the state contracts out governmental functions to industry (such as in mental health care, prisons, or child welfare services). Or it can happen indirectly, when the state withdraws financial and political support for critical agency functions, cooperates with industry in setting and enforcing standards, or simply allows companies to self-regulate.

Agency Incapacity

Government can avoid stringent regulation simply by starving agencies of funds or making them rely on industry largess for resources. The FDA offers a classic case study of how the White House and Congress can weaken a once powerful agency. The FDA is responsible for the safety of approximately 80 percent of food sold and all human drugs, vaccines, and medical devices. . . . Yet Congress has steadily either reduced funding or held it constant, even as the FDA's functions have expanded vastly. . . . The FDA's resource shortfalls have resulted in inadequate inspections, a dearth of scientists, inability to speed the development of new therapies, and neglect of food and drug imports. For example, the FDA now carries out 78 percent fewer food inspections than thirty-five years ago and inspects food manufacturers on average only once every ten years. . . . The FDA is also hampered by the lack of clear regulatory authority, organizational problems, and a scarcity of postapproval data about drugs' risks and benefits. Just as troubling, the FDA's major source of funding for drug approvals is user fees from pharmaceutical companies, which invites criticism about the agency's close relationship with industry.

Self-Policing

As part of the trend against state regulation, agencies have developed self-policing programs that shift the burden of regulatory compliance from government to industry. The Occupational Safety and Health Administration's "Voluntary Protection Program" exempts participating firms from routine inspection and eschews formal adjudication. With the virtual nonenforcement of violations under this program, industry's abysmal record of safety compliance is not surprising. OSHA has repeatedly failed to prosecute firms with a long history of safety violations, even in the face of debilitating injuries and deaths caused by employer negligence. Similarly, the Department of Veterans Affairs' "Medical Errors" program asks hospitals to self-disclose dangerous forms of malpractice, and the EPA's "Greenlights" recognizes and rewards firms for self-disclosing and correcting safety violations. But industry has only mild incentives to self-police, and researchers say they do so only if agencies increase inspections and compliance.

Self-Regulation

In an increasingly deregulated state, industry representatives, rather than government, have initiated much contemporary "regulatory" activity, [including] codes of conduct, collaborative agreements, accreditation, information disclosure, and

ratings.... Perhaps the most prominent recent illustration of self-regulation is
the decision by food and beverage manufacturers to limit sales in schools and curb
advertising to children. But more often than not, self-regulation occurs in response
to pressure by government or advocacy groups. For example, the food and beverage
industries announced their schools and advertising policies shortly after the publication of Federal Trade Commission reports highlighting their deceptive practices
and the risks of obesity. Because they are not in a position to defend themselves and
their families, members of society need the protection of the state. If the government drastically reduces regulation and enforcement and leaves core government
duties to the private sector, current and future generations will suffer. Indeed, it
was in recognition of the palpable harms of the free market that health, safety, and
environmental regimes and civil justice systems emerged. They have evolved over
a long period to work synergistically in their protective effect; the whole system is
now under serious threat.

RECOMMENDED READINGS

Limits of Administrative Power: When Can an Agency Act?

Gostin, Lawrence O. 2006. Physician-assisted suicide: A legitimate medical
    practice? *JAMA* 296: 1941–43. (Argues that *Gonzales v. Oregon* affirms
    the ability of states to regulate medical practice and that this ability may
    promote the easing of end-of-life suffering)
Sunstein, Cass R. 2006. *Chevron* step zero. *Virginia Law Review* 92: 187–
    249. (Argues that the initial question of whether *Chevron* applies is overly
    complex and must be simplified in order to broaden the *Chevron* test's use)

Obligations of Administrative Agencies: When Regulatory Action Must Be Taken

McMichael, Anthony, and Rosalie Woodruff. 2004. Climate change and risk
    to health: The risk is complex, and more than a sum of risks due to individ-
    ual climatic factors. *British Medical Journal* 329: 1416–17. (Links climate
    change and its effects on human health, and emphasizes the need for sus-
    tainable ways of living)
Vladeck, David C. 2006. Unreasonable delay, unreasonable intervention: The
    battle to force regulation of ethylene oxide. In *Administrative Law Stories*,
    ed. Peter L. Strauss, 191–226. New York: Foundation Press. (Details the
    seven-year battle to force OSHA to regulate ethylene oxide and describes
    the legal strategy of unreasonable delay litigation)

Deregulation and New Governance Theory

Freeman, Jody. 2003. Public values in an era of privatization: Extending public
    law norms through privatization. *Harvard Law Review* 116: 1285–1352.

(Argues that privatization is not a shrinking of government but a way to expand government's reach into traditionally private sectors of life)

Lobel, Orly. 2004. The renew deal: The fall of regulation and the rise of governance in contemporary legal thought. *Minnesota Law Review* 89: 262–390. (Argues that there is a sea change occurring in the legal field, as the traditional regulatory model is shifting to a framework that is based on governance)

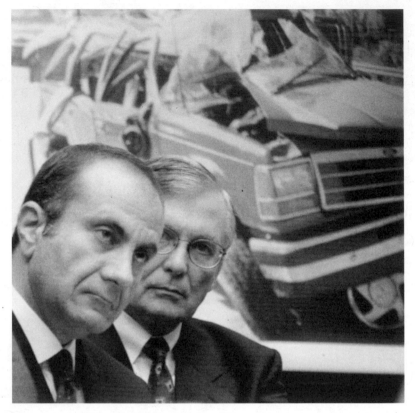

Photo 11. With a photograph of a wrecked Ford Explorer in the background, Ford Motor Company executives listen to testimony on Capitol Hill in September 2000 as part of a House committee investigation of a national recall of Firestone tires. The tires, which Ford installed on many of its Explorers, had manufacturing defects. More than 140 individuals were killed in auto accidents allegedly caused by the defective tires. Reproduced by permission, © Dennis Cook/AP/Wide World Photos, September 6, 2000.

SIX

Tort Law and the Public's Health

Indirect Regulation

When functioning well, a regulatory system prevents injury and rewards innovation. But too often there are regulatory gaps that jeopardize public safety. Since the founding of our Republic, tort liability has filled those gaps.

David C. Vladeck, 2005

The levers of public health regulation are often viewed as being in the hands of legislatures and executive agencies. However, attorneys general and private citizens possess a powerful means of indirect regulation through the tort system. Tort litigation can be an effective method for reducing the burden of injury and disease. The courts help redress harms caused by pollution, toxic substances, unsafe pharmaceuticals or vaccines, and defective or hazardous consumer products. Figure 8 provides an image of how tort law serves as a tool for reducing a variety of harms to the population's health.

The goals of tort law, though often imperfectly achieved, are frequently consistent with public health objectives. The tort system aims to hold individuals and businesses accountable for their dangerous activities, compensate persons who are harmed, deter unreasonably hazardous conduct, and encourage innovation in product design, labeling, and advertising to reduce the risk of injury or disease. Civil litigation, therefore, can provide potent incentives for people and manufacturers to engage in safer, more socially conscious behavior.

Tort law can be an effective method of advancing the public's health,

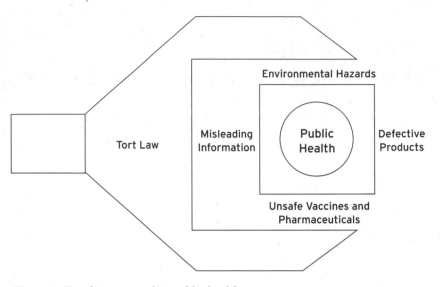

Figure 8. Tort law as a tool in public health.

but like any form of regulation, it is not an absolute good. The tort system imposes economic costs and personal burdens on individuals and businesses, including transaction expenses (e.g., court costs and attorneys' fees) and monetary awards (both compensatory and punitive). Society may not be any the poorer if tort costs make it difficult for dangerous, socially unproductive enterprises (e.g., the tobacco and firearms industries) to operate within the market. However, tort costs may be just as high for socially advantageous goods and services such as vaccines, pharmaceuticals, and medical devices. In such cases, litigation may help ensure safety and efficacy, but it also risks hampering development and production.

Tort litigation, moreover, can be seen as antidemocratic and unfair. Critics argue that the political branches of government, not the judicial branch, should set health policy. Even though redress through the courts is an important right in a constitutional democracy, some observers do not believe that judges and juries should award substantial punitive damages against manufacturers. Critics also claim that often the chief beneficiaries of the tort system are a few plaintiffs and their attorneys, rather than the entire population that has been harmed. For example, some tobacco litigation has imposed substantial penalties on manufacturers but has disproportionately rewarded a relatively small number of smokers and trial lawyers.

Litigation as a form of regulation, then, holds enormous potential for improving the public's health, but also entails economic costs and unjust distribution of benefits and burdens. As in any form of regulation, we balance the public goods resulting from civil litigation against the burdens and inequities.

This chapter takes a look at tort litigation as a tool of public health. (For those who are unfamiliar with the major theories of tort law, it will be helpful to read chapter 6 in the companion text.) First, it discusses tort law generally as a prevention strategy. Second, it explores the complex problems involving science and epidemiology in the courtroom. The courts have long struggled to determine what types of scientific evidence and "proof" should be admissible in public health litigation. Finally, the chapter examines litigation against tobacco companies, the fast-food industry, and medical device and pharmaceutical manufacturers. These cases may suggest new strategies and frameworks for addressing other sets of public health issues. However, tort litigation has its limitations as well; it may increase costs for consumers and may stifle promising research and development.

I. MAJOR THEORIES OF TORT LITIGATION

This section provides a general overview of tort litigation for the public's health and highlights the unique role of the courts in public health regulation. The fundamental questions are, how should public health policy be constructed, and by which institutions—the market, the political system (i.e., the legislative and executive branches of government), or the courts? The two brief selections, by noted public health lawyers, show the courts' unique role in public health regulation and discuss both the advantages and disadvantages of policy making by the courts. As originally published, they use specific types of cases to illustrate particular public health problems. Stephen P. Teret emphasizes air bag, cigarette, and firearm litigation; Wendy E. Parmet and Richard A. Daynard explain a matrix of the forms of legal action used in cases involving tobacco, firearms, and lead paint. Although those illustrations are largely absent from the abridged versions below, this chapter ends by providing updates on tobacco, firearm, and medical device litigation.

LITIGATING FOR THE PUBLIC HEALTH*

Stephen P. Teret

Vector control has long been one of the basic tools of public health. When it was learned that rodents, mosquitoes, and other living organisms transmitted to man the etiologic agents for disease, the public health response was to control those vectors of disease. Today, the vehicles for injury and disease are often manmade products, frequently transmitting energy as the etiologic agent of injury. The public health response should similarly be the control of these vehicles by use of the law. But unlike rodents and mosquitoes, the modern day vehicles of injury and disease have vested interests, lobbyists and political action committees that sometimes thwart effective legislative and regulatory attempts to enhance the public's health. When this happens, public health advocates have turned to the third branch of government, the judiciary, to seek relief from juries.

Product liability litigation is now being used as an effective tool for public health advocacy. Its use is based on the premise that substantial settlements and verdicts against the manufacturer of an unnecessarily dangerous product will ultimately cause that manufacturer to invest in prevention rather than pay the penalty for neglect. Manufacturers, responding to the negative effect which large damage awards have on corporate profits and insurance premiums, have recalled and redesigned formerly unsafe products, and have developed testing methods and design strategies aimed at reducing the likelihood that a new product will injure its user.

But product liability litigation, or the specter thereof, may also retard the introduction of innovative products that can be beneficial to the public's health. Some manufacturers suggest that product liability exposure is great enough to warrant the withdrawal of products from the market, even if on balance the benefit of the product to the public clearly outweighs the risk of the product to an individual. . . . Thus, product liability litigation can be seen as a double-edged sword, to be used as a tool of public health under carefully chosen circumstances, when more conventional forms of advocacy have not proven fruitful. . . .

Cars, cigarettes and guns have presented sizable problems to the public's health. Together, their annual death toll in the United States approaches half a million people. The fact that each of these products may be susceptible to product liability litigation is a reflection that jurors can find the hazards these products pose as unacceptable. Cigarettes and guns can be seen as low-benefit, high-risk products. Cars, although of great social benefit, are inadequately crashworthy with regard to foreseeable risk.

The solution to liability exposure should be the marketing of safe products. For some products, this may mean modification by the use of already existing devices such as air bags. For other products such as cigarettes, it may mean the end of manufacturing and marketing of the product altogether.

But instead of product changes, the perceived crisis of litigation has led many,

*Reprinted from *American Journal of Public Health* 76 (1986): 1027–29.

under the banner of tort reform, to propose limiting monetary recoveries for people damaged from products. Some aspects of these proposals may have merit, particularly with regard to products which are now regulated. But for those products which have been able to avoid meaningful regulation, largely due to the political strength of lobbying groups, litigation represents the only *de facto* form of safety regulation. Limitation of the ability of injured and ill persons to seek compensation from the manufacturers of guns and cigarettes, for example, would permit the continuing damage these products cause to the public's health. The crisis involved with these products is not litigation, but the terrible burden of death and disability caused by these vehicles of injury and disease.

THE NEW PUBLIC HEALTH LITIGATION*

Wendy E. Parmet and Richard A. Daynard

One of the most remarkable developments of the last three decades has been the increasing use of litigation as a public health tool. Although courts have long been called on to review matters concerning public health, historically the courtroom was seldom the forum of choice for public health enthusiasts. Instead, it was the place where those who wished to resist public health regulation, be they milk producers, bread makers, or parents who did not want their children to be vaccinated, went in the hope of limiting the authority of public health agencies. Although such litigants were usually not successful, public health had little to gain by the litigation. At best the regulation might be upheld; at worst, the right of the individual or business to refuse compliance might be proclaimed. The courtroom, in short, was a barrier that public health authorities sometimes needed to pass through on their way to protecting the public's health.

In recent years, however, the tables have turned. Increasingly, individuals and organizations concerned about public health have sought to use litigation to further their goals. In other words, courts are now being used affirmatively in an effort to make public health policy. Most notably, the tobacco control movement has pursued a litigation strategy, not simply to obtain compensation for tobacco's victims, but also to achieve a reduction in tobacco use. Likewise, groups concerned about gun violence have chosen to sue the gun industry. In similar fashion, the American Public Health Association has urged the use of litigation to hold paint manufacturers accountable for the injuries caused by lead paint. Litigation has also played a prominent role in the struggle to ensure access to health care for individuals infected with HIV....

TYPOLOGY OF PUBLIC HEALTH LITIGATION

Courts have always played a role in public health enforcement. If a public health agency ordered a warehouse with rotting food to close, the owner could go to court and seek review of the order. Similarly, if a manufacturer wanted to resist a government regulation, it could challenge that regulation in court. In the process of

*Reprinted from *Annual Review of Public Health* 21 (2000): 437–54.

deciding these cases, courts inevitably help delineate the nature and extent of public health authority. . . .

What is different today is the increasing, and sometimes dominant, role played by public health concerns. In [earlier] cases, individuals sought either to limit public health authorities or to achieve monetary relief. The affirmative protection of the public's health was not often one of the plaintiff's major goals. But in the wake of the civil rights and other law reform movements, public health advocates have increasingly turned to the courts to achieve social change. . . .

THE LITERATURE

Much of the literature analyzing the success of reform litigation has focused on litigation that [concerns] cases brought against governmental entities. One leading scholar on the impact of law reform litigation, Rosenberg (1991), has concluded that much of the constitutional reform litigation of the 1950s, 1960s, and 1970s, including the litigation surrounding *Brown v. Board of Education,* resulted in far less change than is generally believed. . . . Other scholars have suggested that reform litigation may have an even more robust effect. The work of McCann (1992) is particularly relevant to a consideration of the impact of public health litigation. McCann believes that Rosenberg has focused too heavily on the impact of judicial decisions themselves rather than on the multidimensional process of litigation. From McCann's perspective, the focus must be not simply on court decisions and their direct impact but also on the litigation process, which may have a constitutive impact and "reshape perceptions of when and how particular values are realistically actionable" (1992, 732).

Other scholars have considered the impact of product liability litigation, which often touches on questions of public health. For the most part, these scholars have used an economic perspective, asking whether such litigation is economically efficient, rather than whether it is capable of improving public health or influencing the public health agenda. Nevertheless, although these scholars have disagreed about the degree of deterrence achieved by product liability litigation, as well as its efficiency as a deterrent or compensation system, they have generally found that it creates some deterrent effect. . . .

[Ed.–The authors discuss the effectiveness of tobacco litigation.]

PUBLIC HEALTH LITIGATION AND DEMOCRATIC THEORY

A commonly made and potent criticism of litigation-centered reform movements is that they are fundamentally antidemocratic. If change is to occur in our laws, so the criticism goes, it should occur via legislation enacted by democratically accountable representatives. Situating policy development reform in the courts bypasses that political accountability in favor of less accountable judges and juries.

In public health litigation, a further related criticism may be made. In our market economy, individuals are presumed to have significant freedom as to what risks they wish to incur. To the extent that public health policies seek to reduce risks beyond the rate individuals would choose in the market, those policies may be described as inherently paternalistic and contrary to the prevailing individualistic/market ethos. When public health advocates seek to reduce those risks and achieve their aims not through legislation but via judicial decrees, they become particularly vulnerable to a charge of paternalism, for they may be seen as trying to force the public to accept what neither it nor its representatives desire. . . .

Several responses may be made to the charge that public health litigation is both antidemocratic and paternalistic. The first and narrowest is that litigation often serves to further a democratically determined policy. Even if we concede that interference with the market should be the exception rather than the norm and that such exceptions should be derived from politically accountable processes, a significant role remains for litigation. Democratically enacted laws still require interpretation and enforcement, and that often requires litigation. . . .

Another response to the antidemocratic critique recognizes that the judicial law making that defines "the common law" has long been an accepted part of our democratic polity. Indeed many public health policies in place today result from an interactive dialog between courts and legislatures. For example, the doctrine of informed consent for medical services originally emerged from litigation in which plaintiffs asked courts to build on common-law doctrines of battery. . . .

A different response goes further to explain the use of litigation not only in enforcing legislation but also in creating new public health policies. This response questions the assumption that the legislative process itself is as democratic as the antidemocratic critique assumes. As the Supreme Court recognized in the reapportionment cases of the 1960s, there are situations in which, absent judicial intervention, structural flaws in our political system prevent the popular will from being enacted as legislation.

This situation has arisen with some public health issues, owing to campaign contributions by special interests. Because these contributions flow overwhelmingly to incumbents, making credible challenges to their seats both difficult and rare, incumbents often refuse to enact serious campaign reform. What the special interests exact in return for their money is a de facto veto over legislation adverse to their interests. Contributions by the tobacco, gun, and health care industries are cases in point. . . .

There is another way in which litigation may be able to force regulation onto the legislative agenda, even if the affected special interest demurs. Litigation makes compelling drama; lawsuits grab headlines, are regularly featured on talk shows, and become part of ordinary conversation. Lawsuits can therefore thwart the desire of the special interest to restrict discussion of issues involving it to the halls of Congress, administrative agencies, and other venues where challenges to established ways of dealing with the issues are unlikely. Once the public and the media are actively engaged in the issue, the political calculus, in Congress and elsewhere, may change. In other words, litigation may be used not only to achieve judicially imposed changes but also to change the political climate in which issues of public health are debated.

At times, the information obtained via civil litigation's discovery process may play a critical role in disclosing information and educating the public about the nature and causes of health risks, thus making the political process itself more informed. In her study of tobacco litigation, Mather (1998) chronicles the vital role that litigation-induced discovery of tobacco industry documents played in shifting the attitudes of both the public and policymakers about tobacco regulation. . . .

THE EFFICIENCY AND EFFICACY OF PUBLIC HEALTH LITIGATION

One of the fundamental goals of civil litigation is the prevention of socially undesirable activities. In public health litigation . . . a key goal is deterring the injury-causing behavior of a private party. In terms of deterrence, product liability law seeks to reduce the cost of product-related injuries, whereas the partially overlapping area of toxic torts is intended to reduce the number and severity of illnesses caused by toxic substances. Product liability and toxic tort laws reduce injuries and illnesses by encouraging manufacturers and polluters either to make their products and by-products safer or to make fewer of them. The encouragement comes from their fear of having to pay large monetary damages if a jury decides they behaved irresponsibly (negligently, recklessly, fraudulently, etc.) in endangering the public. . . .

Some analysts of contemporary product liability law argue that, by awarding judgments to injured consumers, tort law may actually increase injuries by making the general public and potential plaintiffs less careful. It seems, however, extremely unlikely that many would-be reckless or even negligent drivers (or other users of consumer products) are deterred by the prospect that they or their estates may not be able to recover damages for their physical injuries or deaths. More plausible is the possibility that publicity surrounding product liability litigation may help educate the public about the dangers of hazardous products. But even if consumers do not change their behavior, product manufacturers are typically in a better position to anticipate and internalize the costs of accidents than is the consumer who may be harmed.

Other economic concerns arise from the significant transaction costs associated with litigation. In pure dollar terms, there is little doubt that litigation can be expensive. A 1984 RAND Corporation study determined that 61 cents of every dollar spent on the asbestos litigation went to lawyers' fees and expenses. The tobacco litigation has also been a costly affair. Estimates suggest that industry alone has spent at least $600 million a year on lawyers' fees. The multistate settlement reached by the attorneys general will also result in the industry's paying $500 million per year in attorneys' fees to plaintiffs' counsel for many years to come.

Several scholars have contended that the large transaction costs associated with medical malpractice litigation undermine its efficiency as a method for compensating injured patients. The question of litigation's efficiency as a compensation system, however, should not be confused with the question of whether the system can achieve adequate deterrence or public health improvements. Indeed, to some extent, the high costs of litigation can be assumed to abet public health goals because they increase the cost of accidents and add incentives to reduce injurious activities. Of course, this holds true only when the plaintiff or public health advocate can garner sufficient resources to commence and continue the litigation. . . .

There is the paradoxical concern that the very power of litigation to achieve public health goals may lead lawyers and others to forget that lawyers are not, per se, public health experts. The remedies lawyers seek and the settlements they agree to may not always constitute the optimal solution from a public health perspective. [Nevertheless,] public health litigation itself benefits immensely from the expertise and support provided by public health authorities. To the extent that such litigation is successful in the courtroom, it is often only because it has worked in harmony with the policies of public health officials. The tobacco litigation would have been far less effective than it has been were there no Surgeon General's Reports.

PUBLIC HEALTH LITIGATION AND THE NATURE OF RIGHTS

In recent years legal theorists across the political spectrum have questioned our culture's tendency to reduce issues of policy and politics to questions of legal rights. While some of these concerns focus on the capacity of legal decisions to actually effect change, an issue that has been considered previously, others focus on the nature of legal reasoning and the contours of legal doctrine and ask whether they are supportive or destructive of sound public policy and constructive political changes. Several of these concerns appear particularly pertinent to public health litigation. One set of issues relates to the strong preference in legal doctrine for viewing rights, those interests that the law protects, as negative. To a large degree, legal rights require that someone refrain from taking an action, rather than that someone or something undertake an action. Tort law, for example, will generally not hold an individual responsible for failing to come to the aid of another. . . .

CONCLUSION

Advocates for public health are increasingly going to court to advance their concerns. Such affirmative public health litigation faces formidable obstacles and cannot always achieve its aims. Nevertheless, it may play a significant role in the advancement of public health. Public health litigation may form a critical part of a political struggle to achieve a public health agenda. It may also have a powerful deterrent effect on those individuals and organizations that create risks to the public health. Finally, litigation's articulation and recognition of individual rights can serve as a necessary foundation for more fully protecting the public health.

II. SCIENTIFIC CONUNDRUMS IN MASS TORT LITIGATION: EPIDEMIOLOGY IN THE COURTROOM

Litigators using the court system as an instrument of public health advocacy inevitably confront the vexing questions of proof and causation. As Tom Christoffel and Stephen P. Teret explain, problems of proof and causation in mass tort litigation are materially different from those in traditional tort actions, such as motor vehicle accidents. If X hits Y, who then sustains an immediate injury, causality is readily established by a witness who observes the event and a medical expert who testifies that the harm resulted from the impact. But what if a product (P) or activity (A) is associated with an increased rate of harm (H) in the population? How difficult is it to marshal scientific proof that A or P caused H?

A related question is the degree of proof needed to establish causality. If epidemiologists find an association between, say, exposure to a toxic substance and an increased rate of cancer, how do we know that the substance actually caused the harm about which the plaintiffs complain? Sometimes the causative agent of a plaintiff's condition can be identified with near certainty, but it is impossible to link that agent to a specific company's product. David Ozonoff (2005) poses a hypothetical that usefully illustrates this difficulty: consider a worker exposed to asbestos insulation made by two companies, and assume that both types were used interchangeably and both companies were aware of the health risks of their product. Many years later, the worker develops mesothelioma, a cancer almost always caused by asbestos and thus clearly caused by one of the companies' products. But which one? When causation is impossible to prove, which company should be liable?

EPIDEMIOLOGY AND THE LAW: COURTS AND CONFIDENCE INTERVALS*

Tom Christoffel and Stephen P. Teret

The law, wrote Oliver Wendell Holmes, Jr. (1881, 36), "is forever adopting new principles from life at one end, and it always retains old ones from history at the other." The common law (or case law), which was Holmes's subject, is continually recreated as existing legal principles are applied or modified to fit new fact patterns. And because the law deals with real-world facts, the legal system must keep appropriately abreast with new ways of seeing and understanding the world. This means that, as science develops increasingly more sophisticated and precise means of measurement and analysis, the nation's courts must struggle to decide how much legal weight to afford the never-ending stream of new scientific insights and techniques.

Earlier in this century, courts had to decide whether polygraph readings and paternity test results should be admitted as evidence in legal proceedings. Today's legal controversies include the admissibility of such new types of scientific evidence as DNA fingerprinting. In each case, the judicial concern is one of determining if a particular area of science offers results that are valid and reliable enough to meet accepted legal standards of proof.

Epidemiology provides another example of this interaction of law and science. With the swine flu litigation of the early 1980s, epidemiological evidence began to play an increasingly prominent role in helping courts determine whether a plaintiff's disease or other harm was caused by some activity of the defendant. The increasing judicial reliance on epidemiology is dramatic. . . .

THE BASICS OF TORT LAW

The main force driving the increased use of epidemiology in the courtroom has been tort litigation. The law of torts determines when one person (or groups of per-

*Reprinted from *American Journal of Public Health* 81 (1991): 1661–66.

sons, or corporation or government) must pay compensation for civil, noncontrac-
tual wrongs caused to others. The injuries addressed by tort law include specific
types of intentionally inflicted wrongs (such as assault and battery, defamation,
and invasion of privacy), as well as injuries inflicted unintentionally through failure
to exercise the care that could be expected of an ordinarily prudent person [i.e.,
negligence]. . . .

For a claimant to succeed in a lawsuit alleging unintentional, negligent harm, four
requirements must be met. The plaintiff must prove that (1) the defendant owed the
plaintiff a duty to act in a particular way, (2) the defendant failed to fulfill that duty,
(3) the plaintiff suffered harm, and (4) the defendant's breach of duty was the *cause*
of the plaintiff's harm. The plaintiff bears the burden of demonstrating the existence
of all four elements. This need not be proven beyond a reasonable doubt, as in criminal prosecutions, but simply by a preponderance of evidence. If the plaintiff fails to
prove any one of the four required elements by this criterion, the fact that the other
elements have been satisfied will not matter; the plaintiff will lose.

TOXIC TORTS

During most of this century, tort law was concerned predominantly with injuries for
which the cause-effect association was clear-cut: a car ran into a pedestrian, a shop-
per fell on a store's slippery floor, or a baby choked on a toy with small parts. The
injury and the facts surrounding it were evident. More recently, however, tort law has
been used to seek compensation for injuries in which causation is not provable by
mere eyewitness testimony regarding a specific causal event.

At the heart of such litigation has been a new and rapidly growing area of tort law,
usually labeled "toxic torts" but perhaps more appropriately referred to as "mass-
exposure" or "environmental-injury litigation." Exposure to asbestos, toxic waste,
radiation, and pharmaceuticals have led to large numbers of lawsuits in the past 15
years. In a sense, toxic torts could be viewed as one response to the harmful health
effects resulting from the careless or irresponsible use of modern technology.

The common element linking these various lawsuits is that some activity or product of the defendant is alleged to be associated with increased rates of a particular
type of harm, and the causal relationship between the exposure and the harm is not
amenable to eyewitness testimony. Some harmful agents that have been involved in
such lawsuits are dioxin, Agent Orange, low-level radiation, contaminated groundwater, lead paint chips, tampons leading to toxic shock syndrome, asbestos, diethyl-
stilbestrol (DES), and various pharmaceuticals (including polio and flu vaccines as
well as Bendectin).

These noxious agents have several things in common: (1) all have been alleged
to cause harm to humans, (2) this harm has resulted in lawsuits, (3) the causal
connection between the agent and the specific harm has been the subject of some
specific controversy, and (4) this combination of factors has resulted in epidemiology and epidemiologists being brought into the courtroom. Whether the defendant
is selling a pharmaceutical product, is accused of contaminating groundwater, or
is responsible for the release of radioactive debris into the atmosphere, epidemiological evidence may be critical to showing that the defendant's actions are causally
associated with the plaintiff's damage.

Toxic tort lawsuits do not differ fundamentally from the more familiar motor vehicle injury and product liability lawsuits. There is a victim/plaintiff and an allegedly culpable defendant. The harmful outcome was not sought by the plaintiff. Further, in most cases, the injury was the result of exposure to some form of energy: kinetic, chemical, thermal, electrical, or ionizing radiation. . . .

With toxic tort injuries . . . there is usually a latency period between exposure and the development of noticeable harm. When harm becomes apparent decades after a toxic exposure, the documentation of a cause-effect relationship must rely on forms of proof that are new to the law. Greatly compounding this difficulty of proof is that few harms are limited to unique single-cause, single-effect connections. Most toxic tort harms can result from several causes, only one of which may involve the defendant. And the plaintiff may have been exposed to more than one noxious agent (e.g., tobacco and asbestos). Thus, it is not enough for toxic tort plaintiffs to show that factor X is capable of causing harm Y. Plaintiffs must also demonstrate that it is more likely than not that factor X caused their harm Y. The difficulty here is that, even when it is possible to demonstrate that factor X is responsible for a significant percentage of all cases of harm Y, it can rarely be proven that the harm Y suffered by a particular individual, the plaintiff, was one of the cases caused by factor X. This means that, even where it can be demonstrated that the defendant is responsible for a significant number of the cases of a particular harm, no plaintiff can prove that he or she is one of these particular cases.

A few harmful substances are closely associated with certain signature diseases, such as DES and adenocarcinoma; in such cases, the disease is known to occur rarely, if ever, absent the substance. But these cases are the exception. . . .

"REASONABLY EXCLUSIVE FACTUAL CONNECTION"

The legal system has attempted to fit toxic torts into a standard tort framework, but that has proven difficult to do. Even if it can be shown that a defendant is responsible for a doubling or tripling of the number of cases of a particular disease or other harm, it is hard for individual plaintiffs suffering from that harm to demonstrate that theirs is one of the excess cases, rather than one of the cases that would have occurred absent the defendant. . . .

Proving that the defendant had contributed a factor that is directly associated with the type of harm suffered by the plaintiff does not complete the plaintiff's case unless it can also be shown that the factor is both a necessary and sufficient cause of such harm. If the direct association is one in which the defendant's factor is (1) a sufficient but not necessary cause, (2) a necessary but not sufficient cause, or even (3) neither a necessary nor sufficient—but still a possible—cause, the problem for the court is how to deal fairly with both plaintiff and defendant. . . .

WHAT DOES THIS MEAN?

The expanding role of epidemiology in tort litigation serves to highlight an important and interesting contrast between the nature of scientific proof and of legal proof. Science is a matter of probabilities in a universe of randomness and uncertainty. From the scientist's point of view, . . . to demand certainty would be to misunderstand the nature of scientific knowledge. The legal system, on the other hand, seeks finality in the resolution of disputes. Without such finality, the legal process would be one of continual litigation and relitigation. For this reason, concepts of legal causation have favored single-cause explanations. Tort law posits a direct chain of causation, and a tort defendant's conduct is held to be a cause of a particular event if the event would not have occurred "but for" that conduct or if the conduct was a "substantial factor" in bringing the event about. . . .

The job of the court is to come to the peaceful resolution of disputes. The court does not have the luxury of awaiting further scientific studies to approach the truth; it must come to a timely decision for the benefit of the litigants and the judicial system. Certainly the court would like its decision to be based on what it understands to be the truth, but what the true facts are is often exactly what is being contested. In the end, the court must act on uncertainties to resolve the dispute.

The idea of acting on uncertainty may cause discomfort to scientists, whose discipline allows them to admit that they have not yet achieved a complete understanding of the truth and that further investigation is necessary. When the work of scientists is being used as proof in court—for example, the use of epidemiological evidence in toxic tort cases—scientists may complain that undue weight is being attributed to inconclusive findings. The misperception, however, is in thinking that the conclusion sought by the court is the same conclusion sought by the scientist. The scientist's conclusion is achieved when truth is illuminated, and the level of certainty or proof required for this is very high. The court's conclusion is achieved when the best decision, given the weight of the evidence, is made for that case and the litigants' dispute has been resolved in a socially acceptable fashion. For this, the level of certainty need not be that of the scientist. . . .

CONCLUSION

Epidemiologists need to recognize the growing involvement of their profession in complex tort litigation. . . . As a simple first step, epidemiology and the law should become a standard part of health law courses. On a more complex level, if one or two schools of public health established enough of a reputation in some of the areas being confronted by the courts in toxic tort litigation, these institutions could serve as valuable resource centers to the courts. Judges are free to pick court-appointed experts, but in the toxic tort area they most often do not know where to turn. The result is one of "hired guns" providing expertise for one or both sides of the litigation. . . . Whatever course is ultimately charted, it is clear that epidemiology and the law will be working closely together for some time to come.

. . . . .

The problems of causation discussed by Christoffel and Teret can be overcome only if the judge admits scientific evidence into the court proceedings. It therefore becomes important to understand the criteria used by the judiciary to permit its use. In *Frye v. United States*, 293 F. 1013 (D.C. Cir. 1923), a federal appeals court set a standard for the admissibility of scientific evidence that lasted for more than seventy years. *Frye*'s "general acceptance" test permitted into evidence only "a well recognized scientific principle or discovery . . . sufficiently established to have gained general acceptance in the particular field." Thus, establishing a consensus within the scientific community was crucial to the admission of expert testimony. In 1975 Congress enacted the Federal Rules of Evidence, which reflected a more liberal attitude toward the admission of evidence: "If scientific, technical or other specialized knowledge will assist the trier of fact to understand the evidence . . . a witness qualified as an expert . . . may testify." The Federal Rules favor the admission of relevant testimony, relying on the adversarial process to sort out strong from weak evidence.

After 1975, courts began to divide on whether the restrictive *Frye* test, or the permissive Federal Rules test, governed admissibility. This disagreement led to one of the most important Supreme Court cases on the admissibility of scientific evidence, *Daubert v. Merrell Dow Pharmaceuticals, Inc.*

DAUBERT V. MERRELL DOW PHARMACEUTICALS, INC.*
Supreme Court of the United States
Decided June 28, 1993

Justice BLACKMUN delivered the opinion of the Court.

[Petitioners, two minor children and their parents, alleged in their suit against Merrell Dow Pharmaceuticals, Inc., (respondent) that the children's serious birth defects had been caused by the mothers' prenatal ingestion of Bendectin, a prescription drug marketed by respondent. The district court found in favor of Merrell Dow based on a well-credentialed expert's affidavit concluding, upon reviewing the extensive published scientific literature on the subject, that maternal use of Bendectin has not been shown to be a risk factor for human birth defects. Although petitioners had responded with the testimony of eight other well-credentialed experts, who based their conclusion that Bendectin can cause birth defects on animal studies, chemical structure analyses, and the unpublished "reanalysis" of previously published human statistical studies, the court determined that this evidence did not meet the applicable "general acceptance" standard for the admission of expert testimony. The Ninth Circuit Court of Appeals agreed and affirmed, citing *Frye* for the rule that expert opinion based on a scientific technique is inadmissible unless the technique is "generally accepted" as reliable in the relevant scientific community.]

In this case we are called upon to determine the standard for admitting expert scientific testimony in a federal trial. . . .

In the 70 years since its formulation in the *Frye* case, the "general acceptance" test has been the dominant standard for determining the admissibility of novel sci-

*509 U.S. 579 (1993).

entific evidence at trial. Although under increasing attack of late, the rule continues to be followed by a majority of courts, including the Ninth Circuit.

The *Frye* test has its origin in a short and citation-free 1923 decision concerning the admissibility of evidence derived from a systolic blood pressure deception test, a crude precursor to the polygraph machine. In what has become a famous (perhaps infamous) passage, the then Court of Appeals for the District of Columbia described the device and its operation and declared:

> Just when a scientific principle or discovery crosses the line between the experimental and demonstrable stages is difficult to define. Somewhere in this twilight zone the evidential force of the principle must be recognized, and while courts will go a long way in admitting expert testimony deduced from a well-recognized scientific principle or discovery, *the thing from which the deduction is made must be sufficiently established to have gained general acceptance in the particular field in which it belongs. Frye v. United States,* 54 App. D.C. 46, 47 (1923) (emphasis added). . . .

The merits of the *Frye* test have been much debated, and scholarship on its proper scope and application is legion. Petitioners' primary attack, however, is not on the content but on the continuing authority of the rule. They contend that the *Frye* test was superseded by the adoption of the Federal Rules of Evidence. We agree.

We interpret the legislatively enacted Federal Rules of Evidence as we would any statute. Rule 402 provides the baseline: "All relevant evidence is admissible. . . . " "Relevant evidence" is defined as that which has "any tendency to make the existence of any fact that is of consequence to the determination of the action more probable or less probable than it would be without the evidence." Rule 401. The Rule's basic standard of relevance thus is a liberal one. . . .

Here there is a specific Rule that speaks to the contested issue. Rule 702, governing expert testimony, provides:

> If scientific, technical, or other specialized knowledge will assist the trier of fact to understand the evidence or to determine a fact in issue, a witness qualified as an expert by knowledge, skill, experience, training, or education, may testify thereto in the form of an opinion or otherwise.

Nothing in the text of this Rule establishes "general acceptance" as an absolute prerequisite to admissibility. Nor does respondent present any clear indication that Rule 702 or the Rules as a whole were intended to incorporate a "general acceptance" standard. The drafting history makes no mention of *Frye,* and a rigid "general acceptance" requirement would be at odds with the "liberal thrust" of the Federal Rules. . . . Given the Rules' permissive backdrop and their inclusion of a specific rule on expert testimony that does not mention "general acceptance," the assertion that the Rules somehow assimilated *Frye* is unconvincing. *Frye* made "general acceptance" the exclusive test for admitting expert scientific testimony. That austere standard, absent from, and incompatible with, the Federal Rules of Evidence, should not be applied in federal trials.

That the *Frye* test was displaced by the Rules of Evidence does not mean, however, that the Rules themselves place no limits on the admissibility of purportedly scientific evidence. Nor is the trial judge disabled from screening such evidence. To the contrary, under the Rules the trial judge must ensure that any and all scientific testimony or evidence admitted is not only relevant, but reliable.

The primary locus of this obligation is Rule 702, which clearly contemplates some degree of regulation of the subjects and theories about which an expert may testify. "If scientific, technical, or other specialized knowledge will assist the trier of fact to understand the evidence or to determine a fact in issue" an expert "may testify thereto." (Emphasis added.) The subject of an expert's testimony must be "scientific . . . knowledge." The adjective "scientific" implies a grounding in the methods and procedures of science. Similarly, the word "knowledge" connotes more than subjective belief or unsupported speculation. The term "applies to any body of known facts or to any body of ideas inferred from such facts or accepted as truths on good grounds." (*Webster's* 1986, 1252.) Of course, it would be unreasonable to conclude that the subject of scientific testimony must be "known" to a certainty; arguably, there are no certainties in science. But, in order to qualify as "scientific knowledge," an inference or assertion must be derived by the scientific method. Proposed testimony must be supported by appropriate validation—i.e., "good grounds," based on what is known. In short, the requirement that an expert's testimony pertain to "scientific knowledge" establishes a standard of evidentiary reliability.

Rule 702 further requires that the evidence or testimony "assist the trier of fact to understand the evidence or to determine a fact in issue." This condition goes primarily to relevance, [which has been described as] . . . one of "fit." "Fit" is not always obvious, and scientific validity for one purpose is not necessarily scientific validity for other, unrelated purposes. . . . Rule 702's "helpfulness" standard requires a valid scientific connection to the pertinent inquiry as a precondition to admissibility.

That these requirements are embodied in Rule 702 is not surprising. Unlike an ordinary witness, an expert is permitted wide latitude to offer opinions, including those that are not based on firsthand knowledge or observation. Presumably, this relaxation of the usual requirement of firsthand knowledge . . . is premised on an assumption that the expert's opinion will have a reliable basis in the knowledge and experience of his discipline.

Faced with a proffer of expert scientific testimony, then, the trial judge must determine at the outset, pursuant to Rule 104(a), whether the expert is proposing to testify to (1) scientific knowledge that (2) will assist the trier of fact to understand or determine a fact in issue. This entails a preliminary assessment of whether the reasoning or methodology underlying the testimony is scientifically valid and of whether that reasoning or methodology properly can be applied to the facts in issue. We are confident that federal judges possess the capacity to undertake this review. . . . Some general observations are appropriate.

Ordinarily, a key question to be answered in determining whether a theory or technique is scientific knowledge that will assist the trier of fact will be whether it can be (and has been) tested. . . .

Another pertinent consideration is whether the theory or technique has been subjected to peer review and publication. . . . Submission to the scrutiny of the scientific community is a component of "good science," in part because it increases the likelihood that substantive flaws in methodology will be detected. The fact of publication (or lack thereof) in a peer reviewed journal thus will be a relevant, though not dispositive, consideration in assessing the scientific validity of a particular technique or methodology on which an opinion is premised.

Additionally, in the case of a particular scientific technique, the court ordinarily should consider the known or potential rate of error, and the existence and maintenance of standards controlling the technique's operation.

Finally, "general acceptance" can yet have a bearing on the inquiry. A "reliability assessment does not require, although it does permit, explicit identification of a relevant scientific community and an express determination of a particular degree of acceptance within that community." *United States v. Downing*, 753 F.2d 1224, 1238 (3d Cir. 1985). Widespread acceptance can be an important factor in ruling particular evidence admissible, and "a known technique which has been able to attract only minimal support within the community," *Downing*, 753 F.2d, at 1238, may properly be viewed with skepticism. . . .

We conclude by briefly addressing what appear to be two underlying concerns of the parties and amici in this case. Respondent expresses apprehension that abandonment of "general acceptance" as the exclusive requirement for admission will result in a "free-for-all" in which befuddled juries are confounded by absurd and irrational pseudoscientific assertions. In this regard respondent seems to us to be overly pessimistic about the capabilities of the jury and of the adversary system generally. Vigorous cross-examination, presentation of contrary evidence, and careful instruction on the burden of proof are the traditional and appropriate means of attacking shaky but admissible evidence. . . .

Petitioners and, to a greater extent, their amici . . . suggest that recognition of a screening role for the judge that allows for the exclusion of "invalid" evidence will sanction a stifling and repressive scientific orthodoxy and will be inimical to the search for truth. It is true that open debate is an essential part of both legal and scientific analyses. Yet there are important differences between the quest for truth in the courtroom and the quest for truth in the laboratory. Scientific conclusions are subject to perpetual revision. Law, on the other hand, must resolve disputes finally and quickly. The scientific project is advanced by broad and wide-ranging consideration of a multitude of hypotheses, for those that are incorrect will eventually be shown to be so, and that in itself is an advance. Conjectures that are probably wrong are of little use, however, in the project of reaching a quick, final, and binding legal judgment—often of great consequence—about a particular set of events in the past. We recognize that, in practice, a gatekeeping role for the judge, no matter how flexible, inevitably on occasion will prevent the jury from learning of authentic insights and innovations. That, nevertheless, is the balance that is struck by Rules of Evidence designed not for the exhaustive search for cosmic understanding but for the particularized resolution of legal disputes. . . .

. . . The judgment of the Court of Appeals is vacated, and the case is remanded for further proceedings consistent with this opinion.

.   .   .   .   .

The Supreme Court in *Daubert* left an important issue about admissibility unclear—whether the standards of reliability and relevancy apply only to the expert's methodology or also to her conclusions. In other words, must the trial court blindly accept the anomalous conclusions of an expert who relies on valid studies? In *General Electric Co. v. Joiner,* 522 U.S. 136, 146 (1997), the Supreme Court held that the trial court could critically examine whether the experts' conclusions were supported by the studies they cite: "[C]onclusions and methodology are not entirely distinct from one another. Trained experts commonly extrapolate from existing data. But . . . a district court [is not required] to admit opinion evidence which is connected to the existing data only by the *ipse dixit* of the expert. A court may conclude that there is simply too great an analytical gap between the data and the opinion proffered." Following *Joiner,* the Supreme Court in *Kumho Tire Co., Ltd. v. Carmichael,* 526 U.S. 137 (1999), held that the *Daubert* factors apply not only to scientific experts but to all experts, including engineers. The Court reasoned that no clear line divides scientific knowledge from technical or other specialized knowledge, and there is no convincing need to make such distinctions.

The Supreme Court has progressively tightened the permissive admissibility standard in the Federal Rules, giving trial judges considerable discretion to exclude both scientific methodologies and expert opinions of all kinds that fail to meet tests of reliability and relevance. The Court itself said that the law must make certain that an expert "employs in the courtroom the same level of intellectual rigor that characterizes the practice of an expert in the relevant field" (*Kumho,* 526 U.S. at 152). But the major criticism of the *Daubert* framework is that judges do not possess adequate knowledge or scientific background to effectively assess the validity of theories and data offered by expert witnesses. Another criticism highlights the narrowing effect of *Daubert:* the Supreme Court purported to open courtroom doors to more types of scientific evidence, but the judge's new role as gatekeeper and the general guidelines offered have instead limited the evidence allowed.

Has the Court reached the right balance with respect to the admissibility of scientific evidence? Some authors claim that judges permit the introduction of scientifically unfounded evidence (so-called junk science), with the result that businesses are held liable for harms they did not create. Peter W. Huber, excerpted next, argues that trial lawyers have an incentive to introduce scientific evidence irrespective of its rigor, medical experts are willing to testify for a fee, and juries are prone to decide against defendants with deep pockets.

GALILEO'S REVENGE: JUNK SCIENCE IN THE COURTROOM*

Peter W. Huber

Ever wonder about Princess Di's recent affair with Elvis Presley? You can read all about it on the front page of the supermarket tabloid. Elsewhere on the page appear stories of bizarre accidents and fantastic misadventures. An impact with a car's steering wheel causes lung cancer. Breast cancer is triggered by a fall from a street-car, a slip in a grocery store, an exploding hot-water heater, a blow from an umbrella handle, and a bump from a can of orange juice. Cancer is aggravated, if not actually caused, by lifting a forty-pound box of cheese. Everybody knows, of course, that such stories are fiction. Falls and bumps don't cause cancer.

Other stories tell how a spermicide used with most barrier contraceptives causes birth defects. We know it doesn't. The whooping cough vaccine causes permanent brain damage and death. That's not true either. The swine flu vaccine caused "serum sickness." It didn't. A certain model of luxury car accelerates at random, even as frantic drivers stand on the brakes. Not so. Incompetence by obstetricians is a lead-ing cause of cerebral palsy. It isn't. The morning-sickness drug Bendectin caused an epidemic of birth defects. It didn't. Trace environmental pollutants cause "chemi-cally induced AIDS." They don't.

How can anybody be absolutely, positively certain about these didn'ts, doesn'ts, and don'ts? No one can. But the science that refutes these claims is about as solid as science ever is.

And yet all of these bizarre and fantastic stories—Elvis and Di excepted—are drawn not from the tabloids but from legal reports. They are announced not in smudgy, badly typed cult newsletters but in calf-bound case reports; endorsed not by starry-robed astrologers but by black-robed judges; subscribed to not only by quacks one step ahead of the authorities but by the authorities themselves. They can be found on the dusty shelves of any major law library. The cancer-by-streetcar cases are decades old, but the others are recent.

When they learn of these legal frolics, most members of the mainstream scientific community are astounded, incredulous, and exasperated in about equal measure. . . . Maverick scientists shunned by their reputable colleagues have been embraced by lawyers. Eccentric theories that no respectable government agency would ever fund are rewarded munificently by the courts. Batteries of meaningless, high-tech tests that would amount to medical malpractice or insurance fraud if administered in a clinic for treatment are administered in court with complete impunity by fringe experts hired for litigation. The pursuit of truth, the whole truth, and nothing but the truth has given way to reams of meaningless data, fearful speculation, and fantastic conjecture. Courts resound with elaborate, systematized, jargon-filled, serious-sounding deceptions that fully deserve the contemptuous label used by trial lawyers themselves: *junk science*.

Junk science is the mirror image of real science, with much of the same form but none of the same substance. There is the astronomer, on the one hand, and the

*Reprinted from *Galileo's Revenge: Junk Science in the Courtroom* by permission of Basic Books, a member of Perseus Books, L.L.C. © 1991 by Peter W. Huber.

astrologist, on the other. The chemist is paired with the alchemist, the pharmacologist with the homeopathist. Take the serious sciences of allergy and immunology, brush away the detail and rigor, and you have the junk science of clinical ecology. The orthopedic surgeon is shadowed by the osteopath, the physical therapist by the chiropractor, the mathematician by the numerologist and the cabalist. Cautious and respectable surgeons are matched by some who cut and paste with gay abandon. Further out on the surgical fringe are outright charlatans, well documented in the credulous pulp press, who claim to operate with rusty knives but no anesthesia, who prey on cancer patients so desperate they will believe a palmed chicken liver is really a human tumor. Junk science cuts across chemistry and pharmacology, medicine and engineering. It is a hodgepodge of biased data, spurious inference, and logical legerdemain, patched together by researchers whose enthusiasm for discovery and diagnosis far outstrips their skill. It is a catalog of every conceivable kind of error: data dredging, wishful thinking, truculent dogmatism, and, now and again, outright fraud.

On the legal side, junk science is matched by what might be called liability science, a speculative theory that expects lawyers, judges, and juries to search for causes at the far fringes of science and beyond. The legal establishment has adjusted rules of evidence accordingly, so that almost any self-styled scientist, no matter how strange or iconoclastic his views, will be welcome to testify in court. The same scientific questions are litigated again and again, in one courtroom after the next, so that error is almost inevitable.

Junk science is impelled through our courts by a mix of opportunity and incentive. "Let-it-all-in" legal theory creates the opportunity. The incentive is money: the prospect that the Midas-like touch of a credulous jury will now and again transform scientific dust into gold. Ironically, the law's tolerance for pseudoscientific speculation has been rationalized in the name of science itself. The open-minded traditions of science demand that every claim be taken seriously, or at least that's what many judges have reasoned. A still riper irony is that in aspiring to correct scientific and medical error everywhere else, courts have become steadily more willing to tolerate quackery on the witness stand.

Experienced lawyers now recognize that anything is possible in this kind of system. The most fantastic verdict recorded so far was worthy of a tabloid: with the backing of expert testimony from a doctor and several police department officials, a soothsayer who decided she had lost her psychic powers following a CAT scan persuaded a Philadelphia jury to award her $1 million in damages. The trial judge threw out that verdict. But scientific frauds of similar character if lesser audacity are attempted almost daily in our courts, and many succeed. Most involve real, down-to-earth tragedies like birth defects, cancer, and car accidents. Many culminate in large awards. As the now dimly remembered cancer-by-streetcar cases illustrate, junk science is not an altogether new phenomenon in the courtroom. But its recent and rapid rise is unprecedented in the history of American jurisprudence. Junk science verdicts, once rare, are now common. Never before have so many lawyers grown so wealthy peddling such ambitious reports of the science of things that aren't so.

Yet among all the many refractory problems of our modern liability system, junk science is the most insidious and the least noted. . . . If the operator of a streetcar is to be blamed for cancer, serious science should be on hand to certify the connection. But often it isn't. The rule of law has drifted away from the rule of fact.

What is to be done ... about accidents in court: how [do you] stop legions of case-hardened lawyers from attacking false causes, on behalf of false victims, on the basis of what nobody but a lawyer and his pocket expert call science[?] ...

No one would suggest that junk science should generally be banned or its practitioners silenced. Freedom of speech includes the freedom to say silly and false things, even things that mislead, miseducate, or endanger. But our cherished freedom to say what we like on the front page of the *National Enquirer* need not imply the freedom to say similar things from a witness box in the solemnity of a courtroom. ... It may be funny to see whimsical science in the astrology column next to the comics. It is considerably less funny when something masquerading as science is taken seriously in court, less funny still when millions of dollars change hands on the strength of arrant scientific nonsense, and not funny at all when such awards lead to the disappearance of valuable and perhaps even life-saving products and services.

III. THE PUBLIC HEALTH VALUE OF TORT LITIGATION

A. *The Tobacco Wars: A Case Study*

Recent lawsuits against the tobacco industry have important implications for the public's health, although opinion is divided on the nature of their impact. Some, like Stephen Sugarman (2002), a law professor, believe that the results are mixed and that the future success of these suits remains uncertain. But others champion the potential benefits of tobacco litigation. In the following excerpt, Jon S. Vernick, Lainie Rutkow, and Stephen P. Teret discuss how cases against tobacco manufacturers benefit more than just successful plaintiffs; the larger public also benefits when suits bring information about harmful industry practices into the public eye.

PUBLIC HEALTH BENEFITS OF RECENT LITIGATION AGAINST THE TOBACCO INDUSTRY*

Jon S. Vernick, Lainie Rutkow, and Stephen P. Teret

Litigation against the tobacco industry has met with mixed success. Between 1954 and 1994, private citizens filed more than 800 lawsuits against tobacco manufacturers. The tobacco companies achieved great success in court during this time by

*Reprinted from *JAMA* 298 (2007): 86–89. Copyright © 2007 American Medical Association. All rights reserved.

challenging the science that tied smoking to negative health consequences, by arguing that smokers knew they were taking a risk when they smoked, and by suggesting
that smokers' lifestyles, rather than smoking itself, contributed to their illnesses.
Only 2 courts found in favor of a private citizen, and both of these decisions were
subsequently reversed on appeal.

In the mid-1990s, however, the attorneys general of all 50 states sued several of
the major cigarette manufacturers to recoup health care and other costs incurred
by the states due to smoking-related illnesses. This litigation led to negotiations
between the 4 major tobacco companies and 46 states that resulted in the Master
Settlement Agreement (MSA) in 1997. The MSA required the states to drop any
pending litigation against the 4 companies in exchange for more than $200 billion
to be divided among the states. The MSA also included restrictions on the marketing
and advertising of tobacco products as well as provisions to limit advertising that
targeted youth. The public health benefits of the MSA have been a matter of some
controversy, however, as most states have failed to devote the majority of their
settlement to reducing tobacco consumption.

Recently, a new group of lawsuits has been brought against the industry, often
emphasizing the ways in which tobacco manufacturers have allegedly deceived consumers. Two influential cases decided in 2006 are emblematic of this latest wave of
lawsuits—Engle v. Liggett [945 So. 2d 1246 (Fla. 2006)] and United States v. Philip
Morris [449 F. Supp. 2d 1 (D.C. Cir. 2006)]. Both were widely reported as substantial
victories for the tobacco industry. But a closer examination of the decisions suggests that while they may have provided short-term victories for the industry, the
longer-term effects may well be a boon to public health. . . .

ENGLE V. LIGGETT

In May 1994, 6 individuals with smoking-related health conditions filed a lawsuit in
Florida that may significantly change tobacco litigation and how the tobacco industry does business. In this class action lawsuit against the major domestic cigarette
manufacturers, the named plaintiffs sought to represent "all United States citizens
and residents, and their survivors, who have suffered, presently suffer or have died
from diseases and medical conditions caused by their addiction to cigarettes that
contain nicotine." The case proceeded as a class action lawsuit but the class was
limited to Florida smokers.

The plaintiffs argued that they were "unable to stop smoking because they were
addicted to nicotine and, as a result, developed medical problems ranging from cancer and heart disease to colds and sore throats." They sought compensatory damages for the costs of the harm they had experienced and punitive damages to punish
what they argued was the industry's especially egregious conduct.

After a 2-year trial, the Engle jury concluded that the plaintiffs had proved that
cigarette smoking was addictive, that it caused numerous diseases, and that the
cigarette industry's conduct had given rise to liability for negligence, fraud, and
breach of the product's warranty. The jury awarded the remaining 3 class representatives $12.7 million in compensatory damages, and the class as a whole $145 billion
in punitive damages. The cigarette manufacturers appealed the ruling.

On May 21, 2003, the Florida Court of Appeals reversed the trial court's decision
to allow the case to proceed as a class action lawsuit and overturned the damages

award [*Liggett Group, Inc. v. Engle*, 853 So. 2d 434 (Fla. Dist. Ct. App. 2003)]. The plaintiffs subsequently appealed this decision to the Florida Supreme Court. In December 2006, the Florida Supreme Court issued its landmark ruling, reinstating most of the jury's findings regarding causation and liability but overturning the $145 billion punitive damages verdict. The court upheld the compensatory damages verdict for 2 plaintiffs but decided that the third plaintiff's claim had not been filed in time.

Most importantly, the Florida Supreme Court affirmed the trial court's ruling that smoking cigarettes causes numerous diseases and health conditions, including: "aortic aneurysm, . . . cerebrovascular disease, . . . chronic obstructive pulmonary disease, coronary heart disease, . . . complications of pregnancy, . . . peripheral vascular disease," and many forms of cancer. The court also agreed that "the defendants placed cigarettes on the market that were defective and unreasonably dangerous, . . . [that] nicotine in cigarettes is addictive, . . . [that] the defendants agreed to conceal or omit information regarding the health effects of cigarettes or their addictive nature, . . . [that] all of the defendants sold or supplied cigarettes that were defective, . . . and that all of the defendants were negligent" [945 So. 2d at 1277].

Regarding punitive damages, the Florida Supreme Court concluded that the $145 billion award was excessive. Therefore, entitlement to punitive damages, if any, could only be determined on a case-by-case basis in future individual lawsuits.

UNITED STATES V. PHILIP MORRIS

In 1999, the US government brought a case against the tobacco industry alleging that the companies had, over several decades, repeatedly violated the federal Racketeer Influenced and Corrupt Organizations (RICO) Act. The RICO Act applies to businesses that conspire to and then impact interstate commerce through racketeering activities. The government argued that the tobacco companies engaged in a conspiracy to deny well-established associations between smoking and multiple diseases, the association between second-hand smoke and lung cancer, and the addictive nature of nicotine. The government also alleged that cigarette manufacturers falsely claimed that "low-tar" or "light" cigarettes are less harmful, intentionally marketed tobacco products to persons younger than 21 years, and deliberately concealed evidence to prevent the public from learning about the dangers of smoking.

The government asked that the tobacco industry be prevented from using deceptive marketing practices, and sought the return of $289 billion in past profits that the industry earned through its allegedly illegal, conspiratorial activities. However, a 2005 ruling by a federal appeals court held that under the RICO Act only forward-looking remedies could be imposed on the industry, such as prohibiting future deceptive marketing [396 F.3d 1190 (D.C. Cir. 2005)].

In August 2006, Federal District Court Judge Gladys Kessler issued a 1742-page opinion in *United States v. Philip Morris*, concluding that the industry had indeed violated the RICO Act [449 F. Supp. 2d 1 (D.D.C. 2006)]. The decision proclaims that "[f]rom at least 1953 until at least 2000, each and every one of [the defendant tobacco companies] repeatedly, consistently, and vigorously—and falsely—denied the existence of any adverse health effects from smoking. Moreover, they mounted a coordinated, well-financed, sophisticated public relations campaign to attack and distort the scientific evidence demonstrating the relationship between smoking and disease, claiming that the link between the two was still an 'open question'" [*id*. at 208]. As in *Engle*, the Court's factual findings confirm that the tobacco industry knew of nicotine's addictive nature for decades but tobacco companies "endeavored to keep the extensive research and data they had accumulated out of the public domain and out of the hands of the public health community by denying that such data existed, by refusing to disclose it, and by shutting down or censoring laboratories and research projects which were investigating the mechanisms of nicotine" [*id*. at 307].

The Court used several remedies to punish the industry for its RICO violations, including an injunction that prohibits tobacco companies from using deceptive brand descriptors such as low tar and light. Tobacco companies also must issue statements about the negative health effects of smoking through retail displays and print and television media. In addition, the tobacco companies must disclose their marketing data to the government. [Activities related to defrauding the public that take place outside of the United States are not excluded—see *United States v. Philip Morris USA, Inc.*, 477 F. Supp. 2d 191, 197 (D.D.C. 2007).]

The tobacco companies immediately appealed the decision and on October 31, 2006, a federal appeals court granted a stay of Judge Kessler's decision pending that appeal. [The D.C. Circuit subsequently affirmed most portions of the trial court decision. *United States v. Philip Morris*, No. 06-5267 (D.C. Cir. 2009).]

IMPLICATIONS

When *Engle* was decided, national newspapers described the verdict as a "major legal victory," "highly favorable to cigarette makers," and as lifting "one of the biggest financial clouds over tobacco companies." Similarly, on the day the *Philip Morris* verdict was announced, a Wall Street analyst was quoted as saying, "There's nothing in this ruling that is going to hurt the profitability of the businesses."

Although neither *Engle* nor *Philip Morris* will immediately cost the tobacco industry billions of dollars in punitive damages or require the return of past profits, both cases appear to represent a substantial future threat to the industry and a corresponding potential benefit for the public's health. As a result of *Engle*, individual plaintiffs may now more successfully bring separate lawsuits against the cigarette industry. At those individual trials, the plaintiffs will not have to prove that cigarette smoking is addictive or that cigarettes cause cancer or other health problems. These issues have already been established by *Engle*. Just as important, plaintiffs need not reestablish the legal basis for liability because it will be presumed that the cigarette industry was negligent, engaged in fraud by concealment, and sold defective products.

By thereby reducing the high cost of litigation against the tobacco industry, *Engle* also should make such cases far more attractive for attorneys considering representing sick plaintiffs or their survivors. In fact, major Florida law firms have been actively soliciting clients since *Engle*. As a result, the tobacco industry may be forced to defend thousands of Florida lawsuits without being able to use its usual strategy of denying the health consequences of smoking or the addictive effects of nicotine. . . .

Philip Morris also may have an important impact on industry conduct and upcoming litigation. The opinion presents detailed factual findings documenting decades of illegal industry activity. In addition, the government can now use the tobacco industry's marketing data to monitor the industry's attempts to target youth. If the decision is upheld on appeal, cigarette makers will no longer be allowed to mislead consumers that light or low-tar cigarettes are safe. Research has demonstrated that so-called light cigarettes may encourage some persons to continue smoking but do not lower nicotine and tar intake or reduce the risk of developing smoking-related cancers. Even if *Philip Morris* is reversed on appeal, the opinion provides a roadmap for future litigation based on industry fraud, conspiracy, and misrepresentation.

Despite this markedly improved litigation environment, however, the industry is not without defenses. Each post-*Engle* Florida plaintiff will still have to prove that cigarette smoking caused his or her own illness and the amount of damages he or she experienced. In any individual lawsuit, the industry may try to demonstrate that some other factor was the likely cause of the plaintiff's illness or that the plaintiff should bear some or all of the blame. The tobacco industry has a long-standing policy of using procedural mechanisms to delay the litigation process, hoping that plaintiffs will die, tire, or simply run out of resources.

It is difficult to predict the future effects of any lawsuit. But, *Engle* and *Philip Morris* are in some respects significantly different from prior litigation efforts in that they potentially presage, by their findings, the success of future litigation. This differs sharply from the MSA, which expressly repressed future litigation. Additionally, *Engle* and *Philip Morris* may have other important effects. Publicity associated with these and other recent lawsuits, and the information they have generated, may help to further denormalize smoking and reduce the perceived legitimacy of the tobacco industry. As a result, policymakers may be more willing to seek legislation regulating the industry, such as the Family Smoking Prevention and Tobacco Control Act now pending in Congress. Similarly, the public may be more willing to support restrictions on smoking including efforts to ban smoking in indoor public places. In this changing litigation and regulatory environment, *Engle* and *Philip Morris* can have a greater public health impact than prior litigation.

Ultimately, the tobacco industry may experience an increased cost of doing business as a result of *Engle, Philip Morris,* and litigation and/or regulation likely to follow. Costs of litigation and regulation are generally passed on to consumers in the form of higher prices. Research indicates that higher prices can result in less cigarette consumption, especially among more price-sensitive young people. Therefore, if future lawsuits are more likely to be brought and to succeed as a result of *Engle* and *Philip Morris*, some of the more than 400,000 smoking-related deaths in the United States each year might be prevented.

B. Obesity

Litigation against the food industry draws on theories of liability similar to those used in the tobacco lawsuits, giving hope that obesity-related lawsuits might likewise engender certain public health benefits.

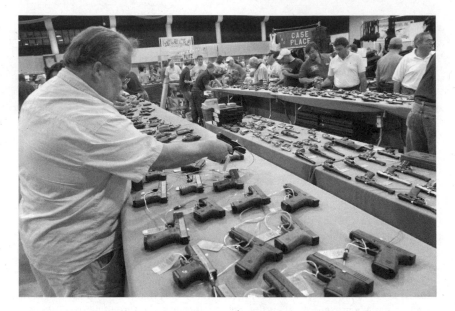

Photo 12. A potential buyer peruses the supply of handguns available at a traveling gun show in Florida. Thirty to 40 percent of American firearms sales take place privately or at gun shows, where private sellers do not have to perform the otherwise-mandatory federal background checks on potential gun purchasers. The two teens responsible for the 1999 Columbine massacre in Littleton, Colorado, purchased the guns they used at a gun show. Reproduced by permission, © Robert Wallis/Corbis, April 9, 2005.

Tobacco litigation brought the harmful effects of smoking to the public's attention, and some believe it is possible that obesity lawsuits can do the same.

It remains to be seen how successful these lawsuits will be in mirroring tobacco litigation and better protecting consumers. In approximately twenty-three states, the passage of what some call "common-sense consumption" laws has severely restricted obesity-related tort litigation. The food and drink industry, using the rhetoric of personal responsibility, continues to lobby strongly for the further adoption of such laws, which generally ban claims "arising out of weight gain, obesity, a health condition associated with weight gain or obesity, or other generally known condition allegedly caused by or allegedly likely to result from long-term consumption of food" (National Restaurant Association 2006). In 2005, federal limitations on obesity-related tort

BOX 5

FIREARMS AND TORT LITIGATION

The firearms industry was largely immunized from litigation with the 2005 passage of the Protection of Lawful Commerce in Arms Act (PLCAA). An individual may no longer bring suit against gun sellers and manufacturers for injuries from the unlawful use of a firearm, unless the suit falls under one of six narrow exceptions. Before the PLCAA was enacted, four main theories of liability were employed in firearm suits: manufacturing defects, design defects, negligent entrustment, and public nuisance.

A recent firearm case, brought under a public nuisance theory, seemed to have a chance of success. In *New York City v. Beretta*, the city sued the firearms company under the third exception to the PLCAA, alleging that the seller "knowingly violated" New York's criminal nuisance statute by marketing guns to legitimate buyers while knowing that the guns would be diverted to illegal markets and by failing to take reasonable steps to inhibit the flow of guns into illegal markets. As a result, the city alleged, "thousands of guns manufactured or distributed by defendants were used to commit crimes in the City of New York." However, in 2008 the Second Circuit dismissed the claims, ruling that the city's case did not fit the PLCAA exception, because the criminal nuisance law at issue was not adequately applicable to the purchase and sale of firearms (*New York City v. Beretta*, 524 F.3d 384 [2d Cir. 2008]).

Although the use of tort law in firearms cases no longer seems to be a viable strategy for preventing gun violence, the *Beretta* case provides an interesting example of employing tort law to promote the public's health. Other areas of litigation, such as obesity lawsuits, have taken up this challenge but their success remains to be seen, and legislation severely restricting tort actions has been passed in a number of jurisdictions.

liability were considered, but the Personal Responsibility in Food Consumption Act of 2005, commonly known as the "Cheeseburger Bill," received no vote in the Senate after its passage in the House.

At the same time, some litigation has progressed. In 2003, two teenagers suffering from obesity and poor health made headlines when they brought suit against McDonald's for false advertising and failure to disclose health risks from eating the chain's food. Their case, *Pelman v. McDonald's*, was dismissed by the district court, but plaintiffs appealed. In 2005, the Second Circuit, in the opinion excerpted below, allowed the claims to go to trial. Regardless of how the plaintiffs fare moving forward, it is unclear whether and to what extent their case will serve as a model for future litigation.

PELMAN V. MCDONALD'S CORP.*
Court of Appeals for the Second Circuit
Decided January 25, 2005

Judge RAKOFF delivered the opinion of the court.

[P]laintiffs Ashley Pelman and Jazlen Bradley, by their respective parents, . . . appeal from the dismissal of Counts I-III of their amended complaint [which allege] . . . that defendant McDonald's Corporation violated both § 349 and § 350 of the New York General Business Law. . . .

Specifically, Count I alleges that the combined effect of McDonald's various promotional representations during this period was to create the false impression that its food products were nutritionally beneficial and part of a healthy lifestyle if consumed daily. Count II alleges that McDonald's failed adequately to disclose that its use of certain additives and the manner of its food processing rendered certain of its foods substantially less healthy than represented. Count III alleges that McDonald's deceptively represented that it would provide nutritional information to its New York customers when in reality such information was not readily available at a significant number of McDonald's outlets in New York visited by the plaintiffs and others. The amended complaint further alleges that as a result of these deceptive practices, plaintiffs, who ate at McDonald's three to five times a week throughout the years in question, were "led to believe[] that [McDonald's] foods were healthy and wholesome, not as detrimental to their health as medical and scientific studies have shown, . . . [and] of a beneficial nutritional value," and that they "would not have purchased and/or consumed the Defendant's aforementioned products, in their entirety, or on such frequency but for the aforementioned alleged representations and campaigns." Finally, the amended complaint alleges that, as a result, plaintiffs have developed "obesity, diabetes, coronary heart disease, high blood pressure, elevated cholesterol intake, related cancers, and/or other detrimental and adverse health effects. . . . " [brackets and ellipses in the original]

What is missing from the amended complaint, however, is any express allegation that any plaintiff specifically relied to his/her detriment on any particular representation made in any particular McDonald's advertisement or promotional material. The district court concluded that, with one exception, the absence of such a particularized allegation of reliance warranted dismissal of the claims under § 350 of the New York General Business Law, which prohibits false advertising. As to the exception—involving McDonald's representations that its French fries and hash browns are made with 100% vegetable oil and/or are cholesterol-free—the district court found that, while the amended complaint might be read to allege implicit reliance by plaintiffs on such representations, the representations themselves were

*396 F.3d 508 (2d Cir. 2005).

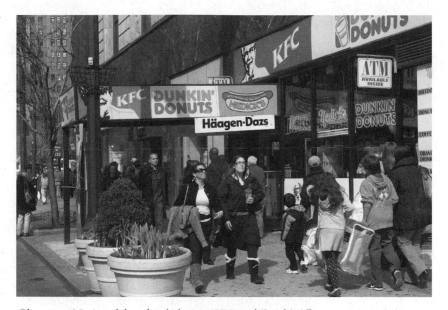

Photo 13. National fast-food chains KFC and Dunkin' Donuts are promi-
nently featured along this New York City sidewalk. The inexpensive, calorie-
dense food available at these and other fast-food outlets contributes to the
growing obesity problem in the United States. Both KFC and McDonald's
have been targeted by lawsuits stemming from the unhealthiness of their food.
Reproduced by permission, © David M. Grossman/The Image Works.

objectively nonmisleading. [Plaintiffs do not challenge the dismissal of their claims
under § 350.]

[Plaintiffs do, however,] challenge the district court's dismissal of the claims
under § 349 of the New York General Business Law, which makes unlawful "deceptive acts or practices in the conduct of any business, trade or commerce or in the
furnishing of any service in this state." Unlike a private action brought under § 350,
a private action brought under § 349 does not require proof of actual reliance.
Additionally, [because a claim of deceptive practices is not an allegation of fraud, an
action under § 349] need only meet the bare-bones notice-pleading requirements of
[the Federal Rules of Civil Procedure].

Although the district court recognized that § 349 does not require proof of reliance, the district court nonetheless dismissed the claims under § 349 because it
concluded that "plaintiffs have failed, however, to draw an adequate causal connection between their consumption of McDonald's food and their alleged injuries." 2003
WL 22052778 at *11 (S.D.N.Y. 2003). Thus, the district court found it fatal that the
complaint did not answer such questions as:

> What else did the plaintiffs eat? How much did they exercise? Is there a family
> history of the diseases which are alleged to have been caused by McDonald's

products? Without this additional information, McDonald's does not have sufficient information to determine if its foods are the cause of plaintiffs' obesity, or
if instead McDonald's foods are only a contributing factor. *Id.*

This, however, is the sort of information that is appropriately the subject of discovery, rather than what is required to satisfy the limited pleading requirements of [the
Federal Rules]. . . . So far as the § 349 claims are concerned, the amended complaint
more than meets the requirements [of the Federal Rules of Civil Procedure].

Accordingly, the district court's dismissal of those portions of Counts I–III of the
amended complaint . . . is vacated, and the case is remanded for further proceedings
consistent with this opinion.

C. Medical Devices and Drugs: Preemption

Several recent and pending cases have dramatically altered the landscape of health-related tort litigation. *Riegel v. Medtronic,* 128 S. Ct.
999 (2008), and *Warner-Lambert Co. v. Kent,* 128 S. Ct. 1168 (2008)
(both discussed in chapter 3), took up the issue of preemption of lawsuits against medical device manufacturers and pharmaceutical companies. The *Riegel* decision has effectively barred plaintiffs from suing
for injuries caused by many medical devices approved by the Food and
Drug Administration. In *Warner-Lambert,* the Court broached the
narrow question of whether a traditional tort action for injuries from
an FDA-approved drug was preempted when state law required plaintiffs to first show fraud-on-the-FDA. The Court was evenly split on the
issue, leaving the Second Circuit's decision intact. *Wyeth v. Levine,* 129
S. Ct. 1187 (2009), addressed the preemption question more broadly. In
Wyeth, the manufacturer faced a suit for failure to warn about the danger of using an "IV push" procedure for a particular antinausea drug.
The company asserted that it could not have warned more effectively,
because the federal Food, Drug, and Cosmetic Act (FDCA) forbids
changes to a drug's labeling without FDA approval. It also argued that
Congress intended drug safety determinations to be made by experts
at the FDA, not by a trial court. The Court disagreed, noting that the
FDCA permits a company to apply for a label change, and that it does
not have to wait for FDA approval to modify the labeling if it wishes
to add a warning. Further, the Court specifically noted that Congress
had the opportunity to add an express preemption provision when it
passed preemption language for medical devices, but chose not to do
so. Thus, while state law claims for failure-to-warn are preempted
for medical devices, they are still available for drugs. In the following

piece, I describe the role of tort litigation as a safety net for claims when regulation has failed to protect the public's health and safety.

THE DEREGULATORY EFFECTS OF PREEMPTING TORT LITIGATION*
Lawrence O. Gostin

Charles Riegel underwent coronary angioplasty in 1996, shortly after sustaining a myocardial infarction. Mr. Riegel's physician inserted the Evergreen balloon catheter, a medical device approved by the US Food and Drug Administration (FDA), into his patient's coronary artery in an attempt to dilate the artery, but the catheter ruptured. Mr. Riegel developed complete heart block, was placed on life support, and underwent emergency coronary artery bypass graft surgery. He sued Medtronic, the manufacturer of the device, alleging that the company was liable under New York tort law in designing, testing, inspecting, labeling, and marketing the catheter. On February 20, 2008, the Supreme Court held that the Medical Device Amendments of 1976 (MDA) bars common law claims challenging the safety or effectiveness of a medical device marketed in a form that received premarket approval from the FDA. *Riegel v. Medtronic Inc.* [128 S. Ct. 999 (2008)] has broad implications for patient safety because it removes all means of judicial recourse for most consumers injured by defective medical devices.

THE MDA AND PREEMPTION

The Federal Food, Drug, and Cosmetic Act (FDCA) has long required FDA approval for the introduction of new drugs to the market, but historically states have regulated medical devices. That changed with the enactment of the MDA in 1976 in light of the proliferation of complex devices and high-profile failures. . . . The MDA imposes various levels of FDA oversight [and] expressly preempts any state "requirement which is different from, or in addition to" MDA requirements and that "relate to the safety or effectiveness of the device." The Supreme Court interprets the MDA's preemption in a manner "substantially informed" by FDA regulations, which state that preemption occurs only when the agency has established "specific counterpart regulations" or other specific requirements applicable to that particular device. Justice Scalia, writing for the Court in *Riegel*, found that the MDA preempts Mr. Riegel's tort action because the FDA's premarket approval process establishes specific safety "requirements" and that New York's common law claims impose "different or additional requirements." . . .

Riegel v. Medtronic Inc. leaves most injured patients without a remedy because Congress has not authorized any federal products liability claims or any other type of compensation mechanism, and the Supreme Court has eliminated almost all state claims. . . . In effect, the Supreme Court is authorizing businesses to use federal patient safety legislation as a shield against state tort law designed to safeguard the public's health.

CONGRESS'S INTENT AND FDA'S POLITICAL REVERSAL

Sponsors of the MDA protested that Congress never intended to bar state tort actions. The overriding purpose of the legislation was to provide additional protection to consumers, not to withhold existing safeguards against defectively designed or labeled devices. [Through the preemption provision] Congress sought merely to ban states from implementing their own premarket approval processes, which many states had enacted in response to public revulsion over the Dalkon Shield and other high-profile medical device failures. If states imposed safety requirements that conflicted with FDA rules, the resulting regulatory confusion would thwart national policy. . . .

For 25 years, the FDA had held the view that Congress wanted federal approval and tort liability to operate simultaneously, "each providing a significant, yet distinct, layer of consumer protection" (Porter 1997, 11). The FDA reversed its position in 2004, an action that some charged was a political decision influenced by the White House, intended to give the industry protection from tort litigation. The Court's decision has the "perverse effect" of granting broad immunity "to an entire industry that, in the judgment of Congress, needed more stringent regulation" (*Medtronic v. Lohr*, 518 U.S. 470, 487 [1996]). . . .

THE INCAPACITATION OF AN AGENCY

The Supreme Court characterized the FDA premarket approval process as "rigorous," entailing an average of 1200 hours of review of a device's properties as well as of manufacturing methods and research studies. But the court's confidence that the agency has the expertise, resources, and information necessary to ensure the safety of food, drugs, and medical devices is misplaced. The FDA is responsible for the safety of approximately 80% of food sold and all human drugs, vaccines, and medical devices. . . . Yet Congress has starved the agency of funds, even as the FDA's functions have expanded vastly and public concern for the safety of foods, drugs, and medical devices has increased. . . . These resource deficits have resulted in high-profile regulatory failures involving serious safety risks of recently approved . . . anti-inflammatory drugs and type 2 diabetes medications. Litigation revealed that manufacturers might have known about these risks but did not promptly inform the FDA. The safety risks of medical devices may be higher than those for pharmaceuticals due to the more limited premarket testing of medical devices. In recent years, manufacturers have recalled defibrillators, pacemakers, heart valves, hip and knee prostheses, and heart pumps, "all of which have exacted a serious toll on patients who face the daunting prospect of removal and replacement surgery" (Vladeck 2008, 997).

Furthermore, the premarket approval process can offer, at best, only a modest assurance of long-term safety. At the time of review, the FDA may not have all the information or sufficient human resources needed to assess those data it does have. More importantly, drugs and medical devices have not been widely tested in the population, which can reveal deficiencies in safety and effectiveness that were unknown at the time of approval. Because the agency is unable to require rigorous postmarket surveillance and thereby provide critical ongoing oversight, patients are left unprotected once a device enters the market. Ideally, the FDA would have the power and resources to systematically review and monitor the safety and effectiveness of products over time. But the tort system is currently needed to fill the glaring gaps in agency oversight. . . .

TORT LAW AS A TOOL OF PUBLIC HEALTH

. . . In thinking about tort law as a tool of public health, it is important to emphasize the role of litigation in preventing risk behavior and providing incentives for safer products. State tort law provides a system of civil justice designed to compensate patients, deter unreasonably hazardous conduct, and encourage innovation in product design, packaging, labeling, and advertising. Tort law, therefore, can be seen as closing regulatory gaps in the FDA premarket approval process and providing some much-needed postmarketing surveillance.

Certainly, tort litigation is imperfect, as it can increase industry costs, discourage commercialization, or delay introduction of products onto the market. Nevertheless, the tort system offers several clear benefits for patients and the health system. Tort law assists patients who have been harmed by defective products, providing compensation for medical costs, pain, and disability. Currently there is no government compensation program for patients injured by defective drugs or medical devices similar to the childhood vaccine compensation system. Furthermore, tort law deters industry negligence and deception and encourages disclosure and innovation to improve product safety. Common law failure-to-warn claims, for example, create incentives for companies to revise their labels in light of risks that were unknown at the time of approval or risks that are greater than originally thought, thereby alerting physicians and patients to potential hazards. If corporations know they are immune from lawsuits, they may be less likely to conscientiously monitor a product's safety, disclose health hazards, and promptly recall hazardous devices from the market.

The tort system has another benefit that is not often fully recognized—through the discovery process, it can compel corporations to disclose everything they know, or reasonably should know, about the product's safety and effectiveness. Tort law, therefore, offers a backup system to uncover vital information about industry practices, as it did so successfully with tobacco litigation. The discovery process provides a "feedback loop" to the FDA, which in the past has changed its regulatory decisions in light of information revealed in court. Litigation can thus be socially and politically mobilizing by uncovering poor industry practices, drawing the attention of the public and policy makers, and driving regulatory reform.

FRAUD COMMITTED ON THE FDA

From a common sense perspective, there are deep concerns about the positions staked out by the FDA and the Supreme Court. Is it reasonable for a consumer protection agency, with the concurrence of the nation's highest court, to conclude that injured patients should be effectively barred from recourse against companies that aggressively market hazardous drugs or medical devices knowing the risks? The public might express even greater skepticism if tort immunity were granted to corporations that defraud the agency. But that may be precisely the position of the Supreme Court, which permits a corporation to use FDA approval as a shield against litigation even if it deceived the agency into granting that approval.

... Arguably, fraud should vitiate any protection the industry could gain from FDA approval. Certainly, the FDA has the power to punish fraud against the agency, but that still leaves injured patients without a remedy or compensation for their injuries. In the post-*Riegel* world, moreover, lawsuits likely will be dismissed before plaintiffs' lawyers can use discovery to prove manufacturers deceived the FDA by providing false information or withholding relevant information. The prospect of less discovery is also concerning because the agency is increasingly reliant on the industry's own data and analysis throughout the regulatory process. Notably, for pharmaceuticals, the FDA already relies on industry user fees to fund the agency's review.

In *Warner-Lambert Co. v. Kent,* announced weeks after *Riegel,* the Supreme Court was asked to determine whether a state products liability statute that creates a "safe harbor" from liability for FDA-approved drugs, but that carves out an exception for fraud, was also preempted. The Court was deadlocked in a 4-to-4 vote, which does not create a precedent. The tied vote had the effect of upholding the Second Circuit decision, allowing the suit to proceed because the tort claims "depend primarily on traditional and preexisting tort sources, not at all on fraud-on-the-FDA cause of action" (*Desiano v. Warner-Lambert & Co.,* 467 F.3d 85, 98 [2d Cir. 2006]). Chief Justice Roberts did not participate in the Court's decision, leaving open the possibility that if the issue comes back before the Court, it could be decided in favor of preemption.

THE FUTURE OF TORT LITIGATION

Following *Riegel,* the courts immediately began considering whether to dismiss thousands of claims against medical device manufacturers, involving products ranging from heart valves, artificial hips, spinal disks, and defibrillators to drug-coated heart stents and stimulators to control pain. To avoid dismissal, plaintiffs' lawyers will have to claim that a device was made improperly, in violation of FDA specifications—a so-called manufacturing as opposed to a "design" defect. Going forward, the FDA reviews dozens, if not hundreds, of new devices annually, which could receive protection against liability. The FDA is even more extensively involved in pharmaceutical approvals. If the courts were to grant drugs the same liability protections offered to medical devices, it would have more systemic effects on the health care system.

The MDA preempts state law that conflicts with federal safety requirements, but the FDCA, which regulates pharmaceuticals, has no express preemption clause. During its 2008-2009 term, the Supreme Court will hear *Wyeth v. Levine,* asking whether the FDCA impliedly preempts state products liability claims against pharmaceutical manufacturers....

The FDA is urging the Supreme Court to preempt stronger state regulation of pharmaceuticals. If the FDA's view were to prevail, patients would have no safety net in the likely event that the agency fails to detect and correct safety hazards. After all, there are 11000 FDA-regulated drugs, with nearly 100 more approved each year, making it virtually impossible to monitor comprehensively the performance of all drugs on the market....

In the end, the public is caught in a catch-22. At the same time the FDA is widely perceived as ineffectual and the hazards of widely used drugs and devices are revealed, the Supreme Court is making it more difficult for patients to discover wrongdoing, even fraud, and to be fairly compensated for their avoidable injuries.

D. Limitations of Tort Law: Economic and Social Costs

Although tort litigation can benefit the public's health, legislation and recent court decisions have limited the availability of this tool. Suits against firearm manufacturers are largely preempted by the Protection of Lawful Commerce in Arms Act (PLCAA), and a number of states now have "commonsense consumption" laws that bar obesity lawsuits. After the *Riegel* decision, it will be exceedingly difficult to bring medical device claims, though the Court allowed similar claims for pharmaceuticals to go forward in *Wyeth*.

While these and other limitations may thwart beneficial public health litigation, some restrictions may be warranted to take into account litigation's economic and social costs. The monetary damages generated by tort litigation create a ripple effect, and improving safety may increase production costs. This added cost is passed along to consumers, who must spend more to purchase the goods and services, or to the employees, who may receive fewer benefits or lower wages, or to both. If costs are high enough, funds for research and development may be cut, and fewer new products or drugs will make it to market. Of course, this is the desired result when the products concerned—such as tobacco and firearms—are inherently dangerous. But in other areas (e.g., vaccines), such an outcome is potentially troubling.

Tort litigation provides injured plaintiffs with an avenue of recourse, and may provide benefits to society as a whole. However, innovative models have been proposed to maximize the public health benefits of litigation and equitably balance the needs of injured plaintiffs and society's broader interests. For example, the National Vaccine Injury Compensation Program provides a no-fault alternative to traditional tort litigation for certain individuals harmed by vaccinations. Another suggestion, which is advocated by David Studdert, Michelle Mello, and Troyen Brennan (2003), is to adopt a medical monitoring system, a court-ordered program that would provide diagnostic tests for early detection of illness in individuals exposed to potentially harmful drugs. Both of these may be viable options to meet the twin goals of injury compensation and improved public health.

RECOMMENDED READINGS

Major Theories of Tort Litigation

Jacobson, Peter D., and Soheil Soliman. 2002. Litigation as public health policy: Theory or reality? *Journal of Law, Medicine & Ethics* 30: 224–38. (Discusses whether public health litigation has influenced policy and if litigation is a viable strategy for effecting policy change)

Vladeck, David C. 2005. Preemption and regulatory failure. *Pepperdine Law Review* 33: 95–97. (Discusses preemption and the role that the executive and judiciary branches play in ensuring consumer safety)

Scientific Conundrums in Mass Tort Litigation: Epidemiology in the Courtroom

Heinzerling, Lisa. 2006. Doubting *Daubert. Journal of Law and Policy* 14: 65–83. (Argues that *Daubert* has effectively narrowed rather than expanded the range of expert evidence allowed at trial)

Ozonoff, David. 2005. Legal causation and responsibility for causing harm. *American Journal of Public Health* 95 (S1): S35–S38. (Highlights the difficulty in determining causation)

The Public Health Value of Tort Litigation

Alderman, Jess, and Richard A. Daynard. 2006. Applying lessons from tobacco litigation to obesity lawsuits. *American Journal of Preventive Medicine* 30: 82–88. (Discusses the likelihood of tobacco litigation strategies being successfully employed in the context of obesity litigation)

Feldman, Eric A., and Ronald Bayer. 2004. *Unfiltered: Conflicts over Tobacco Policy and Public Health.* Cambridge, MA: Harvard Univ. Press. (Provides an overview and a comparison of tobacco policy in eight countries)

Gostin, Lawrence O. 2007. Law as a tool to facilitate healthier lifestyles and prevent obesity. *JAMA* 297: 87–90. (Explains how legal tools such as disclosure, taxation, and surveillance can be employed to combat obesity and promote healthful eating)

Kessler, David A., and David C. Vladeck. 2008. A critical examination of the FDA's efforts to preempt failure-to-warn claims. *Georgetown Law Journal* 96: 461–95. (Argues that the FDA's push for preemption of failure-to-warn claims threatens public health, because litigation can play an important role in product safety)

Mello, Michelle, David Studdert, and Troyen A. Brennan. 2006. Obesity—the new frontier of health law. *New England Journal of Medicine* 354: 2601–10. (Reviews the potential for a regulatory framework to combat obesity)

Rabin, Robert. 1992. A socio-legal history of the tobacco tort litigation. *Stan-*

ford Law Review 44: 853–78. (Surveys the rise of tobacco lawsuits in the late 1950s and the subsequent waves of litigation that have followed)

Studdert, David, Michelle Mello, and Troyen Brennan. 2003. Medical monitoring for pharmaceutical injuries. *JAMA* 289: 889–94. (Proposes a medical monitoring system as a method of addressing adverse health effects in tort law claims)

Sugarman, Stephen. 2002. Mixed results from recent United States tobacco litigation. *Tort Law Review* 10: 94–126. Available at www.law.berkeley.edu/faculty/sugarmans/#Tobacco. (Argues that the outcomes of recent tobacco cases portend limited future success in this type of litigation)

Sugarman, Stephen, and Nirit Sandman. 2007. Fighting childhood obesity through performance-based regulation of the food industry. *Duke Law Review* 56: 1403–90. (Promotes performance-based regulation, similar to the "No Child Left Behind" framework, for food and drink manufacturers to help lower rates of obesity in children)

Vernick, Jon S., Jason W. Sapsin, Stephen P. Teret, and Julie Samia Mair. 2004. How litigation can promote product safety. *Journal of Law, Medicine & Ethics* 32: 551–55. (Explores how litigation can serve the goal of reducing product-related injuries)

Weeks, Elizabeth A. 2007. Beyond compensation: Using torts to promote public health. *Journal of Health Care Law and Policy* 10: 27–59. (Examines the overlap between the fields of tort law and public health, including theories of tort law and product liability)

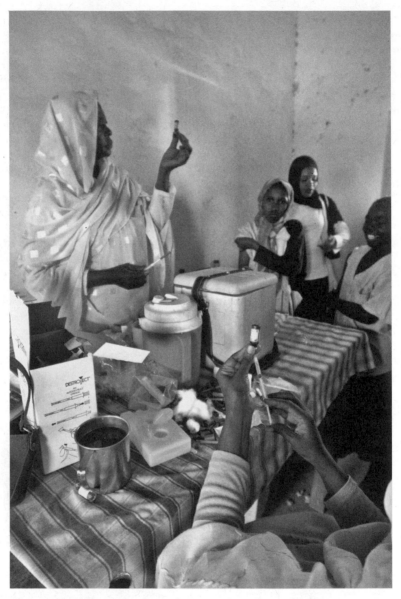

Photo 14. Health workers prepare measles vaccines and vitamin A supplements at a school in South Darfur, Sudan, as part of a 2004 vaccination program launched by the WHO, UNICEF, and the Sudanese Ministry of Health. The program aimed to vaccinate 2.26 million children against measles and to supply children under the age of five with vitamin A supplements. Reproduced by permission, © Christine Nesbitt/africanpictures .net/The Image Works, June 5, 2004.

SEVEN

Global Health Law

Health in a Global Community

Consider three children: one African, one south Asian,
and one European. At birth each, representing the average
for their [region], has life expectancy of less than 50 years.
The African and south Asian figures come from 1970,
the European figure from 1901. Over the past century,
life expectancy for the European child increased by about
30 years, and is still rising. Between 1970 and 2000, the
south Asian child's life expectancy rose by 13 years, whereas
for the child in sub-Saharan Africa, during the same period,
life expectancy rose by 4 months.

> Michael Marmot, on behalf of the Commission on
> Social Determinants of Health, 2007

Scholars view public health law primarily as a domestic field of study.
And constitutional, statutory, administrative, and tort law affecting
the public's health undoubtedly is found mainly at the federal, state,
and local levels. But neither the legal system nor the health system operates in isolation. The forces of globalization heavily influence both,
propelling pathogens, and even behaviors and lifestyles, across national
frontiers. No state, acting alone, can ensure the conditions that will
guarantee the health of its population. This has always been true, but
never as obviously as in today's world. Travel and migration, dense
settlements in urban areas, crowding together of people and livestock,
trade in goods and services, and the dissemination of information and
ideas mean that, more than ever, health is a transnational concern
requiring effective global governance.

This chapter examines the contours of one of the most important
contemporary developments in public international law, an emerging

field called "global health law." The readings in this chapter expand on each of the concepts in the following definition: Global health law is a field that encompasses the legal norms, processes, and institutions needed to create the conditions for people throughout the world to attain the highest possible level of physical and mental health. The field seeks to facilitate health-promoting behavior among the key actors that significantly influence the public's health, including international organizations, governments, businesses, foundations, the media, and civil society. The mechanisms of global health law should stimulate investment in research and development, mobilize resources, set priorities, coordinate activities, monitor progress, create incentives, and enforce standards. Study of the field should be guided by the overarching value of social justice, which requires equitable distribution of health services, particularly to benefit the world's poorest populations.

The domain of global health law is primarily concerned with (1) formal sources of public international law, including, for example, treaties establishing the authority and responsibility of states for the health of their populations and the duties of international cooperation, and (2) formal subjects of international law, including states, individuals, and public international organizations. However, to be an effective global health governance strategy, global health law must evolve beyond these traditional confines. It must foster more effective collective global health action among governments, businesses, civil society, and other actors. Accordingly, my definition of global health law is prescriptive as well as descriptive: it sets out the sort of international legal framework that is needed, but still unavailable, to empower the world community to advance global health in accordance with the value of social justice. Of course, like any legal system, international law tends to evolve slowly in response to developments within the community that creates it and is subject to it. Considerable change in the nature of international law has taken place, for example, as a result of the recognition in the twentieth century of universal human rights. Consequently, the evolution of international law envisioned in this concept of global health law is consistent with the progressive, historical development of international law.

My definition of global health law captures five salient features: namely, its *mission*—ensuring the essential conditions for the public's health; its *key participants*—states, international organizations, private and charitable organizations, and civil society; its *sources*—public international law; its *structure*—innovative mechanisms for global health governance; and its *moral foundations*—the values of social justice, which call for fair distribution of health benefits to the world's most impoverished and least healthy populations.

The mission of global health law is to ensure the conditions necessary for the highest possible level of physical and mental health worldwide. To make a difference for the world's population, the international community should focus on what I call "basic survival needs" (see the final excerpt in this chapter). Basic survival needs focus attention on the major determinants of health—in particular, functioning health systems, sanitation, clean water, uncontaminated food, safe products and services, and access to essential vaccines and pharmaceuticals. My definition posits that legal norms, processes, and institutions can help create the conditions in which people can be healthy.

The key participants in a system of global health governance are the public and private sectors, together with civil society. National governments undoubtedly have, and will continue to have, primary authority and responsibility for the health of their people. However, multiple non-state actors increasingly affect the public's health nationally and internationally. Public international organizations such as the World Health Organization (WHO), the United Nations Development Programme (UNDP), UNICEF (the United Nations Children's Fund), and the World Bank set standards, issue guidance, provide technical assistance, and make loans. Charitable organizations such as the Gates Foundation and Clinton Global Initiative, together with public/private partnerships such as the Global Fund to Fight AIDS, Tuberculosis and Malaria and the International Finance Facility for Immunization, provide resources for research and development, prevention, and treatment; nongovernmental organizations such as Médecins Sans Frontières and Oxfam afford services on the ground; media outlets such as CNN, the BBC, and Al Jazeera influence public perceptions and behaviors; and civil society organizations such as those working on AIDS, mental health, and disability rights offer support and campaign for health reforms.

This chapter proceeds in five sections; its length and the breadth of its topics reflect the broad scope of law in a transnational context. The selections first set forth the global dimensions of health, making clear that globalization is a force that facilitates the spread of infectious and chronic diseases across national borders. Second, the readings examine the growing literature on global health governance, detailing how international law, processes, and institutions can influence health-promoting behavior by a diverse array of stakeholders. Here, the readings discuss the two most important legal instruments in international public health law: the International Health Regulations (IHR) and the Framework Convention on Tobacco Control (FCTC). The next sections examine two bodies of international law that deeply influence global health—human rights and trade law. Human rights law safeguards civil and political rights, but also places duties on states to fulfill social, cultural, and economic rights. The key socioeconomic right for our purposes is the right to health. World trade law governs such important areas as intellectual property (affecting products including vaccines, pharmaceuticals, and medical devices), sanitary and phytosanitary measures (affecting food), and trade in goods (including hazardous products) and services (health care providers). The chapter concludes with a discussion of the future of global health governance, where I make a proposal for an innovative mechanism to facilitate global cooperation—the Framework Convention on Global Health.

I. THE GLOBAL DIMENSIONS OF HEALTH

Many millions of African children and adults die of
malnutrition, pneumonia, motor vehicle accidents
and other largely preventable, if not headline-
grabbing, conditions. One-fifth of all global deaths
from diarrhea occur in just three African countries—
Congo, Ethiopia and Nigeria—that have relatively
low HIV prevalence. Yet this condition, which is not
particularly difficult to cure or prevent, gets scant
attention from the donors that invest nearly $1 billion
annually on AIDS programs in those countries.
    Daniel Halperin, Harvard School of Public Health, 2008

A. Globalization and the Spread of Infectious Diseases: Man-Made and Controllable

The causes of ill health are undeniably global in scope, and thus no state or region acting in isolation can adequately ensure its population's health. The forces of globalization allow infectious diseases to mutate and spread across populations and boundaries. Global climate change creates fertile conditions for the propagation of disease vectors and carriers, such as insects and rodents, and threatens the global food supply (see box 4 and figure 7 in chapter 5). International commerce exposes consumers to the risks of contaminated food, drugs, and consumer products, as imports of toys, toothpaste, and vegetables illustrate.

Global marketing by tobacco companies and food industry conglomerates molds population preferences, fueling tobacco consumption and modifying eating habits across cultures. Bioterrorism is also an omnipresent threat, as individuals and groups intent on political destabilization work to inflict harm on a global scale. These human activities, and many more, have profound health consequences for people everywhere. Members of the world community are interdependent, and they rely on one another for health security.

In the first of a two-part *JAMA* series on global health, I explain why the world's rich should care about the poorest among us. Rich states have a narrow self-interest in helping developing countries because doing so can prevent the transnational spread of infectious diseases; they have an "enlightened" self-interest because poor health contributes to economic decline and political instability; and they have an ethical obligation to ameliorate needless suffering because health is a universal human aspiration and a basic human need.

WHY RICH COUNTRIES SHOULD CARE ABOUT THE WORLD'S LEAST HEALTHY PEOPLE*
Lawrence O. Gostin

Why should rich countries care about the world's least healthy people? ... Rich countries should care because global health serves their national interests, and helping the most disadvantaged is ethically the right thing to do. If international health assistance were structured in a way that was scalable (sufficient to meet deep needs) and sustainable (to create enduring solutions), it would have a dramatic influence on the life prospects of the world's poorest populations.

NATIONAL INTERESTS IN GLOBAL HEALTH

Governments have no choice but to pay close attention to health hazards beyond their borders. [No country can insulate itself from the health effects of people congregating and traveling, living in close proximity to animals, polluting the environment, and relying on overtaxed health systems. The world's communities are interdependent and reliant on one another for health security.] More than 30 infectious diseases have emerged during the last 2 to 3 decades, ranging from hemorrhagic fevers ... to West Nile virus and monkeypox. Vastly increased international trade in fruits, vegetables, meats, and eggs has resulted in major outbreaks of food-borne infections. . . .

Beyond narrow self-interest, are there broader, "enlightened" interests in global health? There is a strong case that a forward-looking foreign policy would seek to redress extremely poor health in the world's most impoverished regions. Epidemic disease dampens tourism, trade, and commerce. . . . Animal diseases [have] severe economic repercussions such as mass cullings of animals and trade bans. Massive economic disruption would ensue from a pandemic of human influenza, with a projected loss of 3% to 6% in global gross domestic product.

In regions with extremely poor health, economic decline is almost inevitable. . . . The World Bank estimates that AIDS has reduced gross domestic product nearly 20% in the most affected countries. AIDS, of course, is only 1 disease in countries experiencing multiple epidemics, starvation and poverty, and regional conflicts.

Countries with extremely poor health become unreliable trading partners without the capacity to develop and export products and natural resources, pay for essential vaccines and medicines, and repay debt. Countries with unhealthy populations require increased financial aid and humanitarian assistance. In short, a foreign policy that seeks to ameliorate health threats in poor countries can benefit the public and private sectors in developed as well as developing countries.

[Poor health can also lead to security concerns.] In its most extreme form, poor health can contribute to political instability, civil unrest, mass migrations, and human rights abuses. . . . Politically unstable states require heightened diplomacy, create political entanglements, and sometimes provoke military responses.

Diseases of poverty overwhelmingly are concentrated in sub-Saharan Africa, and it is no surprise that many of these social and political problems occur in that region. But much of Africa has weak political, military, and economic power, so it can too easily be ignored. The same cannot be said about the burgeoning health crises emerging in pivotal countries in Eurasia, such as China, India, and Russia.

Eurasia has more than 60% of the world's inhabitants; one of the highest combined gross national products; and at least 4 massive armed forces with nuclear capabilities. These countries are in the midst of a "second wave" of HIV/AIDS, with prevalence rates increasing 20-fold in less than a decade. . . . Due to extreme health hazards, Eurasia most likely will experience economic, political, and military decline. Political instability in a region with such geostrategic importance will have major international ramifications.

Governments, therefore, have powerful reasons based on narrow, as well as enlightened, self-interest to ameliorate extreme health hazards beyond their borders. To their credit, . . . developed countries have increased annual global health assistance, from $2 billion in 1990 to $12 billion in 2004. . . . This development assistance may appear substantial but is modest compared with the annual $1 trillion spent globally on military expenditures and $300 billion on agricultural subsidies.

The increase in development assistance, moreover, is largely attributable to extensive resources devoted to a few high-profile problems, such as AIDS, pandemic influenza, and the Asian tsunami. Even factoring in these new investments, most Organisation for Economic Cooperation and Development [OECD] countries have not come close to fulfilling their pledges to donate 0.7% of gross national income per year. . . .

PROFOUND HEALTH INEQUALITIES ARE UNETHICAL

Perhaps it does not, or should not, matter if global health serves the interests of the richest countries. After all, there are powerful humanitarian reasons to help the world's least healthy people. But ethical arguments have failed to capture the full attention of political leaders and the public.

. . . The global burden of disease is shouldered by the poor disproportionately, such that health disparities across continents render a person's likelihood of survival drastically different based on where he or she is born. These inequalities have become so extreme and the resultant effects on the poor so dire that health disparities have become a defining issue of modern society.

The current global distribution of disease has led to radically different health outcomes across the globe. Disparities in life expectancy among rich and poor countries are vast. . . . Although life expectancy in the developed world increased throughout the 20th century, it actually decreased in the least developed countries and in transitional states such as Russia. . . .

Human instinct suggests it is unjust for large populations to have such poor prospects for good health and long life simply by happenstance of where they live. Although almost everyone believes it is unfair that the poor live miserable and short lives, there is little consensus about whether there is an ethical, let alone legal, obligation to help the downtrodden. What do wealthier societies owe as a matter of justice to the poor in other parts of the world?

Perhaps the strongest claim that health disparities are unethical is based on what can be called a theory of human functioning. Health, among all other forms of disadvantage, is special and foundational, in that its effects on human capacities profoundly impact an individual's opportunities in the world. Health is necessary for much of the joy, creativity, and productivity that a person derives from life. . . . Perhaps not as obvious, health also is essential for the functioning of civil societies. Without minimum levels of health, people cannot fully engage in social interactions, participate in the political process, exercise rights of citizenship, generate wealth, create art, and provide for the common security.

The capability to avoid starvation, preventable morbidity, and early mortality is a quality that enriches human life. Depriving individuals of this capability strips them of their freedom to pursue their lives as they wish. Under a theory of human functioning, health deprivations are unethical because they unnecessarily reduce a person's ability to function and the capacity for human agency.

But a theory of human functioning does not answer the more difficult question about who has the corresponding obligation to do something about global inequalities. Even scholars who believe in just distribution of resources frame their claims narrowly and rarely extend them to international obligations of justice. Their theories of justice are "relational" and apply to a fundamental social structure that people share. States may owe their citizens basic health protection by reason of a social compact. However, positing such a relationship among different countries and regions is much more complex.

Increasingly, the global community is sharing a common social, political, and economic structure. International law has established norms in areas ranging from infectious diseases and tobacco use to access to essential vaccines and medicines. . . . Perhaps the international community is moving toward a "global compact on health" in which wealthier countries have an ethical responsibility to serve other countries according to their resources, and poorer countries have expectations to receive help according to their needs.

Political leaders have . . . made numerous pledges of international development assistance, including substantial commitments to the Millennium Development

Goals and the Global Fund to Fight AIDS, Tuberculosis, and Malaria. As mentioned above, many governments also have agreed to spend a certain proportion of their gross national product on foreign assistance. These pledges appear sincere and very specific. [In enacting the] President's Emergency Plan for AIDS Relief (PEPFAR), the United States noted that it "has the capacity" to lead an international response to global AIDS, and that "in an age of miraculous medicines," no person should go without treatment (U.S. Leadership Against HIV/AIDS, Tuberculosis, and Malaria Act of 2003, 22 U.S.C. § 7601 [2003]). . . .

These promises to help others have moral force. Political leaders ought to follow through on their commitments. They appear to be made in good faith, and poor countries rely on the promised assistance for the health and well-being of their populations.

A TIPPING POINT

Politically and economically powerful countries should care about the world's least healthy people. It may be a matter of national interest, [or it] may be ethically the right thing to do to avert an unfolding humanitarian catastrophe. Although no single argument may be definitive in itself, the cumulative weight of the evidence is now overwhelmingly persuasive. Whatever the reasons, perhaps global society is coming to a tipping point where the status quo is no longer acceptable and it is time to take bold action. Global health, like global climate change, may soon become a matter so important to the world's future that it demands international attention, and no state can escape the responsibility to act.

.   .   .   .   .

Securing the basic health needs of the world's poor requires more than persuading key decision makers to prioritize global health spending: while international health assistance is vital, foreign aid and charitable giving do not by themselves improve global health. As Laurie Garrett details, health interventions in resource-poor countries often fail to improve and at times actually worsen public health outcomes. The prevailing philanthropic approach to global health relies largely on disease-specific programs that reflect donor goals rather than local needs and that lack long-term vision. This approach does little to address the underlying factors contributing to the burden of disease in developing countries. Furthermore, because donor funds are not aimed at supporting local solutions or local industries, they contribute to the poorer nations' continuing dependence on foreign aid. Garrett proposes that the world health community address these shortcomings by focusing on the most meaningful health outcomes that can be achieved by systemic improvements in the local public health infrastructure—namely, increased maternal survival rates and improved overall life expectancy.

THE CHALLENGE OF GLOBAL HEALTH*
Laurie Garrett

Less than a decade ago, the biggest problem in global health seemed to be the lack of resources available to combat the multiple scourges ravaging the world's poor and sick. Today, thanks to a recent extraordinary and unprecedented rise in public and private giving, more money is being directed toward pressing heath challenges than ever before. But because the efforts this money is paying for are largely unco-ordinated and directed mostly at specific high-profile diseases—rather than at public health in general—there is a grave danger that the current age of generosity could not only fall short of expectations but actually make things worse on the ground. . . .

[Improving global health requires much more than money.] It takes states, health-care systems, and at least passable local infrastructure to improve public health in the developing world. And because decades of neglect there have rendered local hospitals, clinics, laboratories, medical schools, and health talent dangerously deficient, much of the cash now flooding the field is leaking away without result. . . .

Few of the newly funded global health projects . . . have built-in methods of assessing their efficacy or sustainability. Fewer still have . . . scaled up beyond initial pilot stages. . . . Nearly all have been designed, managed, and executed by residents of the wealthy world (albeit in cooperation with local personnel and agen-cies). . . . Virtually no provisions exist to allow the world's poor to say what they want, decide which projects serve their needs, or adopt local innovations. And nearly all programs lack exit strategies or safeguards against the dependency of local governments.

As a result, the health world is fast approaching a fork in the road. The years ahead could witness spectacular improvements in the health of billions of people, driven by a grand public and private effort[,] . . . or they could see poor societies pushed into even deeper trouble, in yet another tale of well-intended foreign med-dling gone awry. Which outcome will emerge depends on whether it is possible to expand the developing world's local talent pool of health workers, restore and improve crumbling national and global health infrastructures, and devise effective local and international systems for disease prevention and treatment. . . .

PIPE DREAMS

. . . One problem is that not all the funds appropriated end up being spent effectively. [Much of] current aid spending is trapped in bureaucracies and multilateral banks. [A 2006 World Bank report estimated that about half of all funds donated for health efforts in sub-Saharan Africa never reached clinics and hospitals because it went to payments for ghost employees, padded prices, the siphoning off of drugs to the black market, and the sale of counterfeit drugs.]

Another problem is the lack of coordination of donor activities. Improving global health will take more funds than any single donor can provide, and oversight and

*Reprinted by permission of *Foreign Affairs* (86, 2007). Copyright (2007) by the Council on Foreign Relations, Inc. www.ForeignAffairs.org.

guidance require the skills of the many, not the talents of a few compartmentalized in the offices of various groups and agencies. In practice, moreover, donors often function as competitors. . . .

This points to yet another problem; which is that aid is almost always "stove-piped" down narrow channels relating to a particular program or disease. From an operational perspective, this means that a government may receive considerable funds to support, for example, an [antiretroviral]-distribution program for mothers and children living in the nation's capital. But the same government may have no financial capacity to support basic maternal and infant health programs, [leaving mothers without] even the most rudimentary of obstetric and gynecological care or infant immunizations.

Stovepiping tends to reflect the interests and concerns of the donors, not the recipients. . . . Advocacy, the whims of foundations, and the particular concerns of wealthy individuals and governments drive practically the entire global public health effort. Today the top three killers in most poor countries are maternal death around childbirth and pediatric respiratory and intestinal infections leading to death from pulmonary failure or uncontrolled diarrhea. But few women's rights groups put safe pregnancy near the top of their list of priorities, and there is no dysentery lobby or celebrity attention given to coughing babies. . . .

[At the 2006 International AIDS Conference, former president Bill Clinton sug-gested that HIV/AIDS programs would help develop health infrastructure, facilitating broad improvements in health. But this optimistic assessment has not played out. Much of global HIV/AIDS funding goes to stand-alone programs, and, because of HIV-related stigma, countries' public health systems have frequently segregated HIV/AIDS-related programs from general care.] Far from lifting all boats, as Clinton claims, efforts to combat HIV/AIDS have so far managed to bring more money to the field but have not always had much beneficial impact on public health outside their own niche. . . .

BRAIN DRAIN

. . . Health professionals from poor countries worldwide are increasingly abandoning their homes and their professions to take menial jobs in wealthy countries. Morale is low all over the developing world, where doctors and nurses have the knowledge to save lives but lack the tools. Where AIDS and drug-resistant TB now burn through populations like forest fires, health-care workers say that the absence of medicines and other supplies leaves them feeling more like hospice and mortuary workers than healers.

Compounding the problem are the recruitment activities of Western NGOs [non-governmental organizations] and OECD-supported programs inside poor countries, which poach local talent. . . . PEPFAR-funded programs, UN agencies, other rich-country government agencies, and NGOs routinely augment the base salaries of local staff with benefits such as housing and education subsidies, frequently bring-ing their employees' effective wages to a hundred times what they could earn at government-run clinics.

. . . Without tough guidelines or some sort of moral consensus among UN agen-cies, NGOs, and donors, it is hard to see what will slow the drain of talent from already-stressed ministries of health. [The declining number of health care workers is staggering: for example, in Zambia, only 50 of the 600 doctors trained over the past 40 years remain today.]

Donor states need to find ways not only to solve the human resource crisis inside poor countries but also to decrease their own dependency on foreign health-care workers. In 2002, . . . the United Kingdom passed the Commonwealth Code of Practice for the International Recruitment of Health Workers, designed to encourage increased domestic health-care training and eliminate recruitment in poor countries without the full approval of host governments. British officials argue that although the code has limited efficacy, it makes a contribution by setting out guidelines for best practices regarding the recruitment and migration of health-care personnel. No such code exists in the United States, in the EU [European Union] more generally, or in Asia—but it should. . . .

. . . The personnel crisis in the developing world will not be dealt with until the United States and other wealthy nations clean up their own houses. . . . All donor programs in the developing world . . . should have built into their funding parameters ample money to cover the training and salaries of enough new local health-care personnel to carry out the projects in question, so that they do not drain talent from other local needs in both the public and the private sectors.

WOMEN AND CHILDREN FIRST

Instead of setting a hodgepodge of targets aimed at fighting single diseases, the world health community should focus on achieving two basic goals: increased maternal survival and increased overall life expectancy. Why? Because if these two markers rise, it means a population's other health problems are also improving. And if these two markers do not rise, improvements in disease-specific areas will ultimately mean little for a population's general health and well-being. . . .

Maternal mortality data is a very sensitive surrogate for the overall status of health-care systems since pregnant women survive where safe, clean, round-the-clock surgical facilities are staffed with well-trained personnel and supplied with ample sterile equipment and antibiotics. If new mothers thrive, it means that the health-care system is working, and the opposite is also true.

Life expectancy, meanwhile, is a good surrogate for child survival and essential public health services. . . .

The OECD and [NGOs] should thus shift their targets, recognizing that vanquishing AIDS, TB, and malaria are best understood not simply as tasks in themselves but also as essential components of these two larger goals. No health program should be funded without considering whether it could, as managed, end up worsening the targeted life expectancy and maternal health goals, no matter what its impacts on the incidence or mortality rate of particular diseases. . . .

In the current framework, such as it is, improving global health means putting nations on the dole—a $20 billion annual charity program. But that must change. Donors and those working on the ground must figure out how to build not only effective local health infrastructures but also local industries, franchises, and other profit centers that can sustain and thrive from increased health-related spending. For the day will come in every country when the charity eases off and programs collapse, and unless workable local institutions have already been established, little will remain to show for all of the current frenzied activity.

B. The Epidemiologic Transition from Infectious to Chronic Disease: A Double Burden on the Poor

It is not surprising that the spread of infectious diseases is a matter of international concern. But it is less obvious why non-communicable diseases (NCDs) have global dimensions. The world is experiencing an "epidemiological transition" from infectious to chronic diseases, such as cardiovascular diseases, cancers, respiratory conditions, and diabetes. The WHO estimates that NCDs now account for nearly 60 percent of deaths, outstripping infectious diseases and injuries as the leading cause of death and long-term disability worldwide.

In part, the shift toward NCDs is attributable to longer life expectancies and an aging population. As people live longer they are more likely to develop debilitating NCDs. The epidemiologic shift to NCDs is not explained solely by an aging population, however; it is at least partially attributable to the process of globalization. Not only do increased trade and travel contribute to the rapid transmission of infectious disease, but they also facilitate the dissemination of risk factors for various NCDs. Roger S. Magnusson (2007), a leading global health law scholar, explains the root causes for the epidemiological transition from infectious to non-communicable diseases as follows:

> [The shift in disease burden] reflects the rapid rise in behavioural risk factors including smoking and high-sugar, high-fat diets. The "nutrition transition" towards diets that are richer in saturated fats and poorer in complex carbohydrates and dietary fibre, fruit and vegetables; the growth of urban lifestyles involving less physical exertion; and the promotion and rising consumption of tobacco and alcohol, have set the scene for "lifestyle epidemics" to become the greatest health challenge of the 21st century.
>
> While the proximate behavioural risk factors for non-communicable diseases are well-known, the underlying environmental causes are both complex and global in scale. Environmental factors underlying the nutrition transition include the industrialization of food production, the growth of sophisticated supply chain management on a global scale, the expansion of market economies in developing countries, the growing concentration of global food manufacturers as a result of mergers and acquisitions, and the rapid growth of supermarkets in the developing world. Rising incomes, price differentials favouring the cheap production of energy-dense foods, growing urbanization and rapid growth in demand for pre-prepared foods, are also key factors.

Historically, global health policy makers have distinguished between diseases of poverty (acute infectious diseases) and diseases of affluence (chronic NCDs). This distinction is declining in utility as the global burden of disease shifts toward chronic diseases and as chronic disease risk factors become increasingly prevalent in the developing world. Some 80 percent of chronic disease deaths occur in low- and middle-income countries. The epidemiologic shift is particularly problematic in developing countries, where the growing prevalence of NCDs is not offset by a decline in communicable diseases, thereby creating a double burden of disease that strains limited health resources.

Addressing the burden of NCDs in developing countries requires concerted global action. As Derek Yach and colleagues (2004, 2617–18) observe, health policy interventions are integral to such efforts: "[In] the absence of policy actions, consumption of tobacco, alcohol, and foods high in fat and sugar increases along with gross national product, followed by associated increases in chronic diseases decades later. . . . The global challenge policymakers face is how to implement policies now that support continued economic development while simultaneously reducing the rates of chronic diseases." Yet misconceptions regarding NCDs and the health burdens they create present a fundamental barrier to policy action:

> In developed countries, the relationship between socioeconomic inequalities and many chronic diseases and their risk factors are well described. Although the disease burden is more variable in developing countries, the poorest populations, particularly in rapidly growing cities, in many cases already exhibit the highest risks for tobacco use, alcohol use, and physical activity, with evidence emerging for obesity. This will lead to a higher burden of chronic diseases over the long-term. Poverty also leads to greater co-morbidity and decreased access to quality medical care. . . .
>
> Many decision makers mistakenly believe that chronic diseases arise only as a result of the irresponsibility of the individuals who contract them, with the perception that "smoking is a free choice with health consequences." Yet age and uptake of smoking in developing countries are showing a trend toward early teenage years, the stage of life when the addictiveness of tobacco belies freedom of choice. Tobacco marketing is often targeted specifically at children, alcohol advertisements shape young peoples' perceptions and encourage pro-drink attitudes, and food marketing works its way "into the skin" of children and adolescents. . . .
>
> Chronic disease control is not necessarily expensive or ineffective. For example, a recent review of tobacco control [programs] showed that tobacco prevalence can be reduced cost-effectively in high-, middle-, and low-income countries. Several clinical and public health interventions have the potential to reduce the burden of disease from cardiovascular disease, diabetes, and hypertension significantly and at low cost. . . .
>
> The belief that scarce resources should not be used for chronic diseases until infectious diseases are addressed is also fallacious. Several infectious agents cause cancers; tobacco increases deaths from tuberculosis in

already infected populations, and antiretroviral regimens in HIV-infected patients increase the risk of heart disease. (Yach et al. 2004, 2620)

Abdallah S. Daar and colleagues (2007) have proposed strategies for reducing the global burden of chronic NCDs as part of their "grand challenges" series. They hope that focusing on twenty "grand challenges" for NCDs will galvanize health, science, and public policy communities to action. Appropriately, raising the political priority of NCDs is identified as the first grand challenge to reducing chronic NCDs. Daar and colleagues predict that with concerted action, the global community can avert at least 36 million premature deaths by 2015. Building on the "grand challenges" approach, in 2008 the Oxford Health Alliance, a global NGO dedicated to chronic disease prevention, published the Sydney Resolution, which is discussed in box 6.

Given current trends, it is particularly urgent for the global community to prioritize NCDs, undertake appropriate policy interventions, and allocate sufficient resources. Without such action, we will soon live in "a world in which all major diseases are the diseases of the poor" (Ezzati et al. 2005, 3133).

II. INTERNATIONAL PUBLIC HEALTH LAW

The readings above make clear that international health assistance is often chaotic and ineffective. The past decade has seen an explosion of new philanthropists and service organizations engaging in global health, joining a plethora of well-established state and United Nations agencies. There is considerable confusion about how all the various actors and their interventions fit together. Despite the propagation of creative ideas and the influx of resources, there is no architecture of global health. The global community needs effective methods of governing the diverse, fragmented activities on the ground. The WHO has sought to meet this governance challenge by adopting two major international public health instruments—the IHR and the FCTC.

A. *The International Health Regulations: A Historic Development*

The World Health Assembly adopted the new IHR on May 23, 2005, following a decade-long revision process. The severe acute respiratory syndrome (SARS) outbreaks in 2003 provided the major impetus for a global consensus on the need for more coherent regulation of public health hazards of international concern. In some ways, the IHR are

BOX 6

At its 2008 summit, the Oxford Health Alliance, whose membership includes academics, activists, and health care providers, finalized the Sydney Resolution—a global call to action on chronic diseases. The resolution, which has been endorsed by the World Health Federation, aims to inspire diverse stakeholders to take "urgent action to halt the devastating global impact of chronic diseases" in ways that "will promote economic and environmental sustainability."

The resolution focuses on heart disease/stroke, diabetes, chronic lung disease, and cancer—four preventable chronic diseases that account for 50 percent of the world's deaths—and their underlying causes: tobacco use, physical inactivity, and poor diet. "These preventable chronic diseases are at epidemic proportions. They are increasingly affecting younger people and cause physical disability, depression, and early death. There are immense costs to society in lost productivity and increased use of health services. The epidemic threatens economic stability in developed and developing countries alike." In arguing for global action on chronic diseases, the Sydney Resolution declares: "There is a clear way forward.... The development of how we live as societies, share opportunities, interact with the natural environment and how we design our cities, transport systems, food systems, work places and housing will fundamentally determine future patterns of health and disease. We need health services focused on prevention as well as cures and we need our world free of tobacco. We must fundamentally reshape our social and physical environments so that they are aligned with eradicating this epidemic of chronic disease." Five core needs are enumerated in the resolution's call to action:

- Healthy places—designing towns, cities, and rural areas that are smoke-free, and where it is easy to walk, cycle, and play, with unpolluted open spaces and safe local areas that foster social interaction.
- Healthy food—making healthy food affordable, and available to all.
- Healthy business—engaging business in the agendas of promoting healthy people, healthy places, and a healthy planet and making good health good business.
- Healthy public policy—formulating comprehensive, innovative, and "joined-up" legislation and social and economic policies that promote health.
- Healthy societies—addressing equity and socioeconomic disadvantage.

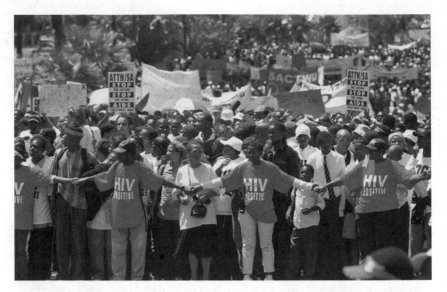

Photo 15. Thousands of protesters march through the streets of Cape Town, South Africa, in February 2003. Organized by South Africa's Treatment Action Campaign (TAC), the march called on that nation's government to expand funding for HIV treatment to the poor. TAC was successful in a legal battle to require that the South African government develop a plan to provide an HIV drug, nevirapine, to pregnant women to prevent mother-to-child transmission of the virus. Reproduced by permission, © Rodger Bosch/The Image Works, February 14, 2003.

part of a long tradition of infectious disease regulation, with antecedents dating back to nineteenth-century European and Pan-American treaties. But, more fundamentally, the revised IHR offer a powerful new paradigm for global health governance. David Fidler and I describe and analyze the revised IHR in the passage below.

THE NEW INTERNATIONAL HEALTH REGULATIONS: AN HISTORIC DEVELOPMENT FOR INTERNATIONAL LAW AND PUBLIC HEALTH*

David P. Fidler and Lawrence O. Gostin

The new International Health Regulations (IHR) appear at a moment when public health, security, and democracy have become intertwined, addressed at the highest levels of government.... This article analyzes the new IHR and their implications for global health and security in the 21st century....

*Reprinted from *Journal of Law, Medicine & Ethics* 33 (2006): 85–94. (Blackwell Publishing).

THE NEW IHR: AN IMPORTANT DEVELOPMENT IN GLOBAL HEALTH GOVERNANCE

... The purpose of the new IHR is "to prevent, protect against, control and provide a public health response to the international spread of disease in ways that are commensurate with and restricted to public health risks, and which avoid unnecessary interference with international traffic and trade" (International Health Regulations 2005, Article 2). The IHR seek to balance the state's right to protect its people's health with obligations to take health-protecting actions in ways that do not unnecessarily interfere with international trade and travel. ...

... The new IHR expand the scope of the IHR's application, incorporate international human rights principles, contain more demanding obligations for states parties to conduct surveillance and response, and establish important new powers for WHO. ...

SCOPE OF THE NEW IHR: AN ALL-RISKS APPROACH

The old IHR applied only to a short list of infectious diseases whose spread was historically associated with trade and travel (e.g., cholera, plague, and yellow fever). The Regulations now encompass public health risks whatever their origin or source, including: (1) naturally occurring infectious diseases ... ; (2) the potential international spread of non-communicable diseases caused by chemical or radiological agents in products moving in international commerce; and (3) suspected ... releases of biological, chemical, or radiological substances.

This "all-risks" approach embodies an important conceptual shift concerning public health's role in the IHR. Trade calculations determined the old IHR's scope, but risks to human health define the new IHR's scope. The result is a set of rules with more public health legitimacy, flexibility, and adaptability. ...

THE NEW IHR AND GENERAL HUMAN RIGHTS PRINCIPLES

The new IHR proclaim that "[t]he implementation of these Regulations shall be with full respect for the dignity, human rights and fundamental freedoms of persons" (Article 3.1). ... For a public health measure to restrict a civil and political right lawfully, the measure must (1) respond to a pressing public or social need; (2) pursue a legitimate aim; (3) be proportionate to the legitimate aim; and (4) be no more restrictive than is required to achieve the purpose sought by restricting the right. The rights-restricting measure must also be implemented in a non-discriminatory manner. Individuals deprived of liberty must be treated with humanity and respect for the inherent dignity of the human person. ...

The extent to which the new IHR incorporate human rights principles means that international human rights law is relevant to the interpretation and implementation of the new IHR. The Regulations' incorporation of human rights will suffer, however, if states parties do not integrate human rights thinking into the operation of their respective public health systems. ...

[The new IHR also include provisions related to informed consent and privacy. Attention to these concerns represents an improvement over the former IHR, but questions remain about protecting human rights when implementing the Regulations.]

NATIONAL PUBLIC HEALTH CAPACITIES: SURVEILLANCE AND RESPONSE

The new IHR require states parties to develop, strengthen, and maintain core surveillance and response capacities. The old IHR had requirements for public health capabilities only at points of entry and exit. The far-reaching provisions in the new IHR shore up major weaknesses in global strategies created by inadequate national surveillance and response capabilities. . . .

Although the new IHR's provisions on surveillance and response capacities recognize the critical need for capacity building, questions remain about the handling of this issue. [The financial and technical resources needed for national capacity building may not be available, and the WHO suffers from resource constraints.] The new IHR also contain no obligations on states parties to provide financial and technical resources to support capacity building. . . .

NOTIFICATION OBLIGATIONS: REPORTING HEALTH EVENTS TO WHO

The new IHR require states parties to notify WHO of all events within their territories that may constitute a public health emergency of international concern, defined as "an extraordinary event which is determined . . . (i) to constitute a public health risk to other States through the international spread of disease and (ii) to potentially require a coordinated international response" (Article 1.1). A "decision instrument" is used to guide states parties in determining whether a disease event may constitute a public health emergency of international concern.

In keeping with the new IHR's expanded scope, the notification obligations reflect a radically different, and more demanding, approach to addressing the international spread of disease. The notification provisions place a premium on states parties having sufficient surveillance capacities to detect disease incidents, assess them under the decision instrument, and report disease events that may constitute public health emergencies of international concern. [There is a serious question as to whether many countries can develop the necessary surveillance capacities.]

Another problem looms for the new IHR's notification requirements. States parties often violated the old IHR by failing to report cases of diseases subject to the Regulations because they feared other countries would implement economically damaging trade or travel restrictions. [The new IHR contain information supply and verification strategies to help combat this problem.]

DATA AND VERIFICATION PROVISIONS: UNOFFICIAL SOURCES OF INFORMATION

The old IHR limited WHO to officially using information provided by states parties. . . . By contrast, the new IHR allow WHO to "take into account reports from sources other than notifications or consultations" from or with governments and to seek verification of such information from states parties in whose territories the events are allegedly occurring (Articles 9.1 and 10.1). States parties must respond to WHO verification requests. . . .

[Nongovernmental sources of information have been critical to the WHO's Global Outbreak Alert and Response Network (GOARN). Access to nongovernmental information incentivizes compliance and transparency by states.]

DECLARATION AND RECOMMENDATION POWERS

The new IHR grant two other important powers to WHO that never appeared in the old IHR. First, the new IHR accord WHO the authority to determine whether a disease event constitutes a public emergency of international concern. States parties have to notify disease events that may constitute such emergencies, but the DG [director-general] determines if disease events are public health emergencies of international concern. [Therefore,] a state party's refusal to cooperate does not bar WHO action.

Second, if the DG determines that a public health emergency of international concern is occurring, then he or she shall issue non-binding, temporary recommendations to states parties on the most appropriate ways to respond. The DG may also issue non-binding, standing recommendations on routine, periodic application of health measures for specific, ongoing public health risks. . . . These powers allow WHO to provide leadership on what health measures are appropriate from scientific and public health perspectives and on the proper ways to balance health protection with respect for human rights and acknowledgement of trade concerns.

PERMISSIBLE HEALTH MEASURES: LIMITS ON NATIONAL PUBLIC HEALTH INTERVENTIONS

States parties to the new IHR are not legally bound to follow WHO temporary or standing recommendations; but the new IHR contain binding limits on the types of health measures states parties can take against public health risks. . . . Generally, states parties cannot require an invasive medical examination, vaccination or other prophylaxis as a condition of entry for any traveler; nor can a state party require any health document for travelers other than those permitted by the new IHR or recommended by WHO. . . .

The new IHR permit states parties to apply health measures that achieve the same or greater level of health protection than WHO recommendations or that are otherwise prohibited by the IHR. Such health measures must be based on scientific principles, available scientific evidence, relevant guidance or advice from WHO, and cannot be more restrictive of international traffic or more invasive or intrusive to persons than reasonably available alternatives that would achieve the level of health protection sought.

[The lack of enforcement mechanisms for these provisions may be problematic, and the same noncompliance problems that plagued the old IHR may reemerge.]

THE NEW IHR AND THE FUTURE OF GLOBAL HEALTH GOVERNANCE

The new IHR contain an international legal regime unprecedented in the history of the relationship between international law and public health. The revised Regulations promise to become a centerpiece for global health governance in the 21st century. . . . The transformational nature of the new IHR creates a regime that has the potential to contribute significantly to the general global governance mission of improving national and international health. The Regulations provide a framework that supports not only improved international cooperation on health but also the strengthening of national health systems, producing more robust health governance horizontally among states and vertically within them.

The new IHR's novelty should not, however, obscure hard realities facing its future. WHO was systematically using non-governmental surveillance information from GOARN's establishment in 1998, well before the IHR revision process was completed; and this strategy would have continued whether or not the new IHR had been adopted. More difficult issues arise with producing effective responses to identified public health risks. For decades, WHO has issued recommendations on many public health problems; but the mixed record of state compliance with WHO guidance should temper enthusiasm for the new IHR's recommendation provisions. The political controversies that surrounded WHO's more aggressive actions during SARS may deter WHO from taking similar actions under the new IHR. Laments about the erosion of global and local public health capabilities suggest that WHO's decades-long effort to improve health conditions in developing countries has also met with only qualified success. The new IHR will not change this dynamic overnight, particularly when the Regulations generate no fresh financial resources to support capacity building. Compliance with international legal restrictions against the implementation of health measures that unnecessarily restrict trade or infringe on human rights has not, in the past, been stellar, as illustrated by how non-compliance helped destroy the old IHR's effectiveness. Whether the quantity and quality of compliance with the new IHR's rules on health measures are better will not depend on any improved enforcement mechanism because the Regulations do not create one.

The new IHR are no "magic bullet" for global health problems. Previous transformations in international law's relationship with public health have, over time, atrophied into insignificance. The history of the old IHR tells just such a story. . . . Controversies and problems surrounding the threat of avian influenza also suggest that the new IHR do not cut through the tangled knot of very hard political, economic, scientific, and public health choices governments must make to address this public health emergency of international concern.

. . . Harvesting the new IHR's benefits for global health requires understanding not only the difficulties this task faces but also the potential the Regulations represent. . . . The seminal achievement of the new IHR constitutes only the end of the beginning. The hard work of making this transformative revision of global health governance effective for individuals, states, and the international community now begins.

.   .   .   .   .

As the preceding article discussed, for the first time in history, the revised International Health Regulations permit an organized global response within the rule of international law. The April 2009 outbreak of a novel strain of influenza A (H1N1) offered the first test of its effectiveness. Although it remains to be seen how the continuing H1N1 outbreak will unfold, in box 7 I provide a brief, summary time line of the initial stages of the outbreak as well as the corresponding actions taken by the WHO.

B. The Framework Convention on Tobacco Control:
Global Strategies to Reduce Smoking

In the mid-twentieth century, the cigarette was a cultural icon in Western society—tobacco smoking was viewed as chic, promoted ubiquitously,

BOX 7

April 12 — Outbreak of influenza-like illness in Veracruz, Mexico, reported to WHO.

April 15–17 — U.S. CDC laboratories identify two cases of a novel strain of A (H1N1) virus in southern California.

April 23 — Novel strain of A (H1N1) virus infection confirmed in several patients in Mexico.

April 25 — In compliance with the International Health Regulations, WHO convenes a meeting of the Emergency Committee, composed of international experts in a variety of disciplines. Upon its advice, Director-General Margaret Chan (WHO 2009c) declares the outbreak "a public health emergency of international concern" (marking the first time such a declaration had been made under the new regulations).

April 27 — According to its categorizations of pandemic phases (WHO 2009a), WHO declares the situation at Pandemic Phase 4, or sustained human-to-human transmission, in Mexico.

April 29 — After broad transmission is documented in the United States, WHO raises alert to Pandemic Phase 5, which is characterized by human-to-human spread of the virus into at least two countries in the same WHO region.

June 11 — All WHO regions reporting cases of novel strain A (H1N1); WHO raises alert to Pandemic Phase 6, which is characterized by community-level outbreaks in at least one other country in a different WHO region in addition to the criteria defined in Phase 5. Designation indicates that a global pandemic is under way.

SOURCE: Adapted from WHO 2009b.

and portrayed by sports and movie stars as an accoutrement of a good life (Brandt 2007). By the close of the century, public and political perceptions had been transformed by revelations about the tobacco industry's knowledge of the risks of smoking and its intent to deceive. The ensuing regulation and tort litigation in North America and western Europe had a salutary effect, even if smoking remains a pressing public health hazard. But in the twenty-first century, the tobacco industry has quietly moved its locus of activity to lucrative emerging markets—the vast populations of Africa, Asia, eastern Europe, and Latin America. Within these regions live some of the poorest, least educated, and sickest people on earth. "Big Tobacco's" new marketing strategy will cause untold morbidity for the world's most vulnerable populations (Gostin 2007b, Gostin 2007f).

The FCTC, the first convention negotiated under article 19 of the WHO Constitution, was adopted in 2003 and entered into force in 2005. Most countries have ratified the treaty, with three densely populated countries conspicuously missing—Indonesia, Russia, and the United States. The FCTC Conference of Parties, representing 80 percent of the world's population, set regulatory goals in Bangkok, Thailand, in July 2007. The conference established historic guidelines on smoke-free environments, announced future guidelines on cross-border advertising, and began work on the first FCTC protocol on illicit trade in tobacco products.

In the following reading, Allyn L. Taylor and Douglas W. Bettcher argue that the FCTC has the potential to be a global "good" for public health, pointing to the demonstrated successes of other international agreements in the area of global health, most of which address environmental issues. Taylor and Bettcher offer the development of the FCTC as a model for the creation of global health agreements, emphasizing the importance of an evidence-based approach in securing political acceptance.

WHO FRAMEWORK CONVENTION ON TOBACCO CONTROL: A GLOBAL "GOOD" FOR PUBLIC HEALTH*
Allyn L. Taylor and Douglas W. Bettcher

Cigarette smoking is one of the largest causes of preventable death worldwide and the leading cause of premature death in industrialized countries. Currently, cigarette

*Reprinted from *Bulletin of the World Health Organization* 78 (2000): 920–29.

smoking and other forms of tobacco consumption kill four million people per year, with the majority of these deaths already occurring in developing nations. Moreover, the epidemic of tobacco addiction, disease and death is continuing to shift rapidly to the developing and transitional market countries. . . .

A significant contributor to the increased risk of tobacco-related diseases worldwide is the globalization of the tobacco epidemic through the successful efforts of the tobacco industry to expand their global trade and to achieve market penetration in developing countries and transitional market economies. Major transnational tobacco companies targeted growing markets in Latin America in the 1960s, the newly industrializing economies of Asia (Japan, the Republic of Korea, China [Province of Taiwan], and Thailand) in the 1980s, and—in the 1990s and currently—have moved into Africa, China, and eastern Europe, and are increasingly targeting young persons and women. . . .

As the vector of the tobacco epidemic, the tobacco industry is well aware of the characteristics of globalization and is attempting to manipulate globalization trends in its favour. Recently released documents of the multinational tobacco industry concretely indicate that the industry "plans, develops and operates its markets on a global scale" (Yach 1999). For example, a careful review of tobacco industry documents has shown that the industry looks towards the creation of new "global brands" and a "global smoker" as one way of overcoming markets which have thus far resisted the tobacco industry's onslaught. . . .

The dramatic increase in tobacco consumption in the last couple of decades portends public health and economic tragedy for nations worldwide in the 21st century. Much of the potential calamity can be averted, however, through effective implementation of tobacco control strategies. In its recent report, *Curbing the epidemic: governments and the economics of tobacco control,* the World Bank (1999) concluded that tobacco control is highly cost-effective as part of a basic public health package in all countries. . . .

Since many, if not all, of the challenges of tobacco control are increasingly transcending national boundaries, stemming the growth of the tobacco pandemic requires global agreement and action. The globalization of the tobacco pandemic restricts the capacity of countries to unilaterally control tobacco within their sovereign borders. All transnational tobacco control issues—including trade, smuggling, advertising and sponsorship, prices and taxes, control of toxic substances, and tobacco package design and labelling require multilateral cooperation and effective action at the global level. If not attended to, these global aspects of tobacco control can overwhelm the best national tobacco control strategies.

AN INTERNATIONAL EVIDENCE-BASED APPROACH

The WHO Convention is being developed as a scientific, evidence-based approach to global tobacco control, which has the potential to significantly advance national and international efforts to curb the growth of the pandemic. [Ed.—This article was published before the FCTC was adopted and came into force.]

Evidence from other treaty-making processes shows that the institutions and procedural mechanisms established by the WHO Convention can prompt timely consensus and action on cogent implementing protocols and, thus, contribute to the implementation of the Convention and the advancement of the global public good of international tobacco control. For example, environmental framework conventions and protocols are often designed to encourage state parties to adopt implementing protocols by mandating regular and institutionalized meetings of the parties. In the case of some framework conventions, the mandatory provisions for consultation "offer the prospect of a virtually continuous legislative enterprise" (Handl 1992, 62). Rapid implementation of the WHO Convention can also be encouraged by institutions and mechanisms that establish incentives for the parties, such as information, technology, training, technical advice and assistance.

Of course, the effective international lawmaking experiences achieved at times in the environmental areas may not accurately reflect WHO's potential to garner broad support for the development and implementation of a Framework Convention on Tobacco Control and related protocols. The extent to which international agreements are effective—and under what conditions—has been a continuing source of theoretical fascination and dispute among scholars of international relations and international law. Although it is beyond the scope of this article to detail the factors that may contribute to the effective adoption and implementation of the WHO Convention, it may be noted that tobacco control does share the characteristic of "scientific certainty" which has galvanized effective international action in some areas of environmental law. Like the hole in the ozone layer above Antarctica which led to the conclusion of the Montreal Ozone Protocol, the health and economic consequences of tobacco consumption are empirically established. In addition, the use of the framework convention protocol approach will allow countries to undertake added substantive and/or institutional commitments as global consensus for concrete measures on tobacco control develops.

FRAMEWORK CONVENTION ON TOBACCO CONTROL: A GLOBAL PUBLIC "GOOD"

As a rational, evidence-based approach, the WHO Convention holds the potential of dramatically advancing global cooperation for tobacco control and can thus be considered a potential intermediate public health good. The principles, norms and standards ultimately codified in the Convention can legally establish global priorities for national action and multilateral cooperation on tobacco control. The institutions eventually established by the Convention, including—potentially—a financial mechanism, technical advice and assistance programmes, a mechanism to monitor treaty compliance, and provisions for ongoing consultation of the parties, can help contribute to the adoption of effective global tobacco control measures. Overall, by providing an ongoing and institutionalized platform for multilateral consultations on tobacco control, the WHO Convention may be able to promote adoption and implementation of effective tobacco control strategies worldwide.

WHO has the constitutional responsibility and the unique opportunity to propel the development of a Framework Convention on Tobacco Control. Importantly, the sheer process of negotiating and seeking its adoption can also be considered a public good. WHO's efforts to achieve global public support for an international regulatory framework for tobacco control may stimulate national policy change and thus make a dramatic contribution to curtailing the spiraling pandemic well before global consensus on cogent tobacco norms is secured.

III. HUMAN RIGHTS: ADVANCING DIGNITY, JUSTICE, AND SECURITY IN HEALTH

It is not necessary to recount the numerous charters
and declarations . . . to understand human rights. . . .
All persons are born free and equal in dignity and
rights. Everyone . . . is entitled to all the rights and
freedoms set forth in the international human rights
instruments without discrimination, such as the rights
to life, liberty, security of the person, privacy, health,
education, work, social security, and to marry and
found a family. Yet, violations of human rights are a
reality to be found in every corner of the globe.

> Jose Ayala Lasso (former UN high commissioner for
> human rights) and Peter Piot (former executive director
> of UNAIDS), 1997

The language of human rights is used in different ways, though usually
with a common core sense. Some mean by "human rights" a set of
entitlements and obligations under international law. Others apply the
term to a set of ethical standards that stress the paramount importance
of individuals. Still others use human rights language for its aspira-
tional, or rhetorical, qualities.

Although all of these uses are important, I use the term primarily
to refer to a body of international law that arose in response to the
egregious affronts to peace and human dignity committed by the Nazis
during World War II. The main source of human rights law within the
United Nations system is the International Bill of Human Rights, composed of the Charter of the United Nations, the Universal Declaration
of Human Rights (UDHR), and two international covenants on human
rights. Human rights are also protected under regional systems, including those in the Americas, Europe, and Africa.

In its preamble, the United Nations Charter articulates the international community's determination "to reaffirm faith in fundamental
human rights, [and] in the dignity and worth of the human person."
The charter, as a binding treaty, requires member states to promote
universal respect for, and observance of, human rights and fundamental freedoms for all without distinction as to race, sex, language, or
religion (articles 55–56).

The UDHR, adopted in 1948, built on the promise of the charter by identifying specific rights and freedoms to which all human beings are entitled. As a declaration of the UN General Assembly, the UDHR is an expression of global consensus on the lasting importance of human rights. It was the international community's first attempt to establish "a common standard of achievement for all peoples and all nations" in the promotion and protection of human rights (preamble). The UDHR has largely fulfilled the promise of its preamble, becoming the "common standard" for evaluating respect for human rights. Although it was not promulgated to legally bind member states, the UDHR's key provisions have so often been applied and accepted that they are now widely considered to have attained the status of customary international law.

The adoption of the UDHR set the stage for a binding, treaty-based scheme to promote and protect human rights. The International Covenant on Civil and Political Rights (ICCPR) and the International Covenant on Economic, Social, and Cultural Rights (ICESCR) were adopted in 1966 and entered into force in 1976. Together, these covenants convert the UDHR's expression of human rights and freedoms into a set of legal obligations incumbent on states parties. The United States has ratified the ICCPR but not the ICESCR. The rights contained in the ICCPR are principally negative or defensive in character, affording individuals a sphere of protection from government restraint. These rights, which are to be respected without discrimination, include the right to life, liberty, and security of person; the prohibition of slavery, torture, and cruel, inhuman, or degrading treatment; the right to an effective judicial remedy; the prohibition of arbitrary arrest, detention, and exile; freedom from arbitrary interference with privacy, family, or home life; freedom of movement; freedom of conscience, religion, expression, and association; and the right to participate in government.

The UDHR characterizes economic, social, and cultural rights as "indispensable for [a person's] dignity and the development of his personality" (article 22). To oversimplify somewhat, the ICESCR forms the foundation for "positive rights," that is, those requiring affirmative duties of the state to provide services. Such positive rights include the right to social security, the right to education, the right to work, the right to receive equal pay for equal work and to remuneration ensuring "an existence worthy of human dignity," and the right to share in the cultural life of the community and "to share in scientific advancement and its benefits" (articles 22–27). Article 12 of the ICESCR requires governments to recognize "the right of everyone to the highest attainable standard of physical and mental health." Article 25 of the UDHR also expressly recognizes that "everyone has the right to a standard of living adequate for the health and well-being of himself and his family, including . . . medical care and necessary social services." The article further specifies the right to social security and support in times of need.

Human rights law follows a set of internationally agreed-on rules specified in the text of treaties and other instruments, is informed by precedent, and is interpreted by tribunals and commissions. International human rights law seldom provides easy answers; rather, the field struggles to define and enforce human rights in the context of the legitimate powers of governments and the needs of communities.

This section begins with a classic exposition of the relationship between health and human rights by Jonathan M. Mann and colleagues. Mann's work is seminal, forming the basis for modern scholarship and advocacy in the field. Above all, he made an early plea for greater clarity of thought about the meaning of the international right to health. The UN Committee on Economic, Social, and Cultural Rights has responded by publishing General Comment 14 on the right to health, excerpted below. The General Assembly subsequently appointed a special rapporteur, who has also published influential guidance.

HEALTH AND HUMAN RIGHTS*
Jonathan M. Mann et al.

Health and human rights have rarely been linked in an explicit manner. With few exceptions, notably involving access to health care, discussions about health have not included human rights considerations. Similarly, except when obvious damage to health is the primary manifestation of a human rights abuse, such as with torture, health perspectives have been generally absent from human rights discourse.

[Despite the gap that exists between health and human rights, both are] powerful, modern approaches to defining and advancing human well-being. Attention to the intersection of health and human rights may provide practical benefits to those engaged in health or human rights work, may help reorient thinking about major global health challenges, and may contribute to broadening human rights thinking and practice. However, meaningful dialogue about interactions between health and human rights requires a common ground. To this end, following a brief overview of selected features of modern health and human rights, this article proposes a provi-

*Reprinted from *Health and Human Rights* 1 (1994): 6–23.

sional, mutually accessible framework for structuring discussions about research, promoting cross-disciplinary education, and exploring the potential for health and human rights collaboration. . . .

A PROVISIONAL FRAMEWORK: LINKAGES BETWEEN HEALTH AND HUMAN RIGHTS

The goal of linking health and human rights is to contribute to advancing human well-being beyond what could be achieved through an isolated health- or human rights–based approach. This [article] proposes a three-part framework for considering linkages between health and human rights; all are interconnected, and each has substantial practical consequences. . . .

THE FIRST RELATIONSHIP: THE IMPACT OF HEALTH POLICIES, PROGRAMS, AND PRACTICES ON HUMAN RIGHTS

Around the world, health care is provided through many diverse public and private mechanisms. However, the responsibilities of public health are carried out in large measure through policies and programs promulgated, implemented, and enforced by, or with support from, the state. Therefore, this first linkage may be best explored by considering the impact of public health policies, programs, and practices on human rights.

The three central functions of public health are: assessing health needs and problems; developing policies designed to address priority health issues; and assuring programs to implement strategic health goals. Potential benefits to and burdens on human rights may occur in the pursuit of each of these major areas of public health responsibility.

For example, assessment involves collection of data on important health problems in a population. However, data are not collected on all possible health problems, nor does the selection of which issues to assess occur in a societal vacuum. Thus, a state's failure to recognize or acknowledge health problems that preferentially affect a marginalized or stigmatized group may violate the right to nondiscrimination by leading to neglect of necessary services, and in so doing, may adversely affect the realization of other rights, including the right to "security in the event of . . . sickness [or] disability" or to the "special care and assistance" to which mothers and children are entitled (UDHR, art. 25).

Once decisions about which problems to assess have been made, the methodology of data collection may create additional human rights burdens. Collecting [health] information from individuals . . . can clearly burden rights to security of person (associated with the concept of informed consent) and of arbitrary interference with privacy. [In addition, the methods used might compromise the right of nondiscrimination. For example, information gathered by a telephone survey, which excludes households without telephones (usually associated with lower socioeconomic status), might produce a skewed assessment and biased programs or policies.] Also, personal health status or health behavior information (such as sexual orientation or history of drug use) has the potential for misuse by the state, whether directly or if it is made available to others, resulting in grievous harm to individuals and violations of many rights. . . .

The second major task of public health is to develop policies to prevent and control priority health problems. Important burdens on human rights may arise in the policy development process. For example, if a government refuses to disclose the scientific basis of health policy or permit debate on its merits, or in other ways refuses to inform and involve the public in policy development, the rights to "seek, receive and impart information and ideas . . . regardless of frontiers" (UDHR, art. 19) and "to take part in the government . . . directly or through freely chosen representatives" (UDHR, art. 21) may be violated. Then, prioritization of health issues may result in discrimination against individuals, as when the major health problems of a population of a specific sex, race, religion, or language are systematically given lower priority. . . .

The third core function of public health, to assure services capable of realizing policy goals, is also closely linked with the right to nondiscrimination. When health and social services do not take logistic, financial, and sociocultural barriers to their access and enjoyment into account, intentional or unintentional discrimination may readily occur. . . .

It is essential to recognize that in seeking to fulfill each of its core functions and responsibilities, public health may burden human rights. In the past, when restrictions on human rights were recognized, they were often simply justified as necessary to protect public health. Indeed, public health has a long tradition, anchored in the history of infectious disease control, of limiting the "rights of the few" for the "good of the many." . . .

Unfortunately, public health decisions to restrict human rights have frequently been made in an uncritical, unsystematic, and unscientific manner. Therefore, the prevailing assumption that public health, as articulated through specific policies and programs, is an unalloyed public good that does not require consideration of human rights norms must be challenged. For the present, it may be useful to adopt the maxim that health policies and programs should be considered discriminatory and burdensome on human rights until proven otherwise. . . .

The idea that human rights and public health must inevitably conflict is increasingly tempered with awareness of their complementarity. [New approaches in the HIV/AIDS context incorporate public health and human rights goals, and such approaches are possible elsewhere.] At present, an effort to identify human rights burdens created by public health policies, programs, and practices, followed by negotiation toward an optimal balance whenever public health and human rights goals appear to conflict, is a necessary minimum. An approach to realizing health objectives that simultaneously promotes—or at least respects—rights and dignity is clearly desirable.

THE SECOND RELATIONSHIP: HEALTH IMPACTS RESULTING FROM VIOLATIONS OF HUMAN RIGHTS

Health impacts are obvious and inherent in the popular understanding of certain severe human rights violations, such as torture, imprisonment under inhumane conditions, summary execution, and "disappearances." . . .

However, health impacts of rights violations go beyond these issues in at least two ways. First, the duration and extent of health impacts resulting from severe abuses of rights and dignity [such as torture] remain generally underappreciated. [In addition, torture broadly influences mental and social well-being; it] is often used as a political tool to discourage people from meaningful participation in or resistance to government.

Second, and beyond these serious problems, it is increasingly evident that viola-tions of many more, if not all, human rights have negative effects on health. For example, the right to information may be violated when cigarettes are marketed without . . . information regarding the harmful health effects of tobacco smoking [or when governments withhold] valid scientific health information about contraception or measures (e.g., condoms) to prevent infection with a fatal virus (HIV). . . .

A related, yet even more complex problem involves the potential health impact associated with violating individual and collective dignity. The UDHR considers dig-nity, along with rights, to be inherent, inalienable, and universal. While important dignity-related health impacts may include such problems as the poor health status of many indigenous peoples, a coherent vocabulary and framework to character-ize dignity and different forms of dignity violations are lacking. A taxonomy and an epidemiology of violations of dignity may uncover an enormous field of previously suspected, yet thus far unnamed and therefore undocumented damage to physical, mental, and social well-being.

Assessment of rights violations' health impacts is in its infancy. Progress will require: a more sophisticated capacity to document and assess rights violations; [and] the application of medical, social science, and public health methodologies to identify and assess effects on physical, mental, and social well-being. . . .

THE THIRD RELATIONSHIP: HEALTH AND HUMAN RIGHTS–
EXPLORING AN INEXTRICABLE LINKAGE

The proposal that promoting and protecting human rights is inextricably linked to the challenge of promoting and protecting health derives in part from recognition that health and human rights are complementary approaches to the central problem of defining and advancing human well-being. This fundamental connection leads beyond the single, albeit broad mention of health in the UDHR (art. 25) and the specific health-related responsibilities of states listed in Article 12 of the ICESCR. . . .

Modern concepts of health recognize that underlying "conditions" establish the foundation for realizing physical, mental, and social well-being. Given the impor-tance of these conditions, it is remarkable how little priority has been given within health research to their precise identification and understanding of their modes of action, relative importance, and possible interactions.

The most widely accepted analysis focuses on socioeconomic status; the positive relationship between higher socioeconomic status and better health status is well documented. Yet this analysis has . . . important limitations [in that it does not fully explain some persistent health disparities].

A second problem lies in the definition of poverty and its relationship to health status. Clearly, poverty may have different health meanings; for example, distinc-tions between the health-related meaning of absolute poverty and relative poverty have been proposed.

A third, practical difficulty is that the socioeconomic paradigm creates an over-whelming challenge with which health workers are neither trained nor equipped to deal. Therefore, the identification of socioeconomic status as the "essential condi-tions" for good health paradoxically may encourage complacency, apathy, and even policy and programmatic paralysis. . . .

Experience with the global epidemic of HIV/AIDS suggests a further analytic approach, using a rights analysis. For example, married, monogamous women in East Africa have been documented to be infected with HIV. Although these women know about HIV and condoms are accessible in the marketplace, their risk factor is their inability to control their husbands' sexual behavior or to refuse unprotected or unwanted sexual intercourse. Refusal may result in physical harm, or in divorce, the equivalent of social and economic death for the woman. Therefore, women's vulnerability to HIV is now recognized to be integrally connected with discrimination and unequal rights, involving property, marriage, divorce, and inheritance. The success of condom promotion for HIV prevention in this population is inherently limited in the absence of legal and societal changes which, by promoting and protecting women's rights, would strengthen their ability to negotiate sexual practice and protect themselves from HIV infection.

More broadly, the evolving HIV/AIDS pandemic has shown a consistent pattern through which discrimination, marginalization, stigmatization, and, more generally, a lack of respect for the human rights and dignity of individuals and groups heighten their vulnerability to becoming exposed to HIV. In this regard, HIV/AIDS may be illustrative of a more general phenomenon in which individual and population vulnerability to disease, disability, and premature death is linked to the status of respect for human rights and dignity. . . .

. . . The concept of an inextricable relationship between health and human rights also has enormous potential practical consequences. For example, health professionals could consider using the International Bill of Human Rights as a coherent guide for assessing health status of individuals or populations; the extent to which human rights are realized may represent a better and more comprehensive index of well-being than traditional health status indicators. . . .

From the perspective of human rights, health experts and expertise may contribute usefully to societal recognition of the benefits and costs associated with realizing, or failing to respect, human rights and dignity. . . . Collaboration with health experts can help give voice to the pervasive and serious impact on health associated with lack of respect for rights and dignity. In addition, the right to health can be developed and made meaningful only through dialogue between health and human rights disciplines. Finally, the importance of health as a precondition for the capacity to realize and enjoy human rights and dignity must be appreciated. . . . People who are healthy may be best equipped to participate fully and benefit optimally from the protections and opportunities inherent in the International Bill of Human Rights.

THE RIGHT TO THE HIGHEST ATTAINABLE STANDARD OF HEALTH*
United Nations Committee on Economic, Social, and Cultural Rights

Health is a fundamental human right indispensable for the exercise of other human rights. . . . The right to health is closely related to and dependent upon the realization of other human rights . . . including the rights to food, housing, work, education, human dignity, life, non-discrimination, equality, the prohibition against torture,

*Reprinted from *General Comment 14*, CESCR, E/C.12/2000/4 (Nov. 8, 2000).

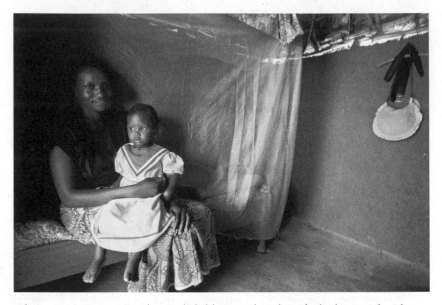

Photo 16. A Kenyan mother and child sit on the edge of a bed covered with
a bed net. Insecticide-treated bed nets are frequently distributed in countries
where malaria is endemic. In Kenya, as many as half of all outpatient visits are
related to malaria. In some areas, each resident may receive between 150 and
300 infective mosquito bites per year. Bed nets, when used consistently and
correctly, are an effective way of preventing nighttime bites. Reproduced by
permission, © Wendy Stone/Corbis, 2004.

privacy, access to information, and the freedoms of association, assembly and
movement....

The right to health is not to be understood as a right to be *healthy.* The right to
health contains both freedoms and entitlements. The freedoms include the right
to control one's health and body, including sexual and reproductive freedom, and
the right to be free from interference, such as the right to be free from torture,
non-consensual medical treatment and experimentation. By contrast, the entitlements include the right to a system of health protection which provides equality of
opportunity for people to enjoy the highest attainable level of health.

The notion of "the highest attainable standard of health" ... takes into account
both the individual's biological and socio-economic preconditions and a State's
available resources.... The right to health must be understood as a right to the
enjoyment of a variety of facilities, goods, services and conditions necessary for the
realization of the highest attainable standard of health....

The Committee interprets the right to health ... as an inclusive right extending
not only to timely and appropriate health care but also to the underlying determinants of health, such as access to safe and potable water and adequate sanitation,
an adequate supply of safe food, nutrition and housing, healthy occupational and
environmental conditions, and access to health-related education and information,
including on sexual and reproductive health....

The right to health . . . contains the following interrelated and essential elements . . . :

Availability

Functioning public health and health-care facilities, goods and services, as well as
programmes, have to be available in sufficient quantity within the State party. The
precise nature of the facilities, goods and services will vary, [but they include] the
underlying determinants of health, such as safe and potable drinking water and
adequate sanitation facilities, hospitals, clinics and other health-related buildings,
trained medical and professional personnel receiving domestically competitive salaries, and essential drugs. . . .

Accessibility

Health facilities, goods and services have to be accessible to everyone without discrimination, within the jurisdiction of the State party. Accessibility has four overlapping dimensions: [(1) non-discrimination—health facilities, goods and services
must be accessible to all without discrimination on any of the prohibited grounds;
(2) physical accessibility—they must be within safe physical reach for all sections of
the population; (3) economic accessibility—they must be affordable to all; and (4)
information accessibility—people should have the right to seek, receive, and impart
information and ideas concerning health issues, while retaining the right to have
personal health data treated with confidentiality].

Acceptability

All health facilities, goods and services must be respectful of medical ethics and
culturally appropriate . . . , as well as being designed to respect confidentiality and
improve the health status of those concerned.

Quality . . .

Health facilities, goods and services must also be scientifically and medically appropriate and of good quality. This requires, *inter alia,* skilled medical personnel, scientifically approved and unexpired drugs and hospital equipment, safe and potable
water, and adequate sanitation.

NON-DISCRIMINATION AND EQUAL TREATMENT

. . . The Covenant proscribes any discrimination in access to health care and underlying determinants of health, as well as to means and entitlements for their pro-
curement, on the grounds of race, colour, sex, language, religion, political or other
opinion, national or social origin, property, birth, physical or mental disability, health
status (including HIV/AIDS), sexual orientation and civil, political, social or other
status. . . . States have a special obligation to provide those who do not have sufficient means with the necessary health insurance and health-care facilities, and to
prevent any discrimination on internationally prohibited grounds in the provision of
health care and health services. . . .

LIMITATIONS

Issues of public health are sometimes used by States as grounds for limiting the
exercise of other fundamental rights. . . . Such restrictions must be in accordance

with the law, including international human rights standards, compatible with the nature of the rights protected by the Covenant, in the interest of legitimate aims pursued, and strictly necessary for the promotion of the general welfare in a democratic society. . . . Limitations must be proportional, i.e. the least restrictive alternative must be adopted where several types of limitations are available. Even where such limitations on grounds of protecting public health are basically permitted, they should be of limited duration and subject to review.

LEGAL OBLIGATIONS

While the Covenant provides for progressive realization and acknowledges the constraints due to the limits of available resources, it also imposes on States parties various obligations which are of immediate effect. States parties have immediate obligations in relation to the right to health, such as the guarantee that the right will be exercised without discrimination of any kind and the obligation to take [deliberate, concrete, and targeted] steps towards the full realization . . . of the right to health. . . .

. . . There is a strong presumption that retrogressive measures taken in relation to the right to health are not permissible. If any deliberately retrogressive measures are taken, the State party has the burden of proving that they have been introduced after the most careful consideration of all alternatives and that they are duly justified by reference to the totality of the rights provided for in the Covenant in the context of the full use of the State party's maximum available resources.

The right to health, like all human rights, imposes three types or levels of obligations on States parties: the obligations to *respect, protect* and *fulfil.* In turn, the obligation to fulfil contains obligations to facilitate, provide and promote. The obligation to *respect* requires States to refrain from interfering directly or indirectly with the enjoyment of the right to health. The obligation to *protect* requires States to take measures that prevent third parties from interfering with article 12 guarantees. Finally, the obligation to *fulfil* requires States to adopt appropriate legislative, administrative, budgetary, judicial, promotional and other measures towards the full realization of the right to health.

INTERNATIONAL OBLIGATIONS

States parties have to respect the enjoyment of the right to health in other countries, and to prevent third parties from violating the right in other countries. . . . Depending on the availability of resources, States should facilitate access to essential health facilities, goods and services in other countries, wherever possible and provide the necessary aid when required. States parties should ensure that the right to health is given due attention in international agreements and . . . ensure that their actions as members of international organizations take due account of the right to health. . . .

VIOLATIONS

In determining which actions or omissions amount to a violation of the right to health, it is important to distinguish the inability from the unwillingness of a State party to comply with its obligations. . . .

Violations of the right to health can occur through the direct action of States or other entities insufficiently regulated by States. The adoption of any retrogressive measures incompatible with the core obligations ... constitutes a violation of the right to health. Violations through *acts of commission* include the formal repeal or suspension of legislation necessary for the continued enjoyment of the right to health or the adoption of legislation or policies which are manifestly incompatible with pre-existing domestic or international legal obligations in relation to the right to health.

Violations of the right to health can also occur through ... *acts of omission*, [which] include the failure to take appropriate steps towards the full realization of everyone's right to [health], the failure to have a national policy on occupational safety and health as well as occupational health services, and the failure to enforce relevant laws. [If resource constraints render it impossible for a State to comply fully with its Covenant obligations, it has the burden of showing that every effort has nevertheless been made to use all available resources at its disposal in order to satisfy, as a matter of priority, these obligations.]

Violations of the Obligation to Respect

Violations of the obligation to respect are those State actions, policies or laws that contravene the standards set out in article 12 of the Covenant and are likely to result in bodily harm, unnecessary morbidity and preventable mortality. [Examples include denying groups access to health facilities, goods, and services through de jure or de facto discrimination and deliberately withholding information vital to health protection or treatment.]

Violations of the Obligation to Protect

Violations of the obligation to protect follow from the failure of a State to take all necessary measures to safeguard persons within their jurisdiction from infringements of the right to health by third parties. [Examples include failures to protect consumers and workers from unhealthy goods and practices; to discourage the production, marketing, and consumption of tobacco; to protect women against violence or prosecute perpetrators; and to enforce environmental laws.]

Violations of the Obligation to Fulfil

Violations of the obligation to fulfil occur through the failure of States parties to take all necessary steps to ensure the realization of the right to health. [Examples include failures to adopt an appropriate national health policy, to provide sufficient public resources for securing the right to health, to monitor realization of the right to health by identifying indicators and benchmarks, and to take measures to reduce inequitable distribution of health facilities, goods, and services.]

IV. WORLD TRADE AND WORLD HEALTH

The very idea of international trade is politically contentious. From a nationalist or populist perspective, trade is responsible for social ills, such as domestic unemployment (outsourcing); unfair/unsafe labor practices abroad (child labor); tainted food, drugs, and consumer goods (unregulated foreign markets); international health care worker migration ("brain drain" from developing to developed countries); and exorbitant prices for essential medicines (access to antiretroviral drugs for the world's poor). From a free market perspective, trade brings innovations in science, increased employment, and greater wealth to all trading partners.

The truth probably lies somewhere between these two extremes. Certainly, to the extent that trade has expanded economies, it has done so primarily in already wealthy countries and has had less benefit, if any, in low-income countries. It has also made it more difficult for the world's poor to gain access to essential medicines, because large corporations rely on laws protecting intellectual property rights to keep prices high. Nonetheless, trade has the potential to improve health and human well-being. As the WHO and the World Trade Organization (WTO) Secretariat's 2002 joint report on trade law and public health notes, there is a "positive link between freer trade and economic growth, which can lead to reduced poverty and higher standards of living, including better health" (23).

Whether and how trade's potential to positively affect global health can be harnessed depends in part on the structure and rules of the international trade system. Since it was created at the conclusion of the Uruguay Round of Multilateral Trade Negotiations in 1995, the World Trade Organization has taken its place at the center of our international trade system. The WTO consists of 151 member states. Each WTO member state is bound by treaties governing *trade in goods* (the most important being the General Agreement on Tariffs and Trade [GATT] and the Agreement on Sanitary and Phytosanitary Measures [SPS]), *trade in services* (the General Agreement on Trade in Services [GATS]), and *intellectual property protections* (the Agreement on Trade-Related Aspects of Intellectual Property Rights [TRIPS]).

The highest governing body of the WTO is the Ministerial Council, which is composed of high-level representatives from each member state. Although the Ministerial Council meets infrequently—typically every two years—it plays a key role in developing WTO trade policy. For example, the 2001 Ministerial Conference in Doha, Qatar, which called for "flexibilities" in access to essential medicines for the poor, has provided health and human rights advocates with a valuable tool for improving global access to HIV/AIDS treatments. Lower-level representatives of WTO states parties also participate in WTO governance through the General Council and specialized councils. The most notable aspect of the WTO's structure is its well-developed and binding dispute settlement system. The dispute settlement process begins with a "consultation" period, which focuses on negotiation, and then proceeds to a kind of trial before panels of trade experts. A panel decision can be appealed to the Appellate Body, a standing body of seven members. Unless WTO member states unanimously vote to overturn it, the decision of the Appellate Body is final and binding.

A cursory examination of the WTO's record on health reveals a troubling trend. When health issues have come before the WTO's dispute settlement organs, countries defending their health-related policies have repeatedly lost. From the 1990 Thailand cigarettes case, which found Thailand's import ban on cigarettes to be unnecessarily restrictive on trade, to the 2007 Brazil tires case (discussed further below), which found Brazil's health-based import ban on tires to have been applied in a way that constituted arbitrary or unjustified discrimination between countries, the resolution of trade disputes appears to have largely favored free trade over health interests.

This story of trade and health is incomplete, however. In the following article, M. Gregg Bloche and Elizabeth R. Jungman contend that a closer examination of WTO rules and jurisprudence reveals that the WTO in fact treats health as an interpretive principle and accords heightened deference to national health policies.

HEALTH POLICY AND THE WTO*
M. Gregg Bloche and Elizabeth R. Jungman

The WTO framers paid little heed to health policy. Over the past several years, however, politics and the AIDS pandemic have pushed health to center stage as a trade issue. The WTO has responded with heightened deference to national authority when member states' health polices conflict with other values protected by trade agreements.

On their face, the principal WTO agreements bearing on health are frustratingly vague in their approach to the task of balancing protection for health against other trade-related concerns. [For example, the TRIPS agreement] contains language that might be read to allow poor countries to elide patents on lifesaving medicines. But TRIPS says little about the prerequisites or procedures for invoking its ambiguous exceptions to patent protection.

Despite this absence of clear direction, the WTO system ... has come to treat protection for health as a *de facto* interpretive principle when disputes arise over the meaning of trade agreements. To be sure, such a principle is nowhere stated in

*Reprinted from *Journal of Law, Medicine & Ethics* 31 (2003): 529–45. (Blackwell Publishing).

WTO associated treaties, declarations, or jurisprudence; nor is health even mentioned as a purpose in the preambles to the major WTO agreements. Yet the special weight accorded to health in WTO decision-making is evident across a broad range of trade issues. . . .

HEALTH AND THE LAW OF THE GATT

. . . Article XX(b) of the GATT . . . allows member states to take actions that restrict trade and that are otherwise proscribed by the GATT if they are "necessary to protect human . . . life or health." Read in conjunction with the WTO standard for reviewing such actions—the requirement that dispute settlement panels "make an objective assessment" of relevant facts and law—this provision appears to permit close scrutiny, by panels and the Appellate Body, of claims of health necessity made to support trade restrictions.

Outside the health context, the Appellate Body has invoked the "objective assessment" standard to support robust scrutiny of member states' trade remedies and restraints. . . .

In sharp contrast, the Appellate Body has been highly deferential to member states' trade restrictions in the GATT Article XX(b) context. Although it has construed the "objective assessment" standard to require that restrictions purportedly "necessary to protect human . . . life or health" be based on some scientific evidence of health risk, it has held that such restrictions need not rest on "majority scientific opinion." In its 2001 decision upholding a French import ban on asbestos-containing products, the Appellate Body stated that "a member may rely, in good faith, on scientific sources which . . . may represent a divergent, but qualified and respected, opinion" (WTO 2001, para. 155). Some have seen this deference to member states' discretion in the face of scientific uncertainty as a step toward WTO adoption of international environmental law's "precautionary principle." Alternatively, this deference follows from treatment of protection for health as an interpretive principle, calling for less onerous standards of proof and review for trade restraints when health is at stake.

Indeed, [in its asbestos opinion, the Appellate Body] announced that "WTO members have a right to determine the level of protection of health that they consider appropriate in a given situation" (WTO 2001, para. 168). France's decision to reduce the risk of new, asbestos-related health risks to zero by barring the manufacture, domestic sale, and import of asbestos-containing products was within this right, the tribunal held. [Allowing national regulators to set a zero-risk goal and to bar imports accordingly constitutes exceptional deference to member states' health policies.]

[The asbestos decision contrasts with the Thailand tobacco opinion—a pre-WTO decision on the requirement that a measure under Article XX(b) be necessary. In that case, a GATT panel found that Thailand's discriminatory taxes on imported cigarettes were proscribed because they failed to meet the necessity test. Thailand, supported by the WHO, argued that enabling foreign competition in the tobacco market would overwhelm the government's antismoking message and boost the incidence of smoking. The panel, however, found that nondiscriminatory taxes on both domestic and foreign cigarettes could achieve the health goals in a more GATT-friendly fashion.]

Whatever the merits of this controversial, pre-WTO ruling, the Appellate Body signaled in its asbestos opinion that member states now have wide latitude to specify health policies that rule out less restrictive alternatives. In response to the exporting country's claim that France could stop the spread of asbestos-related risks through a less restrictive policy of "controlled use" of asbestos-containing construction materials, rather than resorting to an outright ban, the Appellate Body said France's "chosen level of health protection"—no asbestos-related risk—precluded any alternative to an outright ban. The countervailing health risks posed by substitute, non-asbestos building materials were of no moment, from this perspective, since France had specified its health policy more narrowly, as the elimination of asbestos related risks.

. . . The Asbestos opinion's discussion of the Article XX(b) necessity test is striking for its emphasis on the high weight to be given to health, in comparison with other goals. The more "vital or important" the ends at issue, "the easier it [is] to accept as 'necessary' measures designed to achieve those ends." And health, the opinion holds, is "both vital and important in the highest degree" (WTO 2001, para. 172).

HEALTH RISKS FROM FOOD: THE SPS AGREEMENT

In 1998, the Appellate Body ruled that the European Communities' import ban on beef from hormone-fed cattle violated the WTO agreement governing member states' food and agricultural safety regulations. Supporters and critics of this decision agree on its landmark importance as a statement of WTO law governing regulation of food safety. Activists opposed to giving cows growth-promoting hormones condemned the ruling, as did many who worry about the ebb of national authority over food safety more generally. . . .

The EC lost the hormones case on narrow grounds. Applying language in the relevant WTO treaty, the SPS Agreement, requiring regulators to act "based on" a risk assessment, the Appellate Body found that the EC failed to conduct a risk assessment to evaluate its claim that poor control over hormone doses given to animals gives rise to health hazards for humans. Had the EC done such a risk assessment and found dangers of this kind, it could have counted the risk of poor control over hormone administration, the Appellate Body said. This risk, by itself, could have justified the EC's import ban.

Other language in the hormones opinion strongly supports member states' discretion to regulate food and agriculture related health risks. . . . The Appellate Body rejected the proposition that the SPS risk assessment provision requires a showing of a threshold level of risk to justify trade-restricting regulation. The Appellate Body also held that risk assessment can count concerns not reducible to "quantitative analysis" by "laboratory methods." This allows national regulators to weigh subjective factors that influence both the perception and reality of risk. Beyond this, the Appellate Body read the precautionary principle into the SPS provision authorizing countries to regulate "where relevant scientific evidence is insufficient. . . . " In addition, the opinion states that regulators need not show they in fact took into account the risk assessment data and conclusions presented to a WTO panel. This enables member states to present state-of-the-art scientific data when defending their regulations in dispute resolution proceedings, and it eases the administrative (and financial) burden on governments concerned about crafting regulations to survive WTO scrutiny.

Moreover, the opinion treated the SPS mandate that regulation be "based on" a risk assessment as requiring only a "rational relationship" between the regulatory measure and the risk assessment. . . . The Appellate Body allowed for the possibility of "divergent" scientific opinion from "qualified and respected sources." Such opinion [properly supported] could suffice to establish the requisite "rational relationship" between a risk assessment and a regulation. . . .

To sum up, [the] hormones decision requires that there be some empirical substance to claims of health risk if they are to pass muster in the dispute settlement process: subjective perceptions and popular fears are not by themselves enough. But once this low empirical barrier is crossed, emerging SPS jurisprudence protects health to a remarkable degree, through a policy of exceptional deference to member states' assessments of and responses to health risk.

INTELLECTUAL PROPERTY AND LIFESAVING MEDICINES

Nowhere have perceptions of conflict between the WTO system and protection for health been as strong as in the area of trade in lifesaving medications. The AIDS pandemic in sub-Saharan Africa has made WTO treatment of drug companies' intellectual property rights into one of the most visible and poignant international issues of our time. . . .

. . . It is widely held that the Agreement on Trade-Related Aspects of Intellectual Property Rights (TRIPS) makes it more difficult for generic drug makers and "grey market" importers to undercut patent protected prices [for medicines] by exploiting permissive intellectual property law in poor countries. . . .

The Appellate Body has not yet opined on member states' flexibility, under TRIPS, to issue compulsory licenses, permit parallel importing, or import generic drugs manufactured elsewhere. Conflict over these issues has played out within the WTO's political organs. To a remarkable degree, this political process has responded to the desperate medical needs of sub-Saharan Africa and other impoverished regions. In the face of opposition from the pharmaceutical industry and industrialized nations, the WTO's highest governing body, the Ministerial Conference, issued a pronouncement in November 2001 declaring that members have a "right to protect public health, . . . to promote access to medicines for all," and "to use, to the full, the provisions in the TRIPS Agreement, which provide flexibility for this purpose."

This ministerial pronouncement, generally referred to as the Doha Declaration, cleared a path for parallel importing—acquisition of patent-protected drugs at lower prices through arbitrage—by construing TRIPS to allow members to make their own rules for exhaustion of patent rights. It also construed the rather convoluted TRIPS provision on compulsory licensing, or "use without authorization of the right holder," to grant countries several, overlapping "right[s]" [allowing countries greater latitude to use patented products in public health crises]. The Doha Declaration's use of rights language to construe the TRIPS provision on compulsory licensing contrasts with the provision itself, which is framed as a list of constraints on members' authority to issue compulsory licenses. . . .

[To be effective in facilitating access to essential medications, compulsory licensing rules must allow countries to export generic versions of patent-protected drugs to countries that lack generic pharmaceutical industries. The Doha Declaration instructed the TRIPS governing body to "find an expeditious solution to this problem." The resulting 2003 implementation agreement] authorizes individual member states to decide which health problems merit compulsory licenses for export. Critics have expressed concern that the agreement's safeguards against illicit diversion of drugs . . . could slow poor countries' efforts to make legitimate use of its provisions to save lives. . . .

[Nonetheless, the] Doha Declaration and implementation agreement . . . reduced the TRIPS threat to member states' health promotion efforts by construing ambiguous treaty terms in health-friendly fashion. There will be debate over Doha's legal authority, its implications for particular manufacturing and importing scenarios, and whether it should be seen as changing or merely clarifying WTO members' legal obligations. But the Declaration's broad affirmation of members' "right to protect public health" and to "use, to the full," the TRIPS Agreement's "flexibility for this purpose" is consonant with the larger picture we have sketched in this article, of an emerging WTO norm that treats health as reason for special deference to national authority.

CONCLUSION: HEALTH AS AN INTERPRETIVE PRINCIPLE

. . . There is a case to be made for an interpretive principle of protection for health that takes the form of heightened deference to member states' health policies instead of an affirmative transnational duty.

This case rests on the intensely subjective, highly variable nature of people's beliefs about [risks, which] are shaped by our character styles, values and culture, and personal and social experience. These influences tend to be local phenomena. . . . Health policies that fail to take account of these influences risk breaking too sharply with people's subjective needs. And public decision-making mechanisms that fail to offer opportunities for community control, or at least engagement, tend to raise people's anxieties about the risk-benefit judgments reached. Thus health politics is peculiarly local. . . . National, let alone transnational, efforts to systematize and rationalize health policies encounter skepticism and resistance. . . .

One might object that parochial resistance to these rationalizing efforts should not be treated as a challenge to their legitimacy, since these efforts are our best chance to maximize the welfare of the whole. But the more removed these efforts are from democratic oversight, the more tenuous are their claims to political legitimacy in both theory and practice. . . . WTO deference to national health policy is responsive to this challenge. It serves as a steam valve for domestic anxieties about globalization while incorporating protection for health as an interpretive principle.

Protection of health as an interpretive principle, rather than an internationally justiciable right, allows room for national variations in resource availability, perceptions of risk, and balancing between health and other goals. . . .

No WTO organ has explicitly embraced the premise of an international human right to health. For some proponents of such a right, this has been disheartening. Yet the WTO's tacit endorsement of protection for health as an interpretive principle, effected through heightened deference to national health policies, has done as much to establish health as a value in international law as have actions by international bodies more directly focused on health. Indeed, the WTO has arguably done more. Its judicial and ministerial pronouncements have created state practice, through both their legal force and member countries' compliance with them. The WTO has thereby become a prime mover of customary as well as treaty-based international health law. It has recognized a soft, non-justiciable right to health in all but name. Member states, NGOs, and others concerned about the place of health in transnational law should press WTO institutions to make this recognition explicit.

.   .   .   .   .

A recent case decided by the WTO's Appellate Body illustrates both the promise and the shortcomings of WTO jurisprudence on trade and health. In 2006, the European Commission challenged Brazil's ban on the importation of retreaded tires, arguing that it was disguised trade protectionism. Brazil, however, justified its import restrictions on the grounds of environmental and human health, arguing that incinerating tires releases toxic gases and contaminates the soil, water, and air. Mosquitoes also use the tires as breeding grounds, facilitating the transmission of dengue fever, yellow fever, and malaria. In *Brazil—Measures Affecting Imports of Retreaded Tyres,* decided in December 2007, the Appellate Body deferred extensively to Brazil in analyzing the underlying health matters; but in the end, it found the health-based import ban to be an unjustified restriction on trade.

The Appellate Body recognized Brazil's sovereign interest in determining whether the ban on retreaded tires was necessary for health reasons, hinting at its use of health as an interpretive principle. Consider the following passage from its report (WTO 2007, 82–83):

> The issue of whether [Brazil's] Import Ban [on retreaded tires] is necessary within the meaning of Article XX(b) of the GATT 1994 . . . illustrates the tensions that may exist between, on the one hand, international trade and, on the other hand, public health and environmental concerns arising from the handling of waste generated by a product at the end of its useful life. In this respect, the fundamental principle is the right that WTO Members have to determine the level of protection that they consider appropriate in a given context. Another key element of the analysis of the necessity of a measure under Article XX(b) is the contribution it brings to the achievement of its objective. A contribution exists when there is a genuine relationship of ends and means between the objective pursued and the measure at issue. To be characterized as necessary, a measure does not have to be indispensable. However, its contribution to the achievement of the objective must be material, not merely marginal or insignificant, especially if the measure at issue is as trade restrictive as an import ban. Thus, the contribution of the measure has to be weighed against its trade restrictiveness, taking into account the importance of the interests or the values underlying the objective pursued by it. As a key component of a comprehensive policy aimed to reduce the risks arising from the accumulation of waste tyres, the Import Ban produces such a material contribu-

tion to the realization of its objective. [We] consider that this attribution is sufficient to conclude that the Import Ban is necessary, in the absence of reasonably available alternatives. . . .

Accordingly, we uphold the Panel's finding that the Import Ban can be considered "necessary to protect human, animal or plant life or health."

While the Appellate Body's analysis of Brazil's import ban significantly favors the value of health regulations, the ultimate resolution of the case was not in Brazil's favor. The Appellate Body found that because Brazil, in practice, allowed retreaded tires to be imported from other countries and permitted some used tires to be imported for retreading in Brazil, the operation of the import ban actually served to favor trade from certain countries over others and to favor the domestic retreaded tire industry. Therefore the health regulation was, in practice, arbitrarily and unjustifiably discriminating between countries and serving to protect domestic industry from international competition.

Interestingly, the Appellate Body's decision does not prohibit Brazil's import ban. Rather, Brazil can comply with the ruling either by abandoning the import ban or by expanding the ban to operate without exceptions, making it function with more coherence and with a stronger basis in science. Such a development would both improve health and abandon needless favoritism in trade. As the prominent trade law scholars Michael J. Trebilcock and Robert Howse (2005) note, health and environmental concerns are often used as justifications for trade policies that are in fact optimized more to enhance protectionism than to improve health or the environment. Ensuring that health regulations are informed more by science than by protectionist impulses not only would guarantee that the resulting regulations are consistent with the WTO system but would also generate better health outcomes. Such an ideal outcome, however, assumes that we live in a world where policy decisions can be made without the distorting influence of economic protectionism. In reality, the WTO's rules may make adopting and implementing health regulations more difficult; without protectionist incentives to sweeten the deal, it may not be possible to mobilize the political will required to address certain health problems.

V. THE FUTURE OF GLOBAL HEALTH GOVERNANCE

This chapter defined the term "global health law" and discussed the forces of globalization that present health hazards throughout the world. The readings explained the need for an architecture of global health, examining the strengths and weaknesses of existing international law. The chapter concludes here with a proposal for an innovative mechanism for global health governance—the Framework Convention on Global Health.

MEETING THE SURVIVAL NEEDS OF THE WORLD'S LEAST HEALTHY PEOPLE: A PROPOSED MODEL FOR GLOBAL HEALTH GOVERNANCE*
Lawrence O. Gostin

International health assistance is provided in an ineffective way that does not enhance the capability for human functioning. Most funding is driven by emotional, high-visibility events, including large-scale natural disasters such as the Asian tsunami; diseases that capture the public's imagination such as the human immunodeficiency virus and AIDS; or diseases with the potential for rapid global transmission such as hemorrhagic fever, severe acute respiratory syndrome, or pandemic influenza. These funding streams skew priorities and divert resources from building stable local systems to meet everyday health needs....

BASIC SURVIVAL NEEDS

What is truly needed, and what richer countries instinctively (although not always adequately) do for their own citizens, is to meet what can be called "basic survival needs." Basic survival needs include sanitation and sewage, pest control, clean air and water, diet and nutrition, tobacco reduction, essential medicines and vaccines, and well-functioning health systems. Survival needs are laid out in the United Nations' Millennium Development Goals, which call for major improvements in maternal and child health, and the prevention of AIDS, malaria, and other diseases. Meeting everyday survival needs may lack the glamour of high-technology medicine or dramatic rescue, but what they lack in excitement they gain in their potential impact on health, precisely because they deal with the major causes of common disease and disability across the globe. Mobilizing the public and private sectors to meet basic survival needs, comparable to a Marshall Plan, could radically transform prospects for improving health among the world's poorest populations.

... Vast human benefits would accrue from highly cost-effective interventions. For instance, vaccine-preventable diseases are virtually extinct in developed countries but still account for millions of deaths annually in poorer regions. Basic sanitation and water systems would vastly improve global health at minimal cost, such as clean water kits costing as little as $3. An insecticide-treated bed net, which costs roughly $5, is highly effective in reducing malaria, river blindness, elephantiasis, and other insectborne diseases among children. But only about 1 in 7 children in Africa sleep under a bed net, and only 3% of children in sub-Saharan Africa use a net impregnated with insecticide.

The single most important way to ensure basic survival is to build enduring

*Reprinted from *JAMA* 298 (2007): 225–28. Copyright © 2007 American Medical Association. All rights reserved.

health systems in all countries. Health systems include public health agencies with the capacity to identify, prevent, and ameliorate health risks in the population—disease surveillance, laboratories, data systems, and a competent workforce. They also include primary health care, bringing basic medical services (eg, maternal and child health, family planning, and medical treatment) as close as possible to where people live and work. Primary care promotes individual and community self-reliance and participation in the planning, organization, operation, and control of health services, making fullest use of local and national resources. What poor countries need is to gain the capacity to provide essential health services.

PROPOSAL FOR A FRAMEWORK CONVENTION ON GLOBAL HEALTH

If meeting basic survival needs can truly make a difference for the world's population, and if this solution is preferable to other paths, can international law structure legal obligations accordingly? Extant health governance has been lamentably deficient, and a fresh approach is badly needed.

The World Health Organization [WHO] Constitution grants the agency formidable powers, but its potential has never been realized. In 60 years of existence, WHO has enacted only 1 significant regulation (the IHR) and 1 treaty (the FCTC). There is, however, a much larger body of international law that powerfully affects global health in areas ranging from food safety, arms control, and the environment to trade and human rights. The WHO should be a leader in creating, or at least influencing, this body of international law, but that has not happened. The agency has shied away from rulemaking because it has seen itself principally as a scientific, technical agency.

As a result, social activists increasingly have turned to the language of human rights to articulate their aspirations for global health. But recasting the problem of extremely poor health as a human rights violation does not help. The legal obligation to protect the public's health falls primarily on each state (ie, nation-state), but poor countries lack the capacity to do so. Although the International Covenant on Economic, Social, and Cultural Rights posits that all states have duties to cooperate, there are no specific requirements for assisting other countries.

If law is to play a constructive role, new models will be required. One model would be a Framework Convention on Global Health (FCGH). An FCGH is a global health governance scheme that incorporates a bottom-up strategy that strives to do the following: build capacity, so that all countries have enduring and effective health systems; set priorities, so that international assistance is directed to meeting basic survival needs; engage stakeholders, so that a wide variety of state and nonstate participants can contribute their resources and expertise; coordinate activities, so that programs among the proliferating number of participants operating around the world are harmonized; and evaluate and monitor progress, to ensure that goals are met and promises kept.

The framework convention-protocol approach refers to a process of incremental regime development. In the initial stage, participating states would negotiate and agree to the framework instrument, which would establish broad principles for global health governance. In subsequent stages, specific protocols would be developed to achieve the objectives set forth in the original framework. These protocols, organized by key components of the global health strategy, would create more detailed legal norms, structures, and processes. The framework convention-protocol approach has considerable flexibility, allowing participating states to decide the level of specificity that is politically feasible now, saving more complex or contentious issues to be built in later protocols.

The framework convention-protocol approach is becoming an essential strategy of powerful transnational social movements to safeguard health and the environment. [Models for global health governance include the Framework Convention on Tobacco Control as well as environmental treaties like the United Nations Framework Convention on Climate Change.]

An FCGH would represent a historical shift in global health, with broadly imagined global governance. The initial framework would establish the key modalities, with a strategy for subsequent protocols on each of the most important governance parameters. . . .

The framework convention-protocol approach has a number of advantages. The incremental nature of the governance strategy allows the international community to focus on a problem in a stepwise manner, avoiding potential political bottlenecks over contentious elements. The process of creating international norms and institutions also provides an ongoing and structured forum for states and stakeholders to develop a shared humanitarian instinct on global health. A high-profile forum for normative discussion can help educate and persuade participating states, and influence public opinion, in favor of decisive action. And it can create internal pressure for governments and others to actively participate in the framework dialogue. The creation of such a normative community, therefore, may be an essential element of building an international consensus. The imperatives of global health cannot be framed just as a series of isolated problems in far-off places, but rather as a common concern of humankind.

This approach, however, will not be a panacea and cannot easily circumvent many of the seemingly intractable problems of global health governance including the domination of economically and politically powerful countries; the deep resistance to creating obligations to expend, or transfer, wealth; the lack of trust in international legal regimes; and the vocal concerns about the integrity and competency of governments in many of the poorest regions.

But given the dismal nature of extant global health governance, an FCGH is a risk worth taking. It will, at a minimum, identify the genuinely important problems in global health: targeting the major determinants of health, prioritizing and coordinating currently fragmented activities, and engaging a broad range of stakeholders. It also will provide a needed forum to raise visibility for one of the most pressing problems facing humankind.

FAIR TERMS OF INTERNATIONAL COOPERATION ON GLOBAL HEALTH

[A collective international effort is needed to tackle the complex problems of global health.] If all states and stakeholders voluntarily accepted fair terms of cooperation through an FCGH, then [they] could dramatically improve life prospects for millions of people. But it would do more than that. Cooperative action for global health, like action to address global warming, benefits everyone by diminishing collective vulnerabilities.

The alternative to fair terms of cooperation through an FCGH is that everyone would be worse off, particularly those who have compounding disadvantages. Absent a binding commitment to help, rich states might find it politically or economically easier to withhold their fair share of global health assistance, hoping that others will take up the slack. Major outbreaks of infectious disease, including extensively drug-resistant forms, would become increasingly more likely. . . .

If the global community does not accept fair terms of cooperation on global health soon, there is every reason to believe that affluent states, philanthropists, and celebrities simply will move on to another cause. When they do, the vicious cycle of poverty and endemic disease among the world's least healthy people will continue unabated. That is a consequence that no one should be willing to tolerate.

RECOMMENDED READING

The Global Dimensions of Health

Cohen, Jon. 2006. The new world of global health. *Science* 311: 162–67. (Discusses the wave of new global philanthropy and its drawbacks and challenges)

Commission on Social Determinants of Health. 2008. *Closing the Gap in a Generation: Health Equity through Action on the Social Determinants of Health*. Geneva: World Health Organization. (Final report of the Commission on Social Determinants of Health; states that the "toxic combination of bad policies, economics, and politics is, in large measure, responsible for the fact that a majority of people in the world do not enjoy the good health that is biologically possible")

Daar, Abdallah S., et al. 2007. Grand challenges in chronic non-communicable diseases. *Nature* 450: 494–96. (Identifies barriers to solving problems of global non-communicable diseases)

Ezzati, Majid, et al. 2005. Rethinking the "diseases of affluence" paradigm: Global patterns of nutritional risks in relation to economic development. *Public Library of Science Medicine* 2: 404–11. (Posits that cardiovascular disease and other so-called diseases of affluence are likely to dramatically affect the world's poor as well)

Heinzerling, Lisa. 2008. Climate change, human health, and the post-precautionary principle. *Georgetown Law Journal* 96: 445–60. (Suggests two ways of reframing public discourse on climate change: to think of climate change as a public health threat and to stop using the precautionary principle).

Kaul, Inge, Isabelle Grunberg, and Marc A. Stern. 1999. Defining global public goods. *Global Public Goods*, 2–20. Oxford: Oxford Scholarship Online Monographs. (Provides a useful typology of global public goods)

Magnusson, Roger S. 2007. Non-communicable diseases and global health governance: Enhancing global processes to improve health development. *Globalization & Health* 3 (2). (Examines the impact of WHO, World Bank, and UN policies on the development of a global framework for addressing non-communicable diseases)

Taylor, Allyn L. 2004. Governing the globalization of public health. *Journal of Law, Medicine & Ethics* 32: 500–508. (Explains how globalization has created the need for a global health infrastructure)

World Health Organization. 2003. *World Health Report.* Geneva: World Health Organization. (Reports on challenges to increasing health investment and on global health challenges and solutions)

Yach, Derek, Corinna Hawkes, C. Linn Gould, and Karen J. Hofman. 2004. The global burden of chronic diseases: Overcoming impediments to prevention and control. *JAMA* 291: 2616–22. (Discusses potential policy solutions for improving the global response to chronic diseases)

International Public Health Law

Fidler, David P. 2004. *SARS: Governance and the Globalization of Disease.* New York: Palgrave Macmillan. (Recounts the outbreak, explains the implications for global health governance, and makes recommendations for dealing with new infectious diseases such as SARS)

Gostin, Lawrence O., and Allyn L. Taylor. 2008. Global health law: A definition and grand challenges. *Public Health Ethics* 1 (1): 53–63. (Proposes a definition of global health law and a road map for its future)

Roemer, Ruth, Allyn Taylor, and Jean Lariviere. 2005. Origins of the WHO Framework Convention on Tobacco Control. *American Journal of Public Health* 95: 936–38. (Outlines the history of the Framework Convention and its adoption by the WHO)

Human Rights: Advancing Dignity, Justice, and Security in Health

Gruskin, Sofia, ed. 2005. *Perspectives on Health and Human Rights.* New York: Routledge. (Contains readings and materials on health and human rights)

Mann, Jonathan M. 1997. Medicine and public health, ethics, and human rights. *Hastings Center Report* 27 (3): 6–13. (Discusses the relationship and inextricable links between these disciplines)

World Trade and World Health

Sapsin, Jason W., Theresa M. Thompson, Lesley Stone, and Katherine E. DeLand. 2003. International trade, law, and public health advocacy. *Journal of Law, Medicine & Ethics* 31: 546–56. (Examines trade's effect on public health)

Trebilcock, Michael J., and Robert Howse. 2005. *The Regulation of International Trade.* 3d ed. New York: Routledge. (A textbook; provides analysis of the rules and organizations that shape international trade)

United Nations Commission on Human Rights, Economic and Social Council. 2004. *Economic, Social and Cultural Rights: The Right of Everyone to the*

Highest Attainable Level of Physical and Mental Health. Report of the Special Rapporteur, Paul Hunt. Addendum: Mission to the World Trade Organization. UN Doc. E/CN.4/2004/49/Add.1. www.unhchr.ch/Huridocda/ Huridoca.nsf/e06a5300f90fa0238025668700518ca4/5860d7d863239d82c1 256e660056432a/$FILE/G0411390.pdf. (Provides an accessible introduction to technical issues that lie at the intersection of trade and the right to health)

The Future of Global Health Governance

Gostin, Lawrence O. 2008. Meeting basic survival needs of the world's least healthy people: Toward a framework convention on global health. *Georgetown Law Journal* 96: 331–92. (Provides a more detailed examination of the core deficiencies in global health assistance and the proposal for the Framework Convention on Global Health)

Hollis, Aidan, and Thomas Pogge. 2008. *The Health Impact Fund: Making New Medicines Accessible for All.* www.yale.edu/macmillan/igh/hif_book .pdf. (Discusses the current inequitable distribution of medicines; provides a solution in the form of the Health Impact Fund)

Silberschmidt, Gaudenz, Don Matheson, and Ilona Kickbusch. 2008. Creating a Committee C of the World Health Assembly. *Lancet* 371: 1483–86. (Proposes the creation of a Committee C within the World Health Assembly that would serve as a forum for debate of major health initiatives by other key players in the global health arena)

PART THREE

Public Health and Civil Liberties in Conflict

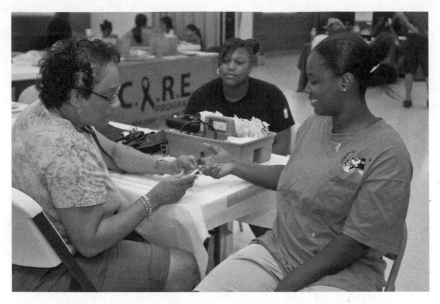

Photo 17. A young woman receives a free diabetes screening at a Texas community center. In much of the country, diabetes rates are alarmingly high. The rising incidence of type II diabetes is linked to the increasing prevalence of obesity. In 2005, New York City's health commissioner, Thomas Frieden, proposed a controversial diabetes surveillance program similar to those typically used for infectious diseases. Reproduced by permission, © Marjorie Kamys Cotera/Daemmrich Photography/The Image Works.

Surveillance and Public Health Research

Privacy and the "Right to Know"

To achieve collective benefits, public health officials systematically collect, store, use, and disseminate vast amounts of personal information, commonly in electronic form. Public health officials monitor health status to identify health problems, diagnose and investigate health hazards, conduct research to understand health problems and find innovative solutions, and disseminate information intended to inform, educate, and empower people in matters related to their health. The data that they collect provide the basic infrastructure necessary to effect many of the common goods of community health. These data are also often personally identifiable and sensitive. Data may reveal information about a person's lifestyle (e.g., sexual orientation), health status (e.g., mental illness, breast cancer, HIV), behaviors (e.g., unsafe sex or needle sharing), and genetics (e.g., family health history).

Society faces hard choices in balancing individual interests in privacy and the collective benefits produced by public health data collection. This chapter explores that tension. The opening section describes public health surveillance from historical and contemporary perspectives, focusing on salient illustrations of health monitoring for infectious diseases (e.g., HIV/AIDS) and chronic diseases (e.g., diabetes). Second, the chapter examines legal and ethical aspects of particular public health practices, with deep historical roots in American public health: the reporting of injuries and diseases to state health departments and partner notification. Third, the chapter explores the difficult, but highly important, distinctions between public health research and practice. Finally, the chapter looks at the right to privacy, which has gained recognition under the Constitution as well as under federal and state statutes. This final section also presents a model public health privacy statute that seeks to reconcile the collective benefits of surveillance with individual interests in privacy.

I. SURVEILLANCE: AN ESSENTIAL PUBLIC HEALTH ACTIVITY, ETHICAL AND RIGHTS-BASED CONCERNS

The population faces numerous health threats, such as contaminated food and water, emerging infections, bioterrorism, and chronic diseases caused by unhealthy lifestyles. Public health agencies cannot avert these threats unless they have a system of early detection and continuous health monitoring. In the absence of a strong public health information infrastructure, communities remain vulnerable to diseases and injuries, particularly those that are novel or not well understood. Surveillance is a fundamental public health activity that yields essential information about patterns of morbidity and mortality in populations. It has also been the source of considerable ethical debate, generated by concerns about privacy and unauthorized use of personal information.

In the following excerpt, the public health professors Ronald Bayer and Amy L. Fairchild offer a brief historical account of the evolution of public health surveillance and ethics, focusing on critical episodes such as the dispute over name-based HIV reporting and the creation of vaccine registries. Bayer and Fairchild use these examples to explain why certain surveillance activities are contested and to highlight the tension between privacy and public health.

PUBLIC HEALTH: SURVEILLANCE AND PRIVACY*
Ronald Bayer and Amy L. Fairchild

It was not until the late 19th century that systematic reporting of infectious diseases began. Surveillance was also undertaken to initiate quarantine, isolation, or vaccination and provoked public and professional concern. Physicians, on occasion, challenged the authority of public health professionals to breach the sanctity of the doctor-patient relationship in the name of surveillance. In New York City, for example, physician outrage over mandatory tuberculosis (TB) reporting beginning in

*Excerpted from *Science* 290 (2000): 1898–99. Reprinted with permission from the American Association for the Advancement of Science.

1897 resulted in an essentially voluntary reporting system in which doctors withheld the names of their private patients and reported the names of their poor, dispensary cases. . . .

Eventually, name-based reporting was extended to a host of other conditions, typically without any sign of protest. But recognizing that resistance could undermine their efforts, public health officials began to develop the legal and organizational capacity for protecting the confidentiality of names.

Nonetheless, in the last part of the 20th century, a protracted and furious debate about surveillance would again surface. The U.S. controversy over HIV name reporting, beginning in 1985, was radically affected by the circumstances under which it emerged, e.g., the special fears surrounding the AIDS epidemic, a transformed conception of the rights of privacy, constitutional limits on state authority exercised for benevolent purposes, the development of a vigorous debate about medical ethics, and the emergence of patient advocacy as a potent social force. An increasing number of public health officials, who believed they could protect the confidentiality of name-based reports, found themselves pitted against AIDS activists and proponents of civil liberties who focused on the potential for discrimination and coercion if names were sent to public health registries.

When it became clear that some form of HIV infection reporting was necessary, the debate shifted to the question of whether relying on unique identifiers in lieu of names could meet surveillance requirements. The coalition opposed to name-based reporting insisted that a uniquely stigmatized disease demanded policies uniquely protective of privacy. Although some public health officials [such as those in Maryland] supported the use of unique identifiers, most remained skeptical. The U.S. Centers for Disease Control and Prevention (CDC) had, by the 1990s, become convinced that name-based reporting was most efficient and accurate. When, in 1999, it mandated that all states adopt some form of HIV surveillance, it only reluctantly acknowledged that, under stringent performance criteria, unique identifiers could serve public health adequately. . . .

Vaccine registries provide a counterpoint to HIV. In response to sporadic disease outbreaks, poor coverage in inner-city communities, increasingly complex vaccine schedules, family mobility, and poor provider and patient awareness of immunization coverage levels, the National Vaccine Advisory Committee (NVAC) recommended in 1999 creation of a nationwide network of state and community immunization registries. . . .

In the face of considerable anxiety, the federal initiative to register immunization coverage put a premium on community participation and cooperation. . . . As a result, a central concern of the NVAC was to protect patient confidentiality. The NVAC report recommended that, at a minimum, registries notify parents of the existence and content of the registry. Critically, it recommended that parents should be permitted to decide whether children would be included in registries. . . .

. . . Vaccine registries thus stand as a challenge to the proposition that only universal, name-based reporting without consent is an adequate basis for surveillance.

CONCLUSIONS

Five themes emerge that help to explain the circumstances under which surveillance is contested and those under which it is accepted without debate.

First, the extent to which surveillance might trigger public health interventions and the way such interventions have been viewed have been central. Fear that those reported would be the targets of coercion or discrimination has energized opposition to name-based reporting. . . .

A second theme is the extent to which proposals for reporting provoke resistance or alarm when they involve diseases carrying social stigma or touch those who view themselves as socially marginalized or vulnerable to social or economic injury. Affected individuals may find pledges that reported information will be protected from unwarranted disclosure hard to believe and, as a consequence, see themselves as endangered.

Third, special populations can elicit special protections. Thus, surveillance regimes involving children and reproduction have put a high premium on both confidentiality and informed consent.

Fourth, although constituencies have sometimes been highly alert to the potential imposition of a surveillance regime, that has not always been the case. In the case of tumor registries, the subjects of reporting remain largely unaware of ongoing reporting requirements. Without such awareness, the possibility of voicing privacy concerns remains out of reach.

Perhaps most important, changes in expectations regarding privacy have had a profound impact on the acceptability of name-based reporting systems and the willingness of policy-makers to consider alternatives. Registries that have developed most recently (particularly birth defects registries and vaccination registries) have been more sensitive to a culture of privacy than older ones, which find themselves challenged. . . .

Every U.S. state has statutes or regulations developed over the course of the 20th century that protect the confidentiality of names reported to disease registries. Nonetheless, existing state laws lack uniformity and make it difficult to define clearly the ways in which they will protect reported data from unwarranted disclosure. That the CDC supported the development of a model state public health privacy act to protect such information underscores the salience of this issue.

This is an opportune moment for analysis of ethical challenges posed by name-based reporting requirements. Such an effort would necessitate recognition that the protection of public health may require some limitations on privacy. The central ethical question posed by name-based reporting is whether an abrogation of medical privacy can be justified by public health benefits. Although medical privacy is a fundamental value, it is not an absolute.

.   .   .   .   .

As disease threats change over time, it is essential that public health surveillance evolve to reflect modern challenges. In the past few decades, non-communicable diseases have emerged as major causes of morbidity and premature mortality. At the same time, new communicable diseases, including AIDS and severe acute respiratory syndrome (SARS), pose serious risks to the public's health. In response to these changes, the New York City Department of Health has taken unprecedented steps to extend the scope and function of its surveillance efforts. In 2005, Health Commissioner Thomas Frieden proposed a diabetes surveillance program, the first of its kind, which would not only track the blood sugar levels of patients in the registry but also inform physicians and patients when blood sugar levels suggest a need for further treatment. In addition, the city proposed, but never implemented, an expansion of HIV testing and surveillance. Both surveillance programs were met with vocal opposition from medical organizations as well as patients, who viewed the efforts to expand surveillance as unwelcome intrusions on the privacy of the doctor-patient relationship. In the following passage, Amy Fairchild, Ronald Bayer, and James Colgrove, all professors of public health, outline the novel New York City diabetes and HIV surveillance programs and the ethical debate that they triggered.

PANOPTIC VISIONS AND STUBBORN REALITIES IN A NEW ERA OF PRIVACY*

Amy L. Fairchild, Ronald Bayer, and James Colgrove

In July 2005, with the fanfare of a new public health campaign, New York City health officials described the dual epidemics of obesity and diabetes. With levels of self-reported diabetes more than doubling between 1994 and 2003, the disease, Frieden said (2006), was "the only major health problem in this country that's getting worse and getting worse quickly." It had accounted for some twenty thousand hospitalizations in 2003.

As a first step in controlling the epidemic, the health department put forward a bold proposal for electronic laboratory-based reporting of hemoglobin tests, an indication of blood sugar levels. Never had a city or state health department initiated ongoing, systematic diabetes surveillance for an entire population. In justifying the new surveillance effort, the health department underscored its legal mandate to prevent and control chronic, as well as communicable, disease. Registries for cancer, dementia, and congenital malformations provided well-established precedents for diabetes surveillance, the department claimed. But more than epidemiological surveillance would come to be involved in the city's plan. Most radically, the health department proposed to use its authority to contact both doctors and patients when [blood tests] suggested the need to review the clinical picture and even to modify the course of treatment if needed. It was that dimension of the proposed effort that would become the object of the most sustained debate. . . .

In response to concerns about stigma and discrimination, Frieden argued that the privacy protections for the registry would be stronger than those for communicable disease reporting. Confidentiality provisions, the department asserted, would explicitly prohibit sharing that might "make it more difficult for persons with diabetes to obtain or renew a driver's license, health insurance, life insurance, etc." (New York City Department of Health and Mental Hygiene 2005). Indeed, even patients themselves would not be able to authorize further disclosure of their registry data.

When the proposal was open for public comment, it attracted scant notice. Those physicians who supported it were all involved in monitoring the quality of care in hospitals. They viewed the surveillance program as an effort to replicate on a citywide basis the system that health care institutions and managed care plans had already put into place. Libertarian physicians' organizations, however, characterized the proposed system as an unwarranted extension of public health authority into the domain of clinical medicine. . . .

Patient opposition to the diabetes proposals centered on privacy and intrusions in the clinical relationship. One patient who testified against the proposal said, "As a diabetic I am not a threat to the city's public health, nor do I wish to be treated as one." Said another opponent, "This isn't smallpox." The health department "does not have a compelling interest in the health of an individual that overrides that individual's right to privacy" (Caruso 2005). . . .

In the era of democratic privacy, none of this language was surprising given the scope of what health officials had proposed and the history of earlier struggles over surveillance. What was striking was how few opponents came forward. Neither the ACLU, its affiliate, nor any of the other groups that had been so engaged in debates about surveillance during the past two decades appeared at the public hearing or submitted formal comments. Nonetheless, the city scaled back its efforts, permitting patients to opt out of health department interventions. Their names, however, would remain in the registry. Further, what had initially appeared to represent a citywide program would begin with a trial in the South Bronx, an impoverished area of the city where diabetes rates were the highest and medical care was inadequate.

Protest broadened only after the Board of Health endorsed Commissioner Frieden's proposals on December 1, 2005. The reaction was fueled in part by city proposals to radically change the scope and function of HIV testing and surveillance. Part of a broader set of moves that included an easing of the informed consent requirements for HIV testing, the HIV surveillance effort sought to give health authorities the ability to intervene with patients whose clinical care appeared to be less than optimal, just as it had proposed to do with diabetes. . . . Of chief concern were patients lost to care, who had "no one responsible, no one accountable" for their medical management. Frieden said that the disparities between whites and people of color infected with HIV represented "a damning indictment of our system" (Santora 2006). He proposed that when officials became aware of someone whose health required a modification of treatment that the department be able to use the information already in hand to contact patients and consult their providers. Further, the health department argued that it was uniquely positioned to refer newly diagnosed cases to clinical services, contacting the patient directly if necessary, and to help physicians contact patients who had dropped out of care. . . .

. . . Organizations that had long been involved in battles of case reporting moved to thwart the health department. In part, opposition centered over disagreements about how to understand the obvious racial disparities in HIV status. [In addition, opponents were concerned about further possible erosions of privacy and liberty (e.g., compulsory treatment and punishment for nonadherence to a treatment regimen) that the program might precipitate.]

To meet the challenge provoked by his proposals, Frieden appeared to modify his stance, as he had in the much less volatile dispute over diabetes surveillance. In contrast to his diabetes program, individuals would have to opt in to the clinical oversight that was at the heart of what he had put forward. "We would reach out to treating doctors, case managers and, *only if there are no viable alternatives,* directly to patients to offer to help link them to existing HIV services." While acknowledging the concerns that such direct intervention would generate, Frieden stressed [to community workers, March 6, 2006], "The epidemic demands effective approaches to reach patients who are not in care."

[These modern surveillance measures have clear antecedents in the nineteenth century. Although framed in the language of quality assurance and Improvement, Frieden's proposals were reminiscent of earlier efforts when health officials sought to oversee the management of tuberculosis by coordinating with a network of nurses and clinics.]

II. TRADITIONAL PUBLIC HEALTH ACTIVITIES: REPORTING AND PARTNER NOTIFICATION

A. *Reporting Injuries and Diseases to the Health Department*

Because few resources are dedicated to public health surveillance, state and local governments rely heavily on clinical reports of disease and injury. Every state requires physicians and laboratories to report certain events that cause harm (e.g., child abuse and gunshot wounds) as well as specified infections (e.g., HIV) and diseases (e.g., hepatitis, rabies, and tuberculosis).

Reporting, although universally mandated, is highly controversial. Daniel M. Fox (1986) has observed that reporting statutes create tensions between physicians, whose primary role is to protect their patients, and public health officials, whose primary role is to protect the population. In particular, physicians defend their confidential therapeutic relationships, whereas public health authorities insist on full reporting.

Public health surveillance has evolved in recent years to include new methods for tracking health measures. Such methods include syndromic surveillance (which uses data that precede diagnosis and signal a sufficient probability of a case or an outbreak to warrant further public health response) and environmental health tracking (which uses data about environmental hazards on an ongoing basis). Despite these advances, clinical reporting remains a critical element in public health surveillance.

In the following reading, Sandra Roush, of the CDC, and colleagues explore the diversity in reporting requirements across the country. Such diversity is a prime example of how social values and priorities influence modern public health surveillance.

MANDATORY REPORTING OF DISEASES AND CONDITIONS BY HEALTH CARE PROVIDERS AND LABORATORIES*

Sandra Roush, Guthrie Birkhead, Denise Koo, Angela Cobb, and David Fleming

Public health surveillance systems in the United States were designed for the reporting of infectious diseases of public health interest, and health care professionals (usually physicians and nurses) have been the primary source of disease reporting. Recently, laboratories have also become an important source of reporting for public health surveillance. Together, health care provider reporting and laboratory reporting may ensure more complete and timely reporting for diseases and conditions recommended to be under national surveillance. The list of diseases and conditions that are recommended for national surveillance is designed to reflect the current needs and priorities for public health surveillance at any given time. . . .

In the United States, the authority to require notification of cases of diseases resides in the respective state legislatures. The states exercise their authority to require reporting by enacting legislation; some state statutes delegate the authority to enumerate the health conditions that are reportable to state or local agencies. Subsequent reporting of morbidity data by the state or territorial health department to CDC is voluntary.

Because of each state's autonomy with regard to morbidity reporting, the list of diseases and conditions that are reported varies by state. [Of the 58 diseases and conditions recommended for national reporting, 35 were reportable in greater than 90 percent of states and territories, 15 were reportable in 75 to 90 percent of the states and territories, and 8 were reportable in less than 75 percent of states and territories. Only 19 (33 percent) of the 58 diseases and conditions were reportable in each of the states and territories.] In addition to the variation among states for the conditions and diseases to be reported, the time frames for reporting, agencies receiving reports, persons required to report, and conditions under which reports are required also may differ among states. In many states, local health departments provide epidemiologic services; as a consequence, health care professionals in many states are encouraged by their public health officials to report diseases directly to local health departments rather than to the state health department. Health care professionals are encouraged to determine the specific requirements in their area by contacting their state health department.

Standardized case definitions for the diseases under national surveillance have been created [by the CDC and the Council of State and Territorial Epidemiologists] to provide uniform criteria for reporting cases. Although the public health case defini-

*Reprinted from *JAMA* 282 (1999): 164–70. Copyright © 1999 American Medical Association. All rights reserved.

tions are useful for surveillance, they are not designed to influence clinical treatment or to delay the reporting of pending case confirmation. . . .

Historically in the United States, infectious disease surveillance has relied primarily on case reports from physicians and other health care professionals. Although these diseases are usually underreported (reporting is estimated at 6%–90% for many of the diseases under national surveillance), if the reporting is consistent over time, these data are a good source of temporal and geographic trends and characteristics of the persons experiencing morbidity. For diseases or other health conditions for which there is a substantial laboratory component included in case diagnosis or definition, laboratory reporting is a useful mechanism to supplement reporting from physicians by clinicians.

Although reporting by clinicians to public health authorities allows immediate public health response, including case investigation, contact prophylaxis, and outbreak control, other methods of surveillance are also necessary to meet the changing needs of public health assessment. Some of these other methods are sentinel surveillance and secondary analysis of hospital discharge or other administrative data sets, prevalence surveys, and vital records. These methods may be used in combination to improve the comprehensiveness of data collection and to provide more complete information to assess local, state, or national goals for public health. . . .

Public health has expanded from its traditional base in infectious disease control, and as the scope of public health expands, the list of diseases and conditions of public health interest will vary between jurisdictions and over time. In the future, greater emphasis should be placed on gathering data electronically from existing sources, including clinical laboratories and computerized medical records. Those concerned about public health will increasingly be required to make the best use of limited resources for surveillance to meet the challenges of a changing medical care system using new information technology.

B. Partner Notification and Contact Tracing

Communicable diseases, particularly those that are sexually transmitted, put sexual partners, family members, and other personal contacts at risk for infection. If the risk is significant, it produces a significant dilemma: whether to safeguard individual privacy or disclose the risk. This tension between privacy and the duty to protect individuals at risk is especially pertinent in partner notification. Partner notification is a complex concept that has at least two distinct, if at times overlapping, meanings: (1) *duty to warn*—the power or duty of private health care professionals to inform their patients' sexual or other partners of foreseeable risks, and (2) *contact tracing*—the statutory power of public health agencies to identify and locate sexual partners and other "contacts" at risk of infection, and to notify them of the risk. In this section, Ronald Bayer, a professor at Columbia University, and Dr. Kathleen Toomey of the CDC discuss these "two faces" of partner notification.

HIV PREVENTION AND THE TWO FACES OF PARTNER NOTIFICATION*
Ronald Bayer and Kathleen E. Toomey

As public health officials confronted the AIDS epidemic in the early 1980s they came to recognize the crucial importance of confidentiality. Only if those at risk for HIV could be convinced that their clinical encounters would not be disclosed without their consent could they be encouraged to undergo counseling and testing. Thus, the CDC, the Surgeon General, the Institute of Medicine, and the Presidential Commission on the HIV Epidemic all came to stress a common point: that the protection of the public's health was not compromised by the protection of confidentiality. On the contrary, the protection of confidentiality was a precondition for the achievement of public health goals.

Although the protection of confidentiality was supported by public health officials, gay rights organizations, and civil liberties groups, the best strategy for reaching those unknowingly placed at risk for infection or those who might inadvertently place others at risk was the subject of profound disagreement.... Deep and sometimes bitter disputes arose over partner notification in the epidemic's first decade.

Disagreements over the scope and limits of the principle of confidentiality, deep distrust over the motives of public health officials, doubts about the relevance and potential efficacy of traditional public health approaches to sexually transmitted diseases in dealing with AIDS, and the enduring suspicions of those who viewed government agencies as a source of endangerment rather than protection were all involved in the controversy. Each of these factors helped to shape the context within which a profound confusion emerged between two very different approaches to informing unsuspecting third parties about their potential exposure to medical risk....

... The first approach, involving the moral "duty to warn," arose out of the clinical setting in which the physician knew the identity of the person deemed to be at risk. This approach provided a warrant for disclosure to endangered persons without the consent of the patient and could involve the revelation of the identity of the "threatening" party (the index patient). The second approach, that of contact tracing, emerged from sexually transmitted disease (STD) control programs in which the clinician typically did not know the identity of those who might have been exposed. This approach was formally predicated upon the voluntary cooperation of the patient in providing the names of contacts, never involved the disclosure of the identity of the index patient, and entailed the protection of the absolute confidentiality of the entire process of notification....

THE TRADITION OF CONTACT TRACING

Clinicians in STD control programs often did not have knowledge of a patient's background or family relationships. To elicit the names of sexual contacts, it was therefore necessary to obtain the cooperation of the index patient, [sometimes through coercion]. To facilitate such cooperation, STD programs promised that the identity

*Reprinted from *American Journal of Public Health* 82 (1992): 1158–64.

of the index patient would never be made available to contacts who were named. The index patient maintained ultimate control over the process, retaining the ability to withhold or provide names. Thus, the tradition of contact tracing was predicated on the voluntary cooperation of index patients and on a striking commitment to the protection of their anonymity. There were, quite obviously, circumstances when the identity of the index patient could be deduced even if he or she was not named, the paradigmatic case being the monogamous partner who was informed that he or she had been exposed to an STD. Yet even in such situations the two central principles of contact tracing remained uncompromised. The public health worker would not confirm the identity of the obvious source of exposure. Even when the index patients themselves requested that their identity be revealed to contacts, no exceptions were to be made.

Despite the four decades of experience with contact tracing, all efforts to undertake such public health interventions in the context of AIDS met with fierce resistance in the first years of the epidemic. Opposition by gay leaders and civil liberties groups had a profound impact on the response of public health officials, especially in states with relatively large numbers of AIDS cases. . . .

Underlying this debate was the fact that in the first years of the AIDS epidemic, no therapy could be offered to asymptomatic infected individuals. Thus, the role of contact tracing in the context of HIV infection differed radically from its role in the context of other STDs. . . . For public health officials, who saw in such information an opportunity to target efforts to foster behavioral changes among individuals still engaging in high-risk behavior that could place both the individual contacted and future partners at risk, that was reason enough to undertake the process. For opponents of contact tracing, the very effort to reach out to such individuals represented a profound intrusion on privacy with little or no compensating benefit. The task of behavioral change, they asserted, could be achieved more effectively and efficiently through general education. . . .

By the late 1980s, the debate over contact tracing had shifted from one centered on the ethical issues of privacy to one focused on efficacy. . . . Early misapprehensions about the extent to which public health officials typically relied on overt coercion in the process, and the degree to which confidentiality might be compromised, had by decade's end all but vanished. With such political concerns allayed, many gay leaders had come to recognize that partner notification, in fact, could be a "useful tool" in efforts to control AIDS. . . .

THE DUTY TO WARN

As physicians were called upon to treat patients with infectious diseases, it was inevitable that they would be confronted by the question of whether the duty to protect the privileged communications within the clinical relationship took priority over the obligation to protect others from their patients' communicable conditions.

A misreading of a number of early 20th century cases has led some commentators to conclude that state courts had established an affirmative duty to breach confidentiality to protect known third parties. Indeed, it was such a misreading that permitted the California Supreme Court to claim the authority of precedent when in 1974 it crafted a doctrine that represented the most striking judicial challenge to the professional discretion of physicians when faced with patients who might endanger

third parties. The "protective privilege ends where the public peril begins," wrote
the majority in *Tarasoff v. Regents of California,* 551 P.2d 332 (Cal. 1976). . . .

[Ed.–In *Tarasoff,* the California Supreme Court held that mental health professionals have a duty to warn identifiable third parties of threats of violence by the
professional's patients. The case involved the murder of Tatiana Tarasoff, who had
a prior casual relationship with Prosenjit Poddar, a mentally deranged patient. In
therapy sessions Poddar indicated to his psychotherapist, Dr. Lawrence Moore, his
intent to kill a girl. Although Poddar did not specifically name Tarasoff, it was evident
to Dr. Moore that she was the intended victim. Dr. Moore did not warn Tarasoff or her
parents, but instead asked the police to pick up Poddar. Although the police detained
Poddar initially, he was later released and advised to stay away from Tarasoff. Two
months later, Poddar murdered Tarasoff. Tarasoff's parents later sued Dr. Moore
on the theory that he had a duty to warn their daughter of the risk that Poddar
presented.]

At the root of the *Tarasoff* decision was an ethical judgment that, although confidentiality was crucial for individual patients' autonomy, the protection of third parties vulnerable to potentially serious harm must be given priority. As a matter of
moral principle, that determination provoked widespread support. What remained a
matter of great controversy, however, was the question of whether such a determination represented wise public policy. Would the recognition of a legal duty to warn or
protect so subvert the trust necessary to the therapeutic relationship that patients
with violent fantasies would be constrained from talking about them with their therapists? Would the reduction in candor ultimately harm the public good by limiting the
capacity of therapists to help their patients control their dangerous behaviors?

The *Tarasoff* doctrine and its ethical underpinnings provided the backdrop to the
disputes that would surface as physicians confronted the dilemma of how to respond
to HIV-infected patients who refused to inform their needle-sharing or sexual partners of their exposure when the clinician knew the identity of the endangered party.
For some the dilemma arose solely in the context of partners who quite obviously
had no reason to suspect that they had been placed at risk, the paradigmatic case
being the female partner of a bisexual man. Other physicians extended their concern
to those who might have reason to know but might nevertheless be ignorant of the
risk to which they had been exposed, for example, the gay male partner in a long-
standing, apparently monogamous relationship. The choices to be made would be all
the more difficult given the extraordinary efforts that had been made to protect the
confidentiality and rights of those infected with HIV. . . .

As public health officials began to consider the issues posed by the warning of
third parties discovered during the clinical work of physicians to be at risk, they
sought to chart a response that was cognizant of both the centrality of confidentiality in the effort to control the spread of HIV infection and the importance of ensuring
that known parties were informed of their possible exposure to HIV. . . . Public health
officials argued for a "privilege to disclose," thus freeing physicians from liability for
either breaching confidentiality or not warning those who were at risk. In so arguing,
these officials were reasserting the principle that had guided public policy in the era
before *Tarasoff* and that historically had guided physician behavior.

The doctrine of the privilege to disclose was a political compromise designed to
meet the concerns of a number of constituencies, not all of whom shared assump-

tions about the appropriate role of physicians in protecting vulnerable third parties from HIV infection. For all clinicians, the doctrine offered the freedom to make
complex ethical judgments without the imposition of state mandates. For clinicians
committed to warning as many unsuspecting partners as possible, it offered the
opportunity to act on their professional obligations without being burdened by the
dictates of the state. For those who believed that breaches of confidentiality were
acceptable only in the rarest of circumstances, the privilege to disclose permitted a
principled recognition that disclosure could be justified without the dangers associated with an overbroad commitment to notification. . . .

CONCLUSIONS

From the perspective of the ethics of the clinical relationship, those who may have
been placed at risk unknowingly have a moral right to [information regarding their
potential infection]. They are entitled to such information so that they may take
steps to protect themselves, so that they can seek HIV testing and clinical evaluation, so that they may commence treatment if necessary, and so that they may avoid
the inadvertent transmission of HIV. The moral claim of those who have unknowingly
been placed at risk entails the correlative moral duty of the clinician to ensure that
the unsuspecting party is informed. Neither the principle of confidentiality nor the
value attached to professional autonomy is an absolute. . . .

If the duty to warn poses difficult ethical questions, contact tracing does not.
Contact tracing typically entails neither disclosure without the consent of the
infected patient nor breaches of confidentiality. In fact, it can be argued that public
health departments have a moral responsibility to undertake efforts modeled on the
tradition of contact tracing programs that can inform individuals at risk about matters crucial to their lives and to the lives of their sexual and needle-sharing partners
without recourse to mandatory measures.

But such a moral injunction may create difficult choices for policymakers, who
must try to balance these activities with other moral claims on limited resources.
Whatever the strengths of contact tracing, it is but one element in a much broader
array of educational and programmatic efforts to limit the spread of HIV infection.
What proportions of the overall prevention efforts should be devoted to this labor-
intensive and inevitably costly strategy? How are limited resources to be allocated
among alternative strategies for achieving behavioral change? To these questions
there can be no universal response. . . . But what an advance it will represent to
face the question of partner notification without the misconception that bedeviled
discussions during the first decade of the AIDS epidemic.

C. Duty to Warn and Right to Know

Bayer and Toomey examine partner notification in terms of the duties
of private health care professionals and governmental health officials.
There is, of course, another potential duty that is equally contested: the
duty placed on contagious persons themselves to disclose the risk to
their sexual or needle-sharing partners.

Significant legal questions arise when partner notification does not occur and infection of a sexual partner results. In *John B. v. Superior Court of L.A. County,* 137 P.3d 153 (Cal. 2006), the Supreme Court of California was presented with a civil suit concerning a husband's liability for infecting his wife with HIV. After testing positive for HIV, the plaintiff was informed by her physician that she had been HIV positive "for a long time," had infected her husband, and had "brought the HIV into the marriage." Her husband was offered treatment, but she was not. A year later, she began to suspect that her husband had been infected with HIV first because he developed AIDS shortly after testing positive for HIV; she later found out that he had also been unfaithful. She sued, alleging that her husband had knowingly infected her with HIV. In considering whether and how the case should proceed, the court asked: "What duty does an HIV-positive individual have to avoid transmitting the virus? What level of awareness should be required before a court imposes a duty of care on an HIV-positive individual to avoid transmission of the virus? What responsibility does the victim have to protect himself or herself against possible infection with the virus?" (137 P.3d at 155).

The court did not answer all of these questions, but it did hold that even when a defendant lacks actual knowledge of his serostatus, he may nonetheless be liable when—given his risk behaviors and symptoms—he should have known of his infection but refused to be tested. The court ruled: "Limiting tort defendants to those who have actual knowledge they are infected with HIV would have perverse effects on the spread of the virus. If only those who have been tested are subject to suit, there may be 'an incentive for some persons to avoid diagnosis and treatment in order to avoid knowledge of their own infection'" (Ibid., 161).

Although courts have recognized the duty to warn sexual partners of known infectious conditions, the Illinois Supreme Court recently declined to extend the duty to third parties. In *Doe v. Dilling,* 888 N.E.2d 24 (Ill. 2008), a woman infected with HIV by her fiancé sued his parents for fraudulently misrepresenting his serostatus to her. She claimed that had his parents not denied his HIV-positive status, she would have sought testing and treatment for HIV. The court refused to extend the tort of fraudulent misrepresentation to encompass cases against third parties, stating that Doe's reliance on the statements made by the parents of her fiancé was unjustifiable and that she "could have easily discovered additional facts if she had not chosen to consciously ignore what was plainly in front of her" (888 N.E.2d at 44).

III. PUBLIC HEALTH RESEARCH AND PRACTICE: UNDERSTANDING THE DISTINCTIONS

Ethical norms and federal law require that in research involving human subjects, including public health research, specific actions must be taken to ensure the well-being of participants, such as the granting of informed consent by study participants and review of the study design by an institutional review board. Public health practice, in contrast, encompasses a wide variety of activities that involve the collection of identifiable health information but are not subject to the same requirements. Some essential public health activities are easily classified as public health practice, such as surveillance through registries and disease-reporting mandates, but others may fall into the realm of research. It is critical that public health practitioners have the ability to distinguish between research and practice before engaging in a given activity so that they can follow the appropriate required procedures. In the following article, James G. Hodge Jr., a professor specializing in public health law, presents a detailed approach to distinguishing public health research from practice. Hodge describes existing guidelines for the classification of research and practice, provides a review of applicable laws, and lays out guidelines for distinguishing between research and practice by considering the essential characteristics of the activities in question.

AN ENHANCED APPROACH TO DISTINGUISHING PUBLIC HEALTH PRACTICE FROM HUMAN SUBJECTS RESEARCH*

James G. Hodge Jr.

What Are the Differences between Public Health Practice and Research? This perplexing question constantly arises in the planning and performance of public health activities involving the acquisition and use of identifiable health information.... These activities include surveillance (e.g., reporting requirements, disease registries, sentinel networks), epidemiological investigations (e.g., to investigate disease outbreaks), and evaluation and monitoring (e.g., public health program development and analysis, oversight functions). Few debate that these essential public health activities, often specifically authorized by law, are classifiable as public health practice.

Other public health activities in which identifiable health data are acquired or

*Reprinted from *Journal of Law, Medicine, & Ethics* 33 (2005): 125–40. (Blackwell Publishing).

used, however, can resemble, include, or constitute human subjects research.... A public health agency may, for example, conduct a double-blinded, controlled study to assess the efficacy of a new vaccine among a randomly-selected group of persons within the affected population. [Such activity constitutes research, and] the public health agency must adhere to a series of protections (e.g., individual informed consent absent a waiver) and procedures (e.g., review by an institutional review board [IRB]) designed to protect the health and safety of human subjects.

Lost in a legal and ethical gray zone are a host of public health activities that are not neatly characterized as either practice or research....

... Clearer distinctions are needed [for activities that are not easily classified] because (1) federal, state, and local laws and ethical principles governing human subjects research can require extensive and burdensome procedures. Misclassification of public health practice activities as research can result in these activities being delayed or conducted less efficiently or at higher costs due to the need to adhere to these procedures; (2) the HIPAA Privacy Rule (and other privacy laws) employ different standards for the disclosure of identifiable health information to public health practitioners (or others) without individual written authorization depending on whether the underlying activity is public health practice or research. In general, it is more difficult to acquire identifiable health data under the Privacy Rule for research purposes; and (3) widespread variation in distinctions between public health practice from research have led to confusion among IRBs and public health agencies, inefficient and duplicative reviews, and infringements on information sharing....

KEY CONCEPTS OF HUMAN SUBJECTS RESEARCH AND PUBLIC HEALTH PRACTICE

The modern definition of human subjects research is a product of its two parts: "research" and "human subjects." The nearly universally-accepted definitions of these terms are found in the Common Rule. Research is defined as "a systematic investigation, including research development, testing, and evaluation, designed to develop or contribute to generalizable knowledge" (32 C.F.R. § 219 [1991])....
A "human subject" is a living individual about whom a researcher obtains (1) data through intervention or interaction with the individual; or (2) individually-identifiable health information. Human subjects research is not limited to any particular actor (e.g., public or private sector individual) or a specific setting (e.g., institution, agency, or corporation). Thus, a public health agency and its representatives may conduct human subjects research even in the pursuit of public health goals and objectives.

[The National Bioethics Advisory Council (NBAC)] and others question whether the common definition of research can or should be applied to public health. Many public health practice activities, such as disease surveillance, are (like research) routinely and systematically carried out, but are not considered research.... A definition of public health research involving human subjects consistent with this approach may be stated as follows: *the collection and analysis of identifiable health data by a public health authority for the purpose of generating knowledge that will primarily benefit those beyond the participating community who bear the risks of participation.*

Public health practice is more difficult to define than research, in part, because public health is so conceptually broad. Public health, according to the Institute of

Medicine (IOM), is what we do collectively to assure the conditions for people to be healthy. . . .

A working definition for public health practice involving identifiable health data builds on the definition for public health research. Public health practice may be defined as: *the collection and analysis of identifiable health data by a public health authority for the purpose of protecting the health of a particular community, where the benefits and risks are primarily designed to accrue to the participating community.* . . .

LEGAL FRAMEWORK UNDERLYING DISTINCTIONS BETWEEN PUBLIC HEALTH PRACTICE AND RESEARCH

Distinctions between public health practice and human subjects research, though complex, are attributable in part to their very different legal and ethical traditions. [While public health practice "is supported by a constitutional, statutory, and regulatory legal environment," ethical and legal principles for human subjects research derive largely from the federal Common Rule.]

Unlike the broad powers to protect the public's health, human subjects research is tightly regulated through federal, state, and local laws, highlighted by the federal Common Rule. The Common Rule, codified in a series of federal regulations, applies to virtually all research involving human subjects that is conducted by (or with funding from) federal agencies. For most activities determined to be human subjects research (as defined above), the Common Rule requires advance review by an IRB or medical ethics board in compliance with various specifications. Among other things, IRBs must assess whether: (1) there is appropriate individual or guardian consent for data collection; (2) the privacy of identifiable information is protected; (3) there exists a sound, safe, and effective research design; (4) research subjects are equitably selected; (5) appropriate data safety monitoring is provided; and (6) vulnerable populations (e.g., children, prisoners, mentally-disabled) are protected. . . .

ENHANCED GUIDELINES TO DISTINGUISH PUBLIC HEALTH PRACTICE AND HUMAN SUBJECTS RESEARCH

. . . This section presents a two-stage process [for distinguishing between public health practice and research].

Regardless of the complexity of the case, this dual stage approach requires public health authorities to honestly describe their intent, motivation, and objectives for their activities by answering some basic questions: (1) what prompted the performance of the activity; (2) on what (or whose) authority is the activity conducted; (3) what do the performers of the activity hope to achieve; (4) how will information from the activity be used; and (5) who will benefit from the activity? . . .

Stage 1—Essential Characteristics of Public Health Practice and Research

The initial step to distinguish public health practice activities from human subjects research activities is to review those parameters that are exclusive to each activity. . . . These essential characteristics, or foundations, of public health practice and research help separate the easy and hard cases, and eliminate some cases altogether from further need for classification.

Essential characteristics of public health practice . . . include:

- Involves specific legal authorization for conducting the activity as public health practice at the federal, state or local levels;
- Includes a corresponding governmental duty to perform the activity to protect the public's health;
- Involves direct performance or oversight by a governmental public health authority (or its authorized partner) and accountability to the public for its performance;
- May legitimately involve persons who did not specifically volunteer to participate (i.e., they did not provide informed consent); and
- Supported by principles of public health ethics that focus on populations while respecting the dignity and rights of individuals.

Essential characteristics of human subjects research . . . include:

- Involves living individuals;
- Involves, in part, identifiable private health information;
- Involves research subjects who voluntarily participate (or participate with the consent of their guardian) absent a waiver of informed consent; and
- Supported by principles of research ethics that focus on the interests of individuals while balancing the communal value of research.

These characteristics distinguish practice from research in many of the easy cases. For example, a public health reporting requirement may be specifically authorized via legislation or administrative regulation. . . .

Stage 2—Enhanced Guidelines

The essential characteristics of public health practice and research suggested in Stage 1 may help resolve the simpler cases, but more complicated scenarios remain. . . . Reviewing the essential characteristics of public health practice or research may not fully allow the practitioner to properly classify this activity. Additional guidance is needed. . . .

The enhanced guidelines, below, provide meaningful bases to distinguish between research and public health practice. . . .

General Legal Authority. Two of the essential characteristics of public health practice (see Stage 1) are that there may be specific legal authority to engage in public health practice and a corresponding duty of public health agencies to fulfill that duty. . . .

. . . While circumstantial analysis of the meaning of the scope and limits of the general legal authorization is necessary to draw firm conclusions, this is a potential factor to consider.

Specific Intent. The CDC and others have focused on the role of intent as a primary factor to distinguish practice and research. . . . The intent of research may be [articulated as *"testing]* a hypothesis and seek[ing] to generalize the findings or acquired knowledge beyond the activity's participants." The intent of public health practice [can be described as *"assuring]* the conditions in which people can be healthy through public health efforts that are primarily aimed at preventing known or suspected injuries, diseases, or other conditions, or promoting the health of a *particular community."* . . . If any intent underlying the activity relates to research, [the activity should] be viewed as research. . . .

Responsibility. In the research context, the focal point of responsibility for the health, safety, and well being of individual participants falls upon a specific individual, typically the principal investigator (PI), as well as those working under the PI's supervision. . . .

Public health practice does not always feature direct individual responsibility for the welfare of participants. . . . Public health practitioners are still accountable for their actions that may impact the health, safety, or welfare of participants in a practice activity, but this does not arise because of a relationship with participants like that of a PI and her subjects. It arises because legal and ethical duties assumed by public health practitioners as governmental representatives require them to promote these interests in the performance of their activities.

Participant Benefits. Public health practice and human subjects research activities both offer the potential to benefit the community through improvements in health outcomes. However, an assessment of the potential (or expectation) of benefits to participants concerning each activity provides an opportunity for drawing better distinctions. Participants in human subjects research may receive (nor expect) no direct benefit from (and may even be harmed by) the activity. . . .

Unlike research, public health practice activities are premised on providing some benefit to participants or the population of which they are members. . . . Public health practice should contribute to improving the health of participants. Research, however, may not. If the activity offers no expectation or prospect of benefit to the participants, then the activity should be classified as research.

Experimentation. There is an experimental quality to research that public health practice does not always share. Research may involve introducing something nonstandard to research subjects or to the analysis of their identifiable health data. . . .

Although innovations are part of public health practice, it is dominated by the use of standard, accepted, and proven interventions to address a known or suspected public health problem. . . . Thus, if any activity involves introduction of non-standard or experimental procedures, the activity is more likely research rather than public health practice.

Subject Selection. . . . Practitioners of public health activities rarely choose participants. Participants are selected because they have or are at risk of, a particular disease or condition and can likely benefit from the activity. Public health practice activities are not designed to test hypotheses but to benefit the participants or their communities. Thus, if an activity utilizes control groups or randomly selects its participants to eliminate bias, the activity is likely research rather than public health practice.

CONCLUSION

Distinguishing between public health practice and research activities conducted or funded by governmental public health authorities is not easy. The similarities of these activities and underlying intents, coupled with a lack of clarification among key legal and ethical policies, makes classification even more difficult. Existing proposals for how to distinguish between practice and research have led to disagreements and incongruous results among public health authorities, IRB members, and others.

Nearly everyone seeks a better way to clarify these concepts. . . . Ultimately, better
distinctions support the overriding objective to perform public health activities that
respect and protect the legal rights and ethical interests of individual participants
while improving or promoting the public's health.

.   .   .   .   .

Serious controversy can arise from public health research that crosses
ethical boundaries. The most egregious and well-known example of
abuse in public health research is the Tuskegee syphilis study. Researchers continued the study even after an effective treatment for syphilis
was available, allowing study participants, African American men in
rural Alabama, to die of syphilis unnecessarily. Such flagrant disregard
for norms of ethical conduct in research and for the essential dignity
of racial and ethnic minorities participating in health studies has generated lasting distrust of physicians and public health practitioners,
particularly among marginalized populations.

The Tuskegee syphilis study may be the most notorious example of
disreputable public health research in modern America, but it is not
unique. During the cold war, vulnerable human subjects were exposed
to radiation without their knowledge or consent. And in the mid-1990s,
the CDC sponsored a study in inner-city Los Angeles that administered
an unlicensed measles vaccine mainly to African American and Latino
children. The children's parents were not informed that the vaccine had
not received FDA approval.

Today, some public health studies continue to elicit controversy.
Particularly contentious are cost-effectiveness studies, which aim to
find the most cost-effective public health interventions for a particular
problem, because some interventions being tested may fail to adequately
protect participants from harm. In one such study, the Kennedy Krieger
Institute sought to discover whether a less expensive approach to lead
paint abatement of houses in poor neighborhoods could successfully
reduce the blood lead levels of children. Parents of children involved in
the study brought suit once the findings were published, and the highest
court of Maryland issued a strongly worded opinion condemning the
researchers for having violated their duties to participants, particularly
the young children studied. In *Grimes v. Kennedy Krieger Institute,
Inc.,* 782 A.2d 807, 812–15 (Md. 2001), the court stated:

> Apparently, it was anticipated that the children . . . would, or at least
> might, accumulate lead in their blood from the dust, thus helping the
> researchers to determine the extent to which the various partial abatement

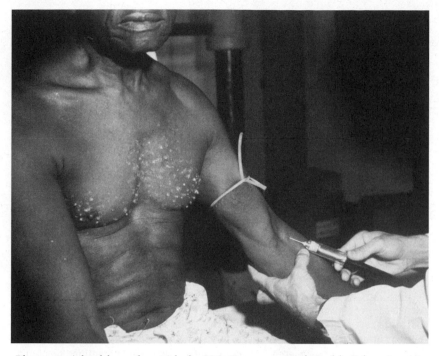

Photo 18. A health worker with the U.S. Department of Health, Education, and Welfare gives an injection to a patient in the infamous Tuskegee study. These experiments, which went on for forty years, left syphilis-infected black men untreated so that researchers could observe the "natural" progression of the disease, even though a cure for the debilitating illness was available. Reproduced by permission, © Corbis Sygma.

methods worked. . . . It can be argued that the researchers intended that the children be the canaries in the mines. . . .

. . . Otherwise healthy children, in our view, should not be . . . intentionally subjected to a research program, which contemplates the probability, or even the possibility, of lead poisoning. . . .

The research relationship proffered to the parents of the children the researchers wanted to use as measuring tools, should never have been presented in a non-therapeutic context in the first instance. Nothing about the research was designed for treatment of the subject children.

In the following excerpt, David Buchanan, a professor of public health, and Franklin Miller, a bioethicist, discuss the Kennedy Krieger lead paint study, analyzing the ethical quandaries presented by the research. They argue that in the face of limited resources, it is unrealistic to require in all circumstances the provision of the most effective interventions and that it is ethically warranted to conduct research that attempts to create incremental improvements in health for populations.

JUSTICE AND FAIRNESS IN THE KENNEDY KRIEGER INSTITUTE LEAD PAINT STUDY: THE ETHICS OF PUBLIC HEALTH RESEARCH ON LESS EXPENSIVE, LESS EFFECTIVE INTERVENTIONS*

David R. Buchanan and Franklin G. Miller

The controversial Kennedy Krieger lead paint abatement study raised serious questions about the ethics of public health research and the relation between research and policies aimed at improving population health. This study tested low-cost lead abatement procedures in housing in Baltimore to determine their effectiveness in reducing blood lead levels in children living in these houses. An impassioned debate has ensued about the role of public health researchers in improving health outcomes, reducing health inequalities, and promoting social justice. . . .

BACKGROUND

The KKI, a children's health facility and research institute affiliated with Johns Hopkins University in Baltimore, MD, conducted research investigating low-cost partial lead abatement procedures to prevent lead poisoning in children living in public housing in inner-city Baltimore between 1993 and 1995. When the research idea was being originated, an estimated 95% of low-income housing in identified neighborhoods in Baltimore was contaminated with lead-based paint. Studies at the time showed that 40% to 50% of the predominantly African American children living in these high-risk neighborhoods had elevated blood lead level. . . . However, because of the high costs of implementing the recommended total lead abatement procedure (approximately $20000 per home), little was being done about the problem. . . .

In the late 1980s, the KKI had tested alternative, less expensive lead reduction methods in empty properties and demonstrated that these techniques reduced ambient lead paint dust by 80% or more. They then proposed a follow-up study to determine if the reduction in lead paint dust in housing that had been abated with these processes would result in lower blood levels in children living in these houses. The study included 108 houses in 5 comparison groups: 3 treatment groups that used the new lead abatement procedures, costing $1650, $3500, and $6500, respectively, and 2 comparison conditions, composed of housing that had been abated by the city of Baltimore and housing built after 1978 that was presumably free of lead paint. By design, the researchers chose not to include a control comparison of existing housing that had received no abatement procedures, because they considered it unethical to follow children who were being exposed to a known health hazard without remediation, despite the fact that this was the condition of the majority of children living in these neighborhoods. . . .

The results of the research showed significant reductions in lead dust in all study

*Reprinted from *American Journal of Public Health* 96 (2006): 781–87.

conditions. Overall, the blood lead levels of children residing in the KKI-treated homes stayed constant or went down, although there were a few cases of increases.

Two families later sued KKI, stating that they were not fully informed of the risks of participation for their children and that KKI failed to inform them in a timely manner of test results. In *Grimes v. Kennedy Krieger Institute, Inc.* [782 A.2d 807 (Md. 2001)], the Maryland Court of Appeals (Maryland's highest court) overturned a lower court's initial ruling to dismiss and reinstated the families' lawsuits. In August 2001, the court of appeals issued a scathing 96-page ruling. . . . The court's remand focused on 3 main issues: (1) informed consent, declaring that parents cannot give consent for their children to enroll in "non-therapeutic" research; (2) a duty to warn because of the "special relationship" between the researchers and participants; and (3) the inadequacies of the institutional review board's review, referring to the Johns Hopkins institutional review board as "in-house organs" who were not "as sufficiently concerned with ethicality of the experiments they review as they are with the success of the experiment."

The judges' remarks made national headlines and spurred a contentious debate about the ethical acceptability of this research. Although concerns were raised about the adequacy of the informed consent process and the timeliness in informing families about blood lead levels, the case was eventually dismissed with prejudice by the lower court. Setting aside these important ethical concerns, we discuss the fundamental question of whether research designed to test less costly interventions that might not be as effective as existing treatments can ever be ethically justified. . . .

ETHICAL CRITIQUE

Since the Maryland Court of Appeals judges' ruling, many commentaries on the case have appeared in public health, legal, medical, and bioethics journals. Critics have questioned the social value of the research and have further questioned whether such research undermines efforts to enforce just social policies. In addition, the critics claim that the research is unfair, because it treats different population groups unequally by providing the research participants with an intervention that is less effective than the best-known treatment available. Finally, they contend that the research exploits the participants by sacrificing their welfare to accomplish the goals of the research.

The first major criticism concerns the social or scientific value of the research, one of the primary ethical requirements for conducting research. . . . According to critics, the conditions that the research was designed to ameliorate should have been remedied not by conducting research aimed at finding a more cost-effective alternative but by providing the most effective extant intervention to those who had not yet received it. . . .

In questioning the value of the research, opponents go even further in alleging that it is a form of capitulation or collusion with status quo conditions of gross social injustice. Several commentators assert that what is needed in these situations is not more knowledge aimed at testing a "feasible" but less costly intervention but the political will to transfer resources to supply a known effective treatment. . . . Critics thus charge the researchers with bad faith and an insincere or indifferent commitment to equality. . . .

Critics also state that this type of research is not fair. These critics assert that by seeking to develop an intervention that may well turn out to be less effective than a currently known treatment, such research creates a double standard that violates the rights and the dignity of disadvantaged populations. Accordingly, research must conform to principles of equity: all people deserve the same treatment, nothing less than the best. . . .

Finally, critics have charged that the welfare of the research participants is being subordinated to social and scientific goals. . . . These critics assert that, because any attendant morbidities could have been prevented by providing the highest standard of care, the participants were being exploited perforce from the outset. . . .

. . . We contend that it is the failure to conduct such research that causes the greater harm, because it limits health interventions to the status quo of those who can afford currently available options and deprives disadvantaged populations of the benefits of imminent incremental improvements in their health conditions. This type of research, however, can be ethically justified only in carefully circumscribed conditions.

To justify public health research aimed at developing less expensive yet less effective interventions, 4 conditions must be met. There must be (1) a large population in need, (2) the existence of a higher standard of treatment that is more effective yet substantially more expensive than a lower standard that would be cheaper but still hypothesized to be significantly effective, (3) resource or political constraints that do not allow full or extensive provision of the higher standard, and (4) a high degree of likelihood that the less costly intervention can and will be implemented on a large scale. Under these conditions, research on less expensive, less effective interventions can be ethically warranted by giving due moral consideration to the feasibility of providing universal public health protections and by the offer of fair terms of cooperation. . . .

. . . In establishing suitable ethical standards for evaluating public health research, it is crucial to recognize that different societal contexts generate different moral obligations. In *Jacobson v. Massachusetts*, 197 U.S. 11 (1905), the U.S. Supreme Court upheld a Massachusetts law that authorized the state board of health to require all citizens to be immunized against smallpox, citing the state's authority to legislate "for the common good, for the protection, safety, prosperity, and happiness of the people."

The Jacobson verdict demonstrates that, outside the doctor's office, the ethical need to protect the population as a whole should take precedence over the individual's right to exercise autonomy. In the context of conducting public health research, there are other valid moral considerations, such as the just distribution of limited resources and equity in access to populationwide protections, that, albeit only under the limited conditions enumerated previously, may supercede an individual's interest in receiving nothing less than the best. . . . It is not compelling to assert that health research can or should be conducted without giving ethically apposite weight to the goal of gaining new knowledge that will benefit society; hence, in the context of conducting public health research, the ethically relevant question is not how an alleged therapeutic obligation can be fulfilled but how the participants can be protected from harm and exploitation. . . .

If it could be anticipated that the participants would be harmed or made worse off, then the terms of research participation would be undeniably unfair and exploitive. Contrary to statements made by the court of appeals judges and others, how-ever, the KKI research cannot be properly characterized as "a non-therapeutic study that promises no medical benefit to the child whatever." Because the participants stood to benefit directly by an environmental intervention hypothesized to effect reduced blood lead levels, the court's assertion reflects a deep misunderstanding of the nature of public health research. Unlike nontherapeutic research designed solely for the sake of advancing medical science, there can be no question that an outcome intrinsic to the KKI research design was the projected benefit to the research par-ticipants of lower blood lead levels.

... It is important to examine the issue of whether the participants were being harmed and treated inequitably by being deprived of a known beneficial treatment....

Critics charge that the KKI participants were treated inequitably, but the com-parison is relative to those better-off individuals who have access to new or refur-bished housing. The comparison is made on the basis of the assumption that the feasibility of universal provision is unproblematic and hence irrelevant. The conduct of public health research, however, introduces valid, ethically germane consider-ation of the feasibility of universal coverage. From a public health perspective, if it is not feasible to extend the current standard of care to the population as a whole, then the appropriate comparison group with respect to the question of inequitable treatment is those who do not now have access to the current standard of care. In the KKI case, it is important to be clear that the children were not being exposed to a risky home environment as a result of their participation in the research. Rather it was the injustice of social conditions that caused their exposure, conditions that the research itself was intended to alleviate. As there was no reason to think that the abatement interventions would increase the lead exposure of the research partici-pants compared with unabated housing, the institutional review board could reason-ably conclude that the participants would not be made worse off as a result of their participation relative to the decision not to participate....

According to the preceding analysis, the KKI study offered a favorable risk-bene-fit ratio both in terms of potential benefits to the participating children, who lived in safer housing, and in terms of the social value of knowledge to be gained regarding cost-effective means of lead abatement. The justification for public health research on less expensive, less effective interventions is based on giving due moral consid-eration to the issue of the feasibility of providing population-wide or population-in-need public health protections, provided that the risks to the research participants are reasonable and proportionately balanced in relation to the prospective health benefits to them and the value of the knowledge to be gained.

CONCLUSIONS

With a range of challenges facing the field of public health—from responding to emerging infectious diseases, to the growing threat of ozone depletion (and conse-quent cancers), to the possibility of new genetic screenings, to treating the growing epidemics of diabetes and hypertension—public health researchers will continue to be confronted with difficult questions about what should be done in situations in which the discovery of a new technology, new drug, or new intervention costs more than it is currently reasonable to expect taxpayers to pay in order to provide population-wide protection. There can be little question that the universal provision

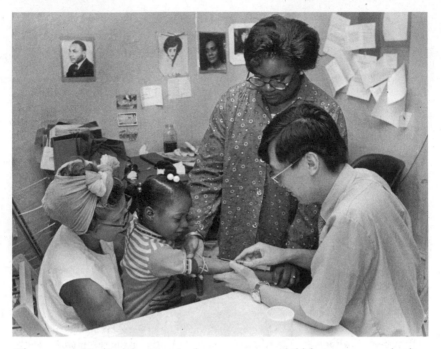

Photo 19. A Harlem physician in the 1970s tests a child for exposure to lead from the paint in her apartment. Before a federal ban went into effect in 1978, paint pigments were largely lead-based. Because lead is highly toxic, the use of such paint in homes posed a significant health hazard. In the controversial study at issue in *Grimes v. Kennedy Krieger Institute,* researchers attempted to determine the most cost-effective methods of lead paint abatement. Reproduced by permission, © Charles Gatewood/The Image Works.

of the most effective intervention—the idea that public health infrastructure could, and therefore should, provide nothing less than the best to everyone—will not always be feasible. In such circumstances, when providing the highest quality of health care to each and every individual is not possible, public health research designed for the purpose of generating alternatives that can realistically be extended to those in need is ethically warranted. The search for interventions that can be provided to substantially greater numbers of people in turn advances a pragmatic understanding of justice. If a less expensive treatment that can reach a greater number of people can be developed, it would yield a net improvement in the health of the population as a whole, and thus it represents substantial progress over status quo conditions that would be likely to persist without a mitigating intervention. Dogmatic stances that preclude research aimed at evaluating cost-effective interventions on grounds of egalitarian justice will result in research paralysis and policy stagnation, thus guaranteeing the continuing neglect of the needs of disadvantaged populations.

IV. INFORMATIONAL PRIVACY: CURRENT PROTECTIONS AND PROPOSED ACTIONS

A. The Constitutional Right to Informational Privacy

Although public health surveillance achieves many common goods, it also invades individual interests in privacy. As the technology of surveillance becomes more advanced, the public is becoming more concerned about how electronic personal information will be used and who will be able to access it.

The Supreme Court, in the foundational case of *Whalen v. Roe,* 429 U.S. 589 (1977), proclaimed a narrow constitutional right to health informational privacy. The Court upheld a New York law that required the reporting of the names and addresses of all persons who have obtained, pursuant to a doctor's prescription, certain drugs for which there is both a lawful and an unlawful market. At the same time, however, the Court noted the strong security protections surrounding the health department's collection and storage of these data.

WHALEN V. ROE*
Supreme Court of the United States
Decided February 22, 1977·

Justice STEVENS delivered the opinion of the Court.

The constitutional question presented is whether the State of New York may record, in a centralized computer file, the names and addresses of all persons who have obtained, pursuant to a doctor's prescription, certain drugs for which there is both a lawful and an unlawful market. . . .

. . . In response to a concern that such drugs were being diverted into unlawful channels, in 1970 the New York Legislature created a special commission to evaluate the State's drug-control laws. The commission found the existing laws deficient in several respects. There was no effective way to prevent the use of stolen or revised prescriptions, to prevent unscrupulous pharmacists from repeatedly refilling prescriptions, to prevent users from obtaining prescriptions from more than one doctor, or to prevent doctors from over-prescribing, either by authorizing an excessive amount in one prescription or by giving one patient multiple prescriptions. . . .

[Ed.—The Court describes the New York statute, which classified drugs according to their potential for abuse, and the filing requirements that compelled physicians to file prescription forms for potentially addictive drugs with the State Department of Health.]

---

*429 U.S. 589 (1977).

With an exception for emergencies, the Act requires that all prescriptions for Schedule II drugs [i.e., the most dangerous and addictive legal drugs] be prepared by the physician in triplicate on an official form. The completed form identifies the prescribing physician; the dispensing pharmacy; the drug and dosage; and the name, address, and age of the patient. One copy of the form is retained by the physician, the second by the pharmacist, and the third is forwarded to the New York State Department of Health in Albany. . . .

. . . About 100,000 Schedule II prescription forms are delivered to a receiving room at the Department of Health in Albany each month. They are sorted, coded, and logged and then taken to another room where the data on the forms is recorded on magnetic tapes for processing by a computer. Thereafter, the forms are returned to the receiving room to be retained in a vault for a five-year period, and then destroyed as required by the statute. The receiving room is surrounded by a locked wire fence and protected by an alarm system. The computer tapes containing the prescription data are kept in a locked cabinet. When the tapes are used, the computer is run "off-line," which means that no terminal outside of the computer room can read or record any information. Public disclosure of the identity of patients is expressly prohibited by the statute and by a Department of Health regulation. Willful violation of these prohibitions is a crime punishable by up to one year in prison and a $2,000 fine. . . .

A few days before the Act became effective, this litigation was commenced by a group of patients regularly receiving prescriptions for Schedule II drugs, by doctors who prescribe such drugs, and by two associations of physicians. After various preliminary proceedings, a three-judge District Court conducted a one-day trial. Appellees offered evidence tending to prove that persons in need of treatment with Schedule II drugs will from time to time decline such treatment because of their fear that the misuse of the computerized data will cause them to be stigmatized as "drug addicts." . . .

Appellees contend that the statute invades a constitutionally protected "zone of privacy." The cases sometimes characterized as protecting "privacy" have in fact involved at least two different kinds of interests. One is the individual interest in avoiding disclosure of personal matters, and another is the interest in independence in making certain kinds of important decisions. Appellees argue that both of these interests are impaired by this statute. The mere existence in readily available form of the information about patients' use of Schedule II drugs creates a genuine concern that the information will become publicly known and that it will adversely affect their reputations. This concern makes some patients reluctant to use, and some doctors reluctant to prescribe, such drugs even when their use is medically indicated. It follows, they argue, that the making of decisions about matters vital to the care of their health is inevitably affected by the statute. Thus, the statute threatens to impair both their interest in the nondisclosure of private information and also their interest in making important decisions independently.

We are persuaded, however, that the New York program does not, on its face, pose a sufficiently grievous threat to either interest to establish a constitutional violation.

Public disclosure of patient information can come about in three ways. Health Department employees may violate the statute by failing, either deliberately or negligently, to maintain proper security. A patient or a doctor may be accused of a violation and the stored data may be offered in evidence in a judicial proceeding. Or, thirdly, a doctor, a pharmacist, or the patient may voluntarily reveal information on a prescription form.

The third possibility existed under the prior law and is entirely unrelated to the existence of the computerized data bank. Neither of the other two possibilities provides a proper ground for attacking the statute as invalid on its face. There is no support in the record, or in the experience of the two States that New York has emulated, for an assumption that the security provisions of the statute will be administered improperly. And the remote possibility that judicial supervision of the evidentiary use of particular items of stored information will provide inadequate protection against unwarranted disclosures is surely not a sufficient reason for invalidating the entire patient-identification program.

Even without public disclosure, it is, of course, true that private information must be disclosed to the authorized employees of the New York Department of Health. Such disclosures, however, are not significantly different from those that were required under the prior law. Nor are they meaningfully distinguishable from a host of other unpleasant invasions of privacy that are associated with many facets of health care. Unquestionably, some individuals' concern for their own privacy may lead them to avoid or to postpone needed medical attention. Nevertheless, disclosures of private medical information to doctors, to hospital personnel, to insurance companies, and to public health agencies are often an essential part of modern medical practice even when the disclosure may reflect unfavorably on the character of the patient. Requiring such disclosures to representatives of the State having responsibility for the health of the community, does not automatically amount to an impermissible invasion of privacy.

Appellees also argue, however, that even if unwarranted disclosures do not actually occur, the knowledge that the information is readily available in a computerized file creates a genuine concern that causes some persons to decline needed medication. The record supports the conclusion that some use of Schedule II drugs has been discouraged by that concern; it also is clear, however, that about 100,000 prescriptions for such drugs were being filled each month prior to the entry of the District Court's injunction. Clearly, therefore, the statute did not deprive the public of access to the drugs. . . .

A final word about issues we have not decided. We are not unaware of the threat to privacy implicit in the accumulation of vast amounts of personal information in computerized data banks or other massive government files. . . . The right to collect and use such data for public purposes is typically accompanied by a concomitant statutory or regulatory duty to avoid unwarranted disclosures. Recognizing that in some circumstances that duty arguably has its roots in the Constitution, nevertheless New York's statutory scheme, and its implementing administrative procedures, evidence a proper concern with, and protection of, the individual's interest in privacy. We therefore need not, and do not, decide any question which might be presented by the unwarranted disclosure of accumulated private data whether intentional or unintentional or by a system that did not contain comparable security provisions. We simply hold that this record does not establish an invasion of any right or liberty protected by the Fourteenth Amendment.

Justice BRENNAN, concurring.

The information disclosed by the physician under this program is made available only to a small number of public health officials with a legitimate interest in the information. As the record makes clear, New York has long required doctors to make this information available to its officials on request, and that practice is not challenged here. Such limited reporting requirements in the medical field are familiar and are not generally regarded as an invasion of privacy. Broad dissemination by state officials of such information, however, would clearly implicate constitutionally protected privacy rights, and would presumably be justified only by compelling state interests.

What is more troubling about this scheme, however, is the central computer storage of the data thus collected. Obviously, as the State argues, collection and storage of data by the State that is in itself legitimate is not rendered unconstitutional simply because new technology makes the State's operations more efficient. However, as the example of the Fourth Amendment shows, the Constitution puts limits not only on the type of information the State may gather, but also on the means it may use to gather it. The central storage and easy accessibility of computerized data vastly increase the potential for abuse of that information, and I am not prepared to say that future developments will not demonstrate the necessity of some curb on such technology.

B. Health Information Privacy Laws: The HIPAA Privacy Rule

The Health Insurance Portability and Accountability Act (HIPAA) of 1996 encouraged the development of electronic patient records. As part of this initiative, Congress authorized the secretary of the Department of Health and Human Services (HHS) to promulgate privacy regulations. The HIPAA Privacy Rule governs the handling of protected health information (PHI). Public health agencies acquire vast amounts of PHI during routine surveillance activities and often obtain such information from entities covered by the Privacy Rule. As a result, the Privacy Rule specifically addresses public health utilization of PHI. In the following excerpt, the relationship between public health and the Privacy Rule is explored in depth by authors from the CDC and HHS.

HIPAA PRIVACY RULE AND PUBLIC HEALTH: GUIDANCE FROM CDC AND THE U.S. DEPARTMENT FOR HEALTH AND HUMAN SERVICES*

Centers for Disease Control and Prevention and Department of Health and Human Services

The HIPAA Privacy Rule (Standards for Privacy of Individually Identifiable Health Information) provides the first national standards for protecting the privacy of health information. The Privacy Rule regulates how certain entities, called covered

*Reprinted from *Morbidity and Mortality Weekly* 52 (2003): S1–S17.

entities [i.e., health plans, health-care clearinghouses, and health-care providers who transmit information in electronic form in connection with certain transactions], use and disclose certain individually identifiable health information, called protected health information (PHI). PHI is individually identifiable health information that is transmitted or maintained in any form or medium (e.g., electronic, paper, or oral), but excludes certain educational records and employment records. . . .

[PHI] must relate to 1) the past, present, or future physical or mental health, or condition of an individual; 2) provision of health care to an individual; or 3) payment for the provision of health care to an individual. If the information identifies or provides a reasonable basis to believe it can be used to identify an individual, it is considered individually identifiable health information. . . .

De-identified data (e.g., aggregate statistical data or data stripped of individual identifiers) require no individual privacy protections and are not covered by the Privacy Rule. . . .

THE PRIVACY RULE AND PUBLIC HEALTH

The Privacy Rule recognizes 1) the legitimate need for public health authorities and others responsible for ensuring the public's health and safety to have access to PHI to conduct their missions; and 2) the importance of public health reporting by covered entities to identify threats to the public and individuals. Accordingly, the rule 1) permits PHI disclosures without a written patient authorization for specified public health purposes to public health authorities legally authorized to collect and receive the information for such purposes, and 2) permits disclosures that are required by state and local public health or other laws. However, because the Privacy Rule affects the traditional ways PHI is used and exchanged among covered entities (e.g., doctors, hospitals, and health insurers), it can affect public health practice and research in multiple ways. . . .

The Privacy Rule permits covered entities to disclose PHI, without authorization, to public health authorities or other entities who are legally authorized to receive such reports for the purpose of preventing or controlling disease, injury, or disability. This includes the reporting of disease or injury; reporting vital events (e.g., births or deaths); conducting public health surveillance, investigations, or interventions; reporting child abuse and neglect; and monitoring adverse outcomes related to food (including dietary supplements), drugs, biological products, and medical devices. . . . To protect the health of the public, public health authorities might need to obtain information related to the individuals affected by a disease. In certain cases, they might need to contact those affected to determine the cause of the disease to allow for actions to prevent further illness. . . .

DISCLOSURES FOR PUBLIC HEALTH PURPOSES

The Privacy Rule allows covered entities to disclose PHI to public health authorities when required by federal, tribal, state, or local laws. . . .

For disclosures not required by law, covered entities may still disclose, without authorization, to a public health authority authorized by law to collect or receive the information for the purpose of preventing or controlling disease, injury, or disability, the minimum necessary information to accomplish the intended public health purpose of the disclosure. . . .

REQUIREMENTS FOR COVERED ENTITIES

Although the Privacy Rule permits disclosures of PHI to public health authorities, covered entities must comply with certain requirements related to these disclosures. [For example, a covered entity must be able to provide an individual, on request, with an accounting of certain disclosures of PHI (e.g., those not made pursuant to the individual's written authorization). Individuals also have the right to adequate notice of the uses and disclosures of PHI that may be made by the covered entity, as well as their rights and the covered entity's legal obligations. Where a disclosure is not required by law or made for treatment purposes, the disclosures must be limited to the minimum amount necessary to achieve the specific goal.]

Public health authorities . . . that perform covered functions (e.g., providing health care or insuring individuals for health-care costs), may be subject to the Privacy Rule's provisions as covered entities. For example, a local public health authority that operates a health clinic providing essential health-care services to low-income persons and performs certain electronic transactions might be . . . a covered entity.

C. Proposed Actions

The HIPAA Privacy Rule safeguards PHI but leaves a great deal of public health data to be protected under state law. As a result, HHS asked the Center for Law and the Public's Health at Georgetown and Johns Hopkins universities to draft a model public health information privacy law with the assistance of an expert national panel. (The full text of the model law can be found at www.publichealthlaw.net.) In the following selection, James G. Hodge Jr., Ronald O. Valdiserri, and I explain the purposes and terms of the model law.

INFORMATIONAL PRIVACY AND THE PUBLIC'S HEALTH: THE MODEL STATE PUBLIC HEALTH PRIVACY ACT*
Lawrence O. Gostin, James G. Hodge Jr., and Ronald O. Valdiserri

Assessing populational health is a core function of state and local public health departments which requires the acquisition, use, and storage of health-related information about individuals. . . .

The accumulation and exchange of these personal data within an increasingly automated public health information infrastructure promises significant public health benefits. Well-planned surveillance helps identify health problems, target interventions, and influence funding decisions. Health information databases facilitate existing and future epidemiologic investigations and research studies. These

*Reprinted from American Journal of Public Health 91 (2001): 1388–92.

essential public health functions rely on the quality and reliability of identifiable health information. . . .

. . . As increasing amounts of identifiable health data are gathered, stored, and exchanged, personal privacy is threatened. Many Americans distrust government agencies and believe the collection of personal data without their explicit permission is morally wrong. If public health authorities disclose intimate information, individuals may suffer embarrassment, stigma, and discrimination in employment, insurance, and government programs. Persons who fear invasions of privacy may avoid clinical tests and treatments, withdraw from research, or provide inaccurate or incomplete health information if they fear invasions of privacy. . . .

Current law and policy often fail to reconcile individual privacy interests with collective public health interests in identifiable health data. Civil libertarians and consumers see informational privacy as a fundamental right and stress the importance of stronger legal safeguards. Public health professionals, on the other hand, strongly assert the need to use data to achieve important public health purposes. To reconcile these 2 divergent approaches, the Georgetown/Johns Hopkins Program on Law and Public Health convened a multidisciplinary team of privacy, public health, and legislative experts to propose a model public health information privacy statute. The Model Act would provide, for the first time, strong and consistent privacy safeguards for public health data, while still preserving the ability of state and local health departments to act for the common good. The Centers for Disease Control and Prevention recommends that states consider adopting the model legislation to "strengthen the current level of protection of public health data" (CDC 1999, 21). . . .

RECONCILING PUBLIC HEALTH AND PRIVACY INTERESTS

. . . The Model Act's approach is to maximize privacy safeguards where they matter most to individuals and facilitate data uses where they are necessary to promote the public's health. This accommodation between privacy and public health balances individual and collective interests.

Consider the sequence of events when a government agency collects public health data through, for example, reporting or other forms of surveillance. [Ed.–See figure 30 in the companion text.] First, the agency *acquires* the data, typically after the patient has given informed consent (usually to a medical care provider) to provide a biologic sample (e.g., blood or urine) or health-related behavioral information (e.g., sexual history or drug use practices). Given that there is a strong public health interest, most people believe that patients should accept this invasion of privacy for the collective good. Next, the agency *uses* the data strictly within the confines of the health department. Again, if the agency has a strong public health interest and the data are shared only with agency officials who have a need to know, data uses should prevail over privacy. When public health authorities acquire and use data strictly within the agency, public health benefits are at their highest and risks to privacy are at their lowest. The agency needs the freedom to use the data to monitor and prevent health risks. . . .

Finally, the agency may be asked or, under unusual circumstances, may seek to disclose personally identifiable information to persons outside the agency—for example, to employers, insurers, commercial marketers, family, or friends. These kinds of disclosures are not very important for the public's health, but they do place patients at considerable risk of embarrassment, stigma, and discrimination. For these reasons, the law ought to provide maximum protection of privacy. The Model Act's approach, therefore, is to give government flexibility to acquire and use data strictly within the mission of the public health agency, providing it can demonstrate an important public health purpose. However, the Model Act affords public health authorities very little discretion to release personally identifiable data outside the agency and imposes serious penalties for disclosures without the patient's informed consent.

THE MODEL STATE PUBLIC HEALTH PRIVACY ACT

The Model Act . . . is based on several core assumptions. . . .

Public health and privacy are synergistic. The debate surrounding public uses of identifiable data and individual privacy assumes that these interests are mutually exclusive. This is not invariably the case, however. Public health agencies have significant interests in protecting the privacy of health-related information. Protecting individual privacy encourages individuals to voluntarily participate in public health and individual health care programs and to freely divulge personal information, thus improving the reliability and quality of data. Privacy advocates (and others) benefit from a well-functioning, efficient public health system that works to improve population health outcomes. In these ways, public health and privacy are synergistic, thus suggesting that the Model Act, if passed, would actually improve public health outcomes, not thwart them.

All identifiable health information deserves legal protection. The Model Act applies to all "protected health information" held by public health agencies. This includes any public health information, whether oral, written, electronic, or visual, that relates to an individual's past, present, or future physical or mental health status, condition, treatment, service, product purchases, or provision of care. This broad definition of protected health information recognizes that any identifiable data (e.g., HIV, STD, or immunization status) can be sensitive.

Nonidentifiable health information requires no protection. The definition of "protected health information" specifically incorporates another core assumption: nonidentifiable health data do not merit privacy protection. Where health data are truly nonidentifiable individual privacy interests are not threatened. . . .

Acquisition and use are contingent upon legitimate public health purposes. The Model Act regulates the ways in which public health agencies acquire, use, disclose, and store protected health information. It safeguards privacy, in part, by requiring public health authorities to demonstrate a legitimate public health purpose for the acquisition and use of data. The act defines "legitimate public health purpose" to mean a population-based activity or individual effort primarily aimed at the prevention of injury, disease, or premature mortality, or the promotion of health in the community. Such efforts include carrying out public health surveillance, conducting epidemiologic research, developing public health policy, and responding to public health needs and emergencies. . . .

In addition to imposing a requirement to justify data acquisition, the Model Act limits the use of identifiable information within the agency. In particular, it specifies that (1) nonidentifiable data must be used whenever possible, (2) the sharing of identifiable data among public health officials must be limited to the minimum amount necessary, (3) public health officials may have access to identifiable data only if they have a demonstrable need to know, and (4) agencies must protect security by maintaining the data in a physically and technologically secure environment.

Disclosures must be strictly limited. While the Model Act affords public health agencies the power to acquire and use health data for important public health purposes, it grants very little authority to disclose identifiable data outside the public health system. The act clarifies that protected health information is not subject to public review (e.g., inspection, dissemination, or investigation by members of the public) and may not be disclosed without the specific informed consent of the individual who is the subject of the information (or the individual's lawful representative), except under narrow circumstances. . . .

[Ed.–The authors describe the circumstances in which disclosures are permitted without informed consent: directly to the individual, to appropriate federal agencies, to health care personnel in a medical emergency, pursuant to a court order, to agencies performing health oversight functions, and to identify a deceased individual.]

Finally, the Model Act permits the exchange of data among public health agencies within the state and outside the state. These information exchanges are viewed as data *acquisitions* or *uses,* not *disclosures.* As such, public health agencies may exchange identifiable health data with other state or local agencies provided the exchanges are necessary for the public's health. . . .

FAIR INFORMATION PRACTICES

Safeguarding privacy requires data holders to engage in a range of fair information practices. These practices assure strong security and privacy of public health information, but do not unreasonably burden public health authorities. The Act incorporates the following fair information practices:

Justifying the need for data collection. Acquiring identifiable data is not an inherent good. Rather, public health authorities must substantiate the need for identifiable data. . . . The Model Act affirms that public health agencies shall only acquire identifiable health information that (a) relates directly to a legitimate public health purpose and (b) is reasonably likely to achieve such a purpose. When information is no longer needed to fulfill the purpose for which it is acquired, it must be expunged or made nonidentifiable.

Informing data subjects. Public health agencies may not acquire identifiable data without public knowledge. Before acquiring such data, public health agencies must provide public notice (through written information distributed in such a way as to reasonably inform the public) concerning their intentions to acquire the data and the purposes for which the data will be used. Individuals are entitled to view records of disclosures of their protected health information, which public health agencies are required to maintain.

Access to one's own data. Subject to reasonable limitations, individuals are entitled to access, inspect, and copy their health data. Public health agencies are required to explain any code, abbreviation, notation, or other marks appearing in the information for the individual's benefit, as well as ensure the accuracy of such data and amend any errors.

Ensuring privacy and security. Public health agencies have a duty to adhere to privacy and security safeguards. Specific protections are administered by a designated health information officer appointed by each public health agency and enforced through significant administrative, criminal, and civil penalties. These protections apply to identifiable health data, regardless of their holder, through various provisions of the act that (a) require an affirmative statement of privacy protections to accompany the disclosure of protected health information and (b) apply similar criminal and civil sanctions for unlawful disclosures to public health officials as well as secondary recipients.

CONCLUSION

Although not perfect, the act provides a balance between the social good of data collection (recognizing its substantial value to community health) and the individual good of privacy (recognizing the normative value of respect for persons). It authorizes public health agencies to acquire, use, and store identifiable health data for public health purposes while simultaneously requiring them to respect individual privacy and imposing stiff penalties for failure to comply. Individuals are empowered with various privacy rights and remedies for breaches of these duties. The community generally is sympathetic to data collection for public health purposes, but it seeks strong legal protection against potentially harmful uses of personal information. States that adopt the act or laws consistent with its structure can stabilize and modernize public health information practices. If the act serves as a model across multiple jurisdictions, it could reduce the variability of existing protections among states, allow for the responsible exchange of health data within a national public health information infrastructure, and ultimately improve public health outcomes.

RECOMMENDED READINGS

Surveillance: An Essential Public Health Activity, Ethical and Rights-Based Concerns

Fairchild, Amy L., and Ava Alkon. 2007. Back to the future? Diabetes, HIV, and the boundaries of public health. *Journal of Health Politics, Policy, and Law* 32: 561–93. (Provides a detailed narrative outlining the debate surrounding New York City's proposed expansion of its surveillance programs to encompass diabetes and to more closely monitor HIV)

Fairchild, Amy L., and Ronald Bayer. 2004. Ethics and the conduct of public health surveillance. *Science* 303: 631–32. (Explores the idea that public health surveillance may require increased ethical oversight, but that existing research guidelines may not be practicable in the context of public health surveillance)

Fox, Daniel M. 1986. From TB to AIDS: Value conflicts in reporting disease. *Hastings Center Report* 16 (6): 11–16. (Explains that reporting statutes create tensions between physicians, whose primary role is to protect their patients' interests, and public health authorities, whose primary role is to protect the population's interests)

Frieden, Thomas R., Moupali Das-Douglas, Scott E. Kellerman, and Kelly J. Henning. 2005. Applying public health principles to the HIV epidemic.

New England Journal of Medicine 353: 2397–2402. (Advocates a comprehensive approach to controlling HIV that utilizes public health activities such as systemic treatment and case management)

Gostin, Lawrence O. 2007. Police powers and public health paternalism: HIV and diabetes surveillance. *Hastings Center Report* 37 (2): 9–10. (Supports New York City's efforts to expand surveillance of HIV and implement surveillance of diabetes)

Traditional Public Health Activities: Reporting and Partner Notification

Hogben, Matthew. 2007. Partner notification for sexually transmitted diseases. *Clinical Infectious Diseases* 44 (Supp. 3): S160–S174. (Outlines new and efficacious developments in methods of partner notification)

Public Health Research and Practice: Understanding the Distinctions

Advisory Committee on Human Radiation Experiments. 1996. *Final Report.* Washington, DC: Department of Energy. (Discusses the findings of the committee commissioned to investigate the thousands of radiation experiments performed by the U.S. government on human subjects between 1944 and 1974)

Brandt, Allan M. 1978. Racism and research: The case of the Tuskegee syphilis study. *Hastings Center Report* 8 (6): 21–29. (Describes the Tuskegee syphilis study in detail and criticizes the report on the study issued by the Department of Health, Education, and Welfare)

King, Patricia A. 2004. Reflections on race and bioethics in the United States. *Health Matrix* 14: 149–53. (Encourages scholars in the field of bioethics to reflect on the historical role of race in health research and confront the role that race will play in the future)

Mastroianni, Anna C., and Jeffrey P. Kahn. 2002. Risk and responsibility: Ethics, *Grimes v. Kennedy Krieger,* and public health research involving children. *American Journal of Public Health* 92: 1073–76. (Proposes that current research oversight systems are not inherently defective, but warrant greater attention and commitment to regain the public's trust)

Informational Privacy: Current Protections and Proposed Actions

Sobel, Richard. 2007. The HIPAA paradox: The privacy rule that's not. *Hastings Center Report* 37 (4): 40–50. (Argues that the HIPAA Privacy Rule undermines patient confidentiality by allowing for easy disclosure and dissemination of personal medical information)

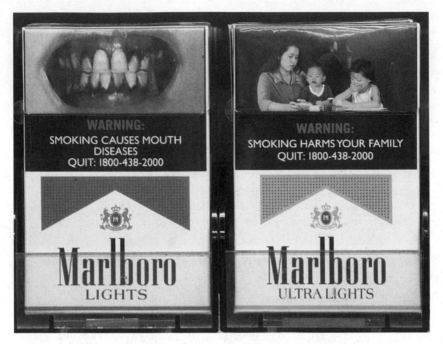

Photo 20. Marlboro cigarettes are displayed in a Singapore supermarket. Singapore law requires tobacco companies to include pictorial health warnings on cigarette packs like the ones shown above. These graphic warnings are far more effective at communicating the health risks of smoking than traditional, text-based warnings. The European Union mandates similar warnings on cigarettes sold in its member countries, but the United States requires only text. Reproduced by permission, © Hanns-Peter Lochmann/dpa/Corbis, March 5, 2006.

Health, Communication, and Behavior

Public health authorities recognize behavior as an important determinant of health in the community. This idea is reflected mostly in modern discourse about the roles of smoking, diet, and sedentary lifestyle in the development of chronic disease, but the influence of behavior in transmitting infection (e.g., sexual or needle-sharing behavior) or causing injury (e.g., use of automobiles and firearms) is also well recognized. Researchers seek to identify effective techniques for changing people's behavior to achieve reductions in chronic and infectious diseases, as well as in injuries. Public health assessments and interventions occur at the point of human contact, whether at the individual, group, or organizational level.

Human behavior is highly complex and influenced by numerous social and environmental factors, but one prerequisite for change is information. The population must at least be aware of the health consequences of risk behaviors to make informed decisions. The public is inundated with messages about health and behavior from the media, businesses, religious and charitable organizations, family, and peers. Perhaps the most important goal of health promotion is to alter the informational environment so that the public can hear the messages conducive to its health and avoid those that encourage risk behavior.

As figure 9 suggests, public health authorities have many tools at their disposal to construct a favorable informational environment, even though, in practice, they may not be particularly adept or successful

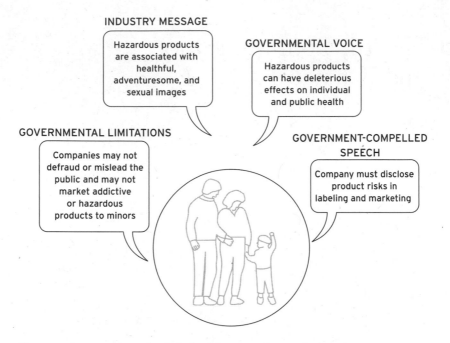

Figure 9. A governmental role in health promotion and education.

at using them. Government can add its voice to the marketplace of ideas by delivering health messages directly or providing incentives for others to do so. Government can also constrain the speech of others by limiting the advertising and promotion of hazardous products. Finally, government can compel businesses to reveal health and safety risks through disclosure and labeling requirements.

The readings in this chapter discuss the goals and techniques of health promotion and health communication. The first section both considers the ethical aspects of health communication and introduces the government as a provider of health information. The second section examines the government's role in restricting private messages that encourage unhealthy behaviors, such as tobacco advertising that encourages youth smoking. The excerpted Supreme Court cases deal with the protection afforded to advertising and promotion by the First Amendment. The third section discusses instances in which the government compels another entity to speak, such as mandatory health and safety disclosures. And the final section applies the issues of commercial speech and compelled speech to a major public health problem—obesity.

I. AN ETHIC FOR HEALTH PROMOTION

Health education is often a preferred public health strategy and is in many respects unobjectionable, especially in comparison with more invasive forms of public health protection. In health communication campaigns, public health practitioners attempt to persuade individuals to alter risk behaviors. Education campaigns are designed to provide information about activities that promote health and well-being and those that are potentially harmful without placing actual restrictions on individuals' health choices.

As public health authorities have become more sophisticated and interdisciplinary in crafting their public health messages, the style of communication campaigns has evolved. The following selection addresses the use of social marketing campaigns to influence health behaviors. Social marketing for public health employs many of the same advertising strategies used to market unhealthful products to the public; it thus embraces the idea of a "free marketplace of ideas" in which public health authorities peddle their health-promoting messages alongside other marketing messages. Sonya Grier and Carol A. Bryant introduce the concept of social marketing for public health promotion and examine the ethical implications of such campaigns.

SOCIAL MARKETING IN PUBLIC HEALTH*

Sonya Grier and Carol A. Bryant

Societies worldwide face an ever-increasing array of health challenges, heightening the importance of social change efforts. Social marketing, the use of marketing to design and implement programs to promote socially beneficial behavior change, has grown in popularity and usage within the public health community. In recent years, the Centers for Disease Control and Prevention (CDC), the U.S. Department of Agriculture (USDA), the U.S. Department of Health and Human Services (USDHHS), and other governmental and nonprofit organizations have used social marketing to increase fruit and vegetable consumption, promote breastfeeding, decrease fat consumption, promote physical activity, and influence a wide variety of other preventive health behaviors. State and local communities are using social marketing to increase utilization of the Supplemental Food and Nutrition Program for Women, Infants, and Children (WIC), prenatal care, low cost mammograms, and other health services. Internationally, social marketing has been used to improve access to potable water, eliminate leprosy in Sri Lanka, increase tuberculosis medicine adherence, and promote immunizations and universal iodization legislation, among other applications....

*Reprinted from *Annual Review of Public Health* 26 (2005): 319–39.

The widespread adoption of social marketing in public health has garnered important successes. Among these is VERB™, a national, multicultural, social marketing program coordinated by CDC. The VERB™ program encourages "tweens" (young people ages 9–13) to be physically active every day. The program was based on extensive marketing research with tweens, their parents, and other influencers. Results were used to design an intervention that combines mass-media advertising, public relations, guerrilla (i.e., interpersonal) marketing, and partnership efforts with professional sports leagues and athletes, as well as well-known sporting-goods suppliers and retailers, to reach the distinct audiences of tweens and adult influencers. VERB™ also partners with communities to improve access to outlets for physical activity and capitalize on the influence parents, teachers, and other people have on tweens' lives. After just one year, this award-winning program resulted in a 34% increase in weekly free-time physical activity sessions among 8.6 million children ages 9–10 in the United States. In communities that received higher levels of VERB™ interventions, the increases in physical activity were more dramatic. Another well-known example is the TRUTH™ campaign, which contributed to the reduction of smoking among teenagers nationwide. . . .

DEFINING SOCIAL MARKETING

. . . Social marketing is typically defined as a program-planning process that applies commercial marketing concepts and techniques to promote voluntary behavior change. Social marketing facilitates the acceptance, rejection, modification, abandonment, or maintenance of particular behaviors by groups of individuals, often referred to as the target audience. . . .

. . . Marketing attempts to influence voluntary behavior by offering or reinforcing incentives and/or consequences in an environment that invites voluntary exchange. Exchange theory views consumers acting primarily out of self-interest as they seek ways to optimize value by doing what gives them the greatest benefit for the least cost. . . . In public health situations, there is rarely an immediate, explicit payback to target audiences in return for their adoption of healthy behavior. Nevertheless, exchange theory reminds social marketers that they must (a) offer benefits that the consumer (not the public health professional) truly values; (b) recognize that consumers often pay intangible costs, such as time and psychic discomfort associated with changing behaviors; and (c) acknowledge that everyone involved in the exchange, including intermediaries, must receive valued benefits in return for their efforts. . . .

COMPARING MARKETING TO OTHER BEHAVIOR MANAGEMENT TOOLS

Social marketing can also be understood by comparing it with other approaches to managing behavior change [including education and law]. . . . Education informs and persuades people to adopt healthy behaviors voluntarily by creating awareness of the benefits of changing. . . . Citizens have free choice in how they respond, and society accepts the costs when some people continue to practice undesirable behaviors. Education is most effective when the goals of society are consistent with those of the target audience, the benefits of behavior change are inherently attractive, immediate, and obvious, the costs of changing are low, and the skills and other resources needed to change are readily available (e.g., putting a baby to sleep on its back to prevent sudden infant death syndrome [SIDS]).

Law or policy development uses coercion or the threat of punishment to manage behavior. Legislation is the most effective tool for public health when society is not willing to pay the costs associated with continued practice of an unhealthy or risky behavior (e.g., drunk driving) yet citizens are unlikely to find it in their immediate self-interest to change.

In contrast, marketing influences behavior by offering alternative choices that invite voluntary exchange. Marketing alters the environment to make the recommended health behavior more advantageous than the unhealthy behavior it is designed to replace and then communicates the more favorable cost-benefit relationship to the target audience. Marketing is the most effective strategy when societal goals are not directly and immediately consistent with people's self-interest but citizens can be influenced to change by making the consequences more advantageous. Like education, marketing offers people freedom of choice; but unlike education, it alters the behavioral consequences rather than expects individuals to make a sacrifice on society's behalf. Education and policy changes are often components in a social marketing intervention; however, marketing also creates an environment more conducive for change by enhancing the attractiveness of the benefits offered and minimizing the costs....

CHALLENGES AND MISCONCEPTIONS

... A criticism of social marketing is that it "blames the victim" by focusing on individual behavior rather than on the underlying environmental and social causes of the problems it addresses. [Some argue] that social marketing, like many public health approaches, tries to rescue people from drowning "downstream," when the important work lies "upstream," combating the environmental and social structural factors that create the health problems. There is an element of truth in this criticism: Social marketers have been guilty of relying too heavily on strategies aimed at changing individual behavior and paying too little attention to environmental factors. The field has benefited from this criticism, and today the importance of understanding the social environment and making it more conducive to individual healthy behavior is well established....

Another long-standing complaint against social marketing is that it is manipulative.... Some public health professionals still reject social marketing because of its ties to Madison Avenue–style advertising, a field that has come under increased scrutiny and criticism....

ETHICAL CONSIDERATIONS

... Unlike most commercial marketing, social marketing involves some of our most deeply held beliefs and moral judgments. Recent work on ethics highlights unique issues about the moral justification of social marketing's aims (e.g., individual or social welfare versus individual satisfaction), procedures (e.g., how much disclosure is necessary in the promotion of a contraceptive about product side effects), and outcomes (e.g., moral changes in a community, especially when the social marketers are not members of that community).

Many ethical criticisms of social marketing focus on power differentials that contribute to an unequal playing field between marketers and consumers. Some authors argue that incorporating consumers in the process, from the beginning of the social marketing design to its implementation and evaluation, would help counteract this issue....

Given the ecological nature of most health conditions, efforts to change health behaviors can impact a variety of contextual factors; therefore, it also is important to anticipate any unintended effects social marketing activities may have on target audiences and others. Media messages, for instance, should not reinforce stereotypes or stigmatize population segments (e.g., by presenting smokers as nasty or parents as unfit) or divert program planners from addressing structural factors needed to facilitate change. . . .

THE NEXT STEPS: A VISION FOR THE FUTURE OF SOCIAL MARKETING IN PUBLIC HEALTH

. . . Public health organizations could benefit from viewing the consumer as the center of everything they do, inviting consumers to be true partners in determining how to best meet their health needs. We envision a public health field in which its practitioners, working at all levels, are committed to understanding and responding to the public's desires as well as their needs and routinely use consumer research to make strategic planning decisions about how best to help its consumers solve their problems and realize their aspirations. We believe the marketing mindset will optimize public health's ability to create trusting relationships with consumers and make their lives healthier and more fulfilling.

.   .   .   .   .

While health education campaigns of any type have ethical challenges, special concerns are raised when the government itself speaks on public health issues. The selection that follows acknowledges the good that can come from health information, but it also discusses the potentially problematic aspects of mass health communication campaigns: the intrusion on personal sovereignty and the assignment of blame for unhealthy behaviors. Ruth R. Faden, a noted bioethicist, discusses the morally relevant attributes of health communication campaigns. Although she recognizes their coercive aspects, Faden explains why many government health messages are ethically acceptable.

ETHICAL ISSUES IN GOVERNMENT-SPONSORED PUBLIC HEALTH CAMPAIGNS*
Ruth R. Faden

Questions have been raised about the extent to which [government] health campaigns interfere with free choice and about the general propriety of governmental attempts to direct social values and lifestyles.
    In the case of public health campaigns, and probably in the case of all health

*Reprinted from *Health Education Quarterly* 14 (1987): 27–37.

promotion strategies, [concerns] about efficacy, about justice, and about autonomy . . . are inextricably interrelated. In some cases, there is almost a hydraulic
relationship between these problems. The more one is improved, the more others
are exacerbated. For example, if public health campaigns are made more effective,
some concerns about injustice may be removed. However, the more effective public
health campaigns become, the more one becomes concerned about governmental
interferences with autonomy. . . .

EFFICACY OF HEALTH COMMUNICATION CAMPAIGNS

There are many problems in evaluating the cost and effectiveness of public health
campaigns. One problem is deciding what counts as a successful campaign, that is,
deciding what the criteria for success ought to be. For example, should success be
defined in terms of behavior change or attitude change? How much change must be
achieved before the campaign can be called a success?

Another problem is deciding what counts as a public campaign, for purposes of
evaluation. For example, one of the earliest, if not the first, public health campaigns
conducted in the U.S. was launched by Cotton Mather in 1721. Mather used pam-
phleteering and rhetoric to persuade the citizens of Boston to accept inoculation
at the outbreak of a smallpox epidemic. While this kind of personal crusading is not
usually what we have in mind when we think of public health campaigns, it is true
that until fairly recently public health campaigns were dominated by private citizens
organized into special interest, voluntary organizations. [Smoking and nutrition
campaigns represent areas in which voluntary organizations are still central to public health campaigns.]

Although there have been notable failures of specific, individual campaigns
in the past, recently researchers have pointed to the successful effects of health
campaigns when taken cumulatively and over time. . . . Increasingly, researchers are
becoming optimistic about the potential for success of well-designed and properly
implemented public health campaigns. . . .

AUTONOMY AND HEALTH CAMPAIGNS

[Paradoxically, improving a health campaign's effectiveness may raise] other concerns about the propriety of the campaign. Here we must face the somewhat awk-
ward realization that we are not altogether certain that all government-sponsored
health campaigns ought to succeed. . . .

The central issue here is the compatibility of government-sponsored health campaigns with respect for individual autonomy and related values. [There exists] one
very central problem about health promotion programs generally—namely, whether
government ought to be in the business of promoting certain lifestyles over others,
in the first place. [Certain] characteristics or criteria . . . distinguish those forms of
influence on a person that are compatible with autonomy from those that are not. . . .

Persuasion can be defined as the intentional and successful attempt to induce a
person(s), through appeals to reason, to freely accept—as his or her own—the beliefs,
attitudes, values, intentions, or actions advocated by the influence agent. In persuasion, the influence agent must bring to the persuadee's attention reasons for
acceptance of the desired perspective. . . .

One central feature of persuasion is that the reasons that comprise the persuasive appeal exist independent of the persuader. If the influence agent creates or in some way has control over the contingencies that the agent offers as "reasons," the influence is no longer strictly persuasive, but rather manipulative or even coercive. . . .

Manipulation of information is a deliberate act that successfully influences a person(s) by nonpersuasively altering the person's understanding of the situation, thereby modifying perceptions of the available options. The influence agent does not change the person's actual options; only the person's perception is modified as a result of the manipulation. . . . Manipulation of information compromises autonomy to the extent that it renders people ignorant, thereby causally constraining relevant aspects of their decisions. Manipulation by deception is the most common form of manipulation of information. Deception includes such strategies as lying, withholding of information, and misleading exaggeration where people are led to believe what is false. . . .

. . . Also qualifying as informational manipulations are such interventions as: (1) intentionally overwhelming a person with excessive information so as to induce confusion and a reduction of understanding, (2) intentionally provoking or taking advantage of fear, anxiety, pain, or other negative affective or cognitive states known to compromise a person's ability to process information effectively, and (3) intentionally presenting information in a way that leads the manipulatee to draw certain predictable and misleading influences. . . .

. . . [In contrast to commercial advertising campaigns], health campaigns are rarely (if ever) deceptive, at least in any ordinary or straightforward, intentional sense. If there are any autonomy-related problems with health campaigns, they are apt to be much more subtle and to derive largely from the potential for skillful application of psychological theory. It is often difficult in practice to distinguish between persuasion and certain forms of psychological and informational manipulation. Many social influence attempts, including many health campaigns, contain elements of both persuasion and manipulation. . . .

To the extent that [some] health campaigns . . . involve elements of psychological or informational manipulation, in the strictest sense they violate the principle of respect for individual autonomy. However, . . . the campaign may still be morally justifiable, depending on the seriousness of the violation and on the moral importance of the warrant for conducting the campaign and using the specific strategies that are disrespectful of autonomy. . . .

JUSTICE, AUTONOMY, AND HEALTH CAMPAIGNS

. . . [There are four justifications for government health promotion.] First, it can be argued that the government has a basic responsibility to protect and promote the nation's health—the public health—independent of the preference structure of individual citizens. This position places an intrinsic value on the public's health as expressed through such aggregate indicators as national life expectancy and morbidity data. Second, there is the closely related argument that at least the majority of citizens desire certain kinds of health promotion or protection that can only be achieved through collective state action. . . . The majority of individuals want to have healthier lifestyles but they do not have the resources either to educate themselves or to modify unhealthful habits on their own. A third argument grounds government intervention by appeal to broadly construed third party or state interests. A prime example here is cost containment. Health promotion programs are justified to the extent that they reduce health care costs or sick day losses. The fourth argument justifies government lifestyle programs to the extent that the targeted lifestyle behavior has the effect of harming innocent others.

These four arguments are by no means mutually exclusive. They can obviously be used in concert to justify the same health campaign: Antismoking campaigns are paradigmatic examples of state health promotion efforts that can plausibly appeal to all four arguments for their justification. [There are, however, objections and critiques of each of these justifications.]

... One might view as unjust state lifestyle campaigns that are defended by appeal to the preferences or will of the majority. . . .

Similarly, objections can and have been raised against the public health justification. One can deny that there is any basic or important value to the nation's health, apart from or independent of the value each citizen places on his or her own health. Someone holding this position may interpret an appeal to the state's obligation to protect the public health as a thinly disguised instance of unjustifiable state paternalism when a lifestyle program disregards the value or preference structures of the individual citizens who are its targets.

Objections can also be mounted against the "social harm, cost containment" justification and "the harm to others" justification. Objections to these positions often reflect empirical and moral disputes about the magnitude and acceptability of the harm at issue, as well as disputes about the limits of government in the liberal state to provide harm protection and to make acceptable tradeoffs between highly valued social goods.

There is a direct relationship between the warrants for a particular health campaign and the extent to which it is morally acceptable for the campaign to violate the principle of respect for autonomy. If one finds the justification for conducting a specific state-financed health campaign to be very morally compelling, one would be more likely to view as ethical the campaign's including elements that violate respect for autonomy. . . .

When people oppose government health campaigns on the grounds that the government ought not to interfere with or attempt to shape existing patterns of health behaviors and lifestyles, a standard response is that, if the government does not get into the business of shaping health attitudes and behavior, those attitudes and behavior will be left to be shaped entirely by the short-term contingencies of our market economy. . . . A major justification for government media campaigns is that they are needed to counter commercial advertising. . . . However, those who reject this justification for government media campaigns counter with the argument that if the government is convinced that an industry is marketing an unhealthful product, instead of engaging in counter-advertising, the government should ban all promotional advertising of the product. Better yet, the government should either set standards that make the product healthful, or if that is not possible, make the product illegal. . . .

Implicit in this position is a different set of assumptions about the role of government from that underlying the current federal position on deregulation. Particularly as regards matters of health and safety, collective efficiency arguments favor strong intervention by [federal] agencies. . . .

... Even for those health problems where there is a preferable, alternative solution (for example, through regulatory or legislative engineering or through technological change), there still may be an appropriate role for health campaigns. [Long-term, cumulative changes to the public climate can come from sustained health campaigns.] For example, the current legislative interest in restricting public smoking areas would likely not have been possible without a background of favorable public opinion. . . . It is likely that the antismoking campaigning of the past 20 years has contributed significantly to the current climate of increasing hostility toward smoking. . . .

Real questions remain about whether health campaigns should be conducted for the explicit purpose of modifying public or legislative opinion over time. There are problems about the use of governmental funds to conduct interventions that may influence the legislative process, however subtly or indirectly. Nevertheless, I see this long-term effect of changing public opinion and perceptions about health practices as one of the more viable justifications for continued federal support of health media campaigns.

.   .   .   .   .

The government can be a voice of consumer protection, guiding individuals toward healthy choices; but because it speaks on behalf of the citizenry, the state has a special obligation to act with honesty, integrity, and neutrality. Thus, ethical and constitutional concerns are raised when the government expresses a preference for one ideology over another. However, the Supreme Court has held that the government is free to favor one ideology without giving equal time or funding to another. In upholding a law that forbade family planning clinics from counseling patients about abortions (the so-called gag rule), the Court found that "the Government can, without violating the Constitution, selectively fund a program to encourage certain activities it believes to be in the public interest, without at the same time funding an alternative program which seeks to deal with the problem in another way" (*Rust v. Sullivan*, 500 U.S. 173, 193 [1991]).

In *DKT International, Inc. v. United States Agency for International Development*, 477 F.3d 758 (D.C. Cir. 2007), the court relied on *Rust* to uphold the constitutionality of a requirement under the President's Emergency Plan for AIDS Relief (PEPFAR) that all funding recipients have a policy "explicitly opposing prostitution and sex trafficking." The court reasoned, "When it communicates its message, either through public officials or private entities, the government can—and often must—discriminate on the basis of viewpoint" (*DKT International*, 477 F.3d at 761). Even though DKT International believes that opposition to commercial sex work stigmatizes and alienates the people most vulnerable to HIV/AIDS, the court ruled that it must adopt that policy in order to receive PEPFAR funding (Masenior and Beyrer 2007).

When the government enters into the marketplace of ideas to promote behavior change, there is a danger that the health messages might come across as paternalistic. Consider the controversial remarks of John Reid, then U.K. health secretary (quoted in the *Guardian;* Wintour and Blackstock 2004). Arguing that "empowerment is different from instruction" and that government needs to be "less preachy, less hectoring, less dictatorial [to] achieve success in the field of public health," Reid criticized antismoking campaigns. Much of his argument focuses on what health problems are prioritized and by whom: "I just do not think the worst problem on our sink estates by any means is smoking, but is an obsession of the learned middle class. . . . Be very careful, that you do not patronize people because . . . people from those lower socio-economic backgrounds have very few pleasures and one of them is smoking. I worry slightly about the unanimity of the middle class professional activists on this."

In addition to being patronizing, government health information campaigns also threaten to assign personal responsibility for behaviors that are largely the result of more complex social and environmental factors. Individuals who engage in less-healthy behaviors may, as a result, be blamed for their illnesses and risk losing social sympathy and support. Their self-image may also be damaged, and they may suffer psychological harm. As Grier and Bryant note in their article excerpted above, health messages may be particularly problematic when they associate certain behaviors with unattractive characteristics, causing stigma and embarrassment. For example, a message that young women are less attractive if they smoke or overeat may be effective, but it sends a worrying signal about self-image.

Truthful government speech, while perhaps patronizing or stigmatizing, is less troubling than truth-distorting government speech. When the government distorts the truth for public health purposes, its legitimacy is called into question. In 1999, the U.S. Postal Service reproduced a pose of the famous abstract expressionist Jackson Pollock for a postage stamp, but the image was cleansed by removing the cigarette from Pollock's mouth. Government can deceive in much more subtle ways, and good intentions can make it difficult to determine when the state goes too far in health promotion. What if public health

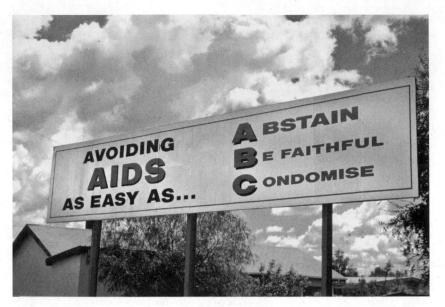

Photo 21. This 2004 image shows an HIV/AIDS awareness billboard in Gaborone, Botswana. The billboard is part of Botswana's "ABC" campaign against HIV/AIDS, which promotes abstinence from sexual activity, faithfulness within relationships, and condom use as the pillars of HIV prevention. In Uganda, a similar ABC campaign and a policy of openness are frequently credited with that country's early success in curbing the epidemic. Reproduced by permission, © Julio Echtart/The Image Works, 2004.

officials act as if there were sound scientific support underlying the health message, even though the data are inconclusive or nonexistent? What if government knowingly exaggerates the risk or underestimates the extent of the behavior change necessary in order to persuade the public to follow public health advice?

This distortion of the truth is even more troubling when it is used not to promote public health but to obfuscate science for other policy objectives. Perhaps worst of all, the government at times actively suppresses, discredits, or alters scientific findings that are inconsistent with its policies. In recent years, the apparently frequent distortion of science for political ends has been deeply troubling to those in public health and to scientists more generally. In 2004, the Union of Concerned Scientists claimed that the Bush administration had allowed policy to trump science on numerous occasions (as described in box 26 of the companion text). The organization asserted that scientific information was ignored, modified, or discredited for political purposes when, for example, the Food and Drug Administration delayed approval of emergency contraceptives against the advice of two advisory panels; the Department of Health and Human Services obscured scientific evaluation of abstinence-only education, pressuring educators to promote abstinence; the Centers for Disease Control and Prevention altered its website to raise doubts about the effectiveness of condoms in preventing HIV transmission; and the Environmental Protection Agency suppressed reports and publicly misrepresented scientific consensus in order to undermine climate change science.

II. COMMERCIAL SPEECH

Public health officials' attempts to control the informational environment are not confined to health education campaigns, of course. Most people understand that government messages have a paltry effect on public attitudes and behaviors. There are just too many voices in the market for those of the government to dominate or, sometimes, even to have a discernible influence. The business community speaks with particular force in the marketplace of ideas. Manufacturers of hazardous products (e.g., cigarettes, alcoholic beverages, and firearms) spend billions of dollars on advertisements and marketing. Public health officials cannot hope to compete with these private purveyors of information through government speech alone. Consequently, restraint of commercial speech is one of the most important strategies to promote health.

For most of the nation's history, the Supreme Court declined to protect commercial speech under the First Amendment of the Constitution. In the mid-1970s, however, the Court began to protect advertisements and product promotions. The early commercial speech cases involved instances when the message itself had public health value: abortion referral services, contraceptive advertisements, or pharmaceutical prices. In *Bigelow v. Virginia*, 421 U.S. 809 (1975), the Court considered whether an advertisement in a Virginia newspaper for abortion services in New York was entitled to protection under the First Amendment. Noting that the editor's interests in conveying the information in the advertisement coincided with the general public's constitutional interests in receiving such information, the Court held that "the fact that the particular advertisement . . . had commercial aspects . . . did not negate all First Amendment guarantees."

Nominally, commercial speech operates as a category of "lower-value" expression, warranting less constitutional protection than social or political discourse. In reality, though, the level of scrutiny given commercial speech has changed over the years and is still in transition. This section explores the evolution of the commercial speech doctrine from the mid-1970s to the present day.

Commercial speech is an expression related solely to the economic interests of the speaker and the audience that does "no more than propose a commercial transaction" (*Virginia State Board of Pharmacy v. Virginia Citizens Consumer Council, Inc.*, 425 U.S. 748, 776 [1976]). The three distinguishing attributes of commercial speech are that it (1) identifies a specific product (i.e., offers a product for sale), (2) is a form of advertising (i.e., is designed to attract public attention to, or patronage for, a product or service, by paid announcements proclaiming its qualities or advantages), and (3) confers economic benefits (i.e., the speaker stands to profit financially).

These criteria appear to be clear, but perplexing issues arise when speech represents "a blending of commercial speech and debate on issues of public importance," as occurred in a case related to labor conditions in Nike's foreign factories (*Nike, Inc. v. Kasky,* 539 U.S. 654, 663 [2003]). Nike had defended itself, via press releases and fact sheets, against accusations from mass media outlets that its products were made with sweatshop labor. A California activist sued Nike, alleging that these statements constituted false advertising. In its defense, Nike asserted that rather than being commercial speech, its press releases about its labor practices were discourse on a matter of public importance and therefore subject to a higher standard of First Amendment review. The Supreme Court heard oral arguments in the case but dismissed its writ of certiorari as being "improvidently granted" (539 U.S. at 655), leaving intact the California Supreme Court's finding that Nike's messages were commercial speech "because the messages . . . were directed by a commercial speaker to a commercial audience, and because they made representations of fact about the speaker's own business operations for the purpose of promoting sales of its products" (*Kasky v. Nike, Inc.,* 45 P.3d 243, 247 [Cal. 2002]).

Once a court finds that a message is "commercial" in nature, it has to decide whether the government may suppress it to achieve a public good. In 1980 the Supreme Court articulated a four-part test to determine the constitutional protection that should be afforded to commercial speech. The criteria laid down in *Central Hudson Gas* &

Electric Corp. v. Public Service Commission, 447 U.S. 557, 566 (1980), are still used today (see figure 33 in the companion text for a graphic representation of the *Central Hudson* test): "For commercial speech to come within [the First Amendment], it at least must concern lawful activity and not be misleading. Next, we ask whether the asserted governmental interest is substantial. If both inquiries yield positive answers, we must determine whether the regulation directly advances the governmental interest asserted, and whether it is not more extensive than is necessary to serve that interest."

In the years following *Central Hudson,* the Supreme Court took a permissive approach to government regulation of commercial speech. For example, in *Posadas de Puerto Rico Associates v. Tourism Co. of Puerto Rico,* 478 U.S. 328 (1986), the Court upheld Puerto Rico's ban on the advertising of casino gambling because there was a substantial state interest and a reasonable belief that advertising would increase such gambling.

In *Posadas,* Justice William Rehnquist (later chief justice) made an argument, now discredited, that the greater power to completely ban a product necessarily includes the lesser power to regulate advertising of that product: "It would . . . surely be a strange constitutional doctrine which would concede to the legislature the authority to totally ban a product or activity, but deny to the legislature the authority to forbid the stimulation of demand for the product or activity" (478 U.S. at 346). This "greater includes the lesser" theory would give the government almost total authority to suppress advertising of tobacco, alcoholic beverages, and gambling. But is Justice Rehnquist correct in assuming that speech restrictions *are* the lesser included power? Arguably, product prohibitions on health or safety grounds would be less offensive to the Constitution than speech prohibitions.

In the mid-1990s, the Court's permissive approach to regulation of commercial speech evolved into "close scrutiny." In *Rubin v. Coors Brewing Co.,* 514 U.S. 476 (1995), the Court insisted that government must have a clear and consistent policy when regulating commercial speech, as it invalidated a federal law prohibiting manufacturers from displaying alcohol content on beer labels. The following year, in *44 Liquormart, Inc. v. Rhode Island,* the Court considered a Rhode Island law that prohibited the advertisement of alcoholic beverage prices. While all nine justices agreed that the Rhode Island law was an unconstitutional restriction on commercial speech, the multiple concurring opinions in the case reveal the Court's deep divide over the proper legal test. Justice John Paul Stevens's opinion announced the judgment of the Court, but none of the opinions garnered a majority. Stevens's opinion would require that the state affirmatively demonstrate a relationship between regulating commercial speech and attaining an important health objective. His opinion emphasized the "special dangers that attend complete bans on truthful, nonmisleading commercial speech."

44 LIQUORMART, INC. V. RHODE ISLAND*
Supreme Court of the United States
Decided May 13, 1996

Justice STEVENS delivered the opinion of the Court with respect to Parts I, II, and VIII, and issued an opinion with respect to Parts III and V, in which Justices KENNEDY, SOUTER, and GINSBURG join, an opinion with respect to Part VI, in which Justices KENNEDY, THOMAS, and GINSBURG join, and an opinion with respect to part IV, in which Justices KENNEDY and GINSBURG join.

Last Term [in *Rubin v. Coors Brewing Co.*] we held that a federal law abridging a brewer's right to provide the public with accurate information about the alcoholic content of malt beverages is unconstitutional. We now hold that Rhode Island's statutory prohibition against advertisements that provide the public with accurate information about retail prices of alcoholic beverages is also invalid. Our holding rests on the conclusion that such an advertising ban is an abridgment of speech protected by the First Amendment....

I

In 1956, the Rhode Island Legislature enacted two separate prohibitions against advertising the retail price of alcoholic beverages. The first ... prohibits [vendors] from "advertising in any manner whatsoever" the price of any alcoholic beverage offered for sale in the State; the only exception is for price tags or signs displayed with the merchandise within licensed premises and not visible from the street. The second statute applies to the Rhode Island news media. It contains a categorical prohibition against the publication or broadcast of any advertisements—even those referring to sales in other States—that "make reference to the price of any alcoholic beverages." ...

III

Advertising has been a part of our culture throughout our history. Even in colonial days, the public relied on "commercial speech" for vital information about the market. Early newspapers displayed advertisements for goods and services ... , and town criers called out prices in public squares. ...

In accord with the role that commercial messages have long played, the law has developed to ensure that advertising provides consumers with accurate information

*517 U.S. 484 (1996).

about the availability of goods and services. In the early years, the common law, and later, statutes, served the consumers' interest . . . by prohibiting fraudulent and misleading advertising. It was not until the 1970's, however, that this Court held that the First Amendment protected the dissemination of truthful and nonmisleading commercial messages about lawful products and services.

In *Bigelow v. Virginia,* 421 U.S. 809 (1975), we held that it was error to assume that commercial speech was entitled to no First Amendment protection or that it was without value in the marketplace of ideas. The following Term in *Virginia Board of Pharmacy v. Virginia Citizens Consumer Council, Inc.,* 425 U.S. 748 (1976), we . . . held that the State's blanket ban on advertising the price of prescription drugs violated the First Amendment.

Virginia Board of Pharmacy reflected the conclusion that the same interest that supports regulation of potentially misleading advertising, namely, the public's interest in receiving accurate commercial information, also supports an interpretation of the First Amendment that provides constitutional protection for the dissemination of accurate and nonmisleading commercial messages. . . . The opinion further explained that a State's paternalistic assumption that the public will use truthful, nonmisleading commercial information unwisely cannot justify a decision to suppress it. . . .

On the basis of these principles, our early cases uniformly struck down several broadly based bans on truthful, nonmisleading commercial speech, each of which served ends unrelated to consumer protection. . . .

At the same time, our early cases recognized that the State may regulate some types of commercial advertising more freely than other forms of protected speech. Specifically, we explained that the State may require commercial messages to "appear in such a form, or include such additional information, warnings, and disclaimers, as are necessary to prevent its being deceptive," *Virginia Board of Pharmacy,* 425 U.S., at 772, and that it may restrict some forms of aggressive sales practices that have the potential to exert "undue influence" over consumers.

Virginia Board of Pharmacy attributed the State's authority to impose these regulations in part to certain "commonsense differences" that exist between commercial messages and other types of protected expression. 425 U. S., at 771, n. 24. Our opinion noted that the greater "objectivity" of commercial speech justifies affording the State more freedom to distinguish false commercial advertisements from true ones, *ibid.,* and that the greater "hardiness" of commercial speech, inspired as it is by the profit motive, likely diminishes the chilling effect that may attend its regulation, *ibid.* . . .

In *Central Hudson Gas & Elec. Corp. v. Public Serv. Comm'n of N.Y.,* 447 U.S. 557 (1980), we took stock of our developing commercial speech jurisprudence. In that case, we considered a regulation "completely" banning all promotional advertising by electric utilities. Our decision acknowledged the special features of commercial speech but identified the serious First Amendment concerns that attend blanket advertising prohibitions that do not protect consumers from commercial harms. . . .

IV

As our review of the case law reveals, Rhode Island errs in concluding that *all* commercial speech regulations are subject to a similar form of constitutional review simply because they target a similar category of expression. The mere fact that messages propose commercial transactions does not in and of itself dictate the constitutional analysis that should apply to decisions to suppress them.

When a State regulates commercial messages to protect consumers from misleading, deceptive, or aggressive sales practices, or requires the disclosure of beneficial consumer information, the purpose of its regulation is consistent with the reasons for according constitutional protection to commercial speech and therefore justifies less than strict review. However, when a State entirely prohibits the dissemination of truthful, nonmisleading commercial messages for reasons unrelated to the preservation of a fair bargaining process, there is far less reason to depart from the rigorous review that the First Amendment generally demands. . . .

The special dangers that attend complete bans on truthful, nonmisleading commercial speech cannot be explained away by appeals to the "commonsense distinctions" that exist between commercial and noncommercial speech. *Virginia Board of Pharmacy*, 425 U.S. at 771. Regulations that suppress the truth are no less troubling because they target objectively verifiable information, nor are they less effective because they aim at durable messages. As a result, neither the "greater objectivity" nor the "greater hardiness" of truthful, nonmisleading commercial speech justifies reviewing its complete suppression with added deference. *Ibid.*

It is in the State's interest in protecting consumers from "commercial harms" that provides "the typical reason why commercial speech can be subject to greater governmental regulation than noncommercial speech." *Cincinnati v. Discovery Network, Inc.*, 507 U.S. 410, 426 (1993). Yet bans that target truthful, nonmisleading commercial messages rarely protect consumers from such harms. Instead, such bans often serve to obscure an "underlying government policy" that could be implemented without regulating speech. . . .

Precisely because bans against truthful, nonmisleading commercial speech rarely seek to protect consumers from either deception or overreaching, they usually rest solely on the offensive assumption that the public will respond "irrationally" to the truth. The First Amendment directs us to be especially skeptical of regulations that seek to keep people in the dark for what the government perceives to be their own good. That teaching applies equally to state attempts to deprive consumers of accurate information about their chosen products. . . .

V

In this case, there is no question that [the] ban constitutes a blanket prohibition against truthful, nonmisleading speech about a lawful product. . . . We must review the price advertising ban with "special care." *Central Hudson*, 447 U. S., at 566, n. 9. . . .

. . . The State bears the burden of showing not merely that its regulation will advance its interest, but also that it will do so "to a material degree." *Edenfield v. Fane*, 507 U.S. 761, 771 (1993). . . . We must determine whether the State has shown that the price advertising ban will *significantly* reduce alcohol consumption.

. . . The State has presented no evidence to suggest that its speech prohibition will *significantly* reduce marketwide consumption [of alcohol, the stated goal of the regulation]. . . .

The State also cannot satisfy the requirement that its restriction on speech be no more extensive than necessary. It is perfectly obvious that alternative forms of regulation that would not involve any restriction on speech would be more likely to achieve the State's goal of promoting temperance. . . .

As a result, even under the less than strict standard that generally applies in commercial speech cases, the State has failed to establish a "reasonable fit" between its abridgment of speech and its temperance goal. *Board of Trustees, State Univ. of N.Y. v. Fox*, 492 U.S. 469, 480 (1989). It necessarily follows that the price advertising ban cannot survive the more stringent constitutional review that *Central Hudson* itself concluded was appropriate for the complete suppression of truthful, nonmisleading commercial speech. . . .

VI

[The State offers three defenses for its advertising ban: (1) that it made a reasonable legislative judgment in enacting the ban, (2) that, under the precedence of *Posadas de Puerto Rico Associates v. Tourism Co. of Puerto Rico*, 478 U.S. 328 (1986), the state can ban price advertising because it could ban the sale of alcohol altogether, and (3) that the Court should give deference to the State's ban because alcohol beverages are "vice" products.]

The State's first argument fails to justify the speech prohibition at issue. Our commercial speech cases recognize some room for the exercise of legislative judgment. However, Rhode Island errs in concluding that . . . *Posadas* establish[ed] the degree of deference that its decision to impose a price advertising ban warrants. . . .

The reasoning in *Posadas* does support the State's argument, but, on reflection, we are now persuaded that *Posadas* erroneously performed the First Amendment analysis. The casino advertising ban was designed to keep truthful, nonmisleading speech from members of the public for fear that they would be more likely to gamble if they received it. As a result, the advertising ban served to shield the State's anti-gambling policy from the public scrutiny that more direct, nonspeech regulation would draw.

Given our longstanding hostility to commercial speech regulation of this type, *Posadas* clearly erred in concluding that it was "up to the legislature" to choose suppression over a less speech-restrictive policy. . . .

Instead, in keeping with our prior holdings, we conclude that a state legislature does not have the broad discretion to suppress truthful, nonmisleading information for paternalistic purposes that the *Posadas* majority was willing to tolerate. . . .

[The Court next considers Rhode Island's argument—based on Justice Rehnquist's "greater includes the lesser" reasoning in *Posadas*—that its authority to ban alcoholic beverages includes the power to restrict advertisements offering them for sale.]

Although we do not dispute the proposition that greater powers include lesser ones, we fail to see how that syllogism requires the conclusion that the State's power to regulate commercial activity is "greater" than its power to ban truthful, nonmisleading commercial speech. Contrary to the assumption made in *Posadas*, we think it quite clear that banning speech may sometimes prove far more intrusive than banning conduct. . . . In short, we reject the assumption that words are necessarily less vital to freedom than actions, or that logic somehow proves that the power to prohibit an activity is necessarily "greater" than the power to suppress speech about it. . . .

... As the entire Court apparently now agrees, the statements in the *Posadas* opinion on which Rhode Island relies are no longer persuasive.

Finally, we find unpersuasive the State's contention that, under *Posadas*, the price advertising ban should be upheld because it targets commercial speech that pertains to a "vice" activity....

... The scope of any "vice" exception to the protection afforded by the First Amendment would be difficult ... to define. Almost any product that poses some threat to public health or public morals might reasonably be characterized ... as relating to "vice activity." Such characterization, however, is anomalous when applied to products ... that may be lawfully purchased on the open market. The recognition of such an exception would also have the unfortunate consequence of ... allowing state legislatures to justify censorship by the simple expedient of placing the "vice" label on selected lawful activities....

VIII

Because Rhode Island has failed to carry its heavy burden of justifying its complete ban on price advertising, we conclude that [the laws and regulations challenged] abridge speech in violation of the First Amendment as made applicable to the States by the Due Process Clause of the Fourteenth Amendment. The judgment of the Court of Appeals is therefore reversed.

. . . . .

Whereas Justice Stevens required the state to demonstrate "that the price advertising ban will significantly reduce alcohol consumption," Justice Sandra Day O'Connor's concurring opinion rejected his refinement of the test for commercial speech restrictions, finding that "because Rhode Island's regulation fails even the less stringent standard set out in *Central Hudson,* nothing here requires adoption of a new analysis for the evaluation of commercial speech regulations" (517 U.S. at 532). In *Greater New Orleans Broadcasting Association v. United States,* the Court declined to resolve the question of whether the state must provide scientific evidence, because flaws in the state's case rendered such an inquiry unnecessary. The Court found that Congress's policy on gambling, which proscribed private casino advertising but promoted gambling on certain Native American land and in state-run lotteries, was "so pierced by exemptions and inconsistencies that the Government cannot hope to exonerate it" (527 U.S. 173, 190 [1999]).

In *Coors Brewing, 44 Liquormart,* and *Greater New Orleans Broadcasting,* the Court had signaled that it would not tolerate restrictions on truthful information that consumers wish to know. In 2001, the Supreme Court reviewed Massachusetts regulations on tobacco advertising in *Lorillard Tobacco Co. v. Reilly.* The regulations prohibited outdoor advertising of tobacco products within 1,000 feet of a public playground or school. In addition, they required that retailers within 1,000 feet of a school or playground place advertisements for tobacco products at least 5 feet from the floor. While the Court held that the Federal Cigarette Labeling and Advertising Act (FCLAA) (see chapter 6) preempted regulation of cigarette advertisements, smokeless tobacco and cigars are outside the act's scope; the stage was thus set for a major First Amendment ruling on tobacco advertising.

LORILLARD TOBACCO CO. V. REILLY*
Supreme Court of the United States
Decided June 28, 2001

Justice O'CONNOR delivered the opinion of the Court.

[In January 1999 the attorney general of Massachusetts promulgated comprehensive regulations governing the advertising and sale of cigarettes, smokeless tobacco, and cigars. Petitioners, a group of cigarette, smokeless tobacco, and cigar manufacturers and retailers, filed suit claiming that the regulations were unconstitutional. The smokeless tobacco and cigar petitioners raise First Amendment challenges to the state's outdoor and point-of-sale advertising regulations. In addition, petitioners claim that certain sales practice regulations for tobacco products violate the First Amendment.]

Petitioners urge us to reject the *Central Hudson* analysis and apply strict scrutiny. Admittedly, several Members of the Court have expressed doubts about the *Central Hudson* analysis and whether it should apply in particular cases. But here, as in *Greater New Orleans*, we see "no need to break new ground. *Central Hudson*, as applied in our more recent commercial speech cases, provides an adequate basis for decision." *Greater New Orleans Broadcasting Assn., Inc. v. United States*, 527 U.S. 173, 184 (1999).

Only the last two steps of *Central Hudson*'s four-part analysis are at issue here. The Attorney General has assumed for purposes of summary judgment that petitioners' speech is entitled to First Amendment protection. With respect to the second step, none of the petitioners contests the importance of the State's interest in preventing the use of tobacco products by minors.

The third step of *Central Hudson* . . . requires that "the speech restriction directly and materially advance the asserted government interest[;] . . . a government body seeking to sustain a restriction on commercial speech must demonstrate that the harms it recites are real and that its restriction will in fact alleviate them to a material degree." *Greater New Orleans*, 527 U.S. at 188. . . .

The last step of the *Central Hudson* analysis "complements" the third step, "asking whether the speech restriction is not more extensive than necessary to serve the interests that support it." *Id.* at 188. We have made it clear that "the least restrictive

*533 U.S. 525 (2001).

means" is not the standard; instead, the case law requires [a reasonable fit between the means and ends]. *Florida Bar v. Went For It, Inc.,* 515 U.S. 618, 632 (1995). . . .

[OUTDOOR ADVERTISING RESTRICTIONS FOR SMOKELESS TOBACCO AND CIGARS]

The outdoor advertising regulations prohibit smokeless tobacco or cigar advertising within a 1,000-foot radius of a school or playground. . . .

The smokeless tobacco and cigar petitioners contend that the Attorney General's regulations do not satisfy *Central Hudson*'s third step. They maintain that although the Attorney General may have identified a problem with underage cigarette smoking, he has not identified an equally severe problem with respect to underage use of smokeless tobacco or cigars. . . . The cigar petitioners catalogue a list of differences between cigars and other tobacco products, including the characteristics of the products and marketing strategies. The petitioners finally contend that the Attorney General cannot prove that advertising has a causal link to tobacco use such that limiting advertising will materially alleviate any problem of underage use of their products.

In previous cases, we have acknowledged the theory that product advertising stimulates demand for products, while suppressed advertising may have the opposite effect. The Attorney General cites numerous studies to support this theory in the case of tobacco products.

The Attorney General relies in part on evidence gathered by the Food and Drug Administration (FDA) in its attempt to regulate the advertising of cigarettes and smokeless tobacco. [Ed.–See chapter 5's discussion of *FDA v. Brown & Williamson Tobacco Corp.* for more on the FDA's efforts.] . . .

The FDA considered several studies of tobacco advertising and trends in the use of various tobacco products. The Surgeon General's report (Department of Health and Human Services 1994) and the Institute of Medicine's report (1994) found that "there is sufficient evidence to conclude that advertising and labeling play a significant and important contributory role in a young person's decision to use cigarettes or smokeless tobacco products." 60 Fed. Reg. 41,332 (1995). . . .

The FDA also made specific findings with respect to smokeless tobacco. The FDA concluded that "the recent and very large increase in the use of smokeless tobacco products by young people and the addictive nature of these products has persuaded the agency that these products must be included in any regulatory approach that is designed to help prevent future generations of young people from becoming addicted to nicotine-containing tobacco products." 60 Fed. Reg. 41,318 (1995). . . .

[The Attorney General also presented evidence that cigar use by minors is increasing and that advertising campaigns increase cigar sales.]

. . . The Attorney General has provided ample documentation of the problem with underage use of smokeless tobacco and cigars. In addition, we disagree with petitioners' claim that there is no evidence that preventing targeted campaigns and limiting youth exposure to advertising will decrease underage use of smokeless tobacco and cigars. On this record and in the posture of summary judgment, we are unable to conclude that the Attorney General's decision to regulate advertising of smokeless tobacco and cigars in an effort to combat the use of tobacco products by minors was based on mere "speculation [and] conjecture." *Edenfield v. Fane,* 507 U.S. 761, 770 (1993).

Whatever the strength of the Attorney General's evidence to justify the outdoor advertising regulations, however, we conclude that the regulations do not satisfy the fourth step of the *Central Hudson* analysis. The final step of the *Central Hudson* analysis requires . . . a reasonable fit between the means and ends of the regulatory scheme. The Attorney General's regulations do not meet this standard. The broad sweep of the regulations indicates that the Attorney General did not "carefully cal-culate the costs and benefits associated with the burden on speech imposed" by the regulations. *Cincinnati v. Discovery Network, Inc.,* 507 U.S. 410, 417 (1993).

. . . In the District Court, petitioners maintained that this prohibition would prevent advertising in 87% to 91% of Boston, Worcester, and Springfield, Massachusetts. The 87% to 91% figure appears to include not only the effect of the regulations, but also the limitations imposed by other generally applicable zoning restrictions. The Attor-ney General disputed petitioners' figures but "conceded that the reach of the regula-tions is substantial." *Lorillard Tobacco Co. v. Reilly,* 218 F.3d 30, 50 (1st Cir. 2000).

The substantial geographical reach of the Attorney General's outdoor advertising regulations is compounded by other factors. "Outdoor" advertising includes not only advertising located outside an establishment, but also advertising inside a store if that advertising is visible from outside the store. The regulations restrict advertise-ments of any size and the term advertisement also includes oral statements.

In some geographical areas, these regulations would constitute nearly a com-plete ban on the communication of truthful information about smokeless tobacco and cigars to adult consumers. The breadth and scope of the regulations, and the process by which the Attorney General adopted the regulations, do not demonstrate a careful calculation of the speech interests involved.

First, the Attorney General did not seem to consider the impact of the 1,000-foot restriction on commercial speech in major metropolitan areas. The Attorney General apparently selected the 1,000-foot distance based on the FDA's decision to impose an identical 1,000-foot restriction when it attempted to regulate cigarette and smokeless tobacco advertising. But the FDA's 1,000-foot regulation was not an adequate basis for the Attorney General to tailor the Massachusetts regulations. . . . The FDA's regulations would have had widely disparate effects nationwide. Even in Massachusetts, the effect of the Attorney General's speech regulations will vary based on whether a locale is rural, suburban, or urban. The uniformly broad sweep of the geographical limitation demonstrates a lack of tailoring.

In addition, the range of communications restricted seems unduly broad. For in-stance, it is not clear from the regulatory scheme why a ban on oral communications is necessary to further the State's interest. Apparently that restriction means that a retailer is unable to answer inquiries about its tobacco products if that communi-cation occurs outdoors. Similarly, a ban on all signs of any size seems ill suited to target the problem of highly visible billboards, as opposed to smaller signs. To the extent that studies have identified particular advertising and promotion practices that appeal to youth, tailoring would involve targeting those practices while permit-ting others. As crafted, the regulations make no distinction among practices on this basis. . . .

The State's interest in preventing underage tobacco use is substantial, and even compelling, but it is no less true that the sale and use of tobacco products by adults is a legal activity. We must consider that tobacco retailers and manufacturers have an interest in conveying truthful information about their products to adults, and adults have a corresponding interest in receiving truthful information about tobacco products. . . .

In some instances, Massachusetts' outdoor advertising regulations would impose particularly onerous burdens on speech. For example, we disagree with the Court of Appeals' conclusion that because cigar manufacturers and retailers conduct a limited amount of advertising in comparison to other tobacco products, "the relative lack of cigar advertising also means that the burden imposed on cigar advertisers is correspondingly small." 218 F.3d at 49. If some retailers have relatively small advertising budgets, and use few avenues of communication, then the Attorney General's outdoor advertising regulations potentially place a greater, not lesser, burden on those retailers' speech. Furthermore, to the extent that cigar products and cigar advertising differ from that of other tobacco products, that difference should inform the inquiry into what speech restrictions are necessary.

In addition, a retailer in Massachusetts may have no means of communicating to passersby on the street that it sells tobacco products because alternative forms of advertisement, like newspapers, do not allow that retailer to propose an instant transaction in the way that onsite advertising does. The ban on any indoor advertising that is visible from the outside also presents problems in establishments like convenience stores, which have unique security concerns that counsel in favor of full visibility of the store from the outside. It is these sorts of considerations that the Attorney General failed to incorporate into the regulatory scheme.

We conclude that the Attorney General has failed to show that the outdoor advertising regulations for smokeless tobacco and cigars are not more extensive than necessary to advance the State's substantial interest in preventing underage tobacco use. . . .

[POINT-OF-SALE ADVERTISING RESTRICTIONS FOR SMOKELESS TOBACCO AND CIGARS]

Massachusetts has also restricted indoor, point-of-sale advertising for smokeless tobacco and cigars. Advertising cannot be "placed lower than five feet from the floor of any retail establishment which is located within a one thousand foot radius of" any school or playground. 940 Code of Mass. Regs. §§ 21.04(5)(b), 22.06(5)(b) (2000). . . .

We conclude that the point-of-sale advertising regulations fail both the third and fourth steps of the *Central Hudson* analysis. . . . The State's goal is to prevent minors from using tobacco products and to curb demand for that activity by limiting youth exposure to advertising. The 5-foot rule does not seem to advance that goal. Not all children are less than 5 feet tall, and those who are certainly have the ability to look up and take in their surroundings. . . .

Massachusetts may wish to target tobacco advertisements and displays that entice children, much like floor-level candy displays in a convenience store, but the blanket height restriction does not constitute a reasonable fit with that goal. . . .

[SALES PRACTICE RESTRICTIONS FOR CIGARETTES, SMOKELESS TOBACCO, AND CIGARS]

. . . The [sales practice] regulations bar the use of self-service displays and require that tobacco products be placed out of the reach of all consumers in a location accessible only to salespersons. . . .

As we read the regulations, they basically require tobacco retailers to place tobacco products behind counters and require customers to have contact with a salesperson before they are able to handle a tobacco product.

... Petitioners contend that "the same First Amendment principles that require invalidation of the outdoor and indoor advertising restrictions require invalidation of the display regulations at issue in this case." Brief for Petitioners Lorillard Tobacco Co., in No. 00-596, 46, n. 7 (2001). ...

We reject these contentions. Assuming that petitioners have a cognizable speech interest in a particular means of displaying their products, these regulations withstand First Amendment scrutiny.

Massachusetts' sales practices provisions regulate conduct that may have a communicative component, but Massachusetts seeks to regulate the placement of tobacco products for reasons unrelated to the communication of ideas. [According to United States v. O'Brien, 391 U.S. 367 (1968), non-content-based government regulation of communicative conduct is valid if (1) it furthers an important government interest, (2) it is unrelated to the suppression of free expression, and (3) the incidental restriction is no greater than essential to the furtherance of that interest.] ...

Unattended displays of tobacco products present an opportunity for access without the proper age verification required by law. Thus, the State prohibits self-service and other displays that would allow an individual to obtain tobacco products without direct contact with a salesperson. It is clear that the regulations leave open ample channels of communication. The regulations do not significantly impede adult access to tobacco products. Moreover, retailers have other means of exercising any cognizable speech interest in the presentation of their products. We presume that vendors may place empty tobacco packaging on open display, and display actual tobacco products so long as that display is only accessible to sales personnel. As for cigars, there is no indication in the regulations that a customer is unable to examine a cigar prior to purchase, so long as that examination takes place through a salesperson. ...

We conclude that the sales practices regulations withstand First Amendment scrutiny. The means chosen by the State are narrowly tailored to prevent access to tobacco products by minors, are unrelated to expression, and leave open alternative avenues for vendors to convey information about products and for would-be customers to inspect products before purchase.

．　．　．　．　．

The courts have also applied the commercial speech doctrine to cases related to the FDA's regulation of dietary supplements and drugs. In 1999, the Court of Appeals for the District of Columbia Circuit invalidated FDA regulations requiring that the agency approve health claims for dietary supplements and that the health claims be supported by "significant scientific evidence" (Pearson v. Shalala, 164 F.3d 650 [D.C. Cir. 1999]). The court found in favor of the government on the second and third prongs of the Central Hudson test, because the government had a substantial interest in preventing the consumer fraud that could result from unverified health claims and because the regulations directly advanced protection against fraud. But the government lost on the fourth prong of *Central Hudson*—there was not a reasonable fit between "the government's goals and the means chosen to advance those goals," since the government could require a disclaimer rather than imposing an outright ban on unapproved health claims (164 F.3d at 657).

The fourth prong of *Central Hudson* has continued to be problematic for public health regulation. In 2002, the Supreme Court held that a law that allowed pharmacists to produce and sell compounded drugs but not to advertise them was an unconstitutional restriction on commercial speech (*Thompson v. Western States Medical Center*, 535 U.S. 357 [2002]). As in *Shalala*, the Court found that the government had failed to show that the speech restrictions were not more extensive than necessary to achieve state interests. Because the speech restrictions were not severable from the rest of the statute, the Court invalidated the entire law allowing the compounding of drugs.

Later, in *Pitt News v. Pappert*, 379 F.3d 96 (3d Cir. 2004), the Third Circuit Court of Appeals struck down as unconstitutional a Pennsylvania ban on alcohol advertising in newspapers affiliated with educational institutions. There too the court, in an opinion written by Samuel Alito (then a circuit judge), held that the restriction was not adequately tailored to achieve the state's objectives. Like the commercial speech cases that came before it, *Pitt News* demonstrates the tension between allowing a "free marketplace of ideas" and restricting advertising to protect consumers from the health harms occasioned by some dangerous products.

III. COMPELLED SPEECH

Public health authorities are concerned not merely with what businesses say but also with what they fail to say. If an industry does not provide accurate explanations of product content, instructions for safe use, and potential hazards, it places consumers at risk. Consequently, the government compels a great deal of speech for public health or consumer protection purposes. First, government requires businesses to *label* their products by specifying their contents or ingredients (e.g., of foods and cosmetics), the potential adverse effects (e.g., of pharmaceuticals and vaccines), and the hazards (e.g., of cigarettes, alcoholic beverages, or pesticides). Second, government provides a *right to know* for consumers (e.g., about the performance of managed care organizations), workers (e.g., about health and safety risks), and the public (e.g., about hazardous chemicals in drinking water). Third, government mandates *counteradvertising* whereby industry or the media must provide health education as a counterbalance to advertisements of hazardous products (e.g., the forced dissemination of antidrinking or antismoking messages).

Government health and safety disclosure laws require businesses to provide certain consumer information. The First Amendment constrains disclosure requirements, however, because it bestows a right not only to speak freely but also to refrain from speaking at all. The compelled speech doctrine protects individuals from being forced to enunciate views that are opposed to their conscience or belief, and it extends as well to some speech by businesses. The framework governing compelled commercial speech, like the commercial speech doctrine, continues to evolve.

The Supreme Court has considered the constitutionality of compelled commercial speech in the form of compelled subsidies. When legislation required fruit and beef producers to contribute funds to federal programs designed to promote their products, the Court found that the subsidy programs did not impermissibly compel speech (*Glickman v. Wileman Bros. & Elliot, Inc.*, 521 U.S. 457 [1997]). But when United Foods, a mushroom producer, challenged a government subsidy program promoting mushrooms, the Court overturned the law on First Amendment grounds (*United States v. United Foods, Inc.*, 533 U.S. 405 [2001]). United Foods objected to the generality of the federal mushroom promotion, wishing instead to promote its own mushrooms as being superior to generic mushrooms. The clearest legal test that emerges from these somewhat contradictory holdings is that when the subsidy and speech are part of some greater regulatory scheme, the law will be upheld, but when no larger regulatory scheme is in place, a compelled subsidy to promote a particular product violates the First Amendment.

The federal courts have also considered laws that mandate disclosure about materials contained in products. In 44 *Liquormart,* we saw that the Court fully protects the right to express truthful, nonmisleading commercial messages about lawful products. How should the courts deal with laws that require companies that wish to be silent to make truthful disclosures about their products to consumers? Consider the case of *International Dairy Foods Association v. Amestoy* (excerpted

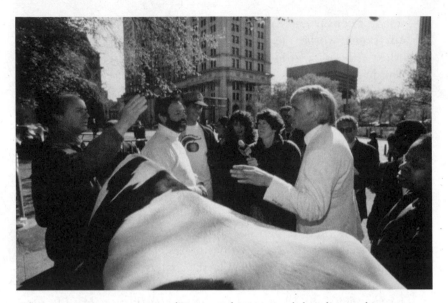

Photo 22. In 1994, a group of Vermont farmers (and their livestock) protest at the state capitol against the use of growth hormones (rBST) in dairy cows. Vermont enacted a statute requiring that milk produced with the use of rBST be so labeled. However, in *International Dairy Foods Association v. Amestoy*, 92 F.3d 67 (2d Cir. 1996), the Second Circuit Court of Appeals found the law to be unconstitutional. Reproduced by permission, © Rick Maiman/Sygma/Corbis, May 3, 1994.

next), which broaches the controversial subject of mandatory disclosure of bovine growth hormone in dairy products.

INTERNATIONAL DAIRY FOODS ASSOCIATION V. AMESTOY*
Court of Appeals for the Second Circuit
Decided August 8, 1996

Circuit Judge ALTIMARI delivered the opinion of the court.

Plaintiffs-appellants [a group of dairy manufacturers] appeal from a decision of the district court denying their motion for a preliminary injunction. The dairy manufacturers challenged the constitutionality of Vt. Stat. Ann. tit. 6, § 2754(c), which requires dairy manufacturers to identify products which were, or might have been, derived from dairy cows treated with a synthetic growth hormone used to increase

*92 F.3d 67 (2d Cir. 1996)

milk production. The dairy manufacturers alleged that the statute violate[s] the . . . First Amendment. . . .

Because we find that the district court abused its discretion in failing to grant preliminary injunctive relief to the dairy manufacturers on First Amendment grounds, we reverse and remand.

BACKGROUND

In 1993, the federal Food and Drug Administration (FDA) approved the use of recombinant Bovine Somatotropin (rBST) (also known as recombinant Bovine Growth Hormone [rGBH]), a synthetic growth hormone that increases milk production by cows. It is undisputed that the dairy products derived from herds treated with rBST are indistinguishable from products derived from untreated herds; consequently, the FDA declined to require the labeling of products derived from cows receiving the supplemental hormone.

In April 1994, defendant-appellee the State of Vermont (Vermont) enacted a statute requiring that "[i]f rBST has been used in the production of milk or a milk product for retail sale in this state, the retail milk or milk product shall be labeled as such." . . . Vermont's Commissioner of Agriculture (Commissioner) subsequently promulgated regulations giving those dairy manufacturers who use rBST four labeling options. . . .

DISCUSSION

[To secure preliminary injunctive relief, the dairy manufacturers must show (a) irreparable harm and (b) likelihood of success on the merits.]

Focusing principally on the economic impact of the labeling regulation, the district court found that appellants had not demonstrated irreparable harm to any right protected by the First Amendment. We disagree. . . .

. . . Because the statute at issue requires appellants to make an involuntary statement whenever they offer their products for sale, we find that the statute causes the dairy manufacturers irreparable harm. . . .

It is not enough for appellants to show, as they have, that they were irreparably harmed by the statute; because the dairy manufacturers challenge government action taken in the public interest, they must also show a likelihood of success on the merits. We find that such success is likely.

In *Central Hudson,* the Supreme Court articulated a four-part analysis for determining whether a government restriction on commercial speech is permissible. We need not address the controversy concerning the nature of the speech in question—commercial or political—because we find that Vermont fails to meet the less stringent constitutional requirements applicable to compelled commercial speech.

Under *Central Hudson,* we must determine: (1) whether the expression concerns lawful activity and is not misleading; (2) whether the government's interest is substantial; (3) whether the labeling law directly serves the asserted interest; and (4) whether the labeling law is no more extensive than necessary. . . .

In our view, Vermont has failed to establish the second prong of the *Central Hudson* test, namely that its interest is substantial. . . . As the district court made clear, Vermont "does not claim that health or safety concerns prompted the passage of the Vermont Labeling Law," but instead defends the statute on the basis of "strong consumer interest and the public's 'right to know.' ... " *International Diary Farmers Ass'n v. Amestoy,* 898 F. Supp. 246, 249 (D. Vt. 1995). These interests are insufficient to justify compromising protected constitutional rights.

Vermont's failure to defend its constitutional intrusion on the ground that it negatively impacts public health is easily understood. After exhaustive studies, the FDA has "concluded that rBST has no appreciable effect on the composition of milk produced by treated cows, and that there are no human safety or health concerns associated with food products derived from cows treated with rBST." *Id.* at 248. Because bovine somatotropin ("BST") appears naturally in cows, and because there are no BST receptors in a cow's mammary glands, only trace amounts of BST can be detected in milk, whether or not the cows received the supplement. Moreover, it is undisputed that neither consumers nor scientists can distinguish rBST-derived milk from milk produced by an untreated cow. Indeed, the already extensive record in this case contains no scientific evidence from which an objective observer could conclude that rBST has any impact at all on dairy products. It is thus plain that Vermont could not justify the statute on the basis of "real" harms.

We do not doubt that Vermont's asserted interest, the demand of its citizenry for such information, is genuine; reluctantly, however, we conclude that it is inadequate. We are aware of no case in which consumer interest alone was sufficient to justify requiring a product's manufacturers to publish the functional equivalent of a warning about a production method that has no discernible impact on a final product.

Although the Court is sympathetic to the Vermont consumers who wish to know which products may derive from rBST-treated herds, their desire is insufficient to permit Vermont to compel the dairy manufacturers to speak against their will. Were consumer interest alone sufficient, there is no end to the information that states could require manufacturers to disclose about their production methods. ...

Because appellants have demonstrated both irreparable harm and a likelihood of success on the merits, the judgment of the district court is reversed, and the case is remanded for entry of an appropriate injunction.

LEVAL, Circuit Judge, dissenting:
    ... The policy of the First Amendment, in its application to commercial speech, is to favor the flow of accurate, relevant information. The majority's invocation of the First Amendment to invalidate a state law requiring disclosure of information consumers reasonably desire stands the Amendment on its ear. In my view, the district court correctly found that plaintiffs were unlikely to succeed in proving Vermont's law unconstitutional. ...

    ... The majority oddly concludes that Vermont's sole interest in requiring disclosure of rBST use is to gratify "consumer curiosity," and that this alone "is not a strong enough state interest to sustain the compulsion of even an accurate factual statement." The majority seeks to justify its conclusion in three ways.

First, it simply disregards the evidence of Vermont's true interests and the district court's findings recognizing those interests. Nowhere does the majority opinion discuss or even mention the evidence or findings regarding the people of Vermont's concerns about human health, cow health, biotechnology, and the survival of small dairy farms.

Second, the majority distorts the meaning of the district court opinion. It relies substantially on Judge Murtha's statement that Vermont "does not claim that health or safety concerns prompted the passage of the Vermont Labeling Law," but "bases its justification . . . on strong consumer interest and the public's 'right to know.'" The majority takes this passage out of context. . . . In the light of the district judge's further explicit findings, it is clear that his statement could not mean what the majority concludes. More likely, what Judge Murtha meant was that Vermont does not claim to *know* whether rBST is harmful. . . .

Third, the majority suggests that, because the FDA has not found health risks in this new procedure, health worries could not be considered "real" or "cognizable." I find this proposition alarming and dangerous; at the very least, it is extraordinarily unrealistic. Genetic and biotechnological manipulation of basic food products is new and controversial. Although I have no reason to doubt that the FDA's studies of rBST have been thorough, they could not cover *long-term* effects of rBST on humans. Furthermore, there are many possible reasons why a government agency might fail to find real health risks, including inadequate time and budget for testing, insufficient advancement of scientific techniques, insufficiently large sampling populations, pressures from industry, and simple human error. To suggest that a government agency's failure to find a health risk in a short-term study of a new genetic technology should bar a state from requiring simple disclosure of the use of that technology where its citizens are concerned about such health risks would be unreasonable and dangerous. . . .

In short, the majority has no valid basis for its conclusion that Vermont's regulation advances no interest other than the gratification of consumer curiosity, and involves neither health concerns nor other substantial interests. . . .

Notwithstanding their self-righteous references to free expression, the true objective of the milk producers is concealment. . . . The question is simply whether the First Amendment prohibits government from requiring disclosure of truthful relevant information to consumers. . . .

The milk producers' invocation of the First Amendment for the purpose of concealing their use of rBST in milk production is entitled to scant recognition. They invoke the Amendment's protection to accomplish exactly what the Amendment opposes. And the majority's ruling deprives Vermont of the right to protect its consumers by requiring truthful disclosure on a subject of legitimate public concern.

. . . . .

The Second Circuit Court of Appeals appears to argue that the power to compel truthful speech is constitutionally permissible only if government has a strong public health interest and that satisfying consumer curiosity is an insufficient governmental objective. Some consumers may feel strongly that they do not wish to buy genetically modified foods, despite being unable to produce conclusive evidence of adverse effects of genetically modified foods on human health or the environment. Should government have the power to compel manufacturers or grocery stores to disclose which foods have been genetically modified?

After *Amestoy,* the Second Circuit heard a similar case regarding a Vermont law that required manufacturers of mercury-containing light-bulbs to disclose the presence of mercury and alert consumers about the proper method for disposing of the product (*National Electrical Manufacturers Ass'n v. Sorrell,* 272 F.3d 104 [2d Cir. 2001]). The court found that the government had a legitimate interest in increasing consumer knowledge and in keeping mercury out of the general waste stream. Instead of applying *Central Hudson*'s more stringent "no more extensive than necessary" test, which is applicable in reviewing laws restricting commercial speech, the court held that the compelled labeling need only be "reasonably related" to the state's interest. In *Amestoy,* in contrast, because the labeling at issue there was aimed only at satisfying consumer interest, it deemed the *Central Hudson* test to be appropriate. The court also noted the "potentially wide-ranging implications" of allowing companies to prevail on First Amendment challenges to the "innumerable federal and state regulatory programs [that] require the disclosure of product and other commercial information" (272 F.3d at 116).

More recent compelled speech issues have arisen out of state and local smoking bans and menu-labeling requirements. The Fifth Circuit Court of Appeals found that the smoking ban imposed by the city of Austin, Texas, did not violate a restaurant's First Amendment right against compelled speech even though the ban would require the restaurant's employees to verbally address a patron's noncompliance (*Roark & Hardee LP v. City of Austin,* 522 F.3d 533 [5th Cir. 2008]). The following section will address growing efforts to combat obesity by, among other strategies, imposing menu-labeling requirements so that more information would be provided.

IV. OBESITY, NUTRITION, AND MARKETING

As the major health risks facing the population shift from infectious diseases (e.g., tuberculosis) to non-communicable diseases (e.g., diabetes, heart disease, and lung cancer), health promotion efforts have evolved to address the growing burden of chronic, non-communicable diseases. In the United States, obesity has garnered a substantial amount of public health and popular attention. While addressing obesity requires a multifaceted approach, a major component has been to alter the food marketing environment. This section first addresses nutrition-labeling requirements for restaurant menus; it then tackles the issue of marketing food to children.

As chapter 6 described, one of the legal community's responses to the obesity epidemic has been tort litigation against producers and purveyors of obesity-producing foods. Consumer protection lawsuits have also been employed as a strategy against fast-food companies. In *Hoyte v. Yum! Brands, Inc.*, 489 F. Supp. 2d 24 (D.D.C. 2007), the plaintiff brought an action against KFC in connection with the restaurant chain's advertising and promotion of foods that contain trans fats. The plaintiff alleged that advertisements stating that KFC served "the best food" and that the foods were "part of a nutritionally healthy lifestyle," without disclosing that they contained trans fats, amounted to deceptive practices by the restaurant chain. The court dismissed the plaintiff's suit because he failed to show actual harm from the foods and because the statements did not speak to the nutritional quality of any individual food item.

As an alternative to tort suits against fast-food companies, states and localities have begun experimenting with unique ways to alter the food environments in their jurisdictions. Tactics include both directly controlling the food environment (e.g., by banning trans fats) and improving consumers' access to health information (e.g., by requiring menus to carry nutrition labels). The latter, health communication–oriented approach focuses on enabling consumers to make better food choices by providing them better information. In a study of consumer knowledge and behavior, Scot Burton and colleagues (2006) found that consumers consistently underestimate the number of calories and the amount of fat in high-caloric foods at restaurants. In addition, when consumers were given menus with nutrition labeling, their expressed preferences and choices changed.

San Francisco and New York City, along with King County, Washington, have taken the lead in using methods consistent with these findings to stem the obesity epidemic in their jurisdictions. The New York City Board of Health's regulations, which were the first to come into effect, require chain restaurants to post nutritional information about their foods on their menus. The New York State Restaurant Association objected to the regulations as impermissibly compelling restaurants to speak on the issue of the link between caloric content and obesity. The Southern District of New York, in the order excerpted below, denied the Restaurant Association's action to enjoin enforcement of the regulations. While the case was on appeal to the Second Circuit, a second order by the Southern District of New York denied the Restaurant Association's motion to stay enforcement of the law until after the appeal (545 F. Supp. 2d 363 [S.D.N.Y. 2008]), thus commencing enforcement in July 2008. Subsequently, in February 2009, the federal court of appeals affirmed the district court's decision, finding, among other issues, that the city's law was reasonably related to its goal of reducing obesity (*New York State Restaurant Association v. New York City Bd. of Health*, 556 F.3d 114 [2009]).

NEW YORK STATE RESTAURANT ASSOCIATION V. NEW YORK CITY BOARD OF HEALTH*

United States District Court for the Southern District of New York
Decided April 16, 2008

United States District Judge HOWELL delivered the opinion of the court.

BACKGROUND

The parties agree that the trend of increasing obesity in the United States poses a health threat to millions of citizens. In New York City, 56.1 percent of the adult population is overweight or obese. Obese and overweight individuals are at a seriously higher risk of heart disease, diabetes, stroke, and cancer, which diseases account for 70 percent of all deaths in the city. . . .

Food served in restaurants plays an increasingly large role in an individual's diet. It is estimated that one-third of daily caloric intake for all Americans comes from foods purchased outside the home. The parties . . . appear to agree that providing nutritional information in restaurants is likely to assist customers to make healthful food choices. Indeed, a number of fast food restaurants already provide a complete nutritional breakdown of their menu items in brochures, on posters, or online. The City has conducted a survey, however, indicating that few customers actually see the nutrient information in fast food restaurants such as McDonald's, Dunkin' Donuts and Burger King that presently disclose such information. To address this perceived deficiency [the New York City Board of Health adopted Regulation 81.50, which] requires covered restaurants to post caloric information on menus and menu boards in a font and format comparable to that used to display the name or price of the menu items. . . . Regulation 81.50 is mandatory for all chain restaurants of a certain size whether or not they presently disclose nutritional information on a voluntary basis. . . .

A. THE PROPER ANALYTICAL FRAMEWORK

NYSRA [the New York State Restaurant Association] argues that Regulation 81.50 violates the First Amendment rights of its members to be free from compelled speech.

The parties concede that Regulation 81.50 implicates only commercial speech, which is subject to "'less stringent constitutional requirements' than other forms

*No. 08-Civ.-1000 (S.D.N.Y. Apr. 16, 2008).

of speech." *National Electric Manufacturers Ass'n v. Sorrell*, 272 F.3d 104, 113 (2d Cir. 2001). Commercial speech is "usually defined as speech that does no more than propose a commercial transaction." *Board of Treasurers of State Univ. of New York v. Fox*, 492 U.S. 469, 473-74 (1989). Regulation 81.50 only requires disclosure of calorie information in connection with a proposed commercial transaction—the sale of a restaurant meal. Thus, the category of speech affected by Regulation 81.50 falls squarely within the traditional definition of commercial speech.

The rationale for extending First Amendment protection to commercial speech is the strong public interest in "intelligent and well informed" economic decisions and the "free flow of commercial information." *Virginia State Board of Pharm. v. Virginia Citizens Consumer Council, Inc.*, 425 U.S. 748, 765 (1976). The Supreme Court, however, has also "recognized the strong government interest in certain forms of economic regulation, even though such regulation may have an incidental effect on rights of free speech and association." *N.A.A.C.P. v. Claiborne Hardware Co.*, 458 U.S. 886, 912 (1982). Moreover, regulations that require disclosure of "factual and uncontroversial" commercial information are subject to "more lenient review" than prohibitions or restrictions on commercial speech, and need only be "reasonably related to the State's interest in preventing deception of consumers." *Sorrell*, 272 F.3d at 113-14 (citing *Zauderer v. Office of Disciplinary Counsel*, 471 U.S. 626, 650, 651 [1985]). As the Second Circuit explained [in *National Electric Manufacturers Ass'n v. Sorrell*],

> Commercial disclosure requirements are treated differently from restrictions on commercial speech because mandated disclosure of accurate, factual, commercial information does not offend the core First Amendment values of promoting efficient exchange of information or protecting individual liberty interests.... Protection of the robust and free flow of accurate information is the principal First Amendment justification for protecting commercial speech, and requiring disclosure of truthful information promotes that goal.... 272 F.3d at 113-14.

[In *Sorrell*, the court held that because factual disclosure requirements do not ordinarily "offend the important utilitarian and individual liberty interests that lie at the heart of the First Amendment," a disclosure requirement need only bear a rational connection to its purpose.] The court went on to find that, while the "overall" purpose of the disclosure was to protect human health and the environment, this goal was "inextricably intertwined with the goal of increasing consumer awareness.... " As such, though the statute was not "intended to prevent 'consumer confusion or deception' per se," its aims were not inconsistent with the rationale for providing First Amendment protection to commercial speech—"[p]rotection of the robust and free flow of accurate information." (*Id.* at 114)....

Zauderer v. Office of Disciplinary Counsel, 471 U.S. 626 (1985), [an earlier Supreme Court case that found compelled disclosures to be constitutional] and *Sorrell* supply the proper standard of review in this case. Like the requirement [in *Sorrell*], Regulation 81.50 compels only the disclosure of "purely factual and uncontroversial" commercial information—the calorie content of restaurant menu items. Furthermore, both Regulation 81.50 and the Vermont statute at issue in *Sorrell* attempt to address a state policy interest by making information available to consumers, consistent with the First Amendment objective, with respect to commercial speech, of providing consumers with "complete and accurate commercial information." *Edenfield v. Fane*, 507 U.S. 761, 766 (1993). Therefore, Regulation 81.50 passes constitutional muster as long as there is a "rational connection" between the disclosure requirement and the City's purpose in imposing it.

NYSRA argues that *Zauderer* and *Sorrell* are inapplicable, and that Regulation 81.50 should be evaluated using the analysis developed for "compelled speech." It is well established that the First Amendment generally does not allow the government to force a speaker to utter a message that is not its own. . . .

. . . NYSRA claims that Regulation 81.50 compels its members to promote the government's messages "that patrons *must* consider the caloric content of food when ordering in a restaurant, and that calories are the only nutritional criterion that patrons need to consider." . . .

. . . Regulation 81.50 does not force any NYSRA member to take a position in any ongoing debate. It does not require any statement, express or implied, regarding the relative nutritional importance of calories or whether a food purchaser ought to consider this information, nor does it prevent any NYSRA member from contesting the City's views on these issues. The City is simply requiring restaurants to report "factual and uncontroversial" information—the number of calories in its products. Of course, it would be possible to recast any disclosure requirement as a compelled "message" in support of the policy views that motivated the enactment of that requirement. However, as discussed above, the mandatory disclosure of "factual and uncontroversial" information is not the same, for First Amendment purposes, as the compelled endorsement of a viewpoint. . . .

NYSRA further argues that [Regulation 81.50] should be analyzed under the four-part test set out in *Central Hudson*, a standard considerably more demanding than the "reasonable relationship" standard. . . . NYSRA seeks to justify increased scrutiny based on the "increasing recognition that commercial speech is of vital importance to First Amendment values." Plaintiff's Reply Mem. 20. . . . The Second Circuit made clear in *Sorrell* that *Central Hudson* is not applied to factual commercial disclosure requirements. The court in *Sorrell* also explained that the use of the *Central Hudson* test in . . . *International Dairy Foods Association v. Amestoy*, was "expressly limited to cases in which a state disclosure requirement is supported by no interest other than the gratification of 'consumer curiosity.'" *Sorrell*, 272 F.3d at 115, n. 6. . . .

. . . *Sorrell* demonstrates that the state's interest in preventing consumer "confusion" and "deception" is not limited to an interest in correcting affirmatively misleading statements and may include an interest in remedying consumers' ignorance or misinformation regarding the products they purchase. . . . Regulation 81.50 is "inextricably intertwined" [*id.* at 115] with the goal of increasing consumer awareness of the calorie content of restaurant meals. The City cites evidence indicating that consumers tend to underestimate the calorie content of restaurant meals, sometimes significantly. . . . The City is attempting to combat obesity by addressing this "information gap"—providing consumers with information about the potential health impact of the products they purchase. The City's method is entirely consistent with First Amendment interests with respect to commercial speech, such as "the discovery of truth," "the efficiency of the 'marketplace of ideas,'" and "[t]he protection of the robust and free flow of accurate information." *Id.* at 114. . . .

B. REGULATION 81.50 IS REASONABLY RELATED TO THE CITY'S INTEREST IN REDUCING OBESITY

... NYSRA does make the argument that the regulation does not directly advance the asserted government interest of reducing obesity, claiming that more research is needed on the relationship between calorie information and consumer behavior and that there is no evidence that Regulation 81.50 will be effective in lowering obesity rates.

The City submitted evidence indicating that weight gain results when calorie intake exceeds calorie expenditure, that the recent rise in obesity is in some part attributable to excess calorie intake, that even modest changes in calorie intake can affect weight, that record-keeping and self-monitoring of food and calorie intake are important components of weight-management programs, and that people tend to underestimate the calorie content of restaurant foods. The City also cites evidence that many consumers report looking at calorie information on packaged foods and changing their purchasing habits based on this information. The City further points out that, after the introduction of mandatory nutrition labeling on packaged foods, food manufacturers began to offer reformulated and "nutritionally improved" products—suggesting that consumer demand for such products is promoted by increased consumer awareness of the nutritional content of available food options.

... One cannot conclude with scientific certainty from the available evidence that that a regulation of this type will ultimately be successful in combating obesity. But ... conclusive proof is not required to establish a reasonable relationship between Regulation 81.50 and the City's interest in reducing obesity. Based on the evidence presented by the City, as well as common sense, it seems reasonable to expect that some consumers will use the [nutrition] information ... to select lower calorie meals when eating at covered restaurants and that these choices will lead to a lower incidence of obesity....

CONCLUSION

For the reasons stated herein, NYSRA has failed to show a likelihood of success on its preemption and First Amendment claims. NYSRA's motion for a preliminary injunction is therefore denied.

. . . . .

More than 9 million children in the United States are obese, and rates of childhood obesity have risen dramatically in past decades (IOM 2005a). The public health community has placed a special emphasis on children in the fight against obesity. The eating habits developed by children follow them into adulthood and influence their future health. While some public health efforts seek to influence parents and children to improve diets, other strategies are directed at changing the food marketing environment. A 2005 Institute of Medicine (2005a, 4) report on food marketing directed at children found that such advertising is pervasive:

> The commercial advertising and marketing of foods and beverages influences the diets and health of children and youth. With annual sales now approaching $900 billion, the food, beverage, and restaurant industries take a central place in the American marketplace. . . .
>
> Children and youth represent a primary focus of food and beverage marketing initiatives. Between 1994 and 2004, the rate of increase in the introduction of new food and beverage products targeted to children and youth substantially outpaced the rate for those targeting the total market. An estimated $10 billion per year is spent for all types of food and beverage marketing to children and youth in America. Moreover, although some very recent public announcements by some in the industry suggest an interest in change, the preponderance of the products introduced and marketed to children and youth have been high in total calories, sugars, salt, and fat, and low in nutrients.

The report detailed the impact of food marketing on children's consumption of junk foods and the effects that poor diets have on the current and future health of children. Significantly, it observed that "before a certain age, children lack the defenses, or skills, to discriminate commercial from noncommercial content, or to attribute persuasive intent to advertising. . . . [Young children have] limited ability to comprehend the nature and purpose of advertising." The current pattern of marketing, it concluded, "represents, at best, a missed opportunity, and, at worst, a direct threat to the health of the next generation" (IOM 2005a, 5, 1).

Many scholars, concerned about the impact of advertising on children who do not understand its intent, see restrictions on child-directed advertising as a policy change that might improve the food environment. A number of countries, from France to Brazil, have proposed or passed laws limiting the amount and type of food advertising aimed at children (Hawkes 2007).

The question of who should be responsible for regulating such practices is a contentious one, however. Should the government restrict the amount and type of food marketing aimed at children, an approach that would raise issues of commercial speech, or should industry groups self-regulate their marketing practices? While reviewing the IOM's 2005 findings, the noted public health and nutrition scholar Marion Nestle (2006, 2529) addressed the inherent problems with expecting industry groups to police themselves:

> The IOM concludes that its data establish a "need and an opportunity [to] . . . turn food and beverage marketing forces toward better diets for American children and youth." This will be no small task. Junk foods are

major sources of revenue for food companies. In response to threats of lawsuits and legislation, companies are scrambling to support health and exercise programs, to announce policies renouncing advertising directed at children under certain ages, and to make their products appear more healthful. Hence: vitamin-enriched candy, whole-grain chocolate cereals, and trans fat–free salty snacks. Yet candies, soft drinks, and snack foods remain the most heavily promoted products.

Companies, says the IOM, must do better, [as they currently] "remain far short of their full potential." If the industry does not change its practices voluntarily, "Congress should enact legislation mandating the shift." Strong words, but the IOM can only advise. . . . Dozens of state legislatures have introduced bills to curb food marketing, and parent and advocacy groups are demanding bans on food marketing in schools.

The Federal Trade Commission (FTC, 2008) reports that food companies spent $1.6 billion to market their products—primarily carbonated beverages, fast foods, and breakfast cereals—to children and teenagers in 2006, relying mainly on television. Stephanie Clifford (2008) notes that both the FTC and the food industry found that self-regulatory industry actions had led to improvements in marketing practices. However, it is reasonable to question the validity of such assessments when the companies themselves define the criteria for healthy foods and police themselves.

Makers of public health policy from a variety of disciplines have proposed myriad options for addressing the obesity epidemic. The two potential solutions addressed above seek to alter the informational environment so that individuals will choose different foods. Forcing restaurants to disclose nutritional information about their products (a form of compelled speech) aids adults in making decisions about their diet. Regulating food marketing to children (a restraint on commercial speech) helps protect children from messages that lead to unhealthy food choices.

V. CONCLUSION

This chapter discussed public health regulation to control the informational environment—government speech, restraints on commercial speech, and mandatory disclosures—and analyzed these regulatory strategies as they apply to the specific issue of obesity and food marketing. The remaining chapters in this part examine more direct public health regulation of individuals and businesses—from compelled medical treatments to administrative searches and seizures.

RECOMMENDED READINGS

An Ethic for Health Promotion

Buchanan, David R. 2000. Disquietudes. In *An Ethic for Health Promotion: Rethinking the Sources of Human Well-Being*, 1–22. Oxford: Oxford Univ. Press. (Examines the science of health promotion and the ethics of interventions to change behavior)

Curtis, Valerie A., Nana Garbrah-Aidoo, and Beth Scott. 2007. Masters of marketing: Bringing private sector skills to public health partnerships. *American Journal of Public Health* 97: 634–41. (Explores the intersection of private marketing and public health promotion in the context of a hand-washing campaign in Ghana)

Guttman, Nurit, and William Harris Ressler. 2001. On being responsible: Ethical issues in appeals to personal responsibility in health campaigns. *Journal of Health Communication* 6: 117–36. (Details the ethical concerns in health promotion campaigns that target individual behavior and assign personal responsibility)

Resnick, David B. 2000. Ethical dilemmas in communicating health information to the public. *Health Policy* 55: 129–49. (Explores scientific uncertainty in health communication and the asymmetry of information between health experts and the lay public)

Commercial Speech

Bayer, Ronald. 2002. Tobacco, commercial speech, and libertarian values: The end of the line for restrictions on advertising? *American Journal of Public Health* 92: 356–59. (Examines the commercial speech doctrine after the Court's decision in *Lorillard Tobacco Co. v. Reilly*)

Carver, Krista Hessler. 2008. A global view of the First Amendment constraints on the FDA. *Food and Drug Law Journal* 63: 151–215. (Examines the intersection of the First Amendment and FDA regulations, including an analysis of *Pearson v. Shalala* and *Thompson v. Western States Medical Center*)

Vladeck, David C., Gerald Weber, and Lawrence O. Gostin. 2004. Commercial speech and the public's health: Regulating advertisements of tobacco, alcohol, high fat foods and other potentially hazardous products. *Journal of Law, Medicine & Ethics* 32: S32–S34. (Provides a short examination of the law governing the advertising of dangerous products)

Compelled Speech

McGarity, Thomas O. 2007. Frankenfood free: Consumer sovereignty, federal regulation, and industry control in marketing and choosing foods in the United States. In *Labeling Genetically Modified Food: The Philosophical and Legal Debate,* ed. Paul Weirich, 128–50. Oxford: Oxford Univ. Press. (Provides an overview of the legal and regulatory climate surrounding genetically modified food in the United States)

Obesity, Nutrition, and Marketing

Burton, Scot, Elizabeth Creyer, Jeremy Kees, and Kyle Huggins. 2006. Attacking the obesity epidemic: The potential health benefits of providing nutrition information in restaurants. *American Journal of Public Health* 96: 1669–75. (Details two studies related to nutritional labeling for menus and consumer behavior)

Hawkes, Corinna. 2007. Regulating food marketing to young people worldwide: Trends and policy drivers. *American Journal of Public Health* 97: 1962–73. (Provides an international perspective on the regulation of food marketing to children)

Institute of Medicine. 2005. *Food Marketing to Children: Threat or Opportunity?* Washington, DC: National Academies Press. (Provides a comprehensive examination of food marketing to children in the United States)

Nestle, Marion. 2006. Food marketing and childhood obesity—a matter of policy. *New England Journal of Medicine* 354: 2527–29. (Provides a review of the 2005 IOM report on food marketing to children and explains its implications for public health)

Parmet, Wendy E., and Jason A. Smith. 2006. Free speech and public health: A population-based approach to the First Amendment. *Loyola of Los Angeles Law Review* 39: 363–446. (Examines public health and the First Amendment in reference to obesity policy, especially in the areas of advertising and promotion)

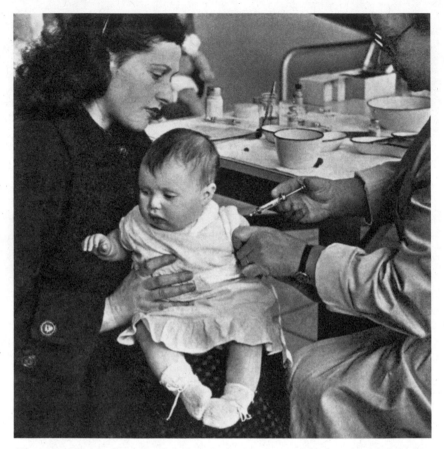

Photo 23. In this photograph, taken in the 1950s, an eight-month-old child receives the diphtheria vaccine while being held by her mother. Before vaccination was widely available, diphtheria was endemic in the United States, and 5 to 10 percent of cases were fatal. Thanks in large part to widespread vaccination, diphtheria is now rare in the United States; for every 100,000 people, fewer than one person per year becomes infected. Reproduced by permission, © Topham/The Image Works.

TEN

Medical Countermeasures for Epidemic Disease

Bodily Integrity

This chapter and the next examine the most ancient and enduring threats to health in the population—infectious diseases. The effects of epidemics on society are as destructive as those of war. For example, the estimated 50 to 100 million deaths from the Spanish influenza pandemic of 1918–20 exceed the number of combatants killed in World War I, World War II, Korea, and Vietnam combined (Johnson and Mueller 2002). And HIV/AIDS has claimed approximately 25 million lives since 1981 (UNAIDS 2008). Not surprisingly, the United States has classified HIV/AIDS as a national security priority, reasoning that it may result in the destabilization of strategic regions such as Africa and Asia.

For most of history, society's only response to epidemics has been the crude separation of persons with disease. But in more recent history, science has developed the biological means to help prevent, detect, and intervene in epidemics. The three major biological approaches are vaccination to prevent outbreaks, screening to identify persons who are infectious, and treatment to alleviate symptoms and reduce infectiousness. The readings in this chapter discuss each of these biological approaches in turn, while the following chapter discusses the separation of exposed or infected individuals from the general population through isolation and quarantine.

The value of biological approaches to infectious diseases cannot be exaggerated. Vaccination programs have eradicated some diseases (e.g., smallpox) and significantly reduced the incidence of others (e.g., polio) that decimated populations in earlier times. Antibiotics and antivirals have been just as important as vaccinations, offering a means to medically treat a wide variety of infectious conditions and reduce contagiousness. Medical treatments for syphilis, tuberculosis, and, more recently, HIV/AIDS have transformed our approach to these and other communicable diseases.

Yet despite the undoubted value of biological approaches, they are neither sufficient nor unambiguously beneficial. Social, economic, and environmental factors may be just as important in controlling the burden and spread of contagious diseases. For example, René and Jean Dubois (1987) demonstrated that improved sanitation, diet, and general economic and social conditions were instrumental in reducing the burden of TB in the mid-twentieth century. Michael Marmot (2004, 147) expanded on their findings, arguing that social status is the key determinant of health: "When tuberculosis was a major cause of death . . . any number of people had been infected with the tubercle bacillus, but they did not die of tuberculosis." After pointing out that social conditions were responsible for such factors as poor nutrition, which contributed to lowered host resistance, he declared: "These social conditions are the cause of death. The tubercle bacillus is [only] the proximate cause."

Scholars have similarly drawn attention to the importance of "ecological" factors such as the physical and social environment in controlling infectious diseases. Overreliance on biological approaches can lead policy makers to neglect social, behavioral, and economic interventions. Sometimes treatment is regarded as a "magic bullet," a view that stifles other kinds of public health innovation (Brandt 1987).

Biological approaches, while exceedingly valuable in public health, do have distinct limitations. Vaccinations can cause infection or other adverse events in previously healthy patients. For example, the swine flu vaccination program was discontinued in the mid-1970s because it was thought to be associated with Guillain-Barré syndrome. Moreover, when antibiotics are prescribed or used inconsistently, pathogens can become resistant. Resistance to medication is one of the most important problems facing medicine today.

Biological approaches can also be intrusive. Vaccination, screening, or treatment imposed without consent invades personal autonomy and bodily integrity. As a result, some people oppose mandatory therapeutic interventions on grounds of conscience, principle, or religion. Even if prophylaxis or treatments for diseases such as TB are beneficial and reduce transmission, individuals claim the freedom to make therapeutic decisions for themselves.

Finally, biological approaches pose social risks. At times, their use disregards privacy, stigmatizes those suffering from an illness, and fuels discrimination. For example, screening reveals intimate personal information that can be used to deny individuals employment or insurance. In addition, when screening primarily targets vulnerable or disfavored populations, it can appear unfair and raise important questions of equity and social justice. But these risks are not inherent and immutable; biological interventions can be tailored to minimize social risks.

The readings in this chapter explore the multiple benefits and drawbacks of biological approaches. When health care or public health professionals act to prevent, identify, or treat an infectious disease, they can improve the health and well-being of individuals and populations. At the same time, however, biological approaches often reduce the resources, or political will, available for broader social, behavioral, and economic interventions. Moreover, biological approaches can diminish individual freedoms and pose risks of invasion of privacy as well as discrimination. These trade-offs—between therapeutic benefits and social risks—are discussed in this chapter's readings.

I. COMPULSORY VACCINATION: IMMUNIZING THE POPULATION AGAINST DISEASE

Vaccinations are among the most cost-effective and widely used public health interventions. The rate of complete immunization of school-age children in the United States (more than 95 percent) is equal to or higher than that in most other developed countries. In addition, vaccination rates for preschool children are improving. As a result, common childhood illnesses such as measles, pertussis, and polio, which once accounted for a large proportion of child morbidity and mortality, have been substantially reduced.

Despite its importance in preventing infectious disease, compulsory immunization sometimes rouses popular resistance. Some people object because they distrust scientists and health officials, fearing that vaccines are ineffective or induce injury; others object on grounds of religion or principle; and still others object to what they view as unwarranted governmental interference with their autonomy and liberty. Angus Dawson (2007, 621–22) reviews three possible rights-based objections to mandatory vaccinations:

> First, it might be argued that it can never be appropriate to overrule parents' decisions about vaccinations, because vaccination is a preventive rather than a therapeutic measure, and in most cases the diseases are trivial and low risk. Invoking the powers of the state to interfere in the family

in such a case, it could be argued, is just inappropriate. However, . . . any attempt to draw a morally significant difference between an action based upon the fact it is either preventive or therapeutic is potentially problematic. . . . Any risks of vaccination of common diseases are low. Whilst the risk of contracting such diseases in the developed world [is] also usually low, if contracted, the potential impact of many of these diseases should not be underestimated. (Neither should it be forgotten that the calculations of such risks and benefits might vary widely depending upon the background societal conditions. In many parts of the developing world childhood diseases are endemic and millions of children die each year from vaccine-preventable diseases.)

Second, it might be argued that parents can invoke a right to refuse this medical intervention. Presumably such a claim would have to involve some kind of justification for seeing this particular right as taking precedence over other rights, including a right of the child to be protected from potential harm. . . . It is worth pointing out that the parents' refusal in this case is not governing their own care, but that of their child. This may make a significant difference to the case. Even if such a right to refuse treatment is held to be central to the debate about vaccinations, it is only likely to block any best interests argument, leaving the harm-to-others argument untouched.

Third, a parent might use another form of appeal to rights. In this case, they may argue that the child has a right to bodily integrity, and that this will be transgressed in the case of compulsory vaccination. Once again, the important thing about rights is that there are many such rights, and that when they are invoked, it is a requirement of their defender to produce an argument not just to say why we have such a right, but explain why that particular right is supposed to take precedence in our moral deliberations. Whilst such an argument can, no doubt, be produced, it can surely be contested. Once again, whilst such a right might, at most, have some claim in relation to arguments about best interests, it is not clear how it might deflect any harm-to-others argument.

Even in light of these arguments, the author ultimately concludes that the potential harm to others that could result from a failure to vaccinate justifies the use of compulsory childhood vaccination, despite the possible objections of parents. The public health benefits of vaccinations supersede the right of an individual parent to govern the treatment of his or her child.

A. The Tragedy of the Commons

In the following selection, Garrett Hardin, a prominent biology professor, contends that individuals acting in their own interests will lead to a "tragedy of the commons." If each person is left free to pursue his or her own personal aspirations, the individual may benefit but the population will suffer. The solution, Hardin argues, is "mutual coercion mutually agreed upon" (i.e., coercion through democratic decision making). Hardin's argument is highly relevant to vaccination policy, as Kevin Malone and Alan Hinman (2007, 339) explain:

> A community free of an infectious disease because of a high vaccination rate can be viewed as a common. As in Hardin's common, the very existence of this common leads to tension between the best interests of the individual and those of the community. Increased immunization rates result in significantly decreased risk for disease. Although no remaining unimmunized individual can be said to be free of risk from the infectious disease, the herd immunity effect generated from high immunization rates significantly reduces these individuals' risk for disease. Additional benefit is conferred on the unimmunized person because avoidance of the vaccine avoids the risk for any adverse reactions associated with the vaccine. As disease rates drop, the risks associated with the vaccine come even more to the fore, providing further incentive to avoid immunization. Thus, when an individual in this common chooses to go unimmunized, it only minimally increases that person's risk for illness, while conferring on that person the benefit of avoiding the risk for vaccine-induced side effects. At the same time, however, this action weakens the herd-effect protection for the entire community. As more and more individuals choose what is in their "best" individual interest, the common eventually fails as herd immunity disappears and disease outbreaks occur. To avoid this "tragedy of the commons," communities (and, in recent times, states) have imposed legal requirements to mandate particular vaccinations.

THE TRAGEDY OF THE COMMONS*
Garrett Hardin

The tragedy of the commons develops in this way. Picture a pasture open to all. It is to be expected that each man will try to keep as many cattle as possible on the commons. Such an arrangement may work reasonably satisfactorily for centuries because tribal wars, poaching, and disease keep the numbers of both man and beast well below the carrying capacity of the land. Finally, however, comes the day of reckoning, that is, the day when the long-desired goal of social stability becomes a reality. At this point, the inherent logic of the commons remorselessly generates tragedy.

As a rational being, each herdsman seeks to maximize his gain. Explicitly or implicitly, more or less consciously, he asks, "What is the utility *to me* of adding one more animal to my herd?" This utility has one negative and one positive component.

(1) The positive component is a function of the increment of one animal. Since

*Reprinted from *Science* 162 (1968): 1234–48. Reprinted with permission from the American Association for the Advancement of Science.

the herdsman receives all the proceeds from the sale of the additional animal, the positive utility is nearly +1.

(2) The negative component is a function of the additional overgrazing created by one more animal. Since, however, the effects of overgrazing are shared by all the herdsmen, the negative utility for any particular decision-making herdsman is only a fraction of -1.

Adding together the component partial utilities, the rational herdsman concludes that the only sensible course for him to pursue is to add another animal to his herd. And another; and another.... But this is the conclusion reached by each and every rational herdsman sharing a commons. Therein is the tragedy. Each man is locked into a system that compels him to increase his herd without limit—in a world that is limited. Ruin is the destination toward which all men rush, each pursuing his own best interest in a society that believes in the freedom of the commons. Freedom in a commons brings ruin to all.

Some would say that this is a platitude. Would that it were! In a sense, it was learned thousands of years ago, but natural selection favors the forces of psychological denial. The individual benefits as an individual from his ability to deny the truth even though society as a whole, of which he is a part, suffers. Education can counteract the natural tendency to do the wrong thing, but the inexorable succession of generations requires that the basis for this knowledge be constantly refreshed....

POLLUTION

In a reverse way, the tragedy of the commons reappears in problems of pollution. Here it is not a question of taking something out of the commons, but of putting something in—sewage, or chemical, radioactive, and heat wastes into water; noxious and dangerous fumes into the air; and distracting and unpleasant advertising signs into the line of sight. The calculations of utility are much the same as before. The rational man finds that his share of the cost of the wastes he discharges into the commons is less than the cost of purifying his wastes before releasing them. Since this is true for everyone, we are locked into a system of "fouling our own nest," so long as we behave only as independent, rational, free-enterprisers.

The tragedy of the commons as a food basket is averted by private property, or something formally like it. But the air and waters surrounding us cannot readily be fenced, and so the tragedy of the commons as a cesspool must be prevented by different means, by coercive laws or taxing devices that make it cheaper for the polluter to treat his pollutants than to discharge them untreated. We have not progressed as far with the solution of this problem as we have with the first. Indeed, our particular concept of private property, which deters us from exhausting the positive resources of the earth, favors pollution. The owner of a factory on the bank of a stream—whose property extends to the middle of the stream—often has difficulty seeing why it is not his natural right to muddy the waters flowing past his door. The law, always behind the times, requires elaborate stitching and fitting to adapt it to this newly perceived aspect of the commons....

MUTUAL COERCION MUTUALLY AGREED UPON

The social arrangements that produce responsibility are arrangements that create coercion, of some sort.... Coercion is a dirty word to most liberals now, but it need not forever be so. As with the four-letter words, its dirtiness can be cleansed away by exposure to the light, by saying it over and over without apology or embarrassment. To many, the word "coercion" implies arbitrary decisions of distant and irresponsible bureaucrats; but this is not a necessary part of its meaning. The only kind of coercion I recommend is mutual coercion, mutually agreed upon by the majority of the people affected.

To say that we mutually agree to coercion is not to say that we are required to enjoy it, or even to pretend we enjoy it. Who enjoys taxes? We all grumble about them. But we accept compulsory taxes because we recognize that voluntary taxes would favor the conscienceless. We institute and (grumblingly) support taxes and other coercive devices to escape the horror of the commons....

Every new enclosure of the commons involves the infringement of somebody's personal liberty. Infringements made in the distant past are accepted because no contemporary complains of a loss. It is the newly proposed infringements that we vigorously oppose; cries of "rights" and "freedom" fill the air. But what does "freedom" mean? When men mutually agreed to pass laws against robbing, mankind became more free, not less so. Individuals locked into the logic of the commons are free only to bring on universal ruin; once they see the necessity of mutual coercion, they become free to pursue other goals. I believe it was Hegel who said, "Freedom is the recognition of necessity."

. . . . . .

Compulsory vaccination (mutual coercion) in a democratic society (mutually agreed on) preserves herd immunity and ensures against the tragedy of the commons. But vaccination carries risks, and these risks are borne by the small group of individuals who suffer the rare adverse reaction. Recognizing that vaccination is a public good, Congress created the National Vaccine Injury Compensation Program (NVICP). The program, which is funded by a vaccine tax, provides no-fault compensation to the families of children who are injured by vaccination. Compensation for those who bear the physical costs of vaccination is just, because it spreads the financial burden of adverse reactions equally among the vaccinated. The NVICP also protects our vaccine supply by shielding vaccine developers and manufacturers from routine tort liability.

B. School Immunization Laws in the Courts

All states, as a condition of school entry, require proof of vaccination against a number of diseases on the immunization schedule, such as diphtheria, measles, and rubella. (A list of currently recommended vaccines has been produced by the Advisory Committee on Immunization Practices, updated at www.cdc.gov/vaccines.) State statutes also often

TABLE 5. Time line of selected federal and state court
decisions on vaccination

Year of Decision	Citation	Major Holding
1830	*Hazen v. Strong*, 2 Vt. 427	Local town council has authority to pay for vaccination of persons exposed, even though there are no cases of smallpox in the community.
1894	*Duffield v. School Dist. of City of Williamsport*, 29 A. 742 (Pa.)	School board regulation that prohibits children not vaccinated for smallpox from attending school is reasonable based on a current outbreak and expert opinions on vaccination's efficacy.
1904	*Viemester v. White*, 84 N.Y.S. 712, aff'd, 72 N.E. 97	No constitutional right to an education exists under the New York Constitution, and thus there is no limit on the type of reasonable regulation (including vaccination requirements) that may be imposed on public education by the legislature.
1905	*Jacobson v. Massachusetts*, 197 U.S. 11	The city of Cambridge may require its citizens to be vaccinated against smallpox, provided the regulations are reasonable and the vaccine does not pose a hazard to the individual.

(continued)

require schools to maintain immunization records and report information to health authorities. Although the exact provisions differ from
state to state, all school immunization laws grant exemptions for children with medical contraindications to immunization. Thus, if a physician certifies that the child is susceptible to adverse effects from the
vaccine, the child is exempt.

The power of states and localities to require children to be vaccinated as a condition of school entrance has been widely accepted
and judicially sanctioned. Building on *Jacobson v. Massachusetts* (excerpted in chapter 4), the Supreme Court established the constitutionality of childhood vaccination laws in the 1922 case of *Zucht v. King*
(excerpted next). Since *Zucht*, the courts have regularly upheld the constitutionality of government mandates for vaccination as a prerequisite
for public school attendance. (For a time line of selected federal and
state court decisions, see table 5.)

TABLE 5. *(continued)*

Year of Decision	Citation	Major Holding
1910	*McSween v. Board of School Trustees,* 129 S.W. 206 (Tex. Civ. App.)	School vaccination laws do not constitute an illegal search and seizure violating the Fourth Amendment.
1913	*Adams v. Milwaukee,* 228 U.S. 572	Vaccination laws do not discriminate against schoolchildren to the exclusion of others in violation of the Equal Protection Clause of the Fourteenth Amendment.
1922	*Zucht v. King,* 260 U.S. 174	States may delegate to a municipality the power to order vaccination, and the municipality may then give broad discretion to the board of health to apply and enforce the regulation.
1927	*Cram v. School Bd. of Manchester,* 136 A. 263 (N.H.)	A father's claim that vaccination of his daughter should not be required because it will "endanger her health and life" by "performing a surgical operation by injecting a poison . . . into [her] blood" is rejected, on the basis of *Jacobson.*
1944	*Prince v. Massachusetts,* 321 U.S. 158	A mother can be prosecuted under child labor laws for using her children to distribute religious literature. The First Amendment's Free Exercise Clause does not allow for the right to expose the community or one's children to harm. The state may restrict parental control to guard the child's well-being. For example, parents cannot claim freedom from compulsory vaccination because of religious objections.
1951	*Seubold v. Fort Smith Special School Sch. Dist.,* 237 S.W.2d 884	Vaccination requirements do not deprive individuals of liberty and property interests without due process of the law.
1963	*State ex rel. Mack v. Board of Educ. of Covington,* 204 N.E.2d 86 (Ohio Ct. App.)	A child does not have an absolute right to enter school without immunization against polio, smallpox, pertussis, and tetanus on the basis of his parents' objections to his vaccination. The school board has authority to make and enforce rules and regulations to secure immunization.

(continued)

TABLE 5. *(continued)*

Year of Decision	Citation	Major Holding
1965	*Wright v. DeWitt Sch. Dist.*, 385 S.W.2d 644 (Ark.)	A compulsory vaccination law with no religious exemption is constitutional, because the right of free exercise is subject to reasonable regulation for the good of the community as a whole.
1968	*McCartney v. Austin*, 293 N.Y.S.2d 188	New York's vaccination statute does not interfere with the freedom to worship in the Roman Catholic faith, because the religion does not proscribe vaccination.
1971	*Dalli v. Board of Educ.*, 267 N.E.2d 219 (Mass.)	State exemption for objectors who believe in the "tenets and practices of a recognized church of religious denomination" violates the Equal Protection Clause, by giving preferential treatment to certain groups over others who have sincere, though unrecognized, religious objections.
1976	*Kleid v. Board of Educ.*, 406 F. Supp. 902 (W.D. Ken.)	Requirement that parents be members of a "nationally recognized and established church or religious denomination" to qualify for religious exemption to vaccination mandate does not violate the Establishment Clause.
1979	*Brown v. Stone*, 378 So. 2d 218 (Miss.), cert. denied, 449 U.S. 887 (1980)	Religious exemption violates the Equal Protection Clause, because it "discriminates against the great majority of children whose parents have no such religious convictions."
1985	*Hanzel v. Arter*, 625 F. Supp. 1259 (S.D. Ohio)	Parents' objections to vaccination based on "chiropractic ethics" do not fall under the protection of the Establishment Clause and, therefore, their children are not exempt from the statutory mandates.
1987	*Shear v. Northmost–East Northmost Union Free Sch. Dist.*, 672 F. Supp. 81 (E.D.N.Y.)	Requirement that parents be "bona fide members of a recognized religious organization" to be exempt on religious grounds from the school vaccination requirement violates the Establishment Clause.
1987	*Maricopa County Health Dept. v. Harmon*, 750 P.2d 1364 (Ariz.)	Health department has authority to exclude unvaccinated children from school even if there are no reported cases of the disease in question and do so without violating the right to public education in the Arizona Constitution.

(continued)

TABLE 5. *(continued)*

Year of Decision	Citation	Major Holding
1988	*Mason v. General Brown Cent. Sch. Dist.*, 851 F.2d 47 (2d Cir.)	Parents' sincerely held belief that immunization is contrary to "genetic blueprint" is a secular, not religious, belief, and thus their children's required vaccination does not violate the Establishment Clause.
1994	*Berg v. Glen Cove City Sch. Dist.*, 853 F. Supp. 651 (E.D.N.Y.)	Jewish parents' religious belief regarding vaccinations was sincere even though nothing in their religion prohibits vaccination.
2000	*Farina v. Board of Educ. of the City of New York*, 116 F. Supp. 2d 503 (S.D.N.Y)	Catholic parents' beliefs regarding vaccinations were personal and medical, and therefore not adequate basis to recover damages from the City Board of Education for its refusal to accept their religious exemption.
2001	*Jones v. State Dep't of Health*, 18 P.3d 1189 (Wyo.)	Health department has no authority to require a student to receive a hepatitis B immunization or to require a student applying for a waiver from immunization requirements to provide a reason for a medical contraindication to immunizations.
2001	*Bowden v. Iona Grammar School*, 726 N.Y.S.2d 685 (App. Div.)	Parents who followed the practices of Temple of the Healing Spirit were entitled to a religious exemption to vaccination requirements for their children because the state statute does not specify which religions are eligible.
2002	*Boone v. Boozman*, 217 F. Supp. 2d 938 (E.D. Ark.).	Statutes that mandate that religious exemptions to vaccination requirements be granted only to adherents of recognized religions violate the First Amendment, but the vaccine mandate itself is constitutional even in the absence of a religious exemption.

ZUCHT V. KING*
Supreme Court of the United States
Decided November 13, 1922

Justice BRANDEIS delivered the opinion of the Court.

Ordinances of the city of San Antonio, Texas, provide that no child or other person shall attend a public school or other place of education without having first presented a certificate of vaccination. Purporting to act under these ordinances, public officials excluded Rosalyn Zucht from a public school because she did not have the required certificate and refused to submit to vaccination. They also caused her to be excluded from a private school. Thereupon Rosalyn brought this suit against the officials in a court of the state. The bill charges that there was then no occasion for requiring vaccination; that the ordinances deprive plaintiff of her liberty without due process of law, by, in effect, making vaccination compulsory; and also that they are void, because they leave to the board of health discretion to determine when and under what circumstances the requirement shall be enforced, without providing any rule by which that board is to be guided in its action, and without providing any safeguards against partiality and oppression. The prayers were for an injunction against enforcing the ordinances, for a writ of mandamus to compel her admission to the public school, and for damages. . . .

Long before this suit was instituted, *Jacobson v. Massachusetts* had settled that it is within the police power of a state to provide for compulsory vaccination. That case and others had also settled that a state may, consistently with the federal Constitution, delegate to a municipality authority to determine under what conditions health regulations shall become operative. And still others had settled that the municipality may vest in its officials broad discretion in matters affecting the application and enforcement of a health law. A long line of decisions by this court had also settled that in the exercise of the police power reasonable classification may be freely applied, and that regulation is not violative of the equal protection clause merely because it is not all-embracing. In view of these decisions we find in the record no question as to the validity of the ordinance. . . . Unlike *Yick Wo v. Hopkins* [see the related case *Jew Ho v. Williamson*, excerpted in chapter 4] these ordinances confer not arbitrary power, but only that broad discretion required for the protection of the public health. . . .

Writ of error dismissed.

. . . . .

In addition to medical exemptions, most states also provide nonmedical exemptions to school-age vaccination requirements. Forty-eight states grant religious exemptions for persons who have sincere religious beliefs in opposition to immunization. (Only Mississippi and West Virginia mandate vaccination of children against the religious beliefs

*260 U.S. 174 (1922).

of their parents.) Twenty-one states also grant exemptions for parents who profess philosophical convictions in opposition to immunization. Table 6 documents school vaccination laws among states (as of August 2006) according to specific diseases, as well as exemptions for each state. In some states, a simple parental signature is sufficient to secure a nonmedical exemption, making it easier to opt out of the vaccination requirement than to fulfill and document it, as required.

In some areas, the ready availability of broad nonmedical exemptions and the ease with which exemptions may be obtained has generated pockets of unvaccinated children. Exemption rates average 2.5 percent in states that allow philosophical exemptions or have simple exemption processes. In some communities, the rate is far higher; for example, in Ashland, Oregon, it is 15 percent.

High exemption rates directly compromise community health by eroding herd immunity. In the first four months of 2008, the Centers for Disease Control and Prevention (CDC) recorded a record-setting sixty-eight cases of measles, all but one of which were in unvaccinated individuals. Such outbreaks of vaccine-preventable diseases are associated with nonmedical exemption laws. States that allow philosophical exemptions have had twice as many cases of whooping cough (pertussis) as those that offer only religious exemptions. And whooping cough incidence is 90 percent higher in states with simple procedures for granting exemptions (Omer et al. 2006).

The widespread use of nonmedical exemptions has provoked concern in the public health community. How should respect for individual beliefs be balanced against community health? In a 2007 editorial in the *Wall Street Journal,* Paul A. Offit declared:

> When it comes to issues of public health and safety, we invariably have laws. Many of these laws are strictly enforced and immutable. We don't allow philosophical exemptions to restraining young children in car seats, to smoking in restaurants or to stopping at stop signs. And the notion of requiring vaccines for school entry, while it seems to tear at the very heart of a country founded on the basis of individual rights and freedoms, saves lives. Given the increasing number of states allowing philosophical exemptions to vaccines, at some point we will to be forced to decide whether it is our inalienable right to catch and transmit potentially fatal infections.

Concerns about the public health impact of nonmedical exemptions aside, these exemptions raise legal questions about whose children should bear the burden of vaccination and how exemptions can be granted without entangling church and state. Most courts have upheld the constitutionality of religious exemptions from compulsory

TABLE 6. School immunization laws, by state

State	Statute	DPT	MMR	Polio	Hib	Hep B	Var	Religious Exemptions	Philosophical Exemptions
Alabama	Ala. Code § 16-30-1	✓	✓	✓	✓		✓	§ 16-30-3	N
Alaska	Alaska Stat. § 14.30.125	✓	✓	✓	✓			§ 14.07.125	N
Arizona	Ariz. Rev. Stat. Ann. § 15-872	✓	✓	✓	✓		✓	§ 15-873	*
Arkansas	Ark. Code Ann. § 6-18-702 MR	✓	✓	✓	✓	✓	✓	§ 6-18-702	Y
California	Cal. Health & Safety Code § 120335	✓	✓	✓	✓	✓	✓	§ 120365	Y
Colorado	Colo. Rev. Stat. § 25-4-902	✓	✓	✓	✓	✓	✓	§ 25-4-903	Y
Connecticut	Conn. Gen. Stat. § 10-204a	✓	✓	✓		✓	✓	§ 10-204a	N
Delaware	Del. Code Ann. Tit. 14, § 131	✓	✓	✓		✓	✓	§ 14-131	N
District of Columbia	D.C. Code Ann. § 38-501	✓	✓	✓		✓		§ 38-506	N
Florida	Fla. Stat. Ann. § 1003.22	✓	✓	✓	✓	✓	✓	§ 1003.22	N
Georgia	Ga. Code Ann. § 20-2-771	✓	✓	✓	✓	✓	✓	§ 20-2-771	N
Hawaii	Haw. Rev. Stat. § 302A-1154	✓	✓	✓	✓	✓	✓	§ 302A-1156	N
Idaho	Idaho Code § 39-4801	✓	✓	✓	✓	✓	✓	§ 39-4802	Y
Illinois	105 Ill. Comp. Stat. § 5/27-8.1	✓	✓	✓	✓	✓	✓	410 ILCS § 315/2	N
Indiana	Ind. Code Ann. § 20-34-4-1	✓	✓MR	✓	✓	✓	✓	§ 20-34-3-2	N
Iowa	Iowa Code Ann. § 139a.8	✓	✓	✓	✓	✓	✓	§ 139A.8	N
Kansas	Kan. Stat. Ann. § 72-5209	✓	✓	✓	✓	✓	✓	§ 72-5209	N
Kentucky	Ky. Rev. Stat. Ann. § 214.034	✓	✓	✓	✓	✓	✓	§ 214.036	N
Louisiana	La. Rev. Stat. Ann. § 17:170(a)	✓	✓	✓	✓	✓	✓	§ 17:170(E)	Y
Maine	Me. Rev. Stat. Ann. Tit. 20-a, § 6355	✓	✓	✓	✓	✓	✓	Tit. 20-A, § 6355	Y
Maryland	Md. Code Ann. Educ. § 7-403	✓	✓	✓		✓	✓	§ 7-403	N
Massachusetts	Mass. Gen. Laws ch. 76, § 15	✓	✓	✓		✓	✓	ch. 76, § 15	N
Michigan	Mich. Comp. Laws ann. § 333.9208	✓	✓	✓		✓	✓	§ 333.9215	Y
Minnesota	Minn. Stat. Ann. § 121A-15	✓	✓	✓	✓	✓	✓	§ 121A.15	Y
Mississippi	Miss. Code Ann. § 41-23-37	✓	✓	✓	✓	✓	✓	N	N

State	Citation	DPT	Polio	MMR	Hib	Hep B	Var	Exempt
Missouri	Mo. Rev. Stat. § 167.181	✓	✓	✓	✓	✓	✓	**
Montana	Mont. Code Ann. § 20-5-403	✓	✓	✓	✓	✓	✓	N
Nebraska	Neb. Rev. Stat. Ann. § 79-217	✓	✓	✓	✓	✓	✓	N
Nevada	Nev. Rev. Stat. § 392.435	✓	✓	✓	✓	✓	✓	N
New Hampshire	N.H. Rev. Stat. Ann. § 141-C:20-a	✓	✓	✓	✓	✓	✓	N
New Jersey	N.J. Stat. Ann. § 26:1A-9	✓	✓	✓	✓	✓	✓	N
New Mexico	N.M. Stat. Ann. § 24-5-1	✓	✓	✓	✓	✓	✓	Y
New York	N.Y. Pub. Health Law § 2164	✓	✓	✓	✓	✓	✓	N
North Carolina	N.C. Gen. Stat. § 130A-155	✓	✓	✓	✓	✓	✓	Y
North Dakota	N.D. Cent. Code § 23-07-17.1	✓	✓	✓	✓	✓	✓	Y
Ohio	Ohio Rev. Code Ann. § 3313.671	✓	✓	✓	✓	✓	✓	Y
Oklahoma	Okla. Stat. Ann. Tit. 70, § 1210.191	✓	✓	✓	✓	✓	✓	N
Oregon	Or. Rev. Stat. § 433.267	✓	✓	✓	✓	✓	✓	N
Pennsylvania	24 Pa. Cons. Stat. Ann. § 13-1303a	✓	✓	✓	✓	✓	✓	N
Rhode Island	R.I. Gen. Laws § 16-38-2	✓	✓	✓	✓	✓	✓	N
South Carolina	S.C. Code Ann. § 44-29-180	✓	✓	✓	✓	✓	✓	N
South Dakota	S.D. Codified Laws § 13-28-7.1	✓	✓	✓	✓	✓	✓	N
Tennessee	Tenn. Code Ann. § 49-6-5001	✓	✓	✓	✓	✓	✓	N
Texas	Tex. Educ. Code Ann. § 38.001	✓	✓	✓ MR	✓	✓	✓	Y
Utah	Utah Code Ann. § 53A-11-301	✓	✓	✓	✓	✓	✓	Y
Vermont	Vt. Stat. Ann. Tit. 18, § 1121	✓	✓	✓	✓	✓	✓	Y
Virginia	Va. Code Ann. § 22.1-271.2	✓	✓	✓	✓	✓	✓	N
Washington	Wash. Rev. Code Ann. § 28A.210.080	✓	✓	✓ MR	✓	✓	✓	Y
West Virginia	W. Va. Code § 16-3-4	✓	✓	✓	✓	✓	✓	N
Wisconsin	Wis. Stat. Ann. § 252.04	✓	✓	✓	✓	✓	✓	Y
Wyoming	Wyo. Stat. Ann. § 21-4-309	✓	✓	✓	✓	✓	✓	N

*Allowed in schools only

**Allowed in child care and Head Start facilities only

ABBREVIATIONS: DPT: Diptheria/pertussis/tetanus vaccine; MMR: Measles-mumps-rubella vaccine; Polio: Poliomyelitis vaccine; Hib: Haemophilus influenzae vaccine; Hep B: Hepatitis B vaccine; Var (varicela): Chicken pox vaccine; MR: Mumps not required vaccination, but the Mississippi Supreme Court in *Brown v. Stone* (excerpted next) found that these exemptions unfairly threaten the health of all school children. More recently, the federal court for the Eastern District of Arkansas in *Boone v. Boozman* (excerpted below) found that the state's religious exemption provision unfairly favored some religious beliefs over others and unnecessarily entangled the state in religious matters. In both *Brown* and *Boone,* the courts found that once the nonmedical exemption provisions were stripped away, the basic compulsory vaccination laws were constitutional. The court decisions, therefore, effectively made childhood vaccination compulsory in Mississippi and Arkansas, even among those with religious or philosophical objections. Although Mississippi still requires vaccination regardless of religious beliefs, Arkansas has amended its laws to allow broader, philosophical exemptions.

*BROWN V. STONE**
Supreme Court of Mississippi
Decided December 19, 1979

Judge SMITH delivered the opinion of the court.
    This is an appeal by Charles H. Brown, father and next friend of Chad Allan Brown, a six-year-old boy, from a [decision] of the Chancery Court of Chickasaw County [denying Brown's request for] injunction to compel the Board of Trustees ... to admit his son as a student without compliance with the immunization requirements of Miss. Code Ann. § 41-23-37 (Supp. 1972). This statute provides (among other things):

> Except as provided hereinafter, it shall be unlawful for any child to attend any school ... unless they shall first have been vaccinated against those diseases specified by the State Health Officer. A certificate of exemption from vaccination for medical reasons may be offered on behalf of a child by a duly licensed physician and may be accepted by the local health officer when, in his opinion, such exemption will not cause undue risk to the community. A certificate of religious exemption may be offered on behalf of a child by an officer of a church of a recognized denomination. This certificate shall certify that parents or guardians of the child are bona fide members of a recognized denomination whose religious teachings require reliance on prayer or spiritual means of healing.

There was filed with the bill the following certificate, signed by a minister of the Church of Christ:

> Be it known that the Church of Christ as a religious body does not teach against the use of medicines, immunizations or vaccinations as prescribed by a duly certified

---
*378 So. 2d 218 (Miss. 1979).

physician. However, Dr. Charles Brown, our local chiropractor, who is a member of the North Jackson Street Church of Christ in Houston, Mississippi, does have strong convictions against the use of any kind of medications and we respect his views.

Charles E. Bland

[Minister Brown's] bill recited (a) that six-year-old Chad Allan Brown was of sufficient age and residence to qualify for admission to the first grade of the Houston Elementary School, but had not been [properly] vaccinated . . . , (b) Charles H. Brown, the father, has not permitted his son to be vaccinated because of "strong and sincere religious beliefs actively practiced and followed" by Charles H. Brown, (c) Charles H. Brown is a member of the Church of Christ, a religious body which does not teach against the use of medicines, immunizations or vaccinations prescribed by a physician, (d) Charles H. Brown has sought a religious exemption from vaccination (of his son) but it was denied because the certificate did not comply with [state law], (e) Chad Allan Brown was denied admission to the school because of the failure to be immunized . . . , (f) . . . Mississippi [laws] are invalid "insofar as they force complainants to join a religious organization in order to practice their religious tenets freely," and the denial of admission of Chad Allan Brown violates complainants' rights protected by the First Amendment to the United States Constitution. . . .

Appellants concede that mandatory immunization against dangerous diseases, without exemptions based on religious beliefs or convictions, has been held constitutionally valid as a reasonable exercise of police power. They contend, however, that the provision for religious exemption violates the First Amendment . . . protecting the free exercise of religion. . . .

The fundamental and paramount purpose of the Mississippi Legislature . . . was to afford protection for school children against crippling and deadly diseases by immunization. That this can be done effectively and safely has been incontrovertibly demonstrated over a period of a good many years and is a matter of common knowledge of which this Court takes judicial notice.

If the religious exemption from immunization is to be granted only to members of certain recognized sects or denominations whose doctrines forbid it, and, as contended by appellants, to individuals whose private or personal religious beliefs will not allow them to permit immunization of their children, . . . the protection of school children generally comprising the school community is defeated.

Is it mandated by the First Amendment . . . that innocent children, too young to decide for themselves, are to be denied the protection against crippling and death that immunization provides because of a religious belief adhered to by a parent or parents? . . . We have concluded that the statute in question, requiring immunization against certain crippling and deadly diseases particularly dangerous to children before they may be admitted to school, serves an overriding and compelling public interest, and that such interest extends to the exclusion of a child until such immunization has been effected, not only as a protection of that child but as a protection of the large number of other children comprising the school community and with whom he will be daily in close contact in the school room. . . . It must not be forgotten that a child is indeed himself an individual, although under certain disabilities until majority, with rights in his own person which must be respected and may be enforced. Where its safety, morals and health are involved, it becomes a legitimate concern of the state.

The protection of the great body of school children attending the public schools in Mississippi against the horrors of crippling and death resulting from poliomyelitis or smallpox or from one of the other diseases against which means of immunization are known and have long been practiced successfully, demand that children who have not been immunized should be excluded from the school community until immunization has been accomplished. That is the obvious overriding and compelling public purpose of [the state's vaccination law]. To the extent that it may conflict with the religious beliefs of a parent, however sincerely entertained, the interests of the school children must prevail.

[The state's vaccination law] is a reasonable and constitutional exercise of the police power of the state insofar as it provides for the immunization of children before they are to be permitted to enter school. The exception, which would provide for the exemption of children of parents whose religious beliefs conflict with the immunization requirements, would discriminate against the great majority of children whose parents have no such religious convictions. To give it effect would result in a violation of the Fourteenth Amendment to the United States Constitution which provides that no state shall make any law denying to any person within its jurisdiction the equal protection of the laws, in that it would require the great body of school children to be vaccinated and at the same time expose them to the hazard of associating in school with children exempted under the religious exemption who had not been immunized as required by the statute. . . . We have no difficulty here in deciding that the statute is "complete in itself" without the provision for religious exemption and that it serves a compelling state interest in the protection of school children.

Therefore, we hold that the provision providing an exception from the operation of the statute because of religious belief is in violation of the Fourteenth Amendment to the United States Constitution and therefore is void. As the United States Supreme Court said in *In re Gault*, 387 U.S. 1, 13 (1967): "Whatever may be their precise impact, neither the Fourteenth Amendment nor the Bill of Rights is for adults alone."

BOONE V. BOOZMAN*

United States District Court for the Eastern District of Arkansas
Decided August 12, 2002

Judge WRIGHT issued the Memorandum Opinion and Order.

Section 6-18-702(a) of the Arkansas Code Annotated provides that no child shall be admitted to school without proof of immunization from certain diseases. . . . Hepatitis B has been designated as one of those diseases from which school children must be immunized. . . . Cynthia Boone brought the present action after the Cabot School District, on or about October 1, 2001, informed her that her daughter, Ashley Boone, could no longer attend Cabot Senior High School because she did not have a Hepatitis B vaccination.

Cynthia Boone sincerely objects to the administration of Hepatitis B vaccine to her daughter for religious reasons and on conscientious grounds which include

*217 F. Supp. 2d 938 (E.D. Ark. 2002).

traditional parenting concerns. The immunization statute does provide a religious exemption; however, the General Assembly limited the exemption as follows:

> The provisions of this section shall not apply if the parents or legal guardian of that child object thereto on the grounds that immunization conflicts with the religious tenets and practices of a *recognized church or religious denomination* of which the parent or guardian is an adherent or member. (Ark. Code Ann. § 6-18-702[d][2] [Repl. 1999] [emphasis supplied]). . . .

SINCERELY HELD RELIGIOUS BELIEFS

A belief must be rooted in religion to be protected by the religion clauses of the First Amendment. However, "religious beliefs need not be acceptable, logical, consistent, or comprehensible to others in order to merit First Amendment protection." *Thomas v. Review Board*, 450 U.S. 707, 714 (1981). [Cynthia Boone has explained that although she was not a member of any church, she was a deeply religious person and felt strongly that Ashley Boone should not have to "defile" her body by injecting it with the Hepatitis B vaccine.]

The Court finds that Cynthia Boone's belief concerning immunization, as divined from her reading of the bible and through God's revelations to her through angels, is rooted in religion and sincere. . . .

STATUTORY EXEMPTION

[The court then analyzed Arkansas' statutory exemption under the Establishment and the Free Exercise Clauses of the First Amendment. The court concluded, "the immunization statute's religious exemption provision, as written and as applied, . . . violates the Establishment Clause" because it has the purpose or effect of advancing or inhibiting religion and results in unnecessary government entanglement with religion. Finding that the statute also violates the Free Exercise Clause, the court said, "Where the State elects to accommodate religion on a particular issue like immunization, it is simply not constitutionally permissible for it to indulge the free exercise rights of some individuals and inhibit the free exercise rights of others on an arbitrary basis."]

In this case, that the statutory exemption has been declared unconstitutional does not dismantle the entire immunization statute. . . . Subsection (d)(2) of Arkansas Code Annotated § 6-18-702 must be stricken as unconstitutional, but the remaining portions of the statute remain in full force and effect. In other words, there now exists no statutory religious exemption to immunization in the State of Arkansas.

FREE EXERCISE CLAUSE—COMPULSORY IMMUNIZATION

Plaintiff challenges the constitutionality of compulsory immunization . . . under the Free Exercise Clause. . . .

This Court has already determined that the statutory religious exemption . . . is unconstitutional, and severed it from the remainder of the immunization statute. Plaintiff cannot now rely on an invalidated statutory exemption to determine the standard of review for her general challenge to the power of the State . . . to immunize religious individuals. Rather, plaintiff must direct her challenge at the remainder of the statute that is in effect.

Subsection (a) of the immunization statute does not target religious beliefs or seek to infringe upon or restrict certain practices because of their religious motivation; its "object" is to protect school children against the spread of disease through mandatory immunization. It applies to all school children, save those for whom immunization would endanger their health. Because the immunization statute is a neutral law of general applicability, heightened scrutiny is not required even though compulsory immunization may burden plaintiff's right to free exercise.

It is well established that the State may enact reasonable regulations to protect the public health and the public safety, and it cannot be questioned that compulsory immunization is a permissible exercise of the State's police power. The Supreme Court has long recognized that a state may require public and private school children to be immunized. The constitutionally-protected free exercise of religion does not excuse an individual from compulsory immunization; in this instance, the right to free exercise of religion and parental rights are subordinated to society's interest in protecting against the spread of disease.

Plaintiff seeks to distinguish her case from what she refers to as "this draconian vaccine jurisprudence" by asserting that those cases were decided on the basis of a declared health emergency involving smallpox, while in this case Hepatitis B presents no "clear and present danger." The Court is not persuaded by this argument. . . .

Because the groups at highest risk for Hepatitis B are unlikely to self-identify and pursue the vaccine, immunizing those individuals as children is the recommended strategy to stem the spread of Hepatitis B. Immunization of school children against Hepatitis B has a real and substantial relation to the protection of the public health and the public safety. The Court therefore finds that requiring school children to be immunized against Hepatitis B is a reasonable exercise of the State's police power and is constitutionally permissible even though it affects plaintiff's religious practice. . . .

SUBSTANTIVE DUE PROCESS

. . . The right to refuse medical treatment is assumed to be a part of liberty protected under the Due Process Clause. . . .

Plaintiff complains that "*Jacobson* and *Zucht* are utterly archaic in 14th Amendment substantive due process terms, and worthless as precedent in light of the extensive jurisprudence of the 20th Century." . . .

The question presented in this case is not, as plaintiff suggests, simply whether a parent has a fundamental right to decide whether her child should undergo a medical procedure such as immunization. Carefully formulated, the question presented by the facts of this case is whether the special protection of the Due Process Clause includes a parent's right to refuse to have her child immunized before attending public or private school where immunization is a precondition to attending school. The Nation's history, legal traditions, and practices answer with a resounding "no." . . .

JUDGMENT

In accordance with the Memorandum Opinion and Order entered this date, this case is hereby dismissed; all relief requested by plaintiff is denied with one exception: subsection (d)(2) of Arkansas Code Annotated § 6-18-702 is stricken as unconstitutional.

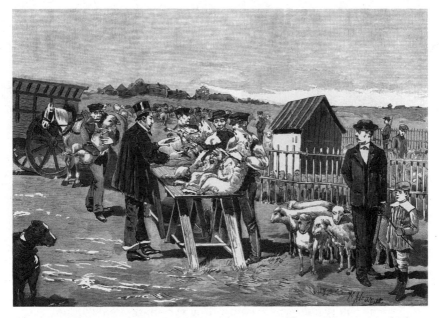

Photo 24. This print depicts Louis Pasteur's 1881 public experiment in which he demonstrated the effectiveness of his anthrax vaccine. He gathered two groups of sheep, vaccinating one group and leaving the other group untouched. Thirty days later, both groups were injected with live anthrax bacteria. All the sheep in the nonvaccinated group died, but the vaccinated sheep survived. Reproduced by permission, © The Pasteur Institute.

C. Current Vaccine Controversies: From Autism to Cervical Cancer

Despite a clear legal justification for vaccine mandates, public health practitioners must take care to use compulsory vaccination powers judiciously and appropriately. They have a wide range of policy options—from merely allowing to encouraging or compelling vaccination—and must balance numerous considerations in choosing the best approach in a particular case. Does the scientific evidence of a particular vaccine's risks and benefits support its widespread use? Given the public health evidence, what policy would make the best use of scarce resources? How does the evidence of individual risks and population-level benefits (e.g., herd immunity) affect the balance between personal autonomy, parental rights, and community welfare? Finally, how will popular perception of a vaccination policy (particularly a coercive policy) affect its ultimate effectiveness and the public's trust in health practitioners and the government more generally?

Examining the controversy surrounding attempts to mandate human papillomavirus (HPV) vaccination provides insight into the complex process attending a decision to mandate vaccination. The vaccine, approved in 2006, prevents the four most prevalent strains of HPV, the most common sexually transmitted infection. Infection with certain strains of the virus can result in cervical cancer. Prevention can therefore significantly improve public health. Yet HPV is not airborne, and vaccination will not create herd immunity. Moreover, regular screening can detect and prevent cervical cancer.

In a 2007 article, *JAMA*'s editor-in-chief Catherine DeAngelis and I argued against mandating HPV vaccination for eleven- and twelve-year-old girls. We determined that in the absence of long-term data on safety and effectiveness (including how long immunity lasts), authorities should wait for more information before mandating vaccination. The limitations of the data are particularly significant given the high cost of the vaccine: a mandatory program might so strain public health budgets that cuts in other programs would be necessary. There are also underlying equity concerns in compelling vaccination only within a certain group (i.e., young girls). Trials are ongoing to determine whether the vaccine is effective in boys as well as girls. If it is, any mandate should apply equally to both sexes.

Finally, we were also concerned that Merck, the company that markets the vaccine, had lobbied heavily in support of mandates in several state legislatures. Such efforts to sway policy makers threaten to compromise the decisions made about public health, which should be based on evidence. Perhaps more significantly, they fuel the perception among vaccination skeptics that government is in bed with industry and thereby damage public trust in the public health system.

> Maintaining the public's trust is vital—both for HPV vaccination in particular and for school-based vaccination programs more generally. Legislation to make HPV vaccine mandatory has undermined public confidence and created a backlash among parents. There is nothing more important to the success of public health policies than to ensure community acceptability. In the absence of an immediate risk of serious harm, it is preferable to adopt voluntary measures, making state compulsion a last resort. (Gostin and DeAngelis 2007, 1922)

Rather than urging a direct jump to a mandate, we argued for comprehensive screening and prevention programs targeted at populations in which cervical cancer is most problematic.

In the piece excerpted below, the public health historian James

Colgrove examines several controversies surrounding vaccination that emerged at the turn of the twenty-first century, focusing particularly on the debate over a hypothesized linkage between the measles, mumps, and rubella (MMR) vaccine and autism. Colgrove's work on vaccination history highlights the frequent disconnect between popular perceptions and scientific assessments of safety and efficacy. The judicious use of compulsory powers in a transparent manner and the use of effective health communication tools can go a long way toward limiting popular resistance to vaccination and fostering greater public trust in health authorities.

EXPANSION AND BACKLASH: VACCINATION AT THE TURN OF THE TWENTY-FIRST CENTURY*
James Colgrove

Vaccination policies and practices in the United States at the turn of the twenty-first century had by many measures achieved remarkable success. Perhaps the most striking achievement, in view of the extended and often acrimonious debates over safety, were record high levels of public acceptance for routine childhood immunization. . . . Disparities in full immunization persisted among children of different racial and ethnic backgrounds, but the gaps in levels of coverage . . . were smaller than those for most other health indicators. Even as the controversy about the alleged connection between measles vaccine and autism crested between 1998 and 2003, and public acceptance of the MMR shot plummeted in the United Kingdom, rates of coverage for the vaccine increased slightly in the United States.

Why the debates over safety had not caused greater public rejection of vaccines in this country remained a matter of speculation. What was clear was that the relationship between vaccine critics and the public health establishment had become increasingly adversarial. Activists who believed that vaccines caused health problems such as autism leveled charges of corruption and bias against immunization proponents. There was an inherent conflict of interest, critics argued, in the fact that the National Immunization Program was responsible both for promoting the use of vaccines and ensuring their safety. It was in response to such criticisms that the CDC announced in February 2005 that it would separate its vaccine advocacy and safety monitoring functions.

By this [time], the evidence against a connection between vaccines and autism had grown. A raft of studies published in 2003 and 2004, conducted in Sweden, Denmark, the United Kingdom, and the United States, using a variety of epidemiological methods, all found no evidence of an association between autism and either the MMR vaccine or vaccines containing the preservative thimerosal. In response

*James Colgrove, *State of Immunity: The Politics of Vaccination in Twentieth-Century America*. © 2006 Regents of the University of California. Published by the University of California Press.

to the new evidence, the Institute of Medicine's immunization safety panel, which had examined both hypothesized links in previous reports, reconvened to conduct an updated evaluation. In May the committee released a new report that reasserted the conclusion of its earlier reviews: that the evidence "favors rejection" of both causal relationships.

The report's language bore imprint of the controversies from which it had emerged. Acknowledging "the anger of some families toward the federal government (particularly the CDC and FDA), vaccine manufacturers, the field of epidemiology, and traditional biomedical research" (IOM 2004, 11), the committee went out of its way to emphasize that autism was a grave problem that imposed enormous burdens on those affected.

But the group insisted that "available funding for research [should] be channeled to the most promising areas" (IOM 2004, 12)—which did not include vaccines. Advocacy organizations for parents of autistic children were not reassured, however. The Coalition for SafeMinds (Sensible Action for Ending Mercury-Induced Neurological Disorders), one of the most vocal parent advocacy groups, slammed the IOM report as "flawed science" that was tainted by "pervasive conflicts of interest" (SafeMinds 2004).

Meanwhile, the disputes over the research of Andrew Wakefield, whose study in *The Lancet* had ignited much of the concern about autism, took an unexpected turn. In early 2004 the journal disclosed allegations of ethical improprieties that had been made against the investigators, including that, at the time the study had been conducted, Wakefield was also gathering evidence for a potential lawsuit by several parents who suspected their children's autism was vaccine-related. In the wake of the accusation of conflict of interest, ten of the original thirteen scientists who had participated in the research retracted their support for the conclusion about the MMR-autism connection. . . .

The issues of risk and compulsion had the potential to undermine the success of the immunization system. So too did structural issues related to supply and financing. The production of vaccines remained concentrated among only a handful of pharmaceutical companies, and the possibility of shortages or interruptions in availability was an ongoing threat. Some new vaccines, including the heptavalent preparation against invasive pneumococcal disease introduced in 2000, were far more expensive than older products, raising questions about benefit ratios and the continuing viability of public- and private-sector funding streams.

The history of vaccination in the twentieth century cannot be viewed as a teleological narrative in which scientific advances produced a steady stream of increasingly sophisticated vaccines, leading to ever-greater levels of infectious disease control. It is clear that whatever new vaccines might emerge in the coming years, a volatile mix of social, political, and legal factors will shape the deployment of those innovations. Declaring in 2004 that "the easy work in vaccine-preventable diseases has been done," three officials with the Institute of Medicine, which had devoted so much study to vaccination over the previous two decades, laid out the challenges for the future:

> How many more vaccinations will parents, physicians and nurses, and insurance providers tolerate? Is the goal to develop vaccines for every infectious disease or

only for serious diseases? How serious should a disease be to warrant a vaccination program? Who is to judge the seriousness of a disease? At some point, this health promotion and disease prevention strategy could wear out its welcome with the population at large. It has done so with some segment of society. The United States lacks a comprehensive scientific and policy approach to explore fully the ramification of the increasing number of vaccines that will soon be available. (Griffin, Stratton, and Chalk 2004, 106)

Vaccination policy underwent numerous transformations over the course of the twentieth century. . . . At the same time, however, fundamental questions have persisted. How should individual liberty be balanced against the need to protect the common welfare? How should authorities act in the face of incomplete or inconsistent scientific information, and how should the public be involved in these decisions? What are the best ways to secure the cooperation of the public in reducing the incidence of disease? Are some or all public health measures inherently, and necessarily, paternalistic? The ways that these questions have been answered by parties to these debates—scientists, physicians, public health officials, parents, legislators, jurists, and activists of all ideological persuasions—have reflected not only their assessment of the value of vaccination but also their views about personal choice and freedom in matters of health and the appropriate role of the state in shaping the decisions of individuals.

II. TESTING AND POPULATION-BASED SCREENING

Although the terms are often used interchangeably, a distinction exists between *testing* and *screening*. *Clinical testing* refers to a medical procedure that determines the presence or absence of disease, or its precursor, in an individual patient. In contrast, *screening* is the systematic application of a medical test to a defined population with the objective of identifying persons with infectious or other diseases. Public health authorities can then offer education, counseling, or treatment. They can also help monitor an epidemic and devise more precisely targeted prevention programs.

Disease screening is a basic tool of modern public health and preventive medicine, but it is not always beneficial—and can be intrusive and unjust. First, screening can be unreliable if the test is technically deficient. If the test instrument is not sufficiently sensitive, it will fail to detect many cases of infection in a population. If the test instrument is not sufficiently specific, it will produce false positives (i.e., persons will test positive although they are not actually infected). Even technically adequate tests will have poor predictive value in populations with a low prevalence of infection. Screening in low-prevalence populations is likely to identify.few cases of infection because relatively few cases exist. (*Predictive value* is explained further in chapter 10 of the companion text.) For example, early in the AIDS epidemic, Illinois mandated HIV screening as a condition of getting a marriage license, but soon discovered that it was highly cost-ineffective, uncovering few true positive and many false positive cases.

Second, screening can be intrusive unless the person is fully informed and provides consent. Screening without informed consent undermines personal autonomy and bodily integrity. In addition, screening reveals sensitive medical information. If this information is then passed on to others without the permission of those screened, their privacy is invaded, and they may also experience discrimination in employment and insurance.

Third, screening can be unjust if it targets vulnerable populations. Suppose TB screening were performed only on the homeless or syphilis screening were performed only on commercial sex workers. The targeted groups could legitimately claim that the screening program was unjust. Even screening programs that target "high-risk" groups may be unjust. For example, the CDC recommends universal HIV screening of pregnant women rather than targeted screening in high-risk communities, because targeted screening would disproportionately burden racial minorities and thus would appear to be unfair. The readings in this section discuss the ethical and legal aspects of screening. Ruth R. Faden, Nancy Kass, and Madison Powers examine the ethical foundations of screening. Thereafter, the section examines the constitutionality of government screening programs.

WARRANTS FOR SCREENING PROGRAMS: PUBLIC HEALTH, LEGAL AND ETHICAL FRAMEWORKS*

Ruth R. Faden, Nancy Kass, and Madison Powers

When a screening program is designed, it is necessary to decide how participation in the program is to be determined. Conventionally, this decision is viewed as a choice between two options: participation in the program is to be either compulsory or voluntary. Often, however, it is difficult to categorize programs simply as one or the other; some elements of the program make participation appear voluntary, while

*Reprinted from *AIDS, Women and the Next Generation: Towards a Morally Acceptable Public Policy for HIV Testing of Pregnant Women and Newborns*, edited by Ruth R. Faden, Gail Geller, and Madison Powers (New York: Oxford Univ. Press, 1991), 3–24.

others seem to include some level of compulsion. As a step toward better organizing this issue for the purpose of analysis, we propose dividing programs into five, rather than two, categories: (1) completely mandatory programs; (2) conditionally mandatory programs; (3) "routine without notification" programs; (4) "routine with notification" programs; and (5) voluntary programs. . . . These categories are not mutually exclusive or exhaustive. . . . Although for government programs these categories may approximate a continuum of legal compulsoriness, they do not necessarily represent a continuum either of autonomous choice on the part of participants or of protection of the public's health, issues to which we will return shortly.

The most stringent level of testing in terms of legal compulsoriness is a *completely mandatory program*, in which, typically, a government agency requires citizens to undergo an intervention, with sanctions imposed on those who do not comply. . . .

In a *conditionally mandatory program*, either government or an institution in the private sector makes access to a designated service or opportunity contingent on participating in the program. These could be rules either established by government (such as having to be screened for syphilis in order to obtain a marriage license . . .), . . . or privately authorized (such as . . . having to undergo a general health screening for certain health or life insurance policies). In each of these instances, the individual has the right not to participate in the activities or services offered by the institution; however, . . . participation in the program is mandatory for eligibility. . . .

In a *routine without notification* program, the intervention is routinely and automatically implemented unless an individual expressly asks that it not be done. However, participants are not notified about the intervention or their right to refuse. Thus as a practical matter, refusals rarely occur. . . .

In a *routine with notification* program, participants are informed of the intervention and their right to refuse before the intervention is implemented. This approach has been proposed for newborn testing for PKU [phenylketonuria, a genetic disorder] but rarely has been adopted.

In a *voluntary* program, the intervention is not implemented without the authorization of participants. In some instances, written informed consent is solicited; in others, authorization or consent is considered to be implied in that participants must ask for or seek out the program. Current examples of voluntary screening programs are programs that screen for the antibody to HIV or those that offer mammograms for screening of breast cancer.

At first, it might appear that these five categories of programs . . . represent a rank ordering, with completely mandatory programs being the most restrictive and voluntary programs being the least restrictive in terms of their impact on autonomous choice. However, depending on the circumstances, conditionally mandatory programs can be as restrictive of choice as completely mandatory ones. The penalties imposed for failing to comply with some completely mandatory programs may be easier to resist than the consequences of forgoing a conditionally mandatory program. For example, in communities where jobs are scarce and needs are great, individuals may have no choice but to submit to preemployment testing. Similarly, routine programs that do not require prior notification may be equally restrictive of choice if they target individuals who are unaware that the interventions are being implemented and thus have no opportunity to choose to refuse. Even routine programs with notification requirements and completely voluntary programs provide no guarantees that participation reflects autonomous choice. Questions of manipulation, understanding, and adequacy of information necessarily remain. Clearly, issues of compulsoriness understood narrowly in terms of legal mandates must be distinguished from the impact of a specific program on issues of choice. . . .

PUBLIC HEALTH FRAMEWORK

Public health is concerned with the prevention and reduction of morbidity and mortality. At the core of a public health framework for evaluating screening programs is a single criterion—the program's harm-to-benefit ratio, where harms and benefits are understood in terms of impact on a community's morbidity and mortality. Although not sufficient in itself, it is always necessary to use the public health framework in assessing the acceptability of a screening program. An acceptable ratio of benefits to harms is, at minimum, a threshold consideration, and, as we shall see, both the legal and ethical frameworks incorporate a public health assessment of harms and benefits in their analyses. No screening program can be justified either legally or morally without first satisfying public health criteria. . . .

Consistently, screening programs have as their goal the reduction of morbidity or mortality in either the general population or a specific population. Screening programs can be justified only if they effect a positive outcome that would not have occurred without the screening. . . . The degree to which a screening program can be successful in reducing morbidity and mortality depends on the prevalence of the condition in the population to be screened, the validity and reliability of the screening tool, the availability of a treatment or intervention for the condition, and the follow-up plans for those detected to be positive. . . . [J.] Wilson and Jungner (1968) [identified] . . . nine specific requirements for the establishment of a screening program: (1) the condition for which the screening is done should be an important health problem; (2) there should be an accepted treatment for patients detected; (3) facilities for diagnosis and treatment should be available; (4) there should be a recognizable latent or early symptomatic stage so that detection can prove beneficial; (5) there should be a suitable screening test; (6) the test should be acceptable to the population; (7) the natural history of the condition should be adequately understood; (8) there should be agreement as to who will treat the patients; [and] (9) the cost of case finding, diagnosis, and treatment should be economically balanced in relation to possible expenditure on medical care as a whole.

Only after a given type of screening program has been thoroughly examined in terms of the degree to which it satisfies the public health criteria is it appropriate to examine the . . . ethical justifications for accepting or rejecting that program as a public policy choice. . . .

ETHICAL FRAMEWORK

Central to [a] framework of ethical analysis is the notion that moral deliberation and justification ordinarily rest on principles, rules, and rights understood as abstract action guides. These action guides, the choice and analysis of which are inherently controversial, together with questions of their relationship both to one another and to a theory of human virtues, constitute the heart of modern ethical theory. . . .

[Ed.–The authors discuss three general moral principles: beneficence, respect for autonomy, and justice.]

BALANCING MORAL PRINCIPLES

Controversial problems about moral principles such as respect for autonomy, beneficence, and justice inevitably arise over how much these principles demand and how to handle situations of conflict among them. Whatever the prominence of these principles, we must acknowledge that if they conflict—as they do on occasion—a serious weighting or priority problem is created. . . . Many problems about policies governing program participation take this form. Primarily they involve whether to override the obligation to respect the autonomy of individuals, as when programs are made completely mandatory. . . .

. . . The decision of whether to implement a screening program requires a balancing of the goals of the three frameworks described. In an important respect, the public health framework is the most fundamental. No screening program can be justified without satisfying at least some public health criteria. . . .

It is our belief that how completely the public health criteria must be satisfied depends on the degree to which the specific type of program proposed compromises other criteria. When a program poses a conflict between public health interests and other interests, greater fulfillment of the public health criteria is necessary in order to justify public health interests taking precedence. For this reason, analyses of the five types of programs must include the degree to which they satisfy public health criteria, understanding that the more programs challenge legal and ethical mandates, the greater will be the requirement that the public health criteria be satisfied.

. . . . .

Because the guarantees of the Constitution principally constrain state actions, the legal battles over screening have centered on government agencies, as well as private entities acting on federal or state rules that require or authorize screening. (There are also separate statutory limits on screening programs. For example, the Americans with Disabilities Act regulates screenings by employers.) The primary constitutional impediment to testing is the Fourth Amendment, which guarantees the right of people to be "secure in their persons" and not subjected to "unreasonable searches and seizures." While the Fourth Amendment is popularly perceived as applying solely to personal or residential searches (for administrative searches, see chapter 12), the Supreme Court has long recognized that the collection and subsequent analysis of biological samples are "searches" (*Schmerber v. California*, 384 U.S. 757 [1966]). Privacy and security interests are generated by the invasion of bodily integrity involved in collecting the sample and the ensuing chemical analysis that extracts personal information. The constitutional issue is whether the analysis of blood, urine, or other tissue is "unreasonable." In the companion cases of *Skinner v. Railway Labor Executives' Association*, 489 U.S. 602 (1989), and *Treasury Employees Union v. Von Raab*, 489 U.S. 656 (1989), the Supreme Court formulated the modern standard of review for screening programs needed for special purposes other than law enforcement.

In criminal cases, a search or seizure is reasonable under the Fourth Amendment only when it is carried out in accordance with a judicial warrant issued upon probable cause (or when the circumstances fall within certain well-defined exceptions). But because most screening programs do not involve law enforcement, a departure from the warrant and probable cause requirements may be justified under the "special needs" doctrine. Under this doctrine, the governmental interests in the screening program and the privacy interests of the individuals are balanced to assess the practicality of the warrant and probable cause requirements. In *Skinner*, the Supreme Court applied the special needs doctrine to uphold the screening of railway employees for drug and alcohol use. The case presented special governmental needs beyond normal law enforcement because the screening program was designed to ensure the safety of the traveling public and employees. In balancing the employees' privacy interests, the Court noted that the employees worked in a highly regulated industry, limiting their reasonable expectation of privacy. Against this backdrop, the government's compelling safety interests outweighed their privacy concerns, making the blood, urine, and alcohol content tests reasonable under the Fourth Amendment.

The special needs doctrine has been applied to other screening programs. For example, courts have upheld compulsory screening for sexually transmitted diseases for persons accused or convicted of sexual assaults (e.g., *Adams v. State*, 498 S.E.2d 268 [Ga. 1998]). The judiciary believes these screening programs to be justified by the "special need" to inform rape victims of their potential exposure to STDs.

Screening programs, even when carried out for public health purposes, may also produce evidence that might be useful in the criminal context—for example, the use of information from a drug screening to prosecute for drug possession. In *Ferguson v. City of Charleston*, the Supreme Court considered the special needs doctrine in an intriguing case involving the drug testing of pregnant women. The screening program was used both to treat pregnant women for drug abuse and to secure criminal convictions.

FERGUSON V. CITY OF CHARLESTON*
Supreme Court of the United States
Decided March 21, 2001

Justice STEVENS delivered the opinion of the Court.

[In 1988 a task force made up of the Medical University of South Carolina (MUSC), police, and local officials developed a policy that set procedures for identifying and testing pregnant patients suspected of drug use without obtaining the individuals' consent. The policy also included police procedures and criteria for arresting patients who tested positive and prescribed prosecutions for drug offenses and/ or child neglect, depending on the stage of the defendant's pregnancy. Petitioners, MUSC obstetrical patients arrested after testing positive for cocaine, filed this suit challenging the policy's validity on the theory that warrantless and nonconsensual drug tests conducted for criminal investigatory purposes were unconstitutional searches. Respondents argued that the searches were reasonable under the "special needs" doctrine, even absent consent, because they were justified by special non-law-enforcement purposes.]

Because the hospital seeks to justify its authority to conduct drug tests and to turn the results over to law enforcement agents without the knowledge or consent of the patients, this case differs from previous cases [including *Skinner*] in which we have considered whether comparable drug tests "fit within the closely guarded category of constitutionally permissible suspicionless searches." *Chandler v. Miller*, 520 U.S. 305, 309 (1997). . . . In those cases, we employed a balancing test that weighed the intrusion on the individual's interest in privacy against the "special needs" that supported the program. As an initial matter, we note that the invasion of privacy in this case is far more substantial than in those cases. . . . The reasonable expectation of privacy enjoyed by the typical patient undergoing diagnostic tests in a hospital is that the results of those tests will not be shared with nonmedical personnel without her consent. In none of our prior cases was there any intrusion upon that kind of expectation.

The critical difference between those [previous] drug-testing cases and this one, however, lies in the nature of the "special need" asserted as justification for the warrantless searches. In each of those earlier cases, the "special need" that was advanced as a justification for the absence of a warrant or individualized suspicion was one divorced from the State's general interest in law enforcement. . . . In this case, however, the central and indispensable feature of the policy from its inception was the use of law enforcement to coerce the patients into substance abuse treatment.

Respondents argue in essence that their ultimate purpose—namely, protecting the health of both mother and child—is a beneficent one. . . . However, we [do] not simply accept the State's invocation of a "special need." Instead, we carry out a "close review" of the scheme at issue before concluding that the need in question was not "special," as that term has been defined in our cases. In this case, a review of

*532 U.S. 67 (2001).

the policy plainly reveals that the purpose actually served by the MUSC searches "is ultimately indistinguishable from the general interest in crime control." *Indianapolis v. Edmond,* 531 U.S. 32, 44 (2000).

In looking to the programmatic purpose, we consider all the available evidence in order to determine the relevant primary purpose.... Tellingly, the document codifying the policy incorporates the police's operational guidelines. It devotes its attention to the chain of custody, the range of possible criminal charges, and the logistics of police notification and arrests. Nowhere, however, does the document discuss different courses of medical treatment for either mother or infant, aside from treatment for the mother's addiction.

Moreover, throughout the development and application of the policy, the Charleston prosecutors and police were extensively involved in the day-to-day administration of the policy. Police and prosecutors decided who would receive the reports of positive drug screens and what information would be included with those reports. Law enforcement officials also helped determine the procedures to be followed when performing the screens. In the course of the policy's administration, they had access to ... medical files on the women who tested positive, routinely attended the substance abuse team's meetings, and regularly received copies of team documents discussing the women's progress. Police took pains to coordinate the timing and circumstances of the arrests with MUSC staff....

While the ultimate goal of the program may well have been to get the women in question into substance abuse treatment and off of drugs, the immediate objective of the searches was to generate evidence for law enforcement purposes in order to reach that goal. The threat of law enforcement may ultimately have been intended as a means to an end, but the direct and primary purpose of MUSC's policy was to ensure the use of those means. In our opinion, this distinction is critical. Because law enforcement involvement always serves some broader social purpose or objective, under respondents' view, virtually any nonconsensual suspicionless search could be immunized under the special needs doctrine by defining the search solely in terms of its ultimate, rather than immediate, purpose. Such an approach is inconsistent with the Fourth Amendment. Given the primary purpose of the Charleston program, which was to use the threat of arrest and prosecution in order to force women into treatment, and given the extensive involvement of law enforcement officials at every stage of the policy, this case simply does not fit within the closely guarded category of "special needs."

The fact that positive test results were turned over to the police does not merely provide a basis for distinguishing our prior cases applying the "special needs" balancing approach to the determination of drug use. It also provides an affirmative reason for enforcing the strictures of the Fourth Amendment. While state hospital employees, like other citizens, may have a duty to provide the police with evidence of criminal conduct that they inadvertently acquire in the course of routine treatment, when they undertake to obtain such evidence from their patients for the specific purpose of incriminating those patients, they have a special obligation to make sure that the patients are fully informed about their constitutional rights, as standards of knowing waiver require.

As respondents have repeatedly insisted, their motive was benign rather than

punitive. Such a motive, however, cannot justify a departure from Fourth Amendment protections, given the pervasive involvement of law enforcement with the
development and application of the MUSC policy.... While respondents are correct
that drug abuse both was and is a serious problem, "the gravity of the threat alone
cannot be dispositive of questions concerning what means law enforcement officers
may employ to pursue a given purpose." Edmond, 531 U.S. at 32-33. The Fourth
Amendment's general prohibition against nonconsensual, warrantless, and suspicionless searches necessarily applies to such a policy.

III. MANDATORY TREATMENT

Medical treatment has transformed public health approaches to disease epidemics. Treatment not only benefits individuals by ameliorating
symptoms but also benefits society by reducing or eliminating infectiousness. But these positive outcomes cannot occur unless individuals take their medication. Moreover, inconsistent treatment can result
in drug resistance, making diseases difficult to cure. Because of the
benefits to individuals and the community, as well as the problem of
drug resistance, public health authorities have an abiding interest in
compulsory treatment. However, mandatory treatment represents a
serious intrusion on a person's bodily integrity. The courts are faced
with the task of balancing the benefits of treatment against the interests
of individuals in their own autonomy.

Most public health statutes authorize mandatory treatment of contagious diseases, whether or not the affected person is competent to make
the decision for herself. The courts consistently affirm the constitutionality of compulsory treatment of persons with infectious diseases (see,
e.g., City of New York v. Antoinette R., 630 N.Y.S.2d 1008 [N.Y. Sup.
Ct. 1995], excerpted in chapter 11).

Although the right to refuse treatment is protected by the Constitution, the Supreme Court balances a person's liberty interests against
relevant state interests. The Court has held that the state may mandate
serious forms of treatment, such as antipsychotic medication, if the person poses a danger to himself or others. The treatment must be medically appropriate so that the person benefits (see, e.g., Washington v.
Harper, 494 U.S. 210 [1990], holding that treatment may be compelled
when a prisoner poses a danger to himself or others and treatment is
in the prisoner's medical interests). The same constitutional standard
would likely apply to mandatory treatment for an infectious disease.
The state could compel such therapy, but only if the treatment reduces

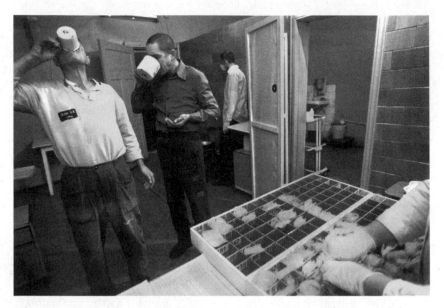

Photo 25. In October 2000, Siberian prisoners receive directly observed therapy (DOT) for tuberculosis. Drug-resistant tuberculosis thrives in Siberian
prisons, and incidence is increasing worldwide. The close living conditions
in institutional settings readily foster tuberculosis transmission. Using DOT
to treat persons in institutions can help prevent the recurrence of active infection and curb the emergence of resistant strains of the disease, as well as preventing new infections. Reproduced by permission, © Karen Kasmauski/
Corbis, October 20, 2000.

a significant risk of transmission and affords medical benefits to the
patient.

A. Directly Observed Therapy

The state's interest in ensuring the completion of treatment may not
always require compulsory hospitalization. Treatment in the community often can be ensured through directly observed therapy (DOT),
commonly used in the management of TB. DOT is a compliance-
enhancing strategy that requires the taking of each dose of medication to be observed by a family member, peer advocate, community
worker, or health care professional. Supervised therapy can take place
in a variety of locations, ranging from a personal residence or place
of employment to a clinic, physician's office, or even a street corner.
Ronald Bayer and David Wilkinson examine the history of DOT.

DIRECTLY OBSERVED THERAPY FOR TUBERCULOSIS: HISTORY OF AN IDEA*

Ronald Bayer and David Wilkinson

DOT has emerged as the standard of care in the treatment of TB in the USA. In response to the dismal record of assuring that those with TB complete their treatment, the problems of TB in persons with HIV infection, and the public alarm that attended the emergence of multidrug-resistant TB in New York, the Advisory Council for the Elimination of Tuberculosis (ACET) has recommended that DOT be considered for all patients in locales that do not achieve at least a 90% completion rate for treatment. What is so striking about these developments in public health practice is that they were so long in coming. Indeed, the idea of using DOT for all, or virtually all, patients with TB emerged more than three decades ago as a result of work in Madras and Hong Kong. [Ed.–The authors discuss the history of DOT in Madras, India, and Hong Kong during the late 1950s and 1960s.] . . .

SUPERVISED THERAPY IN THE USA

While the evidence from abroad suggested that a broad application of supervised therapy was necessary, TB-control efforts in the USA all but ignored the relevance of such findings and remained focused on what insights might be relied upon to predict patient behavior and medication use, and on the importance of fashioning clinical structures and practices that would overcome noncompliance. . . .

DOT remained the exception rather than the rule in the face of evidence to support this approach in problem patients and recommendations from the CDC and the American Thoracic Society that difficult patients be placed on twice weekly supervised therapy.

What accounted for the failure to use directly supervised therapy despite the fact that at least 20–30% of patients throughout the USA failed to complete treatment within 24 months? Many health departments believed that requiring individuals to take their medication in the presence of a responsible party would entail unacceptable assumptions about the prospect of the future behavior of those under care. Rather than a service, DOT was often viewed as an imposition that could be justified only in the presence of evidence that the patient would behave in a way that posed a threat to the public health. At a later date, some argued that widespread application of DOT entailed an inversion of a basic human right by treating TB patients as guilty until proven innocent. But the most important factor was the assumption that the widescale use of supervised therapy would entail an extraordinary and unjustifiable expense. Certainly questions of cost and severe limitations on available resources were among the factors that played a part in the failure of the CDC to press publicly for the wider adoption of DOT as a practice even when some believed such a move would have salutary consequences.

. . . There were, however, examples of successful application of DOT in the 1980s. . . . In Denver, . . . an average of 60% of TB patients treated between 1973

---

*Reprinted from *Lancet* 345 (June 17, 1995): 1545–48. © 1995 by The Lancet, Ltd.

and 1983 were supervised. More striking, there were a few locales where DOT was adopted as a universal or near universal approach in TB. . . . That these developments occurred despite limited support from federal authorities makes clear the fact that resource constraints explained only a part of the resistance in the USA to DOT. Where there was a political commitment to instituting such an approach to TB control it was possible to make substantial changes. Such commitment also required a cultural climate within which supervision of all, or nearly all, patients was not offensive. . . .

The availability of resources and the political and cultural climate surrounding TB control underwent a radical transformation in the early 1990s as a result of a rising number of cases, an increase in drug-resistant disease, and nosocomial outbreaks in hospitals. As a result of the fear that what had been a treatable disease might become an untreatable danger to middle-class populations that had in recent years been spared the threat of TB, concern took hold about the rate at which patients failed to complete their TB therapy in cities such as New York, Chicago, Newark, and Washington. Public concern and a demand for remedial action provoked Congress to greatly increase funding for TB-control efforts. . . . Central to the new commitment was a striking determination to place DOT for most if not all patients at the center of public-health efforts.

When in 1993, the ACET made DOT the standard of care, as a matter of federal policy, it turned from the decades-long efforts to identify individuals at high risk for non-compliance and more recent attempts to designate groups as being at high risk for failure to complete their TB treatment. ACET (1993, 3) stated that "DOT should be considered for all patients because of the difficulty in predicting which patients will adhere to a prescribed regimen. Decisions regarding the use of expanded or universal DOT should be based on a quantitative evaluation of local treatment completion rates." . . .

The embrace of the principle of universal or near-universal DOT by federal, state, and local health departments, has, not surprisingly, provoked opposition from some public-health officials, who believe that their own programs were effective without the need to devote resources to so labor-intensive an effort. More striking has been the criticism from those for whom civil liberties are of pre-eminent importance. Such criticisms have not opposed the universal offer of DOT, making it available to all patients as a service. Nor have they opposed the imposition of DOT by court order after patients have shown that they cannot adhere to the prescribed treatment regimen. What civil liberties groups have found appalling—a violation of the constitutional requirement that the state use the least restrictive alternative in pursuit of public-health goals—is the notion that all or nearly all patients, irrespective of behavior, should be required to ingest their medication in the presence of an observer. The designation of classes of patients—the poor, the homeless, drug users—as being at high risk for noncompliance and as requiring DOT, was viewed as particularly offensive.

Despite such objections we believe that the weight of historical evidence and recent experience make the move to DOT as a standard of care crucial. . . . As DOT programs are started or expanded, it will be necessary to determine the appropriate mix of clinic-based care and care provided by community-based outreach workers; the need for provision of housing for homeless patients; the need for drug and alcohol abuse treatment, and psychiatric services for those who are impaired; the part to be played by financial inducements for remaining in care; and the functions of court mandates and the ultimate threat of compulsory hospitalization for those who refuse to remain in treatment until cured. In short, it will be necessary to examine carefully the role of enablers and incentives. None of these studies will be simple or cheap, and all will require that resources for TB-control remain adequate, even if the number of new cases declines. Recognizing the centrality of DOT is thus just the beginning of the challenge posed by TB.

. . .   .   .

Bayer and Wilkinson discuss DOT in largely favorable terms in this piece. However, Bayer and some of his colleagues later came to feel that public health evidence does not support universal DOT (Bayer, Stayton, et al. 1998, 1056).

Noncompliance with TB treatment regimens persists as a problem even in the DOT context. Some patients, like the patient in *In re Washington* (excerpted below), resist even directly observed therapy. This case concerns Ruby Washington, a patient who, while not necessarily refusing treatment, repeatedly failed to appear for DOT appointments. Enforcement of DOT orders under such circumstances may require more invasive measures, and in the excerpt below, the court considers a liberty-limiting measure—civil confinement—as a method for enforcing mandatory treatment orders. (Civil confinement will be discussed in more detail in the following chapter.) When reading this case, consider whether the two options the court considers, confinement to a hospital or confinement to jail, are equivalently restrictive if the patient is legally prevented from leaving either one.

IN RE WASHINGTON*
Supreme Court of Wisconsin
Decided July 17, 2007

Judge BUTLER delivered the opinion of the Court.

[Ruby Washington, a homeless woman, was diagnosed with tuberculosis in June 2005. She failed to report to a TB clinic for therapy as directed. She checked into a hospital to deliver a baby in August and was served with a court order for DOT. She was released from the hospital in September with the court's permission on the condition that she move in with her sister and appear for therapy regularly. She did not comply; when she was located, she was put in jail. The court declared that she was "a huge health risk" to the community because she failed to take her medication and could become infectious. The judge was reluctant to confine Washington to jail but, citing fiscal concerns, declared that she was unwilling to allow Washington to

*735 N.W.2d 111 (Wis. 2007).

stay in the hospital under guard. The judge told Washington that she would be willing to consider other placements at Washington's suggestion. Washington appeals her confinement.]

[Under the statute allowing confinement of TB patients], the DHFS [Department of Health and Family Services] or local health officer must notify a court in writing of the confinement, and include the following in its filing: (1) A statement of a doctor or advanced practice nurse prescriber that the person has infectious tuberculosis or suspect tuberculosis; (2) evidence that the person has refused to follow a prescribed treatment regimen, or, if the person has suspect tuberculosis, has refused to undergo a medical examination; and (3) a statement that the person poses an imminent and substantial threat to himself or herself or to the public health. . . .

[The DHFS officer must provide documentation of all of the elements above, as well as showing that] . . . "all other reasonable means of achieving voluntary compliance with treatment have been exhausted and no less restrictive alternative exists; or that no other medication to treat the resistant disease is available." . . . A person confined under [the statute] "shall remain confined until the department or local health officer . . . determines that treatment is complete or that the individual is no longer a substantial threat to himself or herself or to the public health." If the person is to be confined for more than six months, "the court shall review the confinement every [six] months." Wisconsin Statute, § 252.07(9)(c). . . .

Washington does not challenge the circuit court's basis for ordering her confinement. . . . She asserts only that the court lacked authority under the statute to order confinement to the [jail].

. . . We conclude that . . . jail [is] a permissible placement option . . . for persons with noninfectious tuberculosis who are noncompliant with a prescribed treatment regimen, provided that "no less restrictive alternative exists" to such placement, and that the particular jail to which a person is to be confined is a place where proper care and treatment will be provided and spread of the disease will be prevented. . . .

Washington contends that because the purpose of confinement for those with tuberculosis who have not complied with a treatment regimen is nonpunitive, . . . confinement to a jail [should be precluded]. We agree that the purpose of any placement is not to punish the noncompliant person for failing to follow a prescribed treatment regimen, but to provide treatment and to prevent him or her from infecting others. The statutory scheme ensures that jail is not a placement of first resort, but rather is permitted only in cases in which no less restrictive alternate placement is available. Additionally, the particular facility to which a person is to be confined, whether a penal institution or other type of facility, must be a place where proper care and treatment will be provided and spread of the disease will be prevented. . . .

. . . If conditions at a particular jail (or other facility) are such that proper care and treatment would be unavailable, or contrary to the prevention of the spread of the disease, such a placement would not be authorized. . . .

Washington next argues that if jail is a permissible place of confinement . . . confinement to jail is not permitted whenever some less restrictive placement is available. . . . We interpret [the statute] to require that "no less restrictive alternative" applies to the place of confinement as well as the fact of confinement.

. . . The local health official petitioning for confinement of a person with tuberculosis who is noncompliant with a treatment regimen must demonstrate "[t]hat all other reasonable means of achieving voluntary compliance with treatment have been exhausted and no less restrictive alternative exists; or that no other medication to treat the resistant disease is available." Wisconsin Statute, § 252(9)(a) 3.

The City argues that the language "no less restrictive alternative exists" applies to the fact of confinement only.... It asserts that the place of confinement need only be ... "a facility where proper care and treatment will be provided and spread of the disease will be prevented." Wisconsin Statute, § 252.07(9)(a)....

In light of the legislature's choice to permit confinement to jail of a person with noninfectious tuberculosis who is noncompliant with a prescribed treatment regimen, we conclude that the ... "no less restrictive alternative" language appl[ies] to the place of confinement as well as the fact of confinement....

[We must therefore determine whether Washington's placement in a jail was necessary under the circumstances.] The circuit court found that Washington posed a "huge health risk" to the community by repeatedly failing to take her medication for tuberculosis. The record shows that Washington had been previously treated for tuberculosis and was therefore at greater risk of developing a more dangerous, drug-resistant strain of the disease. The court concluded that Washington had a history of disappearing from sight, that the Department previously had great difficulty locating her, and that there was nothing in the record to show that she would voluntarily turn herself in to start taking her medicine again. When placed in the community under supervised conditions, Washington walked away from that placement. The court was concerned that Washington "cannot comply with Court orders." It heard testimony that if Washington were to escape custody yet again she would "certainly" become contagious within a month, perhaps in as soon as a week. The court was also concerned that tuberculosis could "become resilient [sic] to medications." ...

Based on these considerations, we conclude that the order confining Washington to jail was not an erroneous exercise of the circuit court's discretion. Washington was at risk to develop a drug-resistant strain of the disease, had a history of disappearing from sight and was belligerent toward officers. The circuit court reasonably concluded from these factors that medical staff would not have been equipped to handle Washington's outbursts, and that the added security of jail was necessary to ensure that she would continue taking her medication and would not escape confinement....

The decision of the court of appeals is affirmed.

B. Mandatory Treatment for Persons Living with HIV/AIDS

Mandatory treatment is widely regarded as lawful and ethical when applied to persons with multidrug-resistant TB. But suppose a person with HIV infection who engages in high-risk sexual activity persistently refuses to adhere to a treatment regimen, and thereby encourages the development of drug-resistant strains. Would compulsory treatment be justified? If not, what distinguishes the case of TB from HIV? Consider these differences: TB is treatable and potentially curable, and a successful therapeutic regimen renders the person noninfectious. In addition, TB is transmitted through the air, whereas HIV is transmitted through blood or other body fluids. How important are these differences? In answering these questions, think about modern treatments for HIV that have the potential to prolong life and reduce infectiousness.

Strong evidence exists that antiretroviral therapy administered to pregnant women can significantly reduce the risk of maternal-to-infant transmission of HIV. Suppose a pregnant woman rejects treatment, placing her fetus at a substantially increased risk of being born with HIV infection. Some ethicists maintain that compulsory treatment of pregnant women for HIV disease violates the principle of consent and therefore is unjustified. In balancing the bodily integrity of the mother with the health benefits to the fetus, whose interests ought to prevail? Is it fair to consider the fetus's interests apart from those of the mother, or are their interests inseparable?

IV. EXPEDITED PARTNER THERAPY

Expedited partner therapy (EPT) recently has emerged as a tool to facilitate the treatment of the sexual partners of individuals known to have a sexually transmitted infection (STI). Notifying and treating the partners of persons with STIs has long been a cornerstone of public health practice. EPT takes this practice one step further by "treating the sex partners of persons with sexually transmitted diseases without an intervening medical evaluation or professional prevention counseling" (CDC 2006, 4). Generally, physicians using EPT provide an extra course of antibiotic therapy when treating a patient with an STI such as chlamydia, gonorrhea, or trichomoniasis so that the patient can provide his or her partner with treatment. This practice is designed to improve treatment rates among the partners of infected patients and decrease the likelihood of reinfection for the person initially treated. When possible, physicians will also contact the patient's partner to discuss treatment and encourage him or her to visit a physician.

Because prescribing laws differ from state to state, the legality of EPT practices may also differ. In the selection below, the public health law professor James Hodge and colleagues examine the legal and ethical issues surrounding the practice. EPT has been shown to reduce reinfection rates, leading to improved health outcomes for the patient. However, the practice prevents the partner from being fully informed about his or her condition and the risks and benefits of treatment. Not seeing a

physician also deprives the partner of continuity of care and the opportunity to be tested for other possible sexually transmitted diseases.

EXPEDITED PARTNER THERAPY FOR SEXUALLY TRANSMITTED DISEASES: ASSESSING THE LEGAL ENVIRONMENT*

James Hodge, Amy Pulver, Matthew Hogben, Dhrubajyoti Bhattacharya, and Erin Fuse Brown

INTRODUCTION

Despite major advances and achievements in the detection, treatment, and prevention of sexually transmitted diseases (STDs) in the United States, infections such
as chlamydia and gonorrhea remain significant public health challenges. The US
Centers for Disease Control and Prevention (CDC) estimates ... that over 700,000
new cases of gonorrhea and 2.8 million new cases of chlamydia occur each year.
To prevent reinfection and curtail further transmission, the CDC recommends that
clinical management of patients with STDs should include treatment of the patients'
current sexual partners....

[One] public health approach is expedited partner therapy (EPT). EPT refers
to the delivery of medications or prescriptions by persons infected with an STD to
their sexual partners without prior clinical assessment of those partners.... After
evaluating multiple studies involving EPT, the CDC concluded that EPT is a "useful
option" to promote partner treatment, particularly for male partners of women with
chlamydial infection or gonorrhea. In August 2006, the CDC recommended EPT as
an option for certain populations with specific conditions.

[The CDC also recognized several issues related to EPT, including concerns about
missed morbidity in unexamined patients, possible adverse reactions to antibiotics,
and the need for widespread coordination of EPT efforts.] In addition, implementation of EPT may raise legal questions and concerns in some settings. Central to these
concerns is the perceived unauthorized distribution of prescriptions or medications
to partners with whom clinicians have not personally evaluated or established a physician–patient relationship....

Beginning in September 2005, to assist state and local STD programs with EPT
implementation efforts, we assessed the legal framework concerning EPT....

BACKGROUND

... Providing access to prescription medications to persons whom a clinician has not
examined or established a professional relationship may be viewed as illegal and unethical.... This basic tenet of health care services helps ensure that individuals do not
gain access to medications they do not need or that could be dangerous to them....

There are, however, exceptions to the general rule. Physicians routinely provide
prescription medications to children or elderly patients through parents or caregivers. Spouses or life partners may be given medications for existing patients.... In

*Reprinted from *American Journal of Public Health* 98 (2008): 238–43.

response to outbreaks of meningococcal meningitis in hospitals, hospital staff and their family members are provided antibiotics without advance clinical diagnosis. . . . Although each of these examples differs from EPT, they share a common purpose: ensuring that safe and effective medications are made available to people who need them, even without direct medical evaluation of the recipients. . . .

Still, health care practitioners may be concerned that they will be subject to sanctions . . . by state licensing boards or civil claims for malpractice for provid-ing prescriptions to nonpatients. . . . State public health laws regulating STDs may condition treatment upon a clinical evaluation and diagnosis of an STD. These provi-sions bolster arguments that EPT violates acceptable clinical standards of care. . . . Clinicians' fears of malpractice or other liability are real, even if there is minimal potential for a sexual partner to suffer serious side effects by taking antibiotics. . . .

Laws concerning the distribution of prescription medicines . . . may not bar EPT, but they can affect whether or how EPT is practiced. Pharmacists may be subject to separate disciplinary action if they dispense a prescription they have reason to know was given outside of a physician–patient relationship or without prior evalu-ation. Other practitioners may be prevented from dispensing (as contrasted with prescribing) drugs to a person who is not the practitioner's patient. . . . Some laws may require information . . . identifying the intended recipient on prescription orders or labels, which could be problematic if the patient does not want to disclose a part-ner's identity. . . .

DISCUSSION

Our assessment suggests that over 75% of the 53 jurisdictions we studied feature laws that either explicitly permit or potentially allow EPT. . . .

Although our analysis suggests a favorable outlook for EPT, the existing legal landscape concerning EPT is ambiguous in a number of states. In most jurisdictions, there is an absence of specific law to authorize, endorse, or support EPT. In some jurisdictions, laws seem to contradict one another. Public health authorities, health care professionals, and policy-makers in these jurisdictions must weigh existing law and policy options and be prepared to seek legal reforms where necessary. Changes in legally binding authorities . . . and the influence of nonbinding legal sources may alter the legal environment. Accordingly, we propose a series of recommendations to facilitate the practice of EPT to protect the interests of clinicians, patients, and their sexual partners.

Laws Expressly Endorsing Expedited Partner Therapy

Laws that expressly endorse EPT should be enacted. . . . [because they] empower physicians and others to practice without fear of sanction. . . . Effective legislation . . . can also help implementation of EPT by broadening the range of diseases that apply to EPT, identifying health care practitioners who may prescribe medications, and expressly authorizing its use amid potential contradictory laws or policies. . . .

Exceptions to Existing Prescription Requirements

Exceptions to existing prescription requirements should be created. Prescription requirements can challenge the implementation of EPT by requiring patient identify-ing information on prescription labels, or by prohibiting the dispensing of drugs to individuals whom the physician has not examined. . . . This requirement may impede EPT because a patient may not know or may be reluctant to share the required information for his or her partner. . . .

Thirteen jurisdictions do not allow pharmacists to dispense medications to individuals who have not undergone a physical examination, have failed to establish a physician-patient relationship, or are not the ultimate user of a prescription. These laws may limit the ability of patients or partners to fill prescriptions written for the partner, if the pharmacist is aware that the partner has not been examined or is not a patient of the prescribing clinician. . . . These prescription requirements should be slightly amended to reflect the greater public health benefits stemming from EPT.

Professional Endorsements

Endorsements from professional boards and associations should be sought. Most jurisdictions' laws do not stipulate that issuing a prescription without prior medical evaluation or outside the physician-patient relationship is a per se instance of physician misconduct, deferring instead to the discretion of medical, nursing, or pharmaceutical licensing authorities or boards at local, state, or national levels. Some state medical boards expressly endorse EPT. On a national level, the American Medical Association has recently endorsed the practice of EPT as applied to chlamydial infection and gonorrhea. . . .

Insurance Reimbursements for Patients and Partners

Insurance reimbursements for STD treatments for patients and partners should be supported. Economic factors have the potential to affect the practice of EPT. . . . For example, who pays for the extra dose of antibiotics distributed to the patient for the partner? Should a patient's health insurance provider cover the costs of 2 doses, even though the partner . . . is the recipient of the extra dose? Denying payment for these medications is antithetical to health promotion because treating the partner of a patient with an STD can be directly tied to improving the health of the patient. Although costs for antibiotics to treat STDs are low . . . , health insurance providers may still seek to deny payment to the patient for the partner's "half." . . . Laws should permit health insurers' payment of the patient's minimal expenses . . . in delivering medications to partners through EPT, but not any additional health care needs of the partner.

CONCLUSIONS

Significant morbidity from STDs in the United States, coupled with diminished resources for traditional partner management practices, requires new public health strategies. By combining patient-based partner notification with clinical treatment through standard prescription antibiotics, EPT offers a promising new tool to improve treatment for some STDs, but its practice may be limited by perceived legal impediments. Our research, however, suggests that laws in most jurisdictions either expressly permit EPT or do not categorically prohibit it. Interpretation of existing laws or additional changes to laws may facilitate the implementation of EPT in many jurisdictions by resolving contradictory licensing, public health, or prescription laws. In turn, EPT may increasingly become an option for treating partners of STD patients and preventing transmission or reinfection from some STDs.

V. CONCLUSION

This chapter has discussed the central importance of biological approaches to the control of infectious disease. Americans have high confidence in the ability of science and technology to solve their most pressing social problems. But, as we have seen, immunization, screening, and treatment are not sterile scientific pursuits: they are highly influenced by politics, law, and values. When these interventions are forced on unwilling individuals or populations, we have to balance public claims to enhance collective well-being against private claims to preserve autonomy and bodily integrity. Similar tensions also arise from the equally contested public health interventions discussed in the next chapter: isolation and quarantine.

RECOMMENDED READINGS

Compulsory Vaccination: Immunizing the Population against Disease

Calandrillo, Steve. 2004. Vanishing vaccinations: Why are so many Americans opting out of vaccinating their children? *University of Michigan Journal of Law Reform* 37: 353–440. (Considers the possible harm that may arise from decreasing adherence to vaccination recommendations and argues for tighter regulation of exceptions to vaccination requirements)

Dawson, Angus. 2007. Vaccination ethics. In *Principles of Health Care Ethics,* ed. Richard E. Ashcroft, Angus Dawson, Heather Draper, and John McMillan, 617–22. 2d ed. Chichester: Wiley. (Discusses ethical arguments for and against compulsory vaccination)

Hodge, James, and Lawrence Gostin. 2002. School vaccination requirements: Historical, social, and legal perspectives. *Kentucky Law Journal* 90: 831–90. (Reviews the history of vaccination and the history and constitutionality of school vaccination mandates)

Malone, Kevin, and Alan Hinman. 2007. Vaccine mandates: The public health imperative and individual rights. In *Law in Public Health Practice,* ed. Richard A. Goodman, Richard E. Hoffman, Wilfredo Lopez, Gene W. Matthews, Mark A. Rothstein, and Karen L. Foster, 338–60. 2d ed. Oxford: Oxford University Press. (Discusses the constitutionality of vaccine mandates in the context of the history, impact, and importance of vaccination)

May, Thomas, and Ross D. Silverman. 2005. Free riding, fairness and the rights of minority groups in exemption from mandatory childhood vaccination. *Human Vaccines* 1 (1): 12–15. (Argues that easily obtained vaccination exemptions will disparately affect minority groups but that more complicated exemptions will disparately burden them, and suggests a remedy for the problem)

Offit, Paul A. 2008. Vaccines and autism revisited—the Hanna Poling case. *New England Journal of Medicine* 358: 2089–91. (Criticizes changes in how the National Vaccine Injury Compensation Program has awarded damages to people claiming vaccine injuries)

Salmon, Daniel A., and Saad B. Omer. 2006. Individual freedoms versus collective responsibility: Immunization decision-making in the face of occasionally competing values. *Emerging Themes in Epidemiology* 3: 13–5. (Balances the necessity of herd immunity for vaccination to succeed against individual autonomy)

Salmon, Daniel A., Jason W. Sapsin, Stephen P. Teret, Richard F. Jacobs, Joseph W. Thompson, Kevin Ryan, and Neal A. Halsey. 2005. Public health and the politics of school immunization requirements. *American Journal of Public Health* 95: 778–83. (Presents options for statutory vaccination exemptions other than religious exemptions)

Testing and Population-Based Screening

Bayer, Ronald, and Amy Fairchild. 2006. Changing the paradigm for HIV testing—the end of exceptionalism. *New England Journal of Medicine* 355: 647–49. (Supports changes in HIV-testing protocols that required counseling and informed consent prior to the test)

Csete, Joanne. 2006. Scaling up HIV testing: Human rights and hidden cost. *HIV/AIDS Policy and Law Review* 11: 1–10. (Argues that HIV stigma persists and that counseling and informed consent should be required with testing)

Gostin, Lawrence O. 2006. HIV screening in health care settings: Public health and civil liberties in conflict? *JAMA* 296: 2023–25. (Examines the implications of a change in CDC-promulgated regulations regarding HIV testing)

Kass, Nancy E. 2000. A change in approach to prenatal HIV screening. *American Journal of Public Health* 90: 1026–27. (Argues that non-universal HIV screening may result in the inappropriate targeting of poor and minority women)

Mandatory Treatment

Bayer, Ronald, and Laurence Dupuis. 1995. Tuberculosis, public health, and civil liberties. *Annual Review of Public Health* 16: 307–26. (Evaluates the problems presented by tuberculosis treatment from a civil liberties perspective)

Farmer, Paul, Fernet Leandre, Joia Mukherjee, Rajesh Gupta, Laura Tarter, and Jim Yong Kim. 2001. Community-based treatment of advanced HIV disease: Introducing DOT-HAART (directly observed therapy with highly active antiretroviral therapy). *Bulletin of the World Health Organization* 79: 1145–51. (Describes the application of the principles of directly observed tuberculosis therapy to highly active antiretroviral therapy for HIV/AIDS)

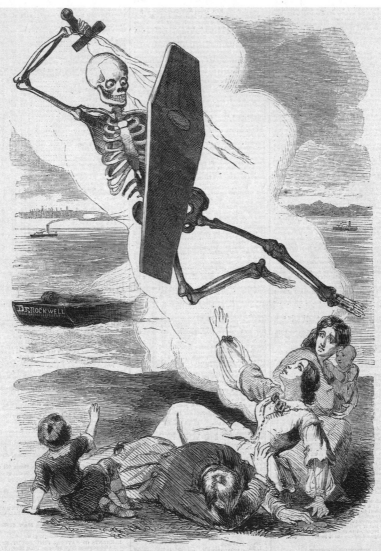

THE QUARANTINE QUESTION.

Photo 26. Since the fourteenth century, ports around the world have used quarantines to stave off epidemics of plague, yellow fever, and other deadly scourges. The caption to this drawing from an 1858 issue of *Harper's Weekly* quotes the dark warning of a certain Dr. Anderson: "While the Angel of Death rides on the fumes of the iron scow, and infected airs are wafted to our shores from the anchorage, we shall have no security against these annual visitations of pestilence." Reproduced from PBS, "The Most Dangerous Woman in America: History of Quarantine," *Nova* (original broadcast date October 12, 2004), www.pbs.org/wgbh/nova/typhoid/quarantine.html.

ELEVEN

Public Health Strategies for Epidemic Disease

Association, Travel, and Liberty

Measures to control communicable diseases are not limited to biological approaches. Societies can also cope with communicable disease epidemics by separating contagious persons from the rest of the population. Public health authorities possess three overlapping powers of detention to help prevent the spread of disease: isolation of known infectious persons, quarantine of healthy persons exposed to disease, and civil commitment (compulsory hospitalization) for care and treatment. (For descriptions of these three forms of detention, see pages 428–36 and table 19 in chapter 11 of the companion text.)

We like to think that the employment of these measures is thoughtful and based solely on the sciences of public health and medicine. But the history of infectious disease control teaches a different lesson. Feelings about infectious disease are sometimes visceral—kindled by fear, stereotype, and enmity. Blamed for epidemics, individuals with disease are viewed as vectors of infection rather than persons in need of care and support. At various times in history disfavored populations— for example, racial or religious minorities, commercial sex workers, injecting drug users, and gay men—have become targets of coercion. Animus toward those with infectious disease can be confounded with deep-seated prejudices against marginalized communities.

Even when compulsory powers must be exercised to prevent the transmission of infectious disease, it is important to consider their effects on individual freedom and dignity. Infectious disease control powers are among society's most coercive measures: isolation and quarantine deprive individuals of their liberty. In a democratic society these coercive powers should be carefully justified. We must balance the public health interests of society against the freedom of the individual.

Decisions about whether to use compulsory powers, and about the groups to which they will apply, are often influenced by social fears and political pressures. It is difficult to exaggerate the dread caused by disease epidemics and their destabilizing effects on people and their communities. The public places intense pressure on elected representatives to "do something" to protect them. The exercise of compulsory powers represents the most visible expression of government's determination to act decisively, whether or not scientific evidence indicates that such action will be effective. When policies are driven by fear, there is great risk that the employment of public health powers might be arbitrary or discriminatory, targeting politically unpopular individuals or groups. Recall the discussion of *Jew Ho v. Williamson* in chapter 4: in 1900, San Francisco health officials quarantined an area of the city where the Chinese American community lived in a purported effort to contain bubonic plague. The city exempted specific homes within the quarantine area that belonged to non-Asians.

Epidemics, and society's response to them, can also powerfully affect businesses and the economy. Quarantines and travel restrictions can significantly impede commerce to and from affected areas. Consider the 2003 outbreak of severe acute respiratory syndrome (SARS), which prompted travel restrictions and advisories that affected several countries. Countries concerned about the economic impacts of travel warnings were reluctant to accurately report on the epidemic's progress.

This chapter will focus on the most ancient and enduring response to communicable disease—crude separation of the sick from the healthy. It reviews the history of infectious disease control, describes the breadth and limits of legal powers relating to civil confinement, and discusses the influence of society, politics, and economics on the implementation and acceptance of personal control measures. Its examples are drawn from our experience with and preparations for outbreaks of SARS, tuberculosis (TB), and pandemic influenza. Personal control measures are highly contentious, and the chapter concludes with a discussion of biosecurity and the debate on the appropriate balance between public health powers and individual freedoms.

I. A BRIEF HISTORY OF THE ANCIENT POWER OF QUARANTINE

Quarantine can be traced back to humanity's early history. As the historian of medicine David F. Musto notes (1986, 97),

> In ancient times citizens noted that occasionally a disease that had appeared in a distant locale was then sweeping toward them from neighboring villages, or that after a ship from a foreign land reached shore with ill persons aboard, people residing in the port city would take ill. Such temporal sequences cannot be ignored and, if the illness is a serious one, fears escalate as the illness comes closer. Knowing the cause of an illness or its mode of transmission provides some rational approach to interrupting the spread of the disease. Prior to the nineteenth century, however, those were unknowns, and so civil authorities were left with whatever means seemed reasonable in the wisdom of the time to fight the spread of diseases. Protective measures were based upon what we would now consider erroneous explanations for contagion. From this era of scant knowledge comes the origin of the familiar word we use to designate attempts to isolate the sick or contagious from the healthy: "Quarantine."

In 2003, during the SARS epidemic, thousands of people were forced into isolation under the authority of quarantine—one of humanity's oldest tools against the spread of disease. Quarantines can be effective, but they are blunt tools that can undermine civil liberties and provoke widespread panic and fear, which themselves can make disease containment more difficult. In the following selection, taken from an informative report commissioned by the United States Public Health and Marine-Hospital Service at the very beginning of the twentieth century, J. M. Eager describes the historical practice of quarantine.

THE EARLY HISTORY OF QUARANTINE: ORIGIN OF SANITARY MEASURES DIRECTED AGAINST YELLOW FEVER*
J. M. Eager

The history of quarantine is closely interwoven with that of medicine in general and of shipping. . . . The story of the beginnings of quarantine is associated particularly with the epidemiology of leprosy, pest, and syphilis. Cholera and yellow fever were later considerations. . . .

*Published by the Government Printing Office, Washington, DC, 1903.

LEPROSY AND LAND QUARANTINES

The first quarantines of which any mention is made in literature were land quarantines used as a protection against leprosy. The ancients regarded this disease as of African origin, and Lucretius states positively that it first came from Egypt. In the Old Testament the first indications are found of precautions taken against contagious maladies. Leviticus, Numbers, and the First Book of Samuel give directions for the sequestration of lepers, first in the desert, then outside the camp, and afterwards without the walls of Jerusalem. In these books the inspection of persons for the detection of leprosy is detailed. Persons afflicted with skin diseases were directed to present themselves before the priests. An observation of each case was made, and, according to minutely described symptoms, isolation of the patients was ordered for a prescribed period.

The crusaders on their arrival outside the walls of Jerusalem found lazarettoes still in existence, and after taking the city from the Mussulmans sent all contagious maladies to these isolated places. The name Hospital of St. Lazarus was given to the place of sequestration. Returning to Europe, the members of the military expeditions brought back with them not only numerous diseases, but also the word "lazaretto," as applied to a place for the isolation of the victims of communicable maladies. As a result lazarettoes were built outside the gates of nearly all the principal cities of Europe. Leprosy itself had, however, been introduced into Europe many centuries earlier. It is spoken of as a foreign disease by the earlier Greek and Latin writers. . . .

Lepers were not strictly confined to the leper houses. They were, however, required to wear a special costume, to limit their walks to certain roads, to give warning of their approach by sounding a clapper, and to forbear communicating with healthy persons and drinking from or bathing in any running stream.

PEST AND EARLY VIEWS OF ETIOLOGY

By the word pest is understood not only bubonic plague, but the different epidemic diseases, whatever they may have been, that were formerly included under that term. . . . The word plague as well as pest was given by ancient medical writers to any epidemic disease that wrought in extensive destruction of life. . . . Throughout all this extensive period notions and practices relating to public sanitation were being evolved in accordance with the prevalent tenets of causation. . . .

MARITIME QUARANTINE

Maritime quarantine originated in connection with the Levantine trade. Its early history is associated with that of shipping in the Mediterranean, especially with that of the traffic of Venice, Genoa, and Marseille. . . . The practice of isolation was first applied against communicable disease by the Hebrews, but the lazarettoes, it appears, were little used in connection with foreign trade, leaving out of the question commerce by sea. . . .

EARLY MARITIME SANITARY LAWS

The Venetians were, it is generally admitted, the first to make provision for maritime sanitation. As far back as the year 1000 there were overseers of public health, but at first the office was not a permanent one. The incumbents were appointed to serve during the prevalence of an epidemic only. The first information we have of this kind of public office is under date of 1348, when . . . overseers of public health [were appointed]. These officers were authorized to spend public money for the purpose of isolating infected ships, goods, and persons at an island of the lagoon. . . .

Neighboring States engaged in commerce in the Mediterranean speedily followed the example of Venice. . . . It was not until 1459 that a public bureau of sanitation existed in the Republic of Venice. In that year officers, called conservators of sanitation, were regularly appointed. . . .

During all this period land quarantines were in operation at times of pest. Offenses against quarantine, both land and maritime, were severely punished. Pietro Follerio, a great Neapolitan jurisconsult of the sixteenth century, mentions whipping, the mill, exile, and death as penalties for infringement of sanitary regulations. . . . Torture, long service in the galleys, and work among the sick in a pest hospital are named among the penalties. . . .

BILLS OF HEALTH

Sanitary bulletins were incident to quarantines and cordons. They were so called because they were stamped with the "bollo" or seal of the authority issuing them. When the system of sanitary bulletins was fully developed these patients, in their connection with ships, were designated as clean, when beyond suspicion; touched, when from a noninfected place in active communication with infected places; suspicious, without sickness aboard, but having received goods from places or from ships or caravans from places where pest prevailed; and dirty, when from a place where disease existed. . . . During the pest at Naples, in the year 1557, citizens, usually merchants, were stationed at the gates of the city to examine bills of health. Corruption and lack of diligence on the part of these persons were punishable by death. Sentinels, some on foot and some on horseback, made a patrol about the city walls to prevent clandestine entrance. Bills of health to be acceptable had to be stamped with the seal of the university of the place from which the traveler came. They gave not only the day but the hour of departure, together with a description of the traveler. Sanitary bulletins were also issued to accompany merchandise, but in times of severe pest all articles except aromatics and medicaments were considered suspicious. . . .

FURTHER HISTORY OF QUARANTINE

. . . Following the discovery by Anthony van Leeuwenhoek, in 1675, of bacteria, called by him "animalcules," there was a wide belief in the casual connection of microscopic creatures with disease, . . . but it was without marked effect on quarantine procedure. The theory, in fact, lost hold on the public and medical minds to such an extent that in the early part of the nineteenth century the doctrine of a living contagion was looked upon as an absurd assumption. It was not until the middle of the last century, following the investigations of Pasteur, Pollender, and Bavaine, that quarantine practice became established on its modern scientific basis. . . .

The international sanitary conferences at Paris in 1851 and 1852, in which participated the different European powers having interests in the Mediterranean, marked the close of the old regime of quarantine. [Lax] regulations were adopted . . . , it being admitted that the efficacy of many measures formerly practiced was doubtful

or negative, science having proclaimed that, for the most part, pestilential maladies
are not contagious. This surprising declaration was followed by a revolution in quarantine methods on the Continent and resulted in the general adoption of practices
based on the limited communicability of epidemic diseases. These changes, with
which the early history of quarantine closes, were brought into effect at the beginning of the new era, during which the doctrine of specific living causes of epidemic
diseases have been built up on the substantial basis of experimental medicine.

II. CONSTITUTIONAL REVIEW OF ISOLATION AND QUARANTINE

A. Pre–Civil Rights Era

As the excerpt by Eager illustrates, the practice of quarantine predates
the founding of the Republic and continues to modern times. In the
early twentieth century, the courts adopted a permissive approach to
quarantine, as the following two state supreme court decisions illustrate. Both cases reveal attitudes based on stereotypes regarding gender
and race.

KIRK V. WYMAN*
Supreme Court of South Carolina
Decided August 19, 1909

Judge WOODS delivered the opinion of the court.
[The city of Aiken, South Carolina, found that Mary Kirk had contagious leprosy
and required her to be isolated in the city hospital for infectious diseases. Kirk
claimed that although she had leprosy, she was not dangerous to the community. In
addition, she complained that the hospital where she was to be placed was really
a "pesthouse, coarse and comfortless" and used for "incarcerating negroes having
small-pox and other dangerous infectious diseases." She further objected to her isolation because of the odors coming from the city dumping ground near the hospital.
She was granted a temporary injunction. The Board of Health appealed, claiming
that she was a danger to community, that they had sought measures to improve the
hospital and would eventually provide a private cottage for her, and that the city
dump was located nearby but did not contain foul deposits.]
    . . . Municipal boards of health . . . are to be considered as deriving their authority
to isolate infected persons . . . from section 1099 of the Civil Code, which provides:

> The said board of health shall have power and it shall be their duty to make and
> enforce all needful rules and regulations to prevent the introduction and spread
> of infectious or contagious diseases by the regulation of intercourse with infected

*65 S.E. 387 (S.C. 1909).

places, by the arrest, separation, and treatment of infected persons, and persons who shall have been exposed to any contagious or infectious diseases.... They shall also have power, with the consent of the town or city council, in case of the prevalence of any contagious or infectious diseases within the town or city, to establish one or more hospitals and to make provisions and regulations for the management of the same....

The principles of constitutional law governing health regulations by statute and municipal ordinance may be thus stated:

First. Statutes and ordinances requiring the removal or destruction of property or the isolation of infected persons, when necessary for the protection of the public health, do not violate the constitutional guaranty of the right of the enjoyment of liberty and property, because neither the right to liberty nor the right of property extends to the use of liberty or property to the injury of others.... The individual has no more right to the freedom of spreading disease by carrying contagion on his person, than he has to produce disease by maintaining his property in a noisome condition.

Second. The state must of necessity lodge the power somewhere to ascertain, in the first instance, and act with promptness, when the public health is endangered by the unhealthful condition of the person or the property of the individual; and the creation by legislative authority of boards of health, with the discretion lodged in them of summary inquiry and action, is a reasonable exercise of the police power....

Third. Arbitrary power over persons and property could not be conferred on a board of health, and no attempt is made in the Constitution or statutes to confer such power.... It is always implied that the power conferred to interfere with these personal rights is limited by public necessity. From this it follows that boards of health may not deprive any person of his property or his liberty, unless the deprivation is ... reasonably necessary to the public health; and such inquiry must include notice to the person whose property or liberty is involved, and the opportunity to him to be heard, unless the emergency appears to be so great that such notice and hearing could be had only at the peril of the public safety.

Fourth. To the end that personal liberty and property may be protected against invasion not essential to the public health—not required by public necessity—the regulations and proceedings of boards of health are subject to judicial review, ... according to the circumstances. In passing upon such regulations and proceedings, the courts consider, first, whether interference with personal liberty or property was reasonably necessary to the public health, and, second, if the means used and the extent of the interference were reasonably necessary for the accomplishment of the purpose to be attained.

Fifth.... The courts must determine whether there is any real relation between the preservation of the public health and the [measure at issue]. If the statute or the regulations made or the proceedings taken under it are not reasonably appropriate to the end in view, the necessity for curtailment of individual liberty, which is essential to the validity of such statutes and regulations and proceedings, is wanting, and the courts must declare them invalid, as violative of constitutional right....

In applying these principles, it is to be borne in mind that the case under consideration is unusual, imposing upon the Aiken board of health a delicate and unpleasant duty. Miss Kirk is not only a lady of refinement, highly esteemed in the community, but she is quite advanced in years. The proceedings of the board show clearly their solicitude to treat Miss Kirk with courtesy and consideration. . . .

That Miss Kirk is afflicted with anaesthetic leprosy contracted while engaged in missionary work in Brazil is admitted. While there is a strong showing that the anaesthetic form of the disease is only slightly contagious, when the distressing nature of the malady is regarded, it is manifest that the board were well within their duty in requiring the victim of it to be isolated. The case then turns on whether, under the principles above stated, . . . the manner of the isolation was so clearly beyond what was necessary to the public protection that the court ought to enjoin it as arbitrary. . . . There is hardly any danger of contagion from Miss Kirk, except by touch, or at least close personal association. What is more important than these opinions is the uncontroverted fact that Miss Kirk has for many years lived in the city of Aiken, attended church services, taught in the Sunday school, mingled freely with the people in social life, resting on the opinion of Dr. Hutchinson, a distinguished London specialist, that her disease was not contagious, and in all that time there has been nothing to indicate that she has imparted the disease to any other person. Was there any necessity to send such a patient to the pesthouse? The board of health had established a strict quarantine of her dwelling, and there was no evidence that Miss Kirk had made any effort to violate it. The maintenance of this quarantine, we cannot doubt, afforded complete protection to the public. It is true the board could not be expected to maintain a permanent quarantine of a house in the heart of the city of Aiken; but the city council had agreed to build for the purpose of isolation a comfortable cottage outside of the city limits, which could have been completed in a short time.

There is some conflict in the affidavits as to the condition of the pesthouse; but it is not denied that it is a structure of four small rooms in a row, with no piazzas, used heretofore for the isolation of negroes with smallpox, situated within a hundred yards of the place where the trash of the city, except its offensive offal, is collected and burned. The smoke from this pile is blown through the house. The board of health, it is true, have made it less uncomfortable by painting and some other work; but, with this improvement, we are forced to the conclusion that even temporary isolation in such a place would be a serious affliction and peril to an elderly lady, enfeebled by disease, and accustomed to the comforts of life. Nothing but necessity would justify the board of health in requiring it, and we think . . . there was no good reason to conclude that such necessity existed.

EX PARTE COMPANY*
Supreme Court of Ohio
Decided December 5, 1922

Judge CLARK delivered the opinion of the court.

[Defendants Martha Company and Irene Irvin were arrested, on separate occa-sions, on the charge of violating § 13031-13 of the Ohio General Code (including

*139 N.E. 204 (Ohio 1922).

prostitution, lewdness, and assignation). While in custody, both were found to have sexually transmitted diseases (syphilis and gonorrhea). The commissioner of health of the city of Akron confined them in their detention home under a quarantine for approximately two months (the time necessary to render each noninfectious through treatment). The defendants filed writs of habeas corpus, protesting that their detention violated their constitutional right to due process. Refusing the writs, the Supreme Court of Ohio upheld the state statute permitting the detention of the defendants as a legitimate exercise of the state's police powers.]

Regulation 2 of the Sanitary Code . . . named, classified, and declared dangerous to the public health certain diseases and disabilities, . . . includ[ing] . . . chancroid, gonorrhea, and syphilis. Regulation 18 of the Sanitary Code declares such diseases to be contagious, infectious, communicable, and dangerous to the public health. Regulation 23 empowers the health commissioner of each city to make examination of persons reasonably suspected of having a venereal disease. All known prostitutes and persons associating with them shall be considered as reasonably suspected of having a venereal disease. Regulation 24 provides that the health commissioner may quarantine any person who has, or is reasonably suspected of having, a venereal disease, whenever in his opinion quarantine is necessary for the protection of the public health. . . .

. . . The right of the state through the exercise of its police power to subject persons and property to reasonable and proper restraints in order to secure the general comfort, health, and prosperity of the state is no longer open to question. In the American constitutional system the power to establish the necessary police regulations has been left with the several states. . . .

The regulations here under consideration, if otherwise lawful, are not in conflict with any provision of the federal or state Constitutions.

It is urged that the Sanitary Code, and the particular regulations in question, are in opposition to and violative of subsection c of § 13031-17:

> Any person charged with a violation of § 13031-13 of the General Code, shall, upon the order of the court having jurisdiction of such case, be subjected to examination to determine if such person is infected with a venereal disease. . . . No person charged with a violation of § 13031-13 of the General Code shall be discharged from custody, paroled or placed on probation if he or she has a venereal disease in an infective stage unless the court having jurisdiction shall be assured that such person will continue medical treatment until cured or rendered noninfectious.

In the cases here considered it is to be observed that both of the petitioners were charged with violations of § 13031-13. Regulation 24 provides that such infected persons shall be subject to quarantine. The statutory provision is that such infected persons shall not be discharged from custody, paroled, or placed on probation. No inconsistency is found as between the regulations complained of and the provisions of subsection c of § 13031-17. In either event quarantine is established. Quarantine in the sense herein used means detention to the point of preserving the infected person from contact with others. The power to so quarantine in proper case and reasonable way is not open to question. It is exercised by the state and the subdivisions of the state daily. The protection of the health and lives of the public is paramount, and those who by conduct and association contract such disease as makes them a menace to the health and morals of the community must submit to such regulation as will protect the public. . . .

It is our conclusion that the provisions of §§ 1232, 1234, 1235, and 1236, General Code, creating a state department of health, a public health council, and authorizing such public health council "to make and amend sanitary regulations to be of general application throughout the state," General Code § 1235, and to provide for the certification, publication, and enforcement of such regulations, is a lawful and valid exercise of legislative power.

．　．　．　．　．

The Ohio Supreme Court upheld a quarantine regulation that "all known prostitutes and people associated with them shall be considered as reasonably suspected of having a venereal disease." "Suspect conduct and association" were deemed sufficient to justify imposing control measures. An Illinois court accepted similarly unfounded assumptions: "suspected" prostitutes were considered "natural subjects and carriers of venereal disease," making it "logical and natural that suspicion be cast upon them" (*People ex rel. Baker v. Strautz*, 54 N.E.2d 441, 444 [Ill. 1944]).

B. Modern Era

In the following case, *City of New York v. Antoinette R.*, a New York trial court authorized the isolation of a woman with TB. Although deferential to public health authorities, the opinion reiterates that states must have a substantial public health interest and afford individuals their due process rights. Such procedural protections are critical to protect individuals from use of the public health power that may be unwarranted or unjustified.

CITY OF NEW YORK V. ANTOINETTE R.*
Supreme Court, Queens County
Decided April 21, 1995

Judge McGANN delivered the opinion of the court.

[The city health commissioner sought enforcement of an order requiring the forcible detention of Antoinette R. in a hospital setting. She had been diagnosed with active, infectious tuberculosis, and the purpose of the detention was to allow for completion of an appropriate regime of medical treatment.]

*630 N.Y.S.2d 1008 (N.Y. Sup. Ct. 1995).

Due to a resurgence of TB, New York City recently revised the Health Code to permit the detention of individuals infected with TB who have demonstrated an inability to voluntarily comply with appropriate medical treatment. Thus, effective April 29, 1993, New York City Health Code § 11.47 was amended to give the Commissioner of Health the authority to issue an order for the removal or detention in a hospital or other treatment facility of a person who has active TB. The prerequisite for an order is that there is a substantial likelihood, based on the person's past or present behavior, that the individual cannot be relied upon to participate in or complete an appropriate prescribed course of medication or, if necessary, follow required contagion precautions for TB. Such behavior may include the refusal or failure to take medication or to complete treatment for TB, to keep appointments for the treatment of TB, or a disregard for contagion precautions.

The statute provides certain due process safeguards when detention is ordered. For example, there are requirements for an appraisal of the risk posed to others and a review of less restrictive alternatives which were attempted or considered. Furthermore, there must be a court review within five days at the patient's request, and court review within sixty days and at ninety-day intervals thereafter. The detainee also has the right to counsel, to have counsel provided, and to have friends or relatives notified. . . .

. . . When [TB] initially becomes active, it is often highly infectious, that is, capable of being transmitted to others. A person with infectious TB can normally be rendered non-infectious within days to weeks. Thereafter, the individual must continue to take a full course of medication, generally for six to nine months, to cure the active TB. If a patient stops taking the appropriate medication before the expiration of these six to nine months, however, that patient will likely become infectious again. Moreover, when the medical regime is interrupted, and the TB resurges in an infectious state, the organisms in the individual's system may eventually mutate and become resistant to the original drugs prescribed. The more times medication is suspended, the more likely is the chance of developing a strain of TB which is resistant to drugs.

These multi-drug resistant [MDR] strains of TB stay infectious and active over longer periods of time and therefore require long-term treatment with more toxic drugs. By comparison, the standard treatment for non-resistant TB consists of administering two drugs, isoniazid and rifampin, for approximately six months until the patient is cured. The cure rate for those completing this treatment is considered 100%. MDR-TB, on the other hand, is resistant to these drugs and to as many as seven other antibiotics. To obtain a cure rate of 60% or less, toxic drugs must be maintained over a minimum period of eighteen to twenty-four months. The most critical characteristic of these MDR strains is that they are capable of being transmitted directly to others during the infectious stage. . . .

. . . The Board recognized that the failure of a TB patient to complete an effective course of therapy creates the likelihood of relapse and facilitates development of drug resistant strains of the disease. The Board therefore decreed that the refusal or failure of TB patients, whether or not infectious, to complete a course of anti-TB therapy creates a significant threat to the public health. Accordingly, the New York City Health Code was amended to allow the Commissioner to issue orders of detention [through] . . . an application to the court for enforcement . . . [based on] clear and convincing evidence [of] the particularized circumstances constituting the necessity for the detention. . . .

The [Commissioner's] request for enforcement of the order . . . is granted. The [Commissioner] has demonstrated through clear and convincing evidence the respondent's inability to comply with a prescribed course of medication in a less restrictive environment. [Antoinette R.] has repeatedly sought medical treatment for the infectious stages of the disease and has consistently withdrawn from medical treatment once symptoms abate. She has also exhibited a pattern of behavior which is consistent with one who does not understand the full import of her condition nor the risks she poses to others, both the public and her family. On the contrary, she has repeatedly tried to hide the history of her condition from medical personnel. Although the court is sympathetic to the fact that she has recently undergone an epiphany of sorts, there is nothing in the record which would indicate that once she leaves the controlled setting of the hospital she would have the self-discipline to continue her cooperation. Moreover, her past behavior and lack of compliance with outpatient treatment when her listed residence was her mother's house, makes it all the more difficult to have confidence that her mother's good intentions will prevail over the respondent's inclinations to avoid treatments. In any event, the court will reevaluate the progress of the respondent's ability to cooperate in a less restrictive setting during its next review of the order in ninety days.

Accordingly, [Antoinette R.] shall continue to be detained in a hospital setting until [she] . . . has completed an appropriate course of medication for TB, or a change in circumstances indicates that the respondent can be relied upon to complete the prescribed course of medication without being in detention.

.   .   .   .   .

Two recent cases underscore the importance of procedural protections for quarantined individuals. In California, Hongkham Souvannarath, a Laotian refugee diagnosed with multidrug-resistant tuberculosis (MDR-TB), received a notice (written in English) requiring her to appear for mandatory examination at the county TB clinic or face isolation and quarantine. After she failed to appear at the clinic, she was taken at gunpoint to the county jail, where the county planned to detain her for the duration of her treatment—up to two years. She was treated as a prisoner and handcuffed to her bed for treatments. Souvannarath challenged her confinement, and a California appellate court ruled that the use of jails for isolation and quarantine violates California law (*Souvannarath v. Hadden*, 116 Cal. Rptr. 2d 7 [Cal. Ct. App. 2002]). In another case, an Arizona man, Robert Daniels, tested positive for MDR-TB and county officials ordered that he be quarantined. Daniels was also treated like a prisoner: he was confined for nine months to a hospital's prisoner unit. The resultant case, *Daniels v. Maricopa County*, No. 2:07-CV-01080 (D. Ariz. filed May 30, 2007), is still pending. *Souvannarath* and *Daniels* underscore the enduring relevance of *Antoinette R.* and the continuing difficulty of balancing public health against individual rights.

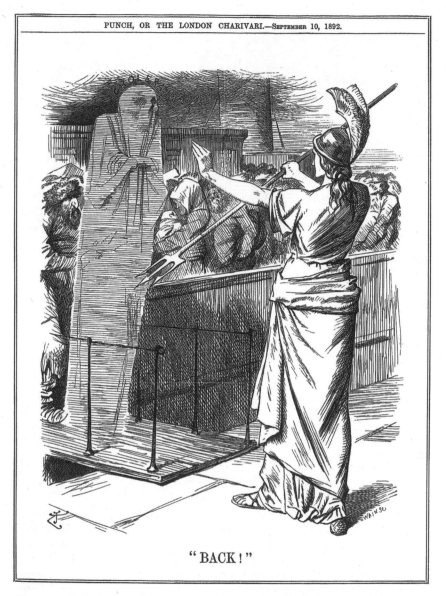

"BACK!"

Photo 27. In this 1892 illustration, Britannia prevents cholera from leaving a ship that has just arrived at a British port. A cholera pandemic claimed 200,000 lives in Russia and almost 1.5 percent of the population in Germany during the early 1890s. Quarantine efforts were integral to preventing cholera from spreading in Britain. Reproduced by permission from *Punch, or the London Chiavari*, © Ann Ronan Picture Library/HIP/The Image Works, September 10, 1892.

III. MEDICAL COUNTERMEASURES AND PUBLIC HEALTH INTERVENTIONS

A. *Severe Acute Respiratory Syndrome*

SARS is a serious form of pneumonia, resulting in acute respiratory distress and sometimes death. The 2003 SARS epidemic provides a dramatic example both of how quickly disease may spread in a globalized world and of the importance of coordinated international efforts to contain disease. Not only did SARS test the limits of national and global health systems, but it also raised critical legal and ethical issues regarding the level of intrusion into personal liberty and privacy that are justified by the specter of an emergent infectious disease. The following excerpt discusses some of these difficult issues and develops principles for acting under situations of scientific uncertainty.

ETHICAL AND LEGAL CHALLENGES POSED BY SEVERE ACUTE RESPIRATORY SYNDROME: IMPLICATIONS FOR THE CONTROL OF SEVERE INFECTIOUS DISEASE THREATS*

Lawrence O. Gostin, Ronald Bayer, and Amy L. Fairchild

Not long after the first reports of [SARS] began to appear in February 2003 and as nations and the international community began to confront the spread of the new disease, it became clear that a host of ethical and legal issues had begun to surface. . . . In several respects, SARS took society back to a pretherapeutic era with no definitive diagnostic test, a nonspecific case definition, and no effective vaccine or treatment. . . .

ETHICAL AND LEGAL RECOMMENDATIONS FOR RESPONDING TO SEVERE INFECTIOUS DISEASE THREATS

. . . We take as a starting point the centrality of the precautionary principle for the ethics of public health. The principle stipulates an obligation to protect populations against reasonably foreseeable threats, even under conditions of uncertainty. First articulated in the context of environmental hazards, the precautionary principle seeks to forestall disasters and guide decision making in the context of incomplete knowledge. Given the potential costs of inaction, it is the failure to implement preventive measures that requires justification. . . .

For nations that share the central values of a liberal democracy, safeguards of individual rights must bound the precautionary principle. Consequently, the least restrictive/intrusive alternative, fairness and justice (both procedural and substan-

*Reprinted from *JAMA* 290 (2003): 3229–37. Copyright © 2003 American Medical Association. All rights reserved.

tive), and transparency provide the basis for effective public health actions that are not unduly burdensome on individual rights.

Requiring the least restrictive/intrusive alternative that can effectively achieve a legitimate public health goal represents a means to impose limits on state interventions consistent with the traditions of privacy, liberty, and freedom of association. The standard does not require public health authorities to adopt measures that are less effective but does require the least invasive intervention that will achieve the objective. How to strike the balance between degrees of efficacy and invasiveness will inevitably remain a matter of controversy.

Justice requires that the benefits and burdens of public health action be fairly distributed, thus precluding the unjustified targeting of already socially vulnerable populations. . . . Procedural justice requires a fair and independent hearing for individuals who are subjected to burdensome public health action. Due process requirements . . . affirm the dignity of the person [and help ensure] accurate decision making.

Finally, transparency requires government officials to make decisions in an open and fully accountable manner. It further demands civic deliberation and public participation in the policy-making process. Individuals should understand the facts and reasons justifying public health interventions, the goals of intervention, and the steps taken to safeguard individual rights. . . .

SURVEILLANCE AND CONTACT TRACING: THE LIMITS OF PRIVACY

Surveillance, as an epidemiological measure and a call to intervene, raises issues regarding the limits of privacy. . . . The absence of legal and ethical challenges to [surveillance] in recent decades—the debates over [name-based reporting of HIV patients] were a striking exception—suggests that name-based surveillance has been recognized as an acceptable limit on privacy. The state, of course, has to meet rigorous standards: demonstrate an important need to know and intervene, make decisions openly, consult with the relevant communities, and use data only for legitimate public health purposes. [Ed.—These ethical and legal limits on surveillance activities are discussed generally in chapter 8.]

ISOLATION AND QUARANTINE: THE LIMITS OF LIBERTY

Isolation and quarantine . . . raise questions about the limits of liberty. Certainly, such separation is warranted to avert significant risks of transmission. But beyond that, there are questions of the level of risk that justifies loss of liberty, the social and economic harms, and potential for using public health as a subterfuge for discrimination. . . . We recommend the following criteria to assess the ethical and legal justification for isolation and quarantine: scientific assessment of risk, targeting restrictive measures, a safe and humane environment, fair treatment and social justice, procedural due process, and the least restrictive alternative.

Scientific Assessment of Risk . . .

Isolation of a confirmed SARS case during the period of infectiousness is firmly supported by legal tradition and ethics. All legal systems, as well as international human rights, permit governments to infringe on personal liberty to prevent a significant risk to the public. . . . Since those with SARS pose a direct threat to close contacts, their liberty can be justifiably restrained. However, if a SARS case is unconfirmed or if the individual simply has been exposed or is suspected of being exposed, the justification for restricting liberty is less clear.

Faced with the prospect of a significant risk—measured in terms of the probability of transmission and the severity of harm—populations should be protected, even in the context of medical uncertainty. The precautionary principle provides a justification for such restrictions: government may act to prevent tangible harms to the population even without complete scientific information. . . .

Targeting Restrictive Measures

In principle, restrictive measures should be limited to those known to be infectious. But in the case of SARS, the uncertainty about how wide to cast the net of quarantine for exposed, asymptomatic individuals is framed by the absence at this juncture of a diagnostic assay that can rapidly distinguish between the infected and merely exposed with high specificity. Were such a test available, it would be possible to screen exposed individuals, subjecting only those who were infected—but not yet symptomatic—to isolation. Under such circumstances, individuals would have the choice of being tested and, if test results are negative, being freed from the burden of quarantine; those choosing not to be tested would be subject to quarantine.

A Safe and Habitable Environment

Since isolation and quarantine are designed to promote well-being and not to punish the individual, public health authorities have the obligation to provide quarters that are decent and not degrading. Jails and prisons are unacceptable settings for confinement. Patients should have adequate health care, protection from further exposure to SARS, the necessities of life such as food and clothing, and means of communication with family, friends, and attorneys. . . . Ideally, patients should be placed in hospitals or other health care settings that offer skilled medical and nursing care, infection control, and isolation facilities. . . .

Contemporary public health practice favors "sheltering in place," preferably in a person's home. Home confinement is less restrictive, more humane, and more likely to achieve public acceptance. Nevertheless, home quarantines can only be morally justified in contexts where residential units permit exposed but asymptomatic individuals to remain confined without imposing risks on those with whom they live. . . .

Fair Treatment and Social Justice

Fairness may require consideration of compensation, particularly for the poor who lose vital income during isolation or quarantine. . . . Such measures were taken in Taiwan where "persons who completed quarantine received the equivalent of US $147" (CDC 2003, 682). . . . Among the possibilities are ensuring that sick pay benefits—where they are contractually available—be guaranteed to those deprived of the ability to work because of quarantine; the provision of basic welfare benefits to those without access to sick pay; and an extension of disaster relief now available to communities faced with flood, storms, and earthquakes. . . .

Procedural Due Process

Due process requires the right to be heard by an independent tribunal in a timely manner with representation by an attorney. The US Supreme Court has noted that civil confinement constitutes "a significant deprivation of liberty" that "can engender adverse social consequences" (*Addington v. Texas*, 441 U.S. 418, 429 [1979]). Although some may argue that home quarantine need not trigger a full-blown hearing, we believe that anyone deprived of liberty under color of law, whatever the place of confinement, should have available a due process hearing. In a public health emergency, it may be necessary to confine individuals before a hearing is held, but a speedy hearing should, if requested, follow. . . .

The Least Restrictive Alternative

Even if all of the foregoing conditions are satisfied, public health authorities should resort to isolation or quarantine only if it is the least restrictive/intrusive alternative. During the first SARS outbreak, broad quarantines were justifiable because of the uncertainties of risk. If careful examination of that experience reveals that more circumscribed measures would serve the public good, more narrowly drawn quarantines would be appropriate.

TRAVEL ADVISORIES AND RESTRICTIONS: LIMITS ON THE FREEDOM OF MOVEMENT

The right to travel within a nation or internationally is vitally important legally, economically, and politically. . . .

International law affords a right to travel within one's country. Individuals also have the human right to leave and return to their country of origin. Yet, these rights may be permissibly restricted on public health grounds. . . .

. . . We maintain that government cannot abridge the right to travel without a legitimate public health purpose and that restrictions must be narrowly drawn and targeted. . . .

Limiting travel is justified by a legitimate public health purpose. Restricting travel by those with SARS, and even those recently exposed to SARS, poses few moral quandaries. There is no right to board conveyances if in so doing one imposes ineliminable risks on others. Nor is there a right of entry into a country if one is sick with an infectious condition marked by high case fatality rates. Consequently, screening passengers before embarkation and at borders is legally and morally appropriate.

The right of return to a person's home country should not be denied. International human rights law entitles individuals to return to their country of citizenship. The reasoning is that people have a right to a place to reside and should not suffer the indignity of forced exclusion from their home country. In emergency situations, however, this principle may be limited when infectious individuals pose a risk to others on international conveyances. As soon as it is safe to do so, individuals infected with or exposed to SARS should be permitted to return to their home countries.

Travel advisories to SARS-affected areas are warranted to accurately inform the public. Travel to areas marked by SARS outbreaks poses a different set of issues. Travel advisories or warnings that inform individuals about the risks of travel to certain locales are not problematic. Indeed, it would represent a failure of public health responsibility not to issue such warnings. . . .

Travel restrictions to SARS-affected areas are justified only where return travel imposes a serious risk to others. More complex and troubling is the imposition of travel restrictions to SARS outbreak areas, such as those that were imposed by some US universities. Competent adults, in general, have the right to assume risks, once informed of the consequences of their decisions. However, when travel to an outbreak area poses a risk of acquiring a fatal illness and where return travel might

impose hazards on others, the case for restrictions is enhanced by the harm principle [and could be justifiable]. . . .

CONCLUSION: ACTING UNDER SCIENTIFIC UNCERTAINTY

There is no way to avoid the dilemmas posed by acting without full scientific knowledge. Failure to move aggressively can have catastrophic consequences. Actions
that prove to have been unnecessary will be viewed as draconian and based on hysteria. The only safeguard is transparency. International and national public health
agencies must be willing to make clear the bases for restrictive measures and openly
acknowledge when new evidence warrants reconsideration of policies. Adoption of
ethical recommendations will be a necessary concomitant of epidemic control in
democratic societies. Public health decisions will reflect in a profound way the manner in which societies both implicitly and explicitly balance values that are intimately
related and inherently in tension.

B. *Tuberculosis*

A scourge thought to be defeated in developed countries decades ago,
TB, or the "white plague," has reemerged since the 1980s as a signifi-
cant threat to global health. Celia W. Dugger, reporting for the *New
York Times* (2008), describes the response in South Africa, where

> The Jose Pearson TB Hospital . . . is like a prison for the sick. It is
> encircled by three fences topped with coils of razor wire to keep patients
> infected with lethal strains of tuberculosis from escaping. . . .
>   "We're being held here like prisoners, but we didn't commit a crime,"
> [said one patient]. "I've seen people die and die and die. The only dis-
> charge you get from this place is to the mortuary." . . .
>   As extensively drug-resistant TB rapidly emerges as a global threat[,] . . .
> South Africa is grappling with a sticky ethical problem: how to balance the
> liberty of individual patients against the need to protect society. . . .
>   [Some argue for isolation in TB hospitals;] other public health experts
> say overcrowded, poorly ventilated hospitals have themselves been a driv-
> ing force in spreading the disease in South Africa. The public would be
> safer if patients were treated at home, they say, with regular monitoring
> by health workers and contagion-control measures for the family. Locking
> up the sick until death will also discourage those with undiagnosed cases
> from coming forward, most likely driving the epidemic underground.

The emergence of MDR-TB and extensively drug-resistant tuberculosis (XDR-TB) has raised questions regarding the adequacy of public
health powers, within the United States as well as in the international
arena. The following excerpt examines some of these limitations
through the lens of the Andrew Speaker incident. In May 2007, Speaker
boarded a plane and flew from Atlanta, Georgia, to Paris, against the
medical advice of county health officials who had diagnosed him with

MDR-TB. He traveled to Greece and then Rome, and then back to the United States through the Czech Republic and Canada. Howard Markel, David P. Fidler, and I argue that Speaker's journey sheds light on some of the notable gaps in our public health powers, particularly with respect to compulsory measures for disease containment. Others contend to the contrary that the incident undermines the case for more expansive use of coercive public health powers (Parmet 2007).

EXTENSIVELY DRUG-RESISTANT TUBERCULOSIS: AN ISOLATION ORDER, PUBLIC HEALTH POWERS, AND A GLOBAL CRISIS*

Howard Markel, Lawrence O. Gostin, and David P. Fidler

. . . Physicians diagnosed Speaker with pulmonary TB in March 2007. . . . Susceptibility testing determined that Speaker's TB was multidrug resistant, which prompted county public health authorities to advise Speaker orally on May 10 not to travel. . . . Instead, Speaker advanced his travel by 48 hours and flew from Atlanta, Georgia, to Paris, France, on May 12. From May 11 through 13, county public health officials tried to deliver written notice to Speaker that travel would be against medical advice and would risk harming others' health. On May 22, the CDC [Centers for Disease Control and Prevention] confirmed that Speaker had XDR-TB. [Ed.–At the time this piece was published, it was thought that Speaker had XDR-TB; later diagnostics confirmed the initial, less serious diagnosis of MDR-TB.]

Speaker's wedding and honeymoon took him to Greece and then Rome, where the CDC contacted him by telephone on May 22 to inform him that he had XDR-TB, should not travel further on commercial airlines, and should report to Italian health authorities while US officials pursued options for his return home. Instead, Speaker flew to Prague, then to Montreal, Canada, and then drove into the United States.

Although the CDC placed Speaker's name on a health surveillance list, a US border guard allowed Speaker into the United States despite seeing the CDC's warning. Once in the country, CDC located Speaker, instructed him to report to Bellevue Hospital in New York City, New York, and indicated that failure to do so would violate federal quarantine law. After 72 hours at Bellevue under a provisional isolation order, Speaker was transported by the CDC to Atlanta and a federal isolation order was issued against him. This order was the first such federal order since a suspected smallpox carrier was quarantined in 1963. . . .

LEGAL AUTHORITY FOR ISOLATION AND QUARANTINE IN THE UNITED STATES

The Complexity of Quarantine Law

Legal authority for public health powers, including isolation and quarantine, exists at local, state, and federal levels. This situation produces problems related to federalism: Which level of government may act? Which laws apply, and in what circumstances? Theoretically, local and state law addresses threats confined to a single

*Reprinted from *JAMA* 298 (2007): 83–86. Copyright © 2007 American Medical Association. All rights reserved.

city, county, or state; federal law applies to diseases arriving from foreign countries or being transmitted across state lines.

Behind that theory lies a complex problem regarding the "lead" government official in any given situation. Public health emergencies require clear lines of authority, and the Speaker case illustrates some breakdowns in this respect: county public health officials were allegedly not clear in their instructions to Speaker because they told him not to travel but that he did not pose a risk to others; and a federal border guard let Speaker into the United States despite being aware of CDC's notification that Speaker should be detained.

State Quarantine Authority

State authority to compel isolation and quarantine derives from the police power. Although all states have authorized isolation and quarantine, these laws vary considerably. Often, different approaches are not a problem, but variation could prevent or delay effective responses to a multistate emergency. Disparate legal structures can also undermine cooperation among state and federal officials. In addition, state quarantine laws are often old and do not reflect contemporary scientific understandings of disease or changes in the protection of civil liberties.

In light of recent threats, states have begun to reconsider quarantine authority within their emergency response systems. [After the 2001 anthrax attacks, President George W. Bush] urged states to review their quarantine authorities as a homeland security priority.... The Speaker case will, again, encourage state governments to revisit their quarantine laws.

Federal Quarantine Authority

Federal quarantine authority grants the secretary of the US Department of Health and Human Services the power to issue regulations to prevent the introduction, transmission, or interstate spread of communicable diseases into or within the United States and to apprehend, detain, or conditionally release individuals infected with "quarantinable diseases" specified by executive order. Infectious TB is a quarantinable disease.

The Speaker case illustrates weaknesses in federal quarantine authority. First, federal powers apply only to a small number of diseases, depriving the CDC of flexibility to respond to novel threats. For a new threat, the president must issue an executive order making the disease quarantinable.... Second, federal rules do not authorize a range of powers, including screening, contact tracing, and directly observed therapy, which may be needed to address certain threats, including XDR-TB. Third, federal quarantine law lacks adequate due process protections [and is arguably unconstitutional] because it does not give affected individuals a right to a fair hearing....

Proposed Revisions to the Federal Quarantine Regulations

Recognizing these problems, the Department of Health and Human Services proposed new regulations in late 2005. The proposed rules would expand the scope of federal power by defining "ill person" to include those with signs or symptoms commonly associated with quarantinable diseases (eg, fever, rash, persistent cough, or diarrhea), thus affording CDC greater flexibility. The proposed regulations would require airlines and other carriers to screen passengers at borders; report cases of illness or death to the CDC; distribute health alert notices to crew and passengers; collect and transmit personal passenger information; order physical examination of exposed persons; and require passengers to disclose information about their contacts, travel itinerary, and medical history. The proposed rules also build more due process protections into federal quarantine law. . . .

The revisions to federal quarantine regulations proved controversial and have not yet been adopted. . . . The travel industry complained about the costs imposed on it to collect passenger data. Civil libertarians argued that the new rules would not protect privacy adequately. Due process advocates criticized the proposal for providing no right to a hearing for "provisional" quarantines lasting up to 3 business days. In addition, the proposal did not address all concerns about due process requirements for full quarantine measures because it required quarantined individuals to request a hearing, provided for informal proceedings, and permitted a CDC employee to preside over the hearing rather than an impartial tribunal. . . .

INTERNATIONAL DIMENSIONS

Speaker's odyssey also reveals the international dimensions of XDR-TB, which highlight questions about how the United States exercises public health powers in a global context, how international law applies to XDR-TB, and what strategies exist to address the global XDR-TB crisis.

Travel Restrictions on Persons Leaving the United States

Speaker's case raises questions about the government's ability to prevent a person who poses a health risk from leaving the United States. County officials orally advised Speaker not to travel, but what government body could have prevented him from traveling to Europe? Given the international context, the federal government is the relevant constitutional authority. Federal law focuses, however, on preventing disease importation and does not mention preventing disease exportation. Neither statutory law nor existing or proposed federal quarantine regulations address the need to prevent persons in the United States who pose a health risk from leaving the country.

Extrajurisdictional Application of US Public Health Law

The CDC advised Speaker to report to Italian authorities, but he did not follow this advice. This raises the question of whether the United States can enforce federal quarantine orders on US citizens in other countries. Federal law does not apply outside the United States unless Congress intends for it to so apply. Congress expressed no such intent in federal public health law, prescribing that federal quarantine regulations " . . . shall be applicable only to individuals coming into a State or possession from a foreign country or a possession" (42 U.S.C. § 264 [2005]).

Screening for Public Health Threats at US Borders

Speaker's entry into the United States focuses attention on screening for health threats at US borders. Unlike Speaker's situation, the typical problems concern the failure or inability of border control systems to identify health threats. . . .

XDR-TB and the New International Health Regulations

Speaker's case also raises broader concerns about the role of international law in addressing XDR-TB. Here, the new International Health Regulations, adopted in May 2005 and entered into force on June 15, 2007 (IHR 2005), deserve attention. [Ed.– see chapter 7 for a discussion of the IHR.] First, public health reactions to Speaker's travels demonstrate that XDR-TB cases may constitute public health emergencies of international concern that must be notified to WHO [the World Health Organization] under the IHR 2005. . . . The United States notified WHO about the Speaker case on May 24 despite the IHR 2005 not being in force. An obligation to report XDR-TB cases could improve global surveillance. . . .

A WHO task force argued that XDR-TB does not constitute a public health emergency of international concern because such a declaration is "really only intended for outbreaks of acute disease, rather than the 'acute-on-chronic' situation of . . . XDR-TB" (WHO Global Task Force on XDR-TB 2007, 5). This interpretation is questionable because the IHR 2005 never uses "acute disease" to define its scope. . . . XDR-TB may be an early test case for how WHO and its member states apply the IHR 2005.

Second, Speaker's isolation order requires examination of whether compulsory measures may be increasingly necessary to contain XDR-TB around the world. The IHR 2005 recognizes the need for such measures but requires that countries apply them in a manner consistent with scientific, public health, and human rights principles.

ADDRESSING THE GLOBAL CRISIS OF XDR-TB

Speaker's travails partially lifted the veil on the global XDR-TB crisis. How do the United States and the international community confront the emergence of XDR-TB around the world? A host of challenges exist, including improving surveillance, designing nonpharmacological interventions that protect public health while respecting human rights, inventing better diagnostics, managing XDR-TB's deadly synergy with HIV/AIDS, creating new antibiotics that are available in developing countries, and building health system capacities to handle the burden of XDR-TB. The grim march of TB from MDR-TB to XDR-TB does not bode well for achieving the changes needed to produce robust global responses to the extremely drug-resistant manifestation of the white plague. XDR-TB threatens global health, challenges the rule of law, and requires improved international cooperation.

C. Pandemic Influenza

The potential threat to human health of pandemic influenza is nothing short of staggering. Scientists fear that the influenza (A) H5N1 strain of bird flu virus could mutate into a form that spreads easily among humans, potentially sparking a pandemic that kills millions. This concern was reinforced when a novel strain of influenza A—H1N1, or swine flu—spread rapidly through Mexico in April 2009 and spread to every part of the globe within months. The global response highlighted enforcement gaps of public health regulatory bodies such as the World Health Organization, despite the new powers granted to it in the recently revised International Health Regulations (described in chapter 7). Moreover, "reminiscent of past responses, many governments [acted] out of fear or economic and political self-interest rather than . . . scientific reason" (Gostin 2009, 2376). Overall, this recent outbreak serves as example of why it is essential to "have an international system guided by science that has adequate funding for research and public health . . . that conforms to the rule of international law" (Gostin 2009, 2378).

In the context of widespread infection and necessary resource constraints, the issue of rationing flu vaccines and antiviral medications will take center stage. It is generally accepted that the social good is served by granting priority access to health workers, defense forces, and emergency workers. But how should priority levels be assigned to other members of the population? Should higher priority be granted to children and the elderly? or to younger, more productive members of the population? The potential for a pandemic to "exacerbate existing social and economic inequalities" has prompted some to take a social justice approach to rationing vaccines in a pandemic, focusing on the needs of disadvantaged groups (Uscher-Pines et al. 2007; quotation, 33). In the following excerpt, the bioethicists Ezekiel J. Emanuel and Alan Wertheimer provide an overview of different ethical frameworks for distributing scarce vaccines.

WHO SHOULD GET INFLUENZA VACCINE WHEN NOT ALL CAN?*
Ezekiel J. Emanuel and Alan Wertheimer

The potential threat of pandemic influenza is staggering: 1.9 million deaths, 90 million people sick, and nearly 10 million people hospitalized, with almost 1.5 million requiring intensive-care units (ICUs) in the United States. The National Vaccine Advisory Committee (NVAC) and the Advisory Committee on Immunization Policy (ACIP) have jointly recommended a prioritization scheme that places vaccine workers, health-care providers, and the ill elderly at the top, and healthy people aged 2 to 64 at the very bottom, even under embalmers. The primary goal informing the recommendation was to "decrease health impacts including severe morbidity and death" (U.S. Department of Health and Human Services 2005a, D-10); a secondary goal was minimizing societal and economic impacts. . . .

THE INESCAPABILITY OF RATIONING

Because of current uncertainty of its value, only "a limited amount of avian influenza A (H5N1) vaccine is being stockpiled" (U.S. Department of Health and Human Services 2005b, S6-5). Furthermore, it will take at least 4 months from identification of a candidate vaccine strain until production of the very first vaccine. At

*Reprinted from *Science* 312 (2006): 854–55.

present, there are few production facilities worldwide that make influenza vaccine, and only one completely in the USA. Global capacity for influenza vaccine production is just 425 million doses per annum, if all available factories would run at full capacity after a vaccine was developed. Under currently existing capabilities for manufacturing vaccine, it is likely that more than 90% of the U.S. population will not be vaccinated in the first year. Distributing the limited supply will require determining priority groups.

Who will be at highest risk? Our experience with three influenza pandemics presents a complex picture. The mortality profile of a future pandemic could be U-shaped, as it was in the mild-to-moderate pandemics of 1957 and 1968 and interpandemic influenza seasons, in which the very young and the old are at highest risk. Or, the mortality profile could be an attenuated W shape, as it was during the devastating 1918 pandemic, in which the highest risk occurred among people between 20 and 40 years of age, while the elderly were not at high excess risk. Even during pandemics, the elderly appear to be at no higher risk than during interpandemic influenza seasons.

... With limited vaccine supply, uncertainty over who will be at highest risk of infection and complications, and questions about which historic pandemic experience is most applicable, society faces a fundamental ethical dilemma: Who should get the vaccine first?

THE NVAC AND ACIP PRIORITY RANKINGS

Many potential ethical principles for rationing health care have been proposed. "Save the most lives" is commonly used in emergencies, such as burning buildings, although "women and children first" played a role on the Titanic. "First come, first served" operates in other emergencies . . . ; "Save the most quality life years" is central to cost-effectiveness rationing. "Save the worst-off" plays a role in allocating organs for transplantation. "Reciprocity"—giving priority to people willing to donate their own organs—has been proposed. "Save those most likely to fully recover" guided priorities for giving penicillin to soldiers with syphilis in World War II. Save those "instrumental in making society flourish" through economic productivity or by "contributing to the well-being of others" has been proposed. . . .

The save-the-most-lives principle was invoked by NVAC and ACIP. It justifies giving top priority to workers engaged in vaccine production and distribution and health-care workers. They get higher priority not because they are intrinsically more valuable people or of greater "social worth," but because giving them first priority ensures that maximal life-saving vaccine is produced so that health care is provided to the sick. Consequently, it values all human life equally, giving every person equal consideration in who gets priority regardless of age, disability, social class, or employment. After these groups, the save-the-most-lives principle justifies priority for those predicted to be at highest risk of hospitalization and dying. We disagree with this prioritization.

LIFE-CYCLE PRINCIPLE

The save-the-most-lives principle may be justified in some emergencies when decision urgency makes it infeasible to deliberate about priority rankings and impractical to categorize individuals into priority groups. We believe that a life-cycle allocation principle . . . based on the idea that each person should have an opportunity to live through all the stages of life is more appropriate for a pandemic. There is great value in being able to pass through each life stage—to be a child, a young adult, and to then develop a career and family, and to grow old—and to enjoy a wide range of the opportunities during each stage.

Multiple considerations and intuitions support this ethical principle. Most people endorse this principle for themselves. We would prioritize our own resources to ensure we could live past the illnesses of childhood and young adulthood and would allocate fewer resources to living ever longer once we reached old age. People strongly prefer maximizing the chance of living until a ripe old age, rather than being struck down as a young person. . . .

THE INVESTMENT REFINEMENT

A pure version of the life-cycle principle would grant priority to 6-month-olds over 1-year-olds who have priority over 2-year-olds, and on. An alternative, the investment refinement, emphasizes gradations within a life span. It gives priority to people between early adolescence and middle age on the basis of the amount the person has invested in his or her life balanced by the amount left to live. Within this framework, 20-year-olds are valued more than 1-year-olds because the older individuals have more developed interests, hopes, and plans but have not had an opportunity to realize them. Although these groupings could be modified, they indicate ethically defensible distinctions among groups that can inform rationing priorities.

One other ethical principle relevant for priority ranking of influenza vaccine during a pandemic is public order. It focuses on the value of ensuring safety and the provision of necessities, such as food and fuel. We believe the investment refinement combined with the public-order principle (IRPOP) should be the ultimate objective of all pandemic response measures, including priority ranking for vaccines and interventions to limit the course of the pandemic, such as closing schools and confining people to homes. These two principles should inform decisions at the start of an epidemic when the shape of the risk curves for morbidity and mortality are largely uncertain.

Like the NVAC and ACIP ranking, the IRPOP ranking would give high priority to vaccine production and distribution workers, as well as health-care and public health workers with direct patient contact. However, contrary to the NVAC and ACIP prioritization for the sick elderly and infants, IRPOP emphasizes people between 13 and 40 years of age. The NVAC and ACIP priority ranking comports well with those groups at risk during the mild-to-moderate 1957 and 1968 pandemics. IRPOP prioritizes those age cohorts at highest risk during the devastating 1918 pandemic. Depending on patterns of flu spread, some mathematical models suggest that following IRPOP priority ranking could save the most lives overall.

CONCLUSIONS

Fortunately, even though we are worried about an influenza pandemic, it is not upon us. Indeed, the current H5N1 avian flu may never develop into a human pandemic. This gives us time both to build vaccine production capacity to minimize the need for rationing and to rationally assess policy and ethical issues about the distribution of vaccines.

IV. BIOTERRORISM

Although many agree that states need to reform their laws to enable public health officials to effectively respond to biological threats, whether these arise from bioterrorism or naturally occurring infectious disease, the question of how proposed legislation should structure an appropriate balance between individual liberties and public health is highly contentious.

Measures designed to control disease invade each of the major spheres of personal liberty: vaccination, physical examination, and medical treatment interfere with bodily integrity (see chapter 10); isolation and quarantine limit freedom of movement and association; and disease surveillance and reporting affect personal privacy (see chapter 8). Regulations designed to safeguard the public's health likewise threaten to impinge on economic interests and freedom of enterprise. Inspections and administrative searches affect commercial privacy interests; permits and licenses affect professional and business pursuits; and nuisance abatements and "takings" (including regulatory takings) affect the right to property (see chapter 12).

Promulgating legislation for emergency public health powers is controversial. Two important values are at stake: individual liberty and public safety. Though security and liberty are sometimes harmonious, they often collide. In the following pieces, George Annas and I tease out these interests, arriving at divergent opinions concerning their proper balance. In order to manage the tension between liberty and safety, each interest must be fully understood, the critical choices must be identified, and then decisions must be made deliberately and with forethought, in advance of a public health emergency. The heated debate over civil and economic liberties in an era in which bioterrorism is a plausible threat can be settled only with a principled framework for balancing individual and collective interests.

PUBLIC HEALTH LAW IN AN AGE OF TERRORISM: RETHINKING INDIVIDUAL RIGHTS AND COMMON GOODS*
Lawrence O. Gostin

This paper explores the appropriate balance between individual interests and common goods. The current focus on individualism should be seen not as fixed and

*Reprinted from *Health Affairs* 21 (November/December 2002): 79–93.

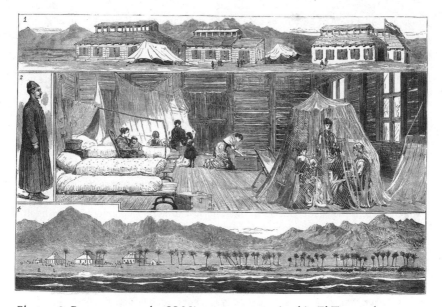

Photo 28. Passengers on the *SS Mira* were quarantined in El Tor on the Arabian coast to prevent the spread of smallpox in 1884. The image shows quarantine sheds used to house the passengers, an Egyptian manservant, the interior of the ladies' quarantine shed, and a view of El Tor from the sea. While this picture depicts a relatively pleasant experience, quarantine conditions among the working poor were often crowded and uncomfortable, and sometimes nearly intolerable. Reproduced by permission from *The Graphic*, © Oxford Science Archive/Heritage-Images/The Image Works, July 19, 1884.

authoritative, but rather as transient and culturally derived. There is, of course, an alternative philosophical tradition that sees individuals primarily as members of communities. This communitarian tradition views individuals as part of social and political networks, with each individual reliant on the others for health and security. Individuals, according to this tradition, gain value from being a part of a well-regulated society that seeks to prevent common risks.

In legal terms, this communitarian tradition is expressed in the "police power" to protect the health, safety, and security of the population. . . .

First, this paper explains modern efforts at public health law reform. Even before September 11, the Robert Wood Johnson Foundation's (RWJF's) Turning Point initiative supported comprehensive reform of antiquated public health laws—the Public Health Statute Modernization Collaborative. After the anthrax outbreak, the Centers for Disease Control and Prevention (CDC) asked the Center for Law and the Public's Health (CLPH) at Georgetown and Johns Hopkins Universities to draft the Model State Emergency Health Powers Act (MSEHPA). [Ed.—As of August 2009, this act has been introduced in whole or part through 171 bills or resolutions in forty-four states and the District of Columbia. Thirty-eight states and the District of Columbia have passed a total of 66 bills or resolutions that include provisions from or closely related to the act.]

Next, the paper shows why existing public health laws provide a weak foundation for public health practice. . . . Finally, the paper offers a systematic defense of MSEHPA. The model act has galvanized the public debate around the appropriate balance between public goods and individual rights. . . . This defense shows how MSEHPA creates strong public health powers while safeguarding individual freedoms—adopting clearer standards and more rigorous procedures than existing statutes do.

TWO NATIONAL PROJECTS FOR PUBLIC HEALTH LAW REFORM

. . . The [RWJF's] Public Health Statute Modernization Collaborative is led by a consortium of states, in partnership with federal agencies and national organizations. . . . It has published a comprehensive assessment of state public health laws, demonstrating the inadequacies of existing law to support modern public health functions. The objective is to ensure that state public health law is consistent with modern constitutional principles and reflects current scientific and ethical values underlying public health practice. . . .

. . . The law-reform process took on new urgency after the terrorist attacks of late 2001. In response, the CLPH drafted MSEHPA . . . in collaboration with members of national organizations representing governors, legislators, public health commissions, and attorneys general. There was also an extensive consultative process involving the major stakeholders such as businesses, public health and civil liberties organizations, scholars, and practitioners. . . .

. . . MSEHPA requires the development of a comprehensive plan to provide a coordinated, appropriate response in the event of a public health emergency. It facilitates the early detection of a health emergency by authorizing the reporting as well as collection and exchange of data. During a public health emergency, state and local officials are authorized to use and appropriate property as necessary for the care, treatment, and housing of patients and to destroy contaminated facilities or materials. They are also empowered to provide care, testing, treatment, and vaccination to persons who are ill or who have been exposed to a contagious disease and to separate affected individuals from the population at large to interrupt disease transmission. At the same time, the act recognizes that a state's ability to respond to a public health emergency must respect the dignity and rights of persons. Guided by principles of justice, state and local governments have a duty to act with fairness and tolerance toward individuals and groups.

INADEQUACY OF EXISTING PUBLIC HEALTH LEGISLATION

. . . Public health legislation is so old that it tells the story of communicable diseases through time, with new layers of regulation with each page in history—from plague and smallpox to tuberculosis and polio, and now HIV/AIDS and West Nile virus. Many laws have not been systematically updated since the early to mid-twentieth century. State laws predate modern public health science and practice. Research demonstrates that existing public health law does not conform to modern ideas relating to the mission, functions, and services of public health agencies. Existing state laws also predate advances in constitutional law and civil liberties (such as privacy and antidiscrimination). For example, many public health laws do not provide rigorous procedural due process protections. Existing laws are so obtuse that few public health practitioners, or even legal counsel, fully understand them. Discussion of law reform, therefore, must take account of the obsolescence and complexity of current legislation.

Public health laws are inconsistent both within states and among them. . . . Inconsistencies among the states and territories lead to profound variation in the structure, substance, and procedures for detecting, controlling, and preventing disease. A certain level of consistency is important in public health because infectious diseases usually occur regionally or nationally, requiring a coordinated approach to surveillance and control.

Many current laws fail to provide necessary authority for each of the key elements for public health preparedness: planning, coordination, surveillance, management of property, and protection of persons. States have not devised clear methods of planning, communication, and coordination among the various levels of government (federal, tribal, state, and local), responsible agencies (public health, law enforcement, and emergency management), and the private sector (food, transportation, and health care). Indeed, because of privacy concerns, many states actually proscribe the exchange of vital information.

Current statutes also do not facilitate surveillance and may even prevent monitoring. For example, many states do not require timely reporting for Category A [i.e., highest-priority] agents of bioterrorism. At the same time, states do not require public health agencies to monitor data held by hospitals, managed care organizations, and pharmacies and may even prohibit them from doing so.

Extant laws usually do provide powers over property and persons, but their scope is limited. Some statutes permit the exercise of certain powers (such as quarantine) but not others (such as directly observed therapy). Other statutes permit the exercise of powers in relation to certain diseases (such as smallpox and tuberculosis) but not others (such as hemorrhagic fevers). There are numerous circumstances that might require management of property in a public health emergency: shortages of vaccines, medicines, hospital beds, or facilities for disposal of corpses. It may even be necessary to close facilities or destroy property that is contaminated or dangerous. There similarly may be a need to exercise powers over individuals to avert a serious threat to the public's health. Vaccination, testing, physical examination, treatment, isolation, and quarantine each may help to contain the spread of communicable diseases. . . .

A DEFENSE OF THE MODEL ACT

Federalism

Critics argue that acts of terrorism are inherently federal matters, so there is no need for expansion of state public health powers. It is certainly true that federal authority is extraordinarily important in responding to catastrophic public health events. . . .

The assertion of federal jurisdiction, of course, does not obviate the need for adequate state and local public health power. States and localities have been the primary bulwark of public health in America. From a historical perspective, local and state public health agencies predated federal agencies. . . .

From a constitutional perspective, states have "plenary" authority to protect the public's health under their reserved powers in the Tenth Amendment. The Supreme Court has made it clear that states have a deep reservoir of public health powers. . . . The Supreme Court, moreover, regards federal police powers as constitutionally limited and has curtailed the expansion of national public health authority.

From an economic and practical perspective, most public health activities take place at the state and local levels: surveillance, communicable disease control, and food and water safety. States and localities probably would be the first to detect and respond to a health emergency and would have a key role throughout. This requires states to have effective, modern statutory powers that enable them to work alongside federal agencies.

Declaration of a Public Health Emergency

Critics express concern that the model act could be triggered too easily, creating a threat to civil liberties. Community-based organizations objected to the idea that a governor might declare a public health emergency for an endemic disease such as HIV/AIDS or influenza. Although this may have been a problem with the act's initial version, the current version expressly states that a governor may not declare a public health emergency for an endemic disease.

. . . The drafters set demanding conditions for a governor's declaration, clearly specifying the level of risk. A public health emergency may be declared only in the event of bioterrorism or a naturally occurring epidemic that poses a high probability of a large number of deaths or serious disabilities. Indeed, the drafters rejected arguments from high-level federal and state officials to set a lower threshold for triggering a health emergency. . . .

Governmental Abuse of Power

Critics argue that governors and public health authorities would abuse their authority and exercise powers without justification. [But the] model act builds in effective protection against governmental abuse. It adopts the doctrine of separation of powers, so that no branch wields unchecked authority. These checks and balances offer a classic means of preventing abuse.

MSEHPA creates several hedges against abuse: (1) The governor may declare an emergency only under strict criteria and with careful consultation with public health experts and the community; (2) the legislature, by majority vote, can override the governor's declaration at any time; and (3) the judiciary can terminate the exercise of power if the governor violates the act's standards or procedures or acts unconstitutionally. . . .

Personal Libertarianism

Critics imply that the model act should not confer compulsory power at all. In particular, they object to compulsory powers to vaccinate, test, medically treat, isolate, and quarantine. Commentators reason that services are more important than power; that individuals will comply voluntarily with public health advice; and that trade-offs between civil rights and public health are not required and even are counterproductive. . . .

First, although the provision of services may be more important than the exercise of power, the state undoubtedly needs a certain amount of authority to protect the public's health. Government must have the power to prevent individuals from endangering others. It is only common sense, for example, that a person who has been exposed to an infectious disease should be required to undergo testing or medical examination and, if infectious, to be vaccinated, treated, or isolated.

Second, although most people can be expected to comply willingly with public health measures because it is in their own interests or desirable for the common welfare, not everyone will comply. Individuals may resist loss of autonomy, privacy, or liberty even if their behavior threatens others. Provided that public health powers are hedged with safeguards, individuals should be required to yield some of their interests to protect the health and security of the community.

Finally, although public health and civil liberties may be mutually enhancing in many instances, they sometimes come into conflict. . . . The history of public health is littered with illustrations of trade-offs between public health and civil liberties. It may be fashionable to argue that there is no tension, but public health officials need to make hard choices, particularly in public health emergencies.

Individuals whose movements pose a serious risk of harm to their communities do not have a "right" to be free of interference necessary to control the threat. There simply is no basis for this argument in constitutional law, and perhaps little more in political philosophy. Even the most liberal scholars accept the harm principle—that government should retain power to prevent individuals from endangering others.

The Supreme Court has been equally clear about the limits of freedom in a constitutional democracy. The rights of liberty and due process are fundamental but not absolute. Justice Harlan in the foundational Supreme Court case of *Jacobson v. Massachusetts* (1905) wrote: "There are manifold restraints to which every person is necessarily subject for the common good. On any other basis organized society could not exist with safety to its members." . . .

Economic Libertarianism

Civil libertarians have not been the only group to criticize MSEHPA. Businesses, as well as law and economic scholars, have complained that it interferes with free enterprise. Most economic stakeholders, including the food, transportation, pharmaceutical, and health care industries, . . . argue that they may have to share data with government, abate nuisances, destroy property, and provide goods and services without their express agreement.

Generally speaking, the model act provides several kinds of powers to regulate businesses: destruction of dangerous or contaminated property, nuisance abatements, and confiscation of property for public purposes. All of these powers have been exercised historically and comply with constitutional and ethical norms. If businesses have property that poses a public threat, government has always had the power to destroy that property. . . . Similarly, if businesses are engaged in an activity that poses a health threat, government has always had the power to abate the nuisance. . . . Finally, government has always had the power to confiscate private property for the public good. In the event of bioterrorism, for example, it may be necessary for government to have adequate supplies of vaccines or pharmaceuticals.

Similarly, government may need to use health care facilities for medical treatment or quarantine of persons exposed to infection.

Businesses argue that government should not have broad powers to control enterprise and property. If these powers have to be exercised, businesses want to ensure that they are compensated according to market values. The model act follows a classical approach to the issue of property rights. Compensation is provided if there is a "taking"—that is, if the government confiscates private property for public purposes (such as the use of a private infirmary to treat or isolate patients). No compensation would be provided for a "nuisance abatement"—that is, if the government destroys property or closes an establishment that poses a serious health threat. This comports with the extant constitutional "takings" jurisprudence of the Supreme Court. . . .

Safeguards of Persons and Property

The real basis for debate over public health legislation should not be that powers are given, because it is clear that power is sometimes necessary. The better question is whether the powers are hedged with appropriate safeguards of personal and economic liberty. The core of the debate over MSEHPA ought to be whether it appropriately protects freedoms by providing clear and demanding criteria for the exercise of power and fair procedures for decision making. It is in this context that the attack on MSEHPA is particularly exasperating, because critics rarely suggest that the act fails to provide crisp standards and procedural due process. Nor do they compare the safeguards in the model act to those in existing public health legislation.

It is important to note that compulsory powers over individuals (testing, physical examination, treatment, and isolation) and businesses (nuisance abatements and seizure or destruction of property) already exist in state public health law. These powers have been exercised since the founding of the Republic. MSEHPA, therefore, does not contain new, radical powers. Most tellingly, the model contains much better safeguards of individual and economic liberty than appear in communicable disease statutes enacted in the early to mid-twentieth century.

Unlike older statutes, MSEHPA provides clear and objective criteria for the exercise of powers, rigorous procedural due process, respect for religious and cultural differences, and a new set of entitlements for humane treatment. First, the criteria for the exercise of compulsory powers are based on the modern "significant risk" standard enunciated in constitutional law and disability discrimination law. The act also requires public health officials to adopt the "least restrictive alternative." Second, the procedures for intervention are rigorous, following the most stringent requirements set by the Supreme Court, including the right to counsel, presentation and cross-examination of evidence, and reasons for decisions. Third, the act shows tolerance of groups through its requirements to respect cultural and religious differences whenever consistent with the public's health. Finally, the act provides a whole new set of rights to care and treatment of persons subject to isolation or quarantine. These include the right to treatment, clothing, food, communication, and humane conditions.

In summary, MSEHPA provides a modern framework for effective identification of and response to emerging health threats, while demonstrating respect for individuals and tolerance of groups. Indeed, the CLPH agreed to draft the law only because a much more draconian approach might have been taken by the federal government and the states acting on their own and responding to public fears and misapprehensions.

RETHINKING THE PUBLIC GOOD

... There are good reasons for believing that resource allocations, ethical values, and law should transform to reflect the critical importance of the health, security, and well-being of the populace. It is not that individual freedoms are unimportant. To the contrary, personal liberty allows people the right of self-determination, to make judgments about how to live their lives and pursue their dreams. Without a certain level of health, safety, and security, however, people cannot have well-being, nor can they meaningfully exercise their autonomy or participate in social and political life.

My purpose is not to assert which are the more fundamental interests: personal liberty or health and security. Rather, my purpose is to illustrate that both sets of interests are important to human flourishing. The Model State Emergency Health Powers Act was designed to defend personal as well as collective interests. But in a country so tied to rights rhetoric on both sides of the political spectrum, any proposal that has the appearance of strengthening governmental authority was bound to travel in tumultuous political waters.

BIOTERRORISM, PUBLIC HEALTH, AND HUMAN RIGHTS*
George J. Annas

A central lesson from 9/11 is that threats to public health are national and global. Unfortunately, public health as a field has an unappealing tendency to look backward when planning for the future.... As Lawrence Gostin's paper outlines, the Centers for Disease Control and Prevention's (CDC's) request to develop a state emergency powers act in the wake of the anthrax attacks reflects this regressive tendency. Its exclusive concentration on the state level misses an important opportunity to exercise national public health leadership and instead promotes a return to the paternalistic pre-human rights days of nineteenth-century public health practices such as forced examination and quarantine....

FEDERAL (AND GLOBAL) PUBLIC HEALTH

State public health laws are often antiquated, but their most antiquated feature is their underlying premise that public health is exclusively a state-level concern. A bioterrorist attack on the United States, for example, is inherently a matter of national security, making it a federal matter.... State laws regarding bioterrorism should be primarily aimed at preparing state and local authorities for their important job of assisting federal agencies, such as the new U.S. Department of Homeland Security, in the response....

At the outset of the twenty-first century, bioterrorism, although only one threat to public health, can be the catalyst to effectively "federalize" and integrate much of what are now uncoordinated and piecemeal state and local public health programs.

*Reprinted from *Health Affairs* 21 (November/December 2002): 94–97.

This should include a renewed effort for national health insurance; national licensure for physicians, nurses, and allied health professionals; and national patient-safety standards. Federal public health leadership will also help us look outward and recognize that prevention of future bioterrorist attacks and even ordinary epidemics will require international cooperation. In this regard, the threat of bioterrorism joins HIV/AIDS and other epidemics to demonstrate the need to globalize public health.

PUBLIC HEALTH AND MEDICINE

A major planning question in responding to a bioterrorist attack is the relationship between medicine and public health. It is almost certain that any attack will first be recognized by physicians working in a hospital emergency room. Therefore, proposals to train emergency room personnel to recognize patients exposed to the most likely bioterrorist agents make perfect sense, as do up-to-date communication systems that can track relevant disease occurrences quickly and accurately (although there is no necessity to report data that identify patients). But who should be in charge after an outbreak has been confirmed?

The suggested act assumes that a state's governor will designate "public health officials" to be in charge and that these officials—who will be issued badges—will be empowered to take over hospitals and order physicians to examine and treat (and quarantine) individuals against their will, even when there is no evidence at all that the individual is either sick or contagious. The act's first draft was even more extreme, making it a crime for any individual to refuse to be examined or treated and a crime for a physician to refuse an order by a public health official to examine or treat a patient. Moreover, should any patient be injured, or even killed, by the treatment (as, for example, immunocompromised individuals could be by smallpox vaccine), the public health officials and state would be immune from lawsuit.

This approach is likely to be counterproductive. Despite its talk about balancing human rights with disease prevention, the suggested act unnecessarily ignores basic human rights. Physicians, on the other hand, have effectively incorporated the doctrine of informed consent into their core medical ethics precepts. Public health still favors legal mandates and government-backed paternalism. Public health should be abandoning paternalism, rather than attempting to use 9/11 to increase it. Public health officials are likely to be much more effective in responding to emergencies if they work with both physicians and the public, rather than trying to exercise arbitrary and unaccountable power over them.

As evidenced by both 9/11 and the anthrax attacks, U.S. hospitals and physicians stand ready to help in any way they can in a mass emergency. The public is also eager—often too eager—to accept medications and line up to seek screening and care at hospitals. The real problem in a bioterrorist event will be supplying medical care, drugs, and vaccines to those who demand them. Nonetheless, the prospect of arbitrary forced treatment and quarantine would rightly engender distrust in government and public health officials and could actually discourage those who might have been exposed from seeking treatment at all—even encourage them to escape to another state....

DEMOCRACY AND PUBLIC HEALTH

The suggested act has been criticized by both civil liberties and libertarian groups. But they are hardly alone....

There is no chance that every state, or even many states, will adopt the suggested act, so if uniformity is seen as necessary, only a federal statute can provide it. [Ed.–At the time of this writing only two states had enacted the MSEHPA. As of August 2009, thirty-eight states and the District of Columbia have passed legislation including provisions from or closely related to the act.]

Under the new Minnesota law [which adopted some MSEHPA provisions "rewritten . . . to be consistent with contemporary medical ethics and constitutional rights"], even in a public health emergency, "individuals have a fundamental right to refuse medical treatment, testing, physical or mental examination, vaccination, participation in experimental procedures and protocols, collection of specimens and preventive treatment programs" (2002 Minnesota Laws 402). Of course there are extreme circumstances under which isolation or quarantine can be employed. But the Minnesota legislature permits such measures only under much more limited conditions. . . . The Minnesota legislature properly recognized that human rights and health are not inherently conflicting goals that must be traded off against each other; they are, as Jonathan Mann and colleagues first articulated in the context of the international HIV/AIDS epidemic, "inextricably linked" (Mann et al. 1994, 19). . . .

Ultimately, public health must rely not on force but on persuasion, and not on blind trust but on trust based on transparency, accountability, democracy, and human rights. There is plenty of time to draft and debate a twenty-first-century federal public health law that takes constitutional rights seriously, unites the public with its medical caretakers, treats medicine and public health as true partners, and moves us in the direction of global cooperation.

RECOMMENDED READINGS

A Brief History of the Ancient Power of Quarantine

Stephenson, Kathryn. 2004. The quarantine war: The burning of the New York Marine Hospital in 1858. *Public Health Reports* 119: 79–92. (Provides a historical account of the 1858 burning of the New York Marine Hospital, a quarantine station for immigrants entering the United States who were suspected of carrying smallpox, yellow fever, or tuberculosis)

Constitutional Review of Isolation and Quarantine

Leavitt, Judith Walzer. 1997. *Typhoid Mary.* Boston: Beacon Press. (Describes the case of Mary Mallon, the real-life "Typhoid Mary," and examines the public health aspects of her experience)

Sciarrino, Alfred J. 2003. The grapes of wrath and the speckled monster (epidemics, biological terrorism, and the early legal history of two major defenses—quarantine and vaccination). *Journal of Medicine and Law* 7: 117–76. (Provides an account of then-existing civil remedies for unjustifiable or unwarranted exercises of the quarantine and isolation power available at the end of the nineteenth century)

Medical Countermeasures and Public Health Interventions

Arras, John D. 2005. Rationing vaccine during an avian influenza pandemic: Why it won't be easy. *Yale Journal of Biology and Medicine* 78: 283–96. (Examines ethical issues and potential courses of action in rationing vaccine supplies during an influenza epidemic)

Fidler, David P. 2003. SARS: Political pathology of the first post-Westphalian pathogen. *Journal of Law, Medicine & Ethics* 31: 485–505. (Examines aspects of global public health and international relations in light of the SARS outbreak)

Gostin, Lawrence O. 2006. Medical countermeasures for pandemic influenza: Ethics and the law. *JAMA* 295: 554–56. (Examines legal and ethical issues in vaccine provision in a pandemic, including those pertaining to intellectual property and regulation)

———. 2006. Public health strategies for pandemic influenza: Ethics and the law. *JAMA* 295: 1700–1704. (Describes the role of public health strategies, including travel restrictions, quarantine, and surveillance, in coping with pandemic flu)

———. 2009. Influenza A(H1N1) and pandemic preparedness under the rule of international law. *JAMA* 301: 2376–78. (Describes the global response to H1N1, notes continued gaps in authority of the WHO and CDC, and argues that the appropriate response to international public health threats must be guided by evidence-based science)

Gostin, Lawrence O., and Benjamin E. Berkman. 2007. Pandemic influenza: Ethics, law, and the public's health. *Administrative Law Review* 59: 121–75. (Provides insights on numerous ethical and legal aspects of responding to pandemic influenza, including vaccine delivery, quarantine, and travel restrictions)

Parmet, Wendy E. 2007. Legal power and legal rights—isolation and quarantine in the case of drug-resistant tuberculosis. *New England Journal of Medicine* 357: 433–35. (Discusses the limitations of coercive public health powers in containing MDR-TB)

Uscher-Pines, Lori, Patrick S. Duggan, Joshua P. Garoon, Ruth A. Karron, and Ruth R. Faden. 2007. Planning for an influenza pandemic: Social justice and disadvantaged groups. *Hastings Center Report* 37 (4): 32–39. (Provides a cross-national comparison and explores the extent to which existing national plans address considerations of social justice)

Bioterrorism

Barbera, Joseph, Anthony Macintyre, Larry Gostin, Tom Inglesby, Tara O'Toole, Craig DeAtley, Kevin Tonat, and Marci Layton. 2001. Large-scale quarantine following biological terrorism in the United States: Scientific examination, logistic and legal limits, and possible consequences. *JAMA* 286: 2711–17. (Expresses skepticism about the efficacy of large-scale quarantines and delineates criteria for invoking a large-scale quarantine: cost-benefit analysis, feasibility, medical necessity)

Fidler, David P., and Lawrence O. Gostin. 2007. Biosecurity and the rule of law. In *Biosecurity in the Global Age: Biological Weapons, Public Health, and the Rule of Law,* 187–218. Stanford: Stanford Univ. Press. (Describes how embedding biosecurity in the rule of law might facilitate effective interventions, protect individual rights and liberties, integrate notions of justice, and ensure transparency and accountability)

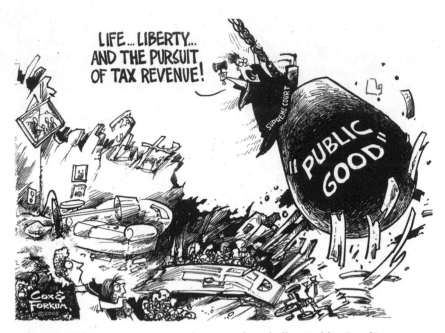

Photo 29. The Supreme Court rides a wrecking ball—"Public Good"—
through a home. Few Supreme Court decisions have aroused the ire generated
by *Kelo v. City of New London,* decided in 2005. In perhaps the most
extreme response, the libertarian property rights activist Logan Darrow
Clements attempted to persuade the town council in Weare, New Hampshire,
to use its eminent domain powers to seize Justice David Souter's home and
replace it with "The Lost Liberty Hotel." Reproduced from Cox and Forkum:
Editorial Cartoons, posted June 23, 2005, www.coxandforkum.com/archives/
000610.html.

TWELVE

Economic Liberty and the Pursuit of Public Health

Previous chapters have focused on the limits on government power to protect personal freedoms: autonomy, privacy, bodily integrity, and liberty. Individuals, however, value not only personal freedom but also economic liberty. They claim the liberty to own and use private property, run businesses, enter into contracts, and pursue trades, livelihoods, or professions.

Market capitalism and the profit incentive are widely valued in modern America. Citizens sometimes see government as an obstacle to achieving their financial dreams. They assert a right to freedom from government bureaucracy, taxation, and burdensome regulation. Some economists believe that regulation, if desirable at all, should redress market failures rather than restrain free enterprise.

Public health advocates strongly oppose unfettered private enterprise and are suspicious of free market solutions to social problems. They see numerous areas of economic life that require careful regulation. For example, public health advocates view regulation as essential to minimizing occupational health and safety risks; improving the safety of food, water, consumer goods, and pharmaceuticals; and preventing degradation of the environment. From a public health perspective, the community can benefit from living in a well-regulated society that promotes health and prevents injury and disease. Although individuals have to forgo a certain amount of economic freedom, they benefit from living in safer and healthier communities.

To achieve communal health and safety, governments have formed specialized agencies. Administrative law, which governs the balance of powers between agencies, the legislature, and the courts, was discussed in chapter 5. In two sections, this chapter focuses on the balance between individual rights and the power of administrative agencies to undertake commercial regulation for the public's health. The first section describes the various techniques of commercial regulation, discussing several public health powers that are integral parts of civil society and staples of public health practice. Public health agencies license professionals, businesses, and institutions to ensure adequate qualifications and standards. They inspect premises and commercial establishments to identify unsanitary conditions, unsafe environments, or dangerous products. Agencies also possess the power to order individuals and companies to abate nuisances that pose unreasonable hazards to members of the community.

Although commercial regulation achieves important societal benefits, it also interferes with a variety of economic freedoms. The second section examines individual claims to economic freedom, reviewing constitutional theories of economic due process, freedom of contract, and government "takings." Those who advocate unfettered free enterprise often turn to the Constitution to justify their libertarian claims. Throughout this chapter, the key issue is the appropriate weight to be afforded to economic freedom. When government acts for the common good, how concerned should we be about impeding commercial and professional opportunities? Are economic freedoms as important as political and civil liberties?

I. REGULATORY TOOLS OF PUBLIC HEALTH AGENCIES

Public health agencies possess ample tools to regulate commercial activities in order to ensure the health and safety of the population. This section examines three of the most common regulatory powers: the authority to license trades, professions, and institutions; to inspect for violations of health and safety standards; and to abate public nuisances.

A. Licenses and Permits

Public health agencies can require persons, businesses, and institutions to obtain a professional or commercial license. A license provides formal permission from the government for a person to perform certain activities, such as practicing a profession (e.g., medicine or nursing), conducting a business (e.g., a restaurant or tattoo parlor), and operating an institution (e.g., a hospital or nursing home). Licenses are part of a regulatory system that sets standards for entering a field and monitors compliance with those standards.

In the following brief excerpt from a late nineteenth-century case, the Supreme Court upheld the licensing of physicians on public health grounds. This ruling is one of the most important precedents for licensing.

DENT V. WEST VIRGINIA*
Supreme Court of the United States
Decided January 14, 1889

Justice FIELD delivered the opinion of the Court.

[The petitioner was indicted for violating a West Virginia statute that requires a practitioner of medicine to obtain a certificate from the state board of health stating that he is a graduate of a reputable medical college, that he has practiced medicine for a specific period of time, or that he has otherwise been examined and found by the board to be qualified to practice medicine. The petitioner claimed that this statute was unconstitutional because it violates his rights to due process under the Fourteenth Amendment.]

. . . The power of the state to provide for the general welfare of its people authorizes it to prescribe all such regulations as in its judgment will secure or tend to secure them against the consequences of ignorance and incapacity, as well as deception and fraud. . . . The nature and extent of the qualifications required must depend primarily upon the judgment of the state as to their necessity. . . . It is only when they have no relation to such calling or profession, or are unattainable by such reasonable study and application, that they can operate to deprive one of his right to pursue a lawful vocation.

Few professions require more careful preparation by one who seeks to enter it than that of medicine. It has to deal with all those subtle and mysterious influences upon which health and life depend. . . . The physician must be able to detect readily the presence of disease and prescribe appropriate remedies for its removal. Everyone may have occasion to consult him, but comparatively few can judge of the qualifications of learning and skill which he possesses. Reliance must be placed upon the assurance given by his license, issued by an authority competent to judge in that respect, that he possesses the requisite qualifications. Due consideration, therefore, for the protection of society may well induce the state to exclude from practice those who have not such a license, or who are found upon examination not

*129 U.S. 114 (1889).

to be fully qualified. The same reasons which control in imposing conditions, upon compliance with which the physician is allowed to practice in the first instance, may call for further conditions as new modes of treating disease are discovered.... It would not be deemed a matter for serious discussion that a knowledge of the new acquisitions of the profession, as it from time to time advances in its attainments for the relief of the sick and suffering, should be required for continuance in its practice, but for the earnestness with which the plaintiff in error insists that by being compelled to obtain the certificate required, and prevented from continuing in his practice without it, he is deprived of his right and estate in his profession without due process of law. We perceive nothing in the statute which indicates an intention of the legislature to deprive one of any of his rights. No one has a right to practice medicine without having the necessary qualifications of learning and skill; and the statute only requires that whoever assumes, by offering to the community his service as a physician, that he possesses such learning and skill, shall present evidence of it by a certificate or license from a body designated by the state as competent to judge of his qualifications....

... It is sufficient, for the purposes of this case, to say that legislation is not open to the charge of depriving one of his rights without due process of law, if it be general in its operation upon the subjects to which it relates, and is enforceable in the usual modes established in the administration of government with respect to kindred matters; that is, by process or proceedings adapted to the nature of the case. The great purpose of the requirement is to exclude everything that is arbitrary and capricious in legislation affecting the rights of the citizen....

There is nothing of an arbitrary character in the provisions of the statute in question. It applies to all physicians, except those who may be called for a special case from another state. It imposes no conditions which cannot be readily met; and it is made enforceable in the mode usual in kindred matters, that is, by regular proceedings adapted to the case.... If, in the proceedings under the statute, there should be any unfair or unjust action on the part of the board in refusing him a certificate, we doubt not that a remedy would be found in the courts of the state. But no such imputation can be made, for the plaintiff in error did not submit himself to the examination of the board after it had decided that the diploma he presented was insufficient....

... The law of West Virginia was intended to secure such skill and learning in the profession of medicine that the community might trust with confidence those receiving a license under authority of the state. Judgment affirmed.

.   .   .   .   .

As the Court suggests in *Dent,* licensing can have important public health benefits because it helps ensure that only qualified individuals engage in a profession. But when the profession being regulated provides needed health services, a licensing regime must strike a balance between quality and access. Strict licensing requirements that limit the scope of practice for health professionals such as registered nurses and

BOX 8
THE LICENSING OF DENTAL HEALTH AIDE THERAPISTS

Currently, over 100 million Americans lack dental insurance; in 2004, more than one in four had untreated cavities. Such inadequate dental care significantly compromises oral health. Among children, dental caries are the most common form of chronic disease: they affect 50 percent of children between the ages of five and nine and 78 percent of children by the age of seventeen. Moreover, evidence is emerging that oral diseases are associated with myriad other conditions, including diabetes, heart disease and stroke, and adverse pregnancy outcomes (U.S. Department of Health and Human Services 2000b), and in rare cases, oral infections can become deadly. In 2007, the family of a twelve-year-old in Maryland, Deamonte Driver, could not afford dental care; he died after a tooth abscess led to a bacterial brain infection.

Midlevel dental health care professionals, akin to nurse practitioners, could provide oral health services to larger numbers of patients (Wendel and Glick 2008), but the proper scope of practice for such practitioners remains hotly debated. For example, among the Alaskan Native population–large numbers of whom have little or no access to licensed dentists–dental health aide therapists (DHATs) are now permitted to provide basic dental care (e.g., treatment of dental caries and uncomplicated tooth removals) after two years of training, though the American Dental Association (ADA) fought the program. Eugene Sekiguchi and colleagues at the ADA (2005, 772) argued that the duties of auxiliary dental personnel should be limited: "The use of DHATs to provide diagnostic and treatment services for caries, tooth removal, and pulpotomies is not a prudent way to meet the dental therapeutic needs of the Alaska Native population. Their educational background, dental training, and experience are very limited.... Most important, patient safety will also be best served if only dentists provide non-reversible treatment." The following year, the ADA filed suit to halt what it alleged to be "unlicensed practice of dentistry." Because the program was administered and authorized under federal law, the trial court found the DHATs' practice lawful, and the ADA settled its suit in July 2007 (Alaska Dental Society 2007).

dental hygienists may improve quality of care, but possibly at a steep social cost—inadequate access to care for significant portions of the population. In box 8, the example of the licensing of dental health aide therapists (DHATs) illustrates this tension.

Approximately fifty countries allow dental therapists to drill and fill dental caries, providing a service that the underserved need. But in most of the United States, state law strictly prohibits anyone but dentists from performing these irreversible procedures; and given the American Dental Association's resistance, adopting a variant of the DHAT program for children nationwide may be difficult. A well-designed licensing scheme for health care practitioners can provide important public health benefits by helping to ensure quality care. Yet if licensing is left to the discretion of officials, they may parcel out privileges unfairly, discriminating against disfavored groups such as racial or religious minorities and women. Social and cultural discrimination need not be blatant to be effective: the poor and minorities may be excluded from professions because they cannot meet educational and qualification standards that are set artificially high.

Consider the impact of licensing requirements on the number of African American physicians during the twentieth century. At the beginning of the century, the United States was a racially segregated society with two national medical associations—the almost exclusively white American Medical Association (AMA) and the predominantly black National Medical Association (NMA). When the AMA took control of medical licensing in the early twentieth century, it forced the closure of many existing medical schools attended by blacks; as a result, the number of African American physicians declined sharply (Kessel 1970). In 1910, an AMA-commissioned report recommended that all but two of the African American medical colleges then in operation be closed (R. Baker et al. 2008). The medical historian Todd L. Savitt (1984, 181–84) tells the story of Leonard Medical School of Shaw University in Raleigh, North Carolina:

> Failure rates on state licensure exams became the measure of a school's worth, once the American Medical Association began publishing this information in 1904. Leonard did not fare so well, either in comparison with other black schools or with other medical students around the country. . . . In the periodic inspections that the American Medical Association's Council on Medical Education made after 1904, Leonard always received C ratings. . . .
>
> . . . The school's administration tried desperately to keep up. . . . But still, at the core, lack of money wore Leonard down. . . . Leonard did not have the growth potential, the financial strength, or the strong faculty to meet the higher educational standards of a new era. . . .
>
> . . . In 1918 Leonard Medical School closed its doors forever.

In July 2008, the AMA issued a formal apology for its "historical antipathy" toward black physicians and expressed regret for a "litany of transgressions" (Watt 2008). As a *New York Times* article (July 11, 2008) noted in reporting on the apology, however, fewer than 2 percent of today's AMA members are black.

B. Administrative Searches and Inspections

States and localities have the power to inspect a product, business, or building to ascertain its authenticity (e.g., possession of a valid license), quality (e.g., purity and fitness for use), or condition (e.g., safety and sanitation). Inspection laws authorize and direct public health authorities to conduct administrative searches to ensure conformity with health and safety standards.

The power of public health authorities to conduct administrative searches or inspections is among the oldest state powers, as it is mentioned expressly in Article I, section 10, clause 2 of the Constitution: states may lay imposts or duties on imports or exports, without the consent of Congress, when "absolutely necessary for executing its Inspections Laws." But inspections also invade a sphere of privacy protected by the Fourth Amendment to the Constitution, which guarantees the "right of people to be secure in their persons, houses, papers, and effects, against unreasonable searches and seizures."

For most of the nation's history, public health inspections were presumed to be constitutional and rarely challenged. However, in 1967 the Supreme Court held in *Camara v. Municipal Court of the City and County of San Francisco* (excerpted next) that public health inspections are governed by the Fourth Amendment and are presumptively unreasonable if conducted without a warrant.

CAMARA V. MUNICIPAL COURT OF THE CITY AND COUNTY OF SAN FRANCISCO*
Supreme Court of the United States
Decided June 5, 1967

Justice WHITE delivered the opinion of the Court.

Appellant brought this action in a California Superior Court alleging that he was awaiting trial on a criminal charge of violating the San Francisco Housing Code [§ 503] by refusing to permit a warrantless inspection of his residence, and that a writ of prohibition should issue to the criminal court because the ordinance authorizing such inspections is unconstitutional on its face....

*387 U.S. 523 (1967).

Appellant has argued throughout this litigation that § 503 is contrary to the Fourth and Fourteenth Amendments in that it authorizes municipal officials to enter a private dwelling without a search warrant and without probable cause to believe that a violation of the Housing Code exists therein. . . .

In *Frank v. State of Maryland,* 359 U.S. 360 (1955), this Court upheld the conviction of one who refused to permit a warrantless inspection of private premises for the purposes of locating and abating a suspected public nuisance. . . .

To the *Frank* majority, municipal fire, health, and housing inspection programs "touch at most upon the periphery of the important interests safeguarded by the Fourteenth Amendment's protection against official intrusion," 359 U.S. at 367, because the inspections are merely to determine whether physical conditions exist which do not comply with minimum standards prescribed in local regulatory ordinances. . . .

We may agree that a routine inspection of the physical condition of private property is a less hostile intrusion than the typical policeman's search for the fruits and instrumentalities of crime. . . . But we cannot agree that the Fourth Amendment interests at stake in these inspection cases are merely "peripheral." . . . Like most regulatory laws, fire, health, and housing codes are enforced by criminal processes. In some cities, discovery of a violation by the inspector leads to a criminal complaint. Even in cities where discovery of a violation produces only an administrative compliance order, refusal to comply is a criminal offense, and the fact of compliance is verified by a second inspection, again without a warrant. Finally, as this case demonstrates, refusal to permit an inspection is itself a crime, punishable by fine or even by jail sentence.

The *Frank* majority suggested, and appellee reasserts, two other justifications for permitting administrative health and safety inspections without a warrant. First, it is argued that these inspections are "designed to make the least possible demand on the individual occupant." 359 U.S. at 367. The ordinances authorizing inspections are hedged with safeguards, and at any rate the inspector's particular decision to enter must comply with the constitutional standard of reasonableness even if he may enter without a warrant. In addition, . . . the warrant process could not function effectively in this field. The decision to inspect an entire municipal area is based upon legislative or administrative assessment of broad factors such as the area's age and condition. Unless the magistrate is to review such policy matters, he must issue a "rubber stamp" warrant which provides no protection at all to the property owner. . . .

. . . Under the present system, when the inspector demands entry, the occupant has no way of knowing whether enforcement of the municipal code involved requires inspection of his premises, no way of knowing the lawful limits of the inspector's power to search, and no way of knowing whether the inspector himself is acting under proper authorization. . . . Yet, only by refusing entry and risking a criminal conviction can the occupant at present challenge the inspector's decision to search. . . . The practical effect of this system is to leave the occupant subject to the discretion of the official in the field. . . . We simply cannot say that the protections provided by the warrant procedure are not needed in this context; broad statutory safeguards are no substitute for individualized review, particularly when those safeguards may only be invoked at the risk of a criminal penalty.

The final justification suggested for warrantless administrative searches is that the public interest demands such a rule: it is vigorously argued that the health and safety of entire urban populations is dependent upon enforcement of minimum fire, housing, and sanitation standards, and that the only effective means of enforcing such codes is by routine systemized inspection of all physical structures.... In assessing whether the public interest demands creation of a general exception to the Fourth Amendment's warrant requirement, the question is not whether the public interest justifies the type of search in question, but whether the authority to search should be evidenced by a warrant, which in turn depends in part upon whether the burden of obtaining a warrant is likely to frustrate the governmental purpose behind the search. It has nowhere been urged that fire, health, and housing code inspection programs could not achieve their goals within the confines of a reasonable search warrant requirement. Thus, we do not find the public need argument dispositive....

There is unanimous agreement among those most familiar with this field that the only effective way to seek universal compliance with the minimum standards required by municipal codes is through routine periodic inspections of all structures. It is here that the probable cause debate is focused, for the agency's decision to conduct an area inspection is unavoidable based on its appraisal of conditions in the area as a whole, not on its knowledge of conditions in each particular building....

... Such programs have a long history of judicial and public acceptance. Second, the public interest demands that all dangerous conditions be prevented or abated, yet it is doubtful that any other canvassing technique would achieve acceptable results.... The warrant procedure is designed to guarantee that a decision to search private property is justified by a reasonable governmental interest. But reasonableness is still the ultimate standard. If a valid public interest justifies the intrusion contemplated, then there is probable cause to issue a suitably restricted search warrant.

· · · · · ·

In a companion case to *Camara*, the Supreme Court held that a fire inspector who searched a business without consent or a warrant violated the Fourth Amendment: "The businessman, like the occupant of a residence, has a constitutional right to go about his business free from unreasonable official entries upon his private commercial property" (*See v. City of Seattle*, 387 U.S. 541, 543 [1967]).

Two decades after *Camara* and *See*, the Supreme Court recognized an exception to the warrant requirement for administrative inspections of closely regulated businesses. In *New York v. Burger*, 482 U.S. 691, 702–03 (1987), the Court held that

Because the owner or operator of commercial premises in a "closely regulated" industry has a reduced expectation of privacy, the warrant and probable cause requirements, which fulfill the traditional Fourth

Amendment standard of reasonableness for a government search, have lessened application. . . .

The warrantless inspection, however, . . . will be deemed to be reasonable only so long as three criteria are met. First, there must be a "substantial" government interest that informs the regulatory scheme pursuant to which the inspection is made.

Second, the warrantless inspections must be "necessary to further [the] regulatory scheme." . . .

Finally, "the statute's inspection program, in terms of the certainty and regularity of its application, [must] provid[e] a constitutionally adequate substitute for a warrant."

Since *Burger,* the courts have permitted public health searches without warrants for a range of heavily regulated (and often hazardous) businesses, such as mines, plants that manufacture firearms, and distilleries that make alcoholic beverages. They also permit inspections without warrants for licensed businesses that bear substantially on public health, such as nursing homes and health care facilities. The judiciary permits administrative searches of pervasively regulated businesses without a warrant because routine inspections are important in enforcing health and safety standards (the advance warning provided by a warrant may enable owners to conceal hazards) and because highly regulated commercial activities have lower expectations of privacy. Today, administrative inspections are used to enforce traditional public health regulations (e.g., meat safety inspections) as well as more modern public health laws (e.g., smoking bans). In the following excerpt, the use of administrative inspections to implement New York City's ban on smoking in bars and restaurants (both heavily regulated businesses) is challenged by a private social club.

PLAYERS, INC. V. CITY OF NEW YORK*
United States District Court for the Southern District of New York
Decided May 20, 2005

MARRERO, District Judge.

This case raises a constitutional challenge to smoking restrictions recently adopted by the City of New York (the "City") and the State of New York (the "State"). . . . The plaintiff . . . is challenging the constitutionality of the smoking bans. . . .

In relevant part, the Fourth Amendment protects "[t]he right of the people to be secure in their persons, houses, and effects, against unreasonable searches and seizures." Players argues that both Local Law 47 and Chapter 13 violate the Fourth

*371 F. Supp. 2d 522 (S.D.N.Y. 2005).

Amendment by authorizing warrantless searches of commercial premises. After reviewing the Smoking Bans, the implementing regulations, and the rules governing the City's authority to secure compliance with health-related laws and regulations, the Court concludes that the statutes and their regulatory schemes do not violate the Fourth Amendment....

The Local Law 47 Regulations and the Middleton Affidavit make clear, however, that the City seeks to enforce the Smoking Bans using the full array of inspection powers available to DHMH [the Department of Health and Mental Hygiene]. As stated above, the Local Law 47 Regulations put the public on notice that the City intends "to utilize the full range of the Department ... and Commissioner's regulatory and enforcement powers" to reduce the harmful effects of second-hand smoke. As relevant to Players' Fourth Amendment challenge, those enforcement powers include powers to inspect commercial establishments for compliance with the Smoking Bans.... DHMH inspectors conduct warrantless inspections of commercial premises under three circumstances: 1) when the premises is open to the public; 2) when permission to enter is given; and 3) if the area being searched is a licensed food service establishment subject to inspection under rules governing those licenses. Health inspectors visiting a food service establishment may now inspect for compliance with the Smoking Bans along with other health laws and regulations....

Inspections without consent conducted in private premises containing licensed food service establishments, however, could raise lesser, but still significant constitutional concerns. Owners and operators of these premises are entitled to the protections of the Fourth Amendment, which traditionally require proof of a warrant and probable cause before a search can be conducted. These traditional criteria, however, have lessened application where the property is being used in a "closely regulated" industry, due to the lessened expectation of privacy associated with operating in that industry. As many courts have held and as Players does not contest, the food industry is a quintessential example of an industry that is "closely regulated."

In [*New York v. Burger*, 482 U.S. 691 (1987),] the Supreme Court held that warrantless inspections were permissible even in the context of a closely regulated business, however, only if three criteria are met: 1) "there must be a substantial government interest that informs the regulatory scheme pursuant to which the inspection is made"; 2) "the warrantless inspections must be necessary to further the regulatory scheme"; and 3) the inspection program, "in terms of the certainty and regularity of its application, must provide a constitutionally adequate substitute for a warrant." *Id.* at 702–03.

The statutes and regulations governing the City's use of its inspection authority to enforce the Smoking Bans in regulated areas of food service establishments satisfy *Burger*'s three-part test. Regarding the first prong, the City clearly has a substantial government interest in ensuring the health of its food supply, and of customers of food service establishments.... Both food safety and the health of food service workers and patrons may be endangered by the consumption of tobacco products in and around food preparation areas; the Court has previously noted that the concern for the safety of individuals exposed to secondhand smoke represented an "important government interest." *NYC C.L.A.S.H., Inc. v. City of New York*, 315 F. Supp. 2d 461, 480 (S.D.N.Y. 2004).

Regarding the second prong of the *Burger* test, the Court concludes that warrantless inspections are necessary to further the regulatory scheme established by the City's health ordinances, including its Smoking Bans, in food service establishments such as Players. As the district court in [*Contreras v. City of Chicago*, 920 F. Supp. 1370 (1996)] stated regarding food inspections, "[a]dvance knowledge of an impending health inspection would provide restaurant owners with the opportunity to take temporary remedial measures designed to mask or conceal violations . . . that would surely undermine the purposes of the City's health and sanitation ordinances." *Id.* at 1390. The City's objectives in applying the Smoking Bans to licensed food service establishments would similarly be frustrated by imposition of a notice or warrant requirement; violators could frustrate the City's objectives in passing Local Law 47 by taking temporary remedial measures that would conceal violations (e.g., by extinguishing and putting away cigarettes) if notice or a warrant were required before entry to those establishments could be gained.

Finally, the third prong of the *Burger* test is satisfied by the comprehensiveness and defined scope of the City's inspection program. *Burger* held that this condition was satisfied if the ordinances are "sufficiently comprehensive and defined that the owner of commercial property cannot help but be aware that his property will be subject to specific inspections undertaken for specific purposes." *Burger,* 482 U.S. at 703. The City's health inspection ordinances and regulations fully satisfy this condition by making clear that food service establishments' receipt of a City license is granted subject to the licensees' agreement to submit to frequent inspections that will secure their compliance with public health–related laws. The New York City Charter explicitly authorizes the Commissioner of DHMH and his or her designees to "at reasonable times, and pursuant to a search warrant when required by law, without fee or hindrance enter, examine and inspect all vessels, premises, grounds, structures, buildings and every part thereof and all underground passages of every sort in the city for compliance with the provisions of law enforced by the department and its rules and regulations. . . . " Owners of premises regulated by DHMH "shall at all reasonable times, when required by any such officers or employees, give them free access thereto." A license will not be granted without a pre-permit inspection and DHMH is explicitly authorized by the code to "inspect any premises, matter or thing within its jurisdiction, including but not limited to any premises where an activity regulated by this Code is carried on, and any record required to be kept pursuant to this Code." . . . Inspectors are limited to searching areas of premises that are covered by the license. Thus, the regulatory scheme also makes clear that the "time, place, and scope of the inspection is limited." *Burger,* 482 U.S. at 711.

Players' counterarguments are unpersuasive. First, Players argues that, because the Smoking Bans are "quasi-criminal," they should be subject to a higher level of scrutiny under the Fourth Amendment. This argument is completely misplaced. *Burger* supplies the relevant test for administrative search schemes related to "closely regulated" industries. There is no further, heightened level of scrutiny to be applied to such schemes where the sanctions for violating the regulatory schemes that the inspections were designed to enforce are "quasi-criminal" or criminal. . . .

Players' second challenge to the statute is similarly unavailing. It argues that, particularly where an administrative search is conducted pursuant to a complaint received by DHMH, an inspection's purpose transforms from an effort to obtain administrative compliance to a "quest for evidence." . . .

But even if this legal proposition is generally valid, there is no evidence here that the challenged inspection scheme is intended to achieve anything other than administrative compliance with the Smoking Bans. The Smoking Bans and their supporting regulations establish civil, rather than criminal, penalties for violations that are intended to secure compliance with a civil administrative scheme established to preserve the public health.... [Players has not] pointed to any action or evidence suggesting that the City's use of its health inspection scheme to enforce the Smoking Bans is intended for any purpose other than to "dissipate, if not eliminate the deadly effects of second-hand smoke." Local Law 47, Regulations 3-4 (2002).

Because the Smoking Bans and their enforcement schemes comply with the requirements of the Fourth Amendment, the Court grants Defendants' summary judgment on Players' Fourth Amendment claim.

C. Nuisance Abatement

Public health authorities have the power to abate public nuisances. At common law, a public nuisance was an act or omission that obstructs or causes inconvenience or damage to the public in the exercise of rights common to all. Nuisance abatement has been one of the most important forms of public health regulation since the earliest days in American history.

In 1999, the attorney general of Rhode Island tested the boundaries of public nuisance law, bringing suit against lead pigment manufacturers for making and selling lead paint before the federal government's 1978 ban. Lead is highly toxic, particularly to children who ingest lead paint chips. Exposure even at fairly low levels can lead to permanent learning disabilities; at higher levels, it can result in convulsions, coma, and even death. As of 2004, 5 percent of Rhode Island children had lead poisoning. After a protracted trial, the jury found the defendants liable, and it appeared that manufacturers might have to pay billions of dollars to clean up contaminated homes. On appeal, however, the Rhode Island Supreme Court reversed the judgment, holding that the case should never have gone to trial as a public nuisance claim (*State v. Lead Industries Association, Inc.*, 951 A.2d 428 [R.I. 2008]).

Rhode Island's common law requires a showing of three principal elements in a public nuisance suit: (1) an unreasonable interference (2) with a right common to the general public (3) by a person or people with control over the nuisance-causing instrumentality when the damage occurred. The court held that the final two elements could not be met by the attorney general. Unlike traditional public rights—air, water, or public rights of way—the right of children not to be poisoned by lead paint is an aggregation of individual rights. According to the court, such individual rights are better addressed through products liability suits (see chapter 6). In addition, there was no public nuisance, because the pigment companies were not in control of the lead paint when it was used in homes, causing damage. Rather, according to the court, the burden of lead paint abatement should rest with landlords and property owners. Chief Justice Frank J. Williams, writing for the court, said, "In reaching this conclusion, we do not mean to minimize the severity of the harm that thousands of children in Rhode Island have suffered as a result of lead poisoning. Our hearts go out to those children whose lives forever have been changed by the poisonous presence of lead. But, however grave the problem of lead poisoning is in Rhode Island, public nuisance law simply does not provide a remedy for this harm" (951 A.2d at 435).

Today, public nuisances are usually defined by the legislature. The legislative or administrative definition is often broad and in effect coterminous with the police power (e.g., "anything which is injurious to health, or indecent or offensive"). Public nuisances include all activities that harm the community or common resources (such as silence, clean air and water, or species diversity).

The judiciary has sustained a wide spectrum of traditional nuisance abatements for such problems as diseased crops, hazardous waste, unsanitary or dangerous buildings, and even public meeting places that increase risks of sexually transmitted diseases. For example, in several cities public health agencies have responded to the HIV epidemic by using nuisance laws to close down bathhouses, believing that they create opportunities for anonymous sex. The courts have usually sustained these closure orders. However, the Florida Supreme Court held that an apartment complex where two cocaine arrests had occurred within six months could not be considered a nuisance, because it was not associated with any "record of persistent drug activity" (*Keshbro, Inc. v. City of Miami*, 801 So. 2d 864, 877 [Fla. 2001]).

In reading *New York v. New St. Mark's Baths* (excerpted next), think about the gay community's argument that the act of closing the baths infringes freedom of association, whereas positive measures, such as education and condom distribution, would help prevent high-risk sexual behavior. Which policy option poses the greater health risk: closure of bathhouses, after which unsafe sex may be practiced in other public gathering places, or regulation of bathhouses, making them places where sex education and condoms are available?

NEW YORK V. NEW ST. MARK'S BATHS*

Supreme Court of New York
Decided June 6, 1986

Judge WALLACH delivered the opinion of the court.

[New York City sought to close a bathhouse as a public nuisance pursuant to state regulation aimed at preventing the spread of AIDS. The court documents the prevalence of AIDS, particularly among gay men, and notes its transmissibility through sexual contact.]

The City has submitted ample supporting proof that high risk sexual activity has been taking place at St. Mark's on a continuous and regular basis. Following numerous on site visits by City inspectors, over 14 separate days, these investigators have submitted affidavits describing 49 acts of high risk sexual activity. . . . This evidence of high risk sexual activity, all occurring either in public areas of St. Mark's or in enclosed cubicles left visible to the observer without intrusion therein, demonstrates the inadequacy of self-regulatory procedures by the St. Mark's attendant staff, and the futility of any less intrusive solution to the problem other than the closure.

With a demonstrated death rate from AIDS . . . plaintiffs and intervening State officers have demonstrated a compelling state interest in acting to preserve the health of the population. Where such a compelling state interest is demonstrated even the constitutional rights of privacy and free association must give way provided, as here, it is also shown that the remedy adopted is the least intrusive reasonably available.

Furthermore, it is by no means clear that defendants' rights will, in actuality, be adversely affected in a constitutionally recognized sense by closure of St. Mark's. The privacy protection of sexual activity conducted in a private home does not extend to commercial establishments simply because they provide an opportunity for intimate behavior or sexual release. . . .

. . . However, the closure of this bath house does not extinguish their opportunities for unrestricted association in establishments which avoid creating a serious risk to the public health. . . .

To be sure, defendants and the intervening patrons challenge the soundness of the scientific judgments upon which the Health Council regulation is based, citing, inter alia, the observation of the City's former Commissioner of Health in a memorandum dated October 22, 1985 that "closure of bathhouses will contribute little if anything to the control of AIDS." Defendants particularly assail the regulation's inclusion of fellatio as a high risk sexual activity, and argue that enforced use of prophylactic sheaths would be a more appropriate regulatory response. They go further and argue that facilities such as St. Mark's, which attempts to educate its patrons with written materials, signed pledges, and posted notices as to the advisability of safe sexual practices, provide a positive force in combating AIDS, and a valuable communication link between public health authorities and the homosexual community. While these arguments and proposals may have varying degrees of merit,

*497 N.Y.S.2d 979 (1986).

they overlook a fundamental principle of applicable law: "It is not for the courts to determine which scientific view is correct in ruling upon whether the police power has been properly exercised . . ." (*Chiropractic Ass'n of New York, Inc. v. Hilleboe,* 12 N.Y.2d 109, 114 [1962]). . . .

Accordingly, defendants' motion to dismiss the complaint is in all respects denied.

II. CONSTITUTIONAL RIGHTS AND NORMATIVE VALUES OF ECONOMIC LIBERTY

The regulatory techniques used by public health agencies (licensing, inspection, and nuisance abatement) do protect the public's health and safety, but they undoubtedly interfere with economic liberties. The Framers clearly intended to protect economic liberties, as evidenced by several constitutional provisions. Notably, the Constitution forbids the state from depriving persons of property (or life or liberty) without due process of law (Fifth and Fourteenth Amendments), from impairing the obligations of contracts (Article 1, section 10), or from taking private property for public use without just compensation (Fifth Amendment).

A. Economic Due Process and Freedom of Contract

Recall the discussion in chapter 4 of the landmark case *Jacobson v. Massachusetts,* in which the Supreme Court held that government has ample authority to safeguard the public's health, even if doing so resulted in a diminution in autonomy and bodily integrity. *Jacobson* was decided in the same term as *Lochner v. New York,* which opened the so-called *Lochner* era in constitutional law—which lasted from 1905 to 1937. During the *Lochner* era, the Supreme Court afforded individuals greater protection in the realm of economic affairs than in personal affairs.

LOCHNER V. NEW YORK*
Supreme Court of the United States
Decided April 17, 1905

Justice PECKHAM delivered the opinion of the Court.
[A New York law prohibited the employment of bakery employees for more than 10 hours a day or 60 hours a week. Lochner was convicted and fined for permitting an employee to work in his Utica, N.Y., bakery for more than 60 hours in one week, or more than 10 hours in one day.]

*198 U.S. 45 (1905).

... When the state, ... in the assumed exercise of its police powers, has passed an act which seriously limits the right to labor or the right of contract in regard to their means of livelihood between persons who are sui juris (both employer and employee), it becomes of great importance to determine which shall prevail—the right of the individual to labor for such time as he may choose, or the right of the State to prevent the individual from laboring ... beyond a certain time prescribed by the State.

This court has ... upheld the exercise of the police powers of the States in many cases which might fairly be considered as border ones, and it [has] been guided by rules of a very liberal nature, the application of which has resulted, in numerous instances, in upholding the validity of state statutes thus assailed....

It must, of course, be conceded that there is a limit to the valid exercise of the police power by the state. There is no dispute concerning this general proposition. Otherwise the 14th Amendment would have no efficacy and the legislatures of the states would have unbounded power, and it would be enough to say that any piece of legislation was enacted to conserve the morals, the health, or the safety of the people; such legislation would be valid, no matter how absolutely without foundation the claim might be. The claim of the police power would be a mere pretext—become another and delusive name for the supreme sovereignty of the state to be exercised free from constitutional restraint. In every case that comes before this court, there-fore, where legislation of this character is concerned, and where the protection of the Federal Constitution is sought, the question necessarily arises: Is this a fair, reason-able, and appropriate exercise of the police power of the state, or is it an unreason-able, unnecessary, and arbitrary interference with the right of the individual to his personal liberty, or to enter into those contracts in relation to labor which may seem to him appropriate or necessary for the support of himself and his family? ...

... There is no reasonable ground for interfering with the liberty of person or the right of free contract, by determining the hours of labor, in the occupation of a baker. There is no contention that bakers as a class are not equal in intelligence and capac-ity to men in other trades or manual occupations, or that they are not able to assert their rights and care for themselves without the protecting arm of the state, inter-fering with their independence of judgment and of action. They are in no sense wards of the state. Viewed in the light of a purely labor law, with no reference whatever to the question of health, we think that a law like the one before us involves neither the safety, the morals, nor the welfare, of the public, and that the interest of the public is not in the slightest degree affected by such an act. The law must be upheld, if at all, as a law pertaining to the health of the individual engaged in the occupation of a baker. It does not affect any other portion of the public than those who are engaged in that occupation. Clean and wholesome bread does not depend upon whether the baker works but ten hours per day or only sixty hours a week. The limitation of the hours of labor does not come within the police power on that ground....

... The mere assertion that the subject relates, though but in a remote degree, to the public health, does not necessarily render the enactment valid. The act must have a more direct relation, as a means to an end, and the end itself must be appro-priate and legitimate, before an act can be held to be valid which interferes with the general right of an individual to be free in his person and in his power to contract in relation to his own labor....

We think that there can be no fair doubt that the trade of a baker, in and of itself, is not an unhealthy one to that degree which would authorize the legislature to interfere with the right to labor, and with the right of free contract on the part of the individual, either as employer or employee. . . . It might be safely affirmed that almost all occupations more or less affect the health. There must be more than the mere fact of the possible existence of some small amount of unhealthiness to warrant legislative interference with liberty. . . . No trade, no occupation, no mode of earning one's living, could escape this all-pervading power, and the acts of the legislature in limiting the hours of labor in all employments would be valid, although such limitation might seriously cripple the ability of the laborer to support himself and his family. . . .

. . . We think that such a law as this, although passed in the assumed exercise of the police power, and as relating to the public health, or the health of the employees named, is not within that power, and is invalid. The act is not, within any fair meaning of the term, a health law, but is an illegal interference with the rights of individuals, both employers and employees, to make contracts regarding labor upon such terms as they may think best. . . .

Mr. Justice HARLAN, joined by Justice WHITE and Justice DAY, dissenting:
It is plain that this statute was enacted in order to protect the physical well-being of those who work in bakery and confectionery establishments. . . .

[A writer describes the health impacts of such labor:] "The constant inhaling of flour dust causes inflammation of the lungs and of the bronchial tubes. The eyes also suffer through this dust, which is responsible for the many cases of running eyes among the bakers. . . . The average age of a baker is below that of other workmen; they seldom live over their fiftieth year, most of them dying between the ages of forty and fifty. During periods of epidemic diseases the bakers are generally the first to succumb to the disease, and the number swept away during such periods far exceeds the number of other crafts in comparison to the men employed in the respective industries." . . .

. . . There are many reasons of a weighty, substantial character, based upon the experience of mankind, in support of the theory that, all things considered, more than ten hours' steady work each day, from week to week, in a bakery or confectionery establishment, may endanger the health and shorten the lives of the workmen, thereby diminishing their physical and mental capacity to serve the state and to provide for those dependent upon them. . . .

. . . Let the state alone in the management of its purely domestic affairs, so long as it does not appear beyond all question that it has violated the Federal Constitution. This view necessarily results from the principle that the health and safety of the people of a state are primarily for the state to guard and protect.

. . . . .

The *Lochner* era caused deep concern among those who realized that much of what public health agencies do interferes with economic freedoms involving contracts, business relationships, the use of property, and the practice of trades and professions. *Lochner,* in the words of

Justice Harlan's dissent, "would seriously cripple the inherent power of the states to care for the lives, health, and well-being of their citizens" (198 U.S. at 73). In the following three decades, the Supreme Court struck down important health and social legislation that set minimum wages for women, protected consumers from hazardous products, and licensed or regulated businesses.

By the time of the New Deal, the laissez-faire philosophy that undergirded *Lochner*-ism was being challenged by those who believed that economic transactions were characterized by relationships of unequal wealth and power. Following the Great Depression, people were looking toward government to actively pursue the values of welfare, health, and greater social and economic equity. It was within this political and social context that the Supreme Court repudiated the principles of *Lochner*: "What is this freedom? The Constitution does not speak of freedom of contract. It speaks of liberty and prohibits the deprivation of liberty without due process of law" (*West Coast Hotel Co. v. Parrish,* 300 U.S. 379, 391 [1937]). The period after the New Deal saw the resurgence of a permissive judicial approach to public health regulation, irrespective of its effects on commercial and business affairs.

B. Regulatory "Takings"

The power of eminent domain allows states and the federal government to confiscate private property for governmental activities. This historic power of sovereign nations is constrained by the Fifth Amendment, which requires the government to give landowners "just compensation" when taking property for public use. The theory behind the takings clause is that individuals should not have to shoulder public burdens that should be borne by the community as a whole.

Government confiscation or physical occupation of property is a "possessory" taking that certainly requires compensation. During the early twentieth century, the Supreme Court held that government regulation that "reaches a certain magnitude" is also a taking that requires compensation (*Pennsylvania Coal Co. v. Mahon,* 260 U.S. 393, 413 [1922]). Initially, this idea of "regulatory" takings was not a problem for public health agencies, because the Court suggested that government need not compensate property owners when it was regulating within the police power. However, regulatory takings took on public health significance in 1992 with the Court's decision in *Lucas v. South Carolina Coastal Council.*

LUCAS V. SOUTH CAROLINA COASTAL COUNCIL*
Supreme Court of the United States
Decided June 29, 1992

Justice SCALIA delivered the opinion of the Court.

In 1986, petitioner David H. Lucas paid $975,000 for two residential lots on the Isle of Palms in Charleston County, South Carolina, on which he intended to build single-family homes. In 1988, however, the South Carolina Legislature enacted the Beachfront Management Act, S.C. Code Ann. § 48-39-250 et seq. (Supp. 1990), which had the direct effect of barring petitioner from erecting any permanent habitable structures on his two parcels. A state trial court found that this prohibition rendered Lucas's parcels "valueless." This case requires us to decide whether the Act's dramatic effect on the economic value of Lucas's lots accomplished a taking of private property under the Fifth and Fourteenth Amendments requiring the payment of "just compensation." . . .

Prior to Justice Holmes's exposition in *Pennsylvania Coal Co. v. Mahon*, 260 U.S. 393 (1922), it was generally thought that the Takings Clause reached only a "direct appropriation" of property, or the functional equivalent. . . . Justice Holmes recognized in *Mahon*, however, that if the protection against physical appropriations of private property was to be meaningfully enforced, the government's power to redefine the range of interests included in the ownership of property was necessarily constrained by constitutional limits. If, instead, the uses of private property were subject to unbridled, uncompensated qualification under the police power, "the natural tendency of human nature [would be] to extend the qualification more and more until at last private property disappear[ed]." *Id.*, at 415. These considerations gave birth in that case to the oft-cited maxim that "while property may be regulated to a certain extent, if regulation goes too far it will be recognized as a taking." *Ibid.*

Nevertheless, our decision in *Mahon* offered little insight into when, and under what circumstances, a given regulation would be seen as going "too far" for purposes of the Fifth Amendment. In 70-odd years of succeeding "regulatory takings" jurisprudence, we have generally eschewed any "set formula" for determining how far is too far, preferring to "engag[e] in . . . essentially ad hoc, factual inquiries." *Goldblatt v. Hempstead*, 369 U.S. 590, 594 (1962). We have, however, described at least two discrete categories of regulatory action as compensable without case-specific inquiry into the public interest advanced in support of the restraint. The first encompasses regulations that compel the property owner to suffer a physical "invasion" of his property. In general (at least with regard to permanent invasions), no matter how minute the intrusion, and no matter how weighty the public purpose behind it, we have required compensation. . . .

The second situation in which we have found categorical treatment appropriate is where regulation denies all economically beneficial or productive use of land. As we have said on numerous occasions, the Fifth Amendment is violated when land-use regulation "does not substantially advance legitimate state interests *or denies an*

---

*505 U.S. 1003 (1992).

owner economically viable use of his land." Agins v. City of Tiburon, 447 U.S. 255, 260 (1980).

We have never set forth the justification for this rule. Perhaps it is simply, as Justice Brennan suggested, that total deprivation of beneficial use is, from the landowner's point of view, the equivalent of a physical appropriation. . . .

. . . Affirmatively supporting a compensation requirement[] is the fact that regulations that leave the owner of land without economically beneficial or productive options for its use—typically, as here, by requiring land to be left substantially in its natural state—carry with them a heightened risk that private property is being pressed into some form of public service under the guise of mitigating serious public harm. . . .

We think, in short, that there are good reasons for our frequently expressed belief that when the owner of real property has been called upon to sacrifice all economically beneficial uses in the name of the common good, that is, to leave his property economically idle, he has suffered a taking. . . .

. . . In [the view of the South Carolina Supreme Court], the Beachfront Management Act was no ordinary enactment, but involved an exercise of South Carolina's "police powers" to mitigate the harm to the public interest that petitioner's use of his land might occasion. . . . In the court's view, [the] petitioner's challenge [came] within a long line of this Court's cases sustaining against Due Process and Takings Clause challenges the State's use of its "police powers" to enjoin a property owner from activities akin to public nuisances. . . .

Where the State seeks to sustain regulation that deprives land of all economically beneficial use, we think it may resist compensation only if the logically antecedent inquiry into the nature of the owner's estate shows that the proscribed use interests were not part of his title to begin with. This accords, we think, with our "takings" jurisprudence, which has traditionally been guided by the understandings of our citizens regarding the content of, and the State's power over, the "bundle of rights" that they acquire when they obtain title to property. It seems to us that the property owner necessarily expects the uses of his property to be restricted, from time to time, by various measures newly enacted by the State in legitimate exercise of its police powers; "as long recognized, some values are enjoyed under an implied limitation and must yield to the police power." *Mahon,* 260 U.S. at 413. And in the case of personal property, by reason of the State's traditionally high degree of control over commercial dealings, he ought to be aware of the possibility that new regulation might even render his property economically worthless (at least if the property's only economically productive use is sale or manufacture for sale). In the case of land, however, we think the notion pressed by the Council that title is somehow held subject to the "implied limitation" that the State may subsequently eliminate all economically valuable use is inconsistent with the historical compact recorded in the Takings Clause that has become part of our constitutional culture.

Where "permanent physical occupation" of land is concerned, we have refused to allow the government to decree it anew (without compensation), no matter how weighty the asserted public interests involved—though we assuredly would permit the government to assert a permanent easement that was a pre-existing limitation upon the landowner's title. We believe similar treatment must be accorded confiscatory regulations, i.e., regulations that prohibit all economically beneficial use of land: Any limitation so severe cannot be newly legislated or decreed (without compensation), but must inhere in the title itself, in the restrictions that background principles of the State's law of property and nuisance already place upon land ownership. A law or decree with such an effect must, in other words, do no more than duplicate the result that could have been achieved in the courts—by adjacent landowners (or other uniquely affected persons) under the State's law of private nuisance, or by the State under its complementary power to abate nuisances that affect the public generally, or otherwise. . . .

. . . In light of our traditional resort to "existing rules or understandings that stem from an independent source such as state law" to define the range of interests that qualify for protection as "property" under the Fifth and Fourteenth Amendments, *Board of Regents of State Colleges v. Roth*, 408 U.S. 564, 577 (1972), this recognition that the Takings Clause does not require compensation when an owner is barred from putting land to a use that is proscribed by those "existing rules or understandings" is surely unexceptional. When, however, a regulation that declares "off-limits" all economically productive or beneficial uses of land goes beyond what the relevant background principles would dictate, compensation must be paid to sustain it.

The "total taking" inquiry we require today will ordinarily entail (as the application of state nuisance law ordinarily entails) analysis of, among other things, the degree of harm to public lands and resources, or adjacent private property, posed by the claimant's proposed activities, the social value of the claimant's activities and their suitability to the locality in question, and the relative ease with which the alleged harm can be avoided through measures taken by the claimant and the government (or adjacent private landowners) alike. The fact that a particular use has long been engaged in by similarly situated owners ordinarily imports a lack of any common-law prohibition (though changed circumstances or new knowledge may make what was previously permissible no longer so). So also does the fact that other landowners, similarly situated, are permitted to continue the use denied to the claimant.

It seems unlikely that common-law principles would have prevented the erection of any habitable or productive improvements on petitioner's land; they rarely support prohibition of the essential use of land. The question, however, is one of state law to be dealt with on remand. . . . South Carolina must identify background principles of nuisance and property law that prohibit the uses he now intends in the circumstances in which the property is presently found. Only on this showing can the State fairly claim that, in proscribing all such beneficial uses, the Beachfront Management Act is taking nothing.

•   •   •   •   •

After *Lucas*, much remains unsettled regarding the reach of the regulatory takings doctrine. Few courts have used *Lucas* to find that a regulation denies a landowner all economically beneficial or productive use of real property and constitutes a *per se* taking. In 1998, a federal district court in Nevada held that the Tahoe Regional Planning Agency had effectuated a *per se* taking under *Lucas* when it temporarily banned development in the Lake Tahoe Basin to preserve the lake's clarity and environmental stability. In important victories for environmental, conservation, and public health advocates, both the Ninth Circuit and the Supreme Court disagreed, holding that a temporary provision could not constitute a *per se* taking (*Tahoe-Sierra Preservation Council, Inc. v. Tahoe Regional Planning Agency,* 535 U.S. 302 [2002]).

Most analyses of regulatory takings rely on the three-factor test of *Penn Central Transportation Co. v. New York City,* 438 U.S. 104 (1978), instead of *Lucas*'s *per se* rule. Under *Penn Central,* courts consider (1) the economic impact of the regulation on the property owner, (2) the extent to which the regulation has interfered with investment-backed expectations, and (3) the character of the governmental action. Unlike *Lucas*'s categorical rule, the third factor of *Penn Central* allows courts to consider the government's interests in protecting public health and safety. Nonetheless, the *Penn Central* test can be used to vigorously protect property rights to the detriment of public health regulation. For example, in *Philip Morris, Inc. v. Reilly,* 312 F.3d 24 (1st Cir. 2002), the United States Court of Appeals for the First Circuit held that a Massachusetts state law requiring cigarette manufacturers to disclose brand-specific ingredient lists to state regulators for eventual public dissemination effects an unconstitutional taking of trade secrets. Moreover, the Supreme Court has expanded the scope of *Penn Central,* holding that a property owner may bring a regulatory takings claim in cases in which the regulation at issue was in effect when the property was acquired (*Palazzo v. Rhode Island,* 533 U.S. 606 [2001]).

Property rights activists claim that an expansive understanding of the regulatory takings doctrine simply allows for the just distribution of a regulation's financial burden among the public as a whole. But in practice, a broader understanding of what constitutes a regulatory taking creates a potentially insurmountable fiscal barrier to implementing needed public health regulations. It remains to be seen whether lower courts will seize on the "property rights" tenor of Justice Antonin Scalia's opinion in *Lucas* to strike down important public health and environmental regulations. And it is unclear how the Supreme Court's regulatory takings jurisprudence will develop under the Roberts Court. Upcoming Supreme Court terms will certainly be key to the future of commercial regulations for public health purposes.

C. Public Use

Physical takings of property must conform to the requirements of the Fifth Amendment: "Nor shall private property be taken for public use, without just compensation." The first of these requirements constrains the uses for which property may be taken, while the second ensures that property owners are properly compensated for their loss. When property is taken for the construction of a school, park, or public right-of-way, the public use requirement is undoubtedly met. And the government clearly cannot take property for the private benefit of a particular private property. But can the government take private property for the creation of retail and office space as part of a larger community development project? In an enormously controversial decision—*Kelo v. City of New London* (excerpted below)—the Supreme Court upheld the city's confiscation of private property for commercial development. Critics vociferously argued that the Court's decision benefited large businesses to the detriment of politically powerless groups unable to effectively advocate for their property rights.

KELO V. CITY OF NEW LONDON*
Supreme Court of the United States
Decided June 23, 2005

Justice STEVENS delivered the opinion of the Court.

In 2000, the city of New London approved a development plan that, in the words of the Supreme Court of Connecticut, was "projected to create in excess of 1,000 jobs, to increase tax and other revenues, and to revitalize an economically distressed city, including its downtown and waterfront areas." 843 A. 2d 500, 507 (2004). In assembling the land needed for this project, the city's development agent has purchased property from willing sellers and proposes to use the power of eminent domain to acquire the remainder of the property from unwilling owners in exchange for just compensation. The question presented is whether the city's proposed disposition of this property qualifies as a "public use" within the meaning of the Takings Clause of the Fifth Amendment to the Constitution. . . .

. . . Decades of economic decline led a state agency in 1990 to designate the City [of New London] a "distressed municipality." . . . In 1998, the City's unemployment rate was nearly double that of the State, and its population of just under 24,000 residents was at its lowest since 1920.

These conditions prompted state and local officials to target New London, and particularly its Fort Trumbull area, for economic revitalization. To this end, respondent New London Development Corporation (NLDC), a private nonprofit entity established some years earlier to assist the City in planning economic development, was reactivated. In January 1998, the State authorized a $5.35 million bond issue to support the NLDC's planning activities and a $10 million bond issue toward the creation of a Fort Trumbull State Park. In February, the pharmaceutical company Pfizer Inc. announced that it would build a $300 million research facility on a site immediately

*545 U.S. 469 (2005).

adjacent to Fort Trumbull; local planners hoped that Pfizer would draw new business to the area, thereby serving as a catalyst to the area's rejuvenation. After receiving initial approval from the city council, the NLDC continued its planning activities and held a series of neighborhood meetings to educate the public about the process. In May, the city council authorized the NLDC to formally submit its plans to the relevant state agencies for review. Upon obtaining state-level approval, the NLDC finalized an integrated development plan focused on 90 acres of the Fort Trumbull area. . . .

The NLDC intended the development plan to capitalize on the arrival of the Pfizer facility and the new commerce it was expected to attract. In addition to creating jobs, generating tax revenue, and helping to "build momentum for the revitalization of downtown New London," the plan was also designed to make the City more attractive and to create leisure and recreational opportunities on the waterfront and in the park.

The city council approved the plan in January 2000, and designated the NLDC as its development agent in charge of implementation. The city council also authorized the NLDC to purchase property or to acquire property by exercising eminent domain in the City's name. The NLDC successfully negotiated the purchase of most of the real estate in the 90-acre area, but its negotiations with petitioners failed. As a consequence, in November 2000, the NLDC initiated the condemnation proceedings that gave rise to this case.

Petitioner Susette Kelo has lived in the Fort Trumbull area since 1997. She has made extensive improvements to her house, which she prizes for its water view. Petitioner Wilhelmina Dery was born in her Fort Trumbull house in 1918 and has lived there her entire life. Her husband Charles (also a petitioner) has lived in the house since they married some 60 years ago. In all, the nine petitioners own 15 properties in Fort Trumbull. . . . There is no allegation that any of these properties is blighted or otherwise in poor condition; rather, they were condemned only because they happen to be located in the development area. . . .

Two polar propositions are perfectly clear. On the one hand, it has long been accepted that the sovereign may not take the property of A for the sole purpose of transferring it to another private party B, even though A is paid just compensation. On the other hand, it is equally clear that a State may transfer property from one private party to another if future "use by the public" is the purpose of the taking; the condemnation of land for a railroad with common-carrier duties is a familiar example. Neither of these propositions, however, determines the disposition of this case.

As for the first proposition, the City would no doubt be forbidden from taking petitioners' land for the purpose of conferring a private benefit on a particular private party. Nor would the City be allowed to take property under the mere pretext of a public purpose, when its actual purpose was to bestow a private benefit. The takings before us, however, would be executed pursuant to a "carefully considered" development plan. . . . All the members of the Supreme Court of Connecticut agreed that there was no evidence of an illegitimate purpose in this case. . . .

On the other hand, this is not a case in which the City is planning to open the condemned land—at least not in its entirety—to use by the general public. Nor will the private lessees of the land in any sense be required to operate like common carriers, making their services available to all comers. . . .

The disposition of this case therefore turns on the question whether the City's development plan serves a "public purpose." Without exception, our cases have defined that concept broadly, reflecting our longstanding policy of deference to legislative judgments in this field.

In *Berman v. Parker,* 348 U.S. 26 (1954), this Court upheld a redevelopment plan targeting a blighted area of Washington, D.C., in which most of the housing for the area's 5,000 inhabitants was beyond repair. Under the plan, the area would be condemned and part of it utilized for the construction of streets, schools, and other public facilities. The remainder of the land would be leased or sold to private parties for the purpose of redevelopment, including the construction of low-cost housing. . . .

In *Hawaii Housing Authority v. Midkiff,* 467 U.S. 229 (1984), the Court considered a Hawaii statute whereby fee title was taken from lessors and transferred to lessees (for just compensation) in order to reduce the concentration of land ownership. We unanimously upheld the statute and rejected the Ninth Circuit's view that it was "a naked attempt on the part of the state of Hawaii to take the property of A and transfer it to B solely for B's private use and benefit." *Hawaii Housing Authority v. Midkiff,* 467 U.S. 229, 235 (1984). . . . Our opinion also rejected the contention that the mere fact that the State immediately transferred the properties to private individuals upon condemnation somehow diminished the public character of the taking. "[I]t is only the taking's purpose, and not its mechanics," *id.* at 244, we explained, that matters in determining public use. . . .

Viewed as a whole, our jurisprudence has recognized that the needs of society have varied between different parts of the Nation, just as they have evolved over time in response to changed circumstances. . . . For more than a century, our public use jurisprudence has wisely eschewed rigid formulas and intrusive scrutiny in favor of affording legislatures broad latitude in determining what public needs justify the use of the takings power.

Those who govern the City were not confronted with the need to remove blight in the Fort Trumbull area, but their determination that the area was sufficiently distressed to justify a program of economic rejuvenation is entitled to our deference. The City has carefully formulated an economic development plan that it believes will provide appreciable benefits to the community, including—but by no means limited to—new jobs and increased tax revenue. As with other exercises in urban planning and development, the City is endeavoring to coordinate a variety of commercial, residential, and recreational uses of land, with the hope that they will form a whole greater than the sum of its parts. To effectuate this plan, the City has invoked a state statute that specifically authorizes the use of eminent domain to promote economic development. Given the comprehensive character of the plan, the thorough deliberation that preceded its adoption, and the limited scope of our review, it is appropriate for us, as it was in *Berman,* to resolve the challenges of the individual owners, not on a piecemeal basis, but rather in light of the entire plan. Because that plan unquestionably serves a public purpose, the takings challenged here satisfy the public use requirement of the Fifth Amendment. . . .

Justice O'CONNOR, with whom Chief Justice REHNQUIST, and Justices SCALIA and THOMAS join, dissenting:
. . . In moving away from our decisions sanctioning the condemnation of harmful

property use, the Court today significantly expands the meaning of public use. It holds that the sovereign may take private property currently put to ordinary private use, and give it over for new, ordinary private use, so long as the new use is predicted to generate some secondary benefit for the public—such as increased tax revenue, more jobs, maybe even aesthetic pleasure. But nearly any lawful use of real private property can be said to generate some incidental benefit to the public. Thus, if predicted (or even guaranteed) positive side-effects are enough to render transfer from one private party to another constitutional, then the words "for public use" do not realistically exclude any takings, and thus do not exert any constraint on the eminent domain power. . . .

It was possible after *Berman* and *Midkiff* to imagine unconstitutional transfers from A to B. Those decisions endorsed government intervention when private property use had veered to such an extreme that the public was suffering as a consequence. Today nearly all real property is susceptible to condemnation on the Court's theory. In the prescient words of a dissenter from the infamous decision in [*Poletown Neighborhood Council v. City of Detroit*], "[n]ow that we have authorized local legislative bodies to decide that a different commercial or industrial use of property will produce greater public benefits than its present use, no homeowner's, merchant's or manufacturer's property, however productive or valuable to its owner, is immune from condemnation for the benefit of other private interests that will put it to a 'higher' use." 304 N.W.2d 455, 464 (Mich. 1981) (Fitzgerald, J., dissenting). This is why economic development takings "seriously jeopardiz[e] the security of all private property ownership." *Id.* at 465 (Ryan, J., dissenting).

Any property may now be taken for the benefit of another private party, but the fallout from this decision will not be random. The beneficiaries are likely to be those citizens with disproportionate influence and power in the political process, including large corporations and development firms. As for the victims, the government now has license to transfer property from those with fewer resources to those with more. The Founders cannot have intended this perverse result. "[T]hat alone is a *just* government," wrote James Madison, "which *impartially* secures to every man, whatever is his *own*." For the National Gazette, Property (Mar. 29, 1792).

. . . . .

Years after *Kelo*, the Court's decision remains controversial. The city has halted plans to evict the plaintiffs, and parts of New London's development project have stalled. A *New York Times* article notes that "investors are concerned about building on land that some people consider a symbol of property rights" (Yardley 2005). But elsewhere, similar projects are moving forward. On June 23, 2008, the Supreme Court declined to hear an appeal concerning Brooklyn's $4 billion Atlantic Yards Project, which centers on a basketball arena intended to house the New Jersey Nets (*Goldstein v. Pataki*, 516 F.3d 50 [2d Cir. 2008], *cert. denied*, 128 S.Ct. 2964 [2008]).

III. CONCLUSION

The court cases discussed in this chapter raise a vital normative issue about the significance of economic liberty in our society. How important is unbridled freedom in property uses, financial relationships, and the pursuit of occupations? A market economy is valued because it increases productivity and raises standards of living. Free enterprise also has public health significance because of the positive association between socioeconomic status and well-being. After all, it is possible to theorize that the free market will create wealth not only for entrepreneurs but for the wider population.

Despite the value of the freewheeling entrepreneur, should we strive for a well-regulated society that deters harmful commercial activities? Surely no one would defend gratuitously burdensome regulation, but government does have an obligation to safeguard the health of its people and their environment. Suppose a manufacturer will gain more profit if it makes a product without a safety feature (e.g., automobiles without air bags) or fails to control its by-products (e.g., toxic waste dumped into a lake). Isn't it within the government's prerogative to regulate such activity? If the legislature makes a social choice that favors communal health and safety over economic freedom, arguably the courts should respect that judgment.

RECOMMENDED READINGS

Regulatory Tools of Public Health Agencies

Baker, Robert B., Harriet A. Washington, Ololade Olakanmi, Todd L. Savitt, Elizabeth A. Jacobs, Eddie Hoover, and Matthew K. Wynia. 2008. African American physicians and organized medicine, 1846–1968: Origins of a racial divide. *JAMA* 300: 306–13. (Details the history of racial bias and segregation in organized medicine and its continuing effects in the United States)

Bohmer, Richard. 2007. The rise of in-store clinics—threat or opportunity? *New England Journal of Medicine* 356: 765–68. (Describes the debate over the relative merits and drawbacks of retail health clinics)

Burris, Scott. 2003. Legal aspects of regulating bathhouses. In *Gay Bathhouses and Public Health Policy,* ed. William J. Woods and Diane Binson, 131–49. New York: Harrington Park Press. (Discusses cases resulting in closure of bathhouses and the utility of closure in discouraging risk behaviors)

Lewin, Nancy L., Jon S. Vernick, Peter L. Beilenson, Julie S. Mair, Melisa M. Lindamood, Stephen P. Teret, Daniel W. Webster, et al. 2005. The Baltimore Youth Ammunition Initiative: A model application of local public health authority in preventing gun violence. *American Journal of Public Health* 95: 762–65. (Details Baltimore's use of public nuisance law to control the sale of ammunition to minors)

Constitutional Rights and Normative Values of Economic Liberty

Gostin, Lawrence O. 2006. Property rights and the common good. *Hastings Center Report* 36 (5): 10–11. (Examines *Kelo* and argues that its impact on the residents of areas slated for redevelopment may be positive)

Kesselheim, Aaron S., and Jerry Avon. 2006. Biomedical patents and the public's health: Is there a role for eminent domain? *JAMA* 295: 434–37. (Analyzes the use of eminent domain in the pharmaceutical industry after *Kelo* affirmed the use of the takings doctrine to serve the greater public good)

Parmet, Wendy E. 1996. From *Slaughter-House* to *Lochner:* The rise and fall of the constitutionalization of public health. *American Journal of Legal History* 40: 476–503. (Provides an in-depth analysis of the role of public health in constitutional law)

PART FOUR

The Future of the Public's Health

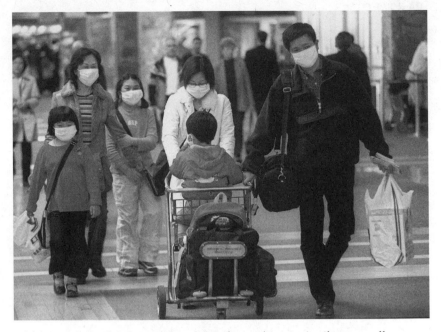

Photo 30. A family of travelers arriving from China in April 2003 walks through Vancouver International Airport wearing surgical masks to protect them from contracting SARS. The 2003 SARS epidemic sickened more than 8,000 people on four continents and killed 774. No serious outbreaks have been reported since the initial emergence of the disease. Reproduced by permission, © Christopher J. Morris/Corbis, April 3, 2003.

THIRTEEN

Concluding Reflections on the Field

Case Studies on Biosecurity, Genomics, and Obesity

The field of public health vastly helped improve the health and well-being of populations during the twentieth century, leading to substantial increases in life expectancy, improved sanitation and living conditions, and reductions in infectious diseases. Nevertheless, major problems, as well as remarkable opportunities, confront the field in a new century.

This chapter offers case studies on three of the most complex and important public health challenges: bioterrorism and biosecurity, public health genomics, and obesity. Each of these challenges raises core questions regarding the proper scope of and ethic for public health, highlights the interconnectedness of domestic and global health, and demonstrates the importance of recognizing and ameliorating underlying inequalities that leave society's most vulnerable to bear the heaviest burden of ill health and premature death.

I. "PUBLIC HEALTH IN REVERSE": BIOTERRORISM AND BIOSECURITY

On September 11, 2001, the United States experienced the devastating effects of terrorist attacks within its borders that led to civilian mass casualties at New York's World Trade Center, at the Pentagon, and in Pennsylvania. One month later, the deliberate dissemination of anthrax spores through the U.S. postal system highlighted the health and security risks posed by the malevolent use of biological agents. These events shocked the country into recognizing the vast challenges of preventing, detecting early, and containing health threats, as well as caring for and treating large populations facing possible injury, disease, and death. As waves of emerging infectious diseases (from severe acute respiratory syndrome, or SARS, to avian flu to H1N1) temporarily—albeit significantly—disrupted the economic activities and health systems of affected areas, the need to incorporate security measures into public health services—"public health preparedness"—began to top the agendas of politicians and public health officials alike.

In response to these threats, public health programs and initiatives have increasingly been "securitized." From laboratories to political fora, greater emphasis has been given to integrating traditional national security measures and public health tools. Biosecurity, this "radical" melding of the security and public health fields, not only embodies "society's collective responsibility to safeguard the population from dangers presented by pathogenic microbes" but also demonstrates that "the policy worlds of public health and security are interdependent" (Fidler and Gostin 2007, 4, 121). As economic globalization and international travel have burgeoned, individual nations—both developed and developing—are affected by other countries' potential health and security problems. Therefore, biosecurity measures must take into account domestic and international factors (e.g., economic instability and social inequities) that contribute to and result from outbreaks of naturally occurring and deliberately released infectious diseases.

This section examines the pressing and important problems of biological warfare and bioterrorism. It then considers the controversies stemming from the securitization of public health in the post-9/11 era. Finally, this section discusses the domestic and international socioeconomic environments that may give rise to bioterrorism, as well as the conditions that may be exacerbated by biological warfare and infectious disease.

A. Biological Warfare and Bioterrorism

Biological warfare is defined as the intentional release of microorganisms or toxins of biological origin against armed forces in a time of war. Bioterrorism is the deliberate release of microorganisms or toxins of biological origin against civilian populations in order to destabilize social and political structures. The U.S. Public Health Service has called biological warfare and bioterrorism "public health in reverse" because of their potentially devastating effects on populations (H. Cohen, Gould, and Sidel 1999).

Biological warfare has evolved from the crude use of cadavers to contaminate water supplies to the development of specialized munitions intended to be employed both on the battlefield and covertly. Documented episodes of bioterrorism, although rare, have been dramatic. In 1995 the Aum Shinrikyo ("Supreme Truth") cult released the chemical agent sarin in a Tokyo subway. In 1984 an Oregon cult allegedly contaminated salad bars with the biological agent salmonella (Cole 1995; MacKenzie 1998). In the aftermath of 9/11, public health and criminal justice authorities investigated—though to date without success—cases of the intentional dispersal of anthrax.

It is all too easy to envision a deadly scenario:

> Imagine a bioterrorist event in Washington, DC with the release of enough smallpox to infect 100 people. For ten days, the victims are unaware of their plight, but on days 11–13 a fever erupts with a violent headache, followed by a rash. If the victims travel to other cities such as New York or Tokyo during early disease, they spread virus particles via saliva from spots developing in the mouth. The red spots on the skin harden into pea-sized bumps that become reeking pustules. On the average, 30 of the original 100 will develop more serious forms of the disease and die: those who survive may be badly scarred or blind. Accurate diagnosis may not occur until the second wave of victims has been infected, and vaccinations may not begin until the third wave. A huge, coordinated public health response would be required to deliver and administer the vaccine needed to contain the epidemic around the world. (Meacham and Croom 2004, 178)

The agents most likely to be used as biological weapons (see table 7) have the potential to be aerosolized and dispersed over a wide geographic area and are resistant to sunlight, desiccation, and heat. They also have the potential to cause lethal or debilitating disease, are transmitted person to person, and are not easily prevented or treated. The agents that best meet these criteria include smallpox, anthrax, plague, viral hemorrhagic fever, and botulism (Leggiadro 2000). With advances in genetic engineering, these biological agents, which are already capable of inflicting devastating morbidity and mortality, could be manipulated to increase their resistance to treatment, their durability, and their contagiousness.

The use of anthrax and smallpox as biological weapons raises particularly fascinating and controversial issues. Even though the Food and

TABLE 7. Five deadliest biological agents

Biological Agent	Description	Symptoms	Fatality Rate	Treatment
Inhalation Anthrax (*Bacillus anthracis*)	Inhaled spores germinate and release toxins, causing swelling in the chest cavity. Possible blood and brain infection.	Fever, fatigue, and malaise, starting within 2 to 46 days; progresses to chest pain, cough, rapid deterioration of health.	Kills more than 85 percent of those it infects, often within 1 to 3 days after symptoms appear.	Antibiotics (preferably ciprofloxacin) should be given before symptoms appear. Vaccine available, though not for civilians.
Smallpox (*Variola* virus)	Very contagious airborne disease.	About 12 to 14 days after infection, fever, aches, vomiting, rash of small red spots that grow into larger painful pustules covering the body.	Fatal in 20 percent of unvaccinated patients.	No treatment. U.S. has vaccine for about 6 million people. Only a fraction of those vaccinated before 1972 still protected.
Pneumonic Plague (*Yersinia pestis*)	Natural, flea-borne form causes bubonic plague. Gravest threat is posed by aerosolized form, leading to pneumonic plague.	High fever, headache, and bloody cough; progresses to labored breathing, bluish-grayish skin color, respiratory failure, and death.	Without treatment, a person with pneumonic plague will almost always die within 1 to 2 days after symptoms begin.	Various antibiotics, including streptomycin and gentamicin. Isolate patients.
Viral Hemorrhagic Fever	Highly infectious RNA viruses including Ebola, Marburg, Lassa, and dengue fever. Spread by rodents, ticks, and mosquitoes.	Vary from one type of VHF to the next. Include fever, muscle aches, exhaustion, internal bleeding.	Varies. Death rate from dengue is as low as 1 percent. Ebola fatality rates have reached 90 percent.	Mainly supporting therapy. Antiviral drug ribavirin useful in treating some viruses but not others (Ebola, Marburg).
Inhalation Botulism (*Clostridium botulinum*)	Produces toxin that blocks nerve signals, inhibits muscle movement. Weapon would most likely aerosolize toxin.	Difficulty swallowing food, mental numbness, muscle paralysis, possible breathing failure.	Unclear; only a handful of cases of the inhalation form have been reported.	Patients with respiratory paralysis should be placed on ventilator. Antitoxin given early may prevent progression.

SOURCE: U.S. Centers for Disease Control and Prevention and U.S. Army Military Research Institute of Infectious Disease.

Drug Administration (FDA) did not approve any anthrax vaccine until December 2003, in 1998 the Department of Defense (DoD) established the Anthrax Vaccine Immunization Program (AVIP), designed to achieve total force protection against anthrax by 2004 (CDC 2000b). Military leaders are worried about the safety of their service members on the battlefield, but the AVIP remains highly controversial. The evidence for the safety and effectiveness of the anthrax vaccine is equivocal. Members of the armed forces are concerned about possible adverse effects in the short and long term, and they question the DoD's decision to compel vaccination against their will. In 2003, service members successfully challenged the AVIP in *Doe v. Rumsfeld*, 297 F. Supp. 2d 119 (D.D.C. 2003). Days after the court halted the program, the FDA published a final rule categorizing the vaccine as safe and effective for use against inhalation anthrax. In doing so, however, the FDA violated its own rules that allow meaningful public comment, so the program was again halted by the court in October 2004 (*Doe v. Rumsfeld*, 341 F. Supp. 2d 1 [D.D.C. 2004]). For the next two years, the program proceeded on a voluntary basis and participation rates did not exceed 50 percent (Weiss, Weiss, and Weiss 2007). After the FDA issued a proper formal ruling that the vaccine safe and effective, the DoD announced on October 15, 2006, that it would resume mandatory anthrax vaccinations.

The public health response to smallpox is equally contested and raises unique issues. Smallpox vaccination is very effective, but most people today have no immunity: mass immunization came to an end more than twenty-five years ago, after smallpox had been eradicated. The World Health Organization (WHO) destroyed most of the remaining vaccine stocks in the early 1990s. The smallpox virus, also known as variola, is now classified as a Biosafety Level 4 hot agent (the most dangerous virus) because it is lethal, airborne, and highly contagious.

At present, variola exists officially in only two repositories—at the laboratories of the Centers for Disease Control (CDC) in Atlanta, Georgia, and at a Russian facility in Novosibirsk, Siberia. However, there is growing suspicion that the virus may also be found in clandestine biowarfare laboratories. The WHO has struggled with the question of whether to destroy the two official stocks of the virus. Experts are concerned about the possible release of the virus, whether accidental or intentional, because the appearance of a single case of smallpox anywhere on earth would become a global health emergency. After the anthrax attacks of 2001, many began to fear that smallpox might be used in an act of bioterror; should such an attack occur, it would be exceedingly difficult to develop a new vaccine if the official stocks of the virus had been eliminated. In November 2001, the United States declared that it would not destroy its supply of smallpox virus.

On December 13, 2002, President George W. Bush announced a multiphase national smallpox vaccination plan, using a new and not yet approved vaccine, with several phases: half a million military personnel would undergo immediate, mandatory vaccination; up to 500,000 health care workers would be vaccinated on a voluntary basis; and members of the public who insist on being vaccinated would eventually have access to vaccine. As explained in box 32 of the companion text, the plan to vaccinate the military went ahead as planned, but the health care worker plan faltered badly and was officially "paused" in June 2003. Many health care workers refused to be vaccinated, weighing the very low risk of a smallpox attack against the possibility that the vaccine might have adverse effects; moreover, no plan was in place to compensate them if they did suffer harm.

In the following section, Donald A. Henderson, a physician and epidemiologist who played a vital role in the international eradication of smallpox, examines the "looming threat" of bioterrorism.

THE LOOMING THREAT OF BIOTERRORISM*
Donald A. Henderson

Of the weapons of mass destruction (nuclear, chemical, and biological), the biological ones are the most greatly feared, but the country is least well prepared to deal with them. Virtually all federal efforts in strategic planning and training have so far been directed toward crisis management after a chemical release or an explosion. Should such an event occur, fire, police, and emergency rescue workers would proceed to the scene and, with the FBI assuming lead responsibility, stabilize the situation, deal with casualties, decontaminate, and collect evidence for identification of a perpetrator. This exercise is not unfamiliar. Spills of hazardous materials, explosions, fires, and other civil emergencies are not uncommon events.

The expected scenario after release of an aerosol cloud of a biological agent is entirely different. The release could be silent and would almost certainly be undetected. The cloud would be invisible, odorless, and tasteless. It would behave much like a gas in penetrating interior areas. No one would know until days or weeks later that anyone had been infected (depending on the microbe). Then patients would begin appearing in emergency rooms and physicians' offices with symptoms of a strange disease that few physicians had ever seen. Special measures would be needed for patient care and hospitalization, obtaining laboratory confirmation

*Reprinted from *Science* 283 (1999): 1279–82. Reprinted with permission from the American Association for the Advancement of Science.

regarding the identity of microbes unknown to most laboratories, providing vaccine or antibiotics to large portions of the population, and identifying and possibly quarantining patients. Trained epidemiologists would be needed to identify where and when infection had occurred, so as to identify how and by whom it may have been spread. Public health administrators would be challenged to undertake emergency management of a problem alien to their experience and in a public environment where pestilential disease, let alone in epidemic form, has been unknown.

The implicit assumption has frequently been that chemical and biological threats and the responses to them are so generically similar that they can be readily handled by a single "chembio" expert, usually a chemist. This is a serious misapprehension. . . .

PROBABLE AGENTS

Any one of thousands of biological agents that are capable of causing human infection could be considered a potential biological weapon. Realistically, only a few . . . can be cultivated and dispersed effectively so as to cause cases and deaths in numbers that would threaten the functioning of a large community. Other factors also determine which microbes are of priority concern: specifically, the possibility of further human-to-human spread, the environmental stability of the organism, the size of the infectious dose, and the availability of prophylactic or therapeutic measures.

A Russian panel of bioweapons experts reviewed the microbial agents and concluded that there were 11 that were "very likely to be used." The top four were smallpox, plague, anthrax, and botulism. Lower on their list were tularemia, glanders, typhus, Q fever, Venezuelan equine encephalitis, and Marburg and influenza viruses. Each of the four top-rated agents is associated with high case fatality rates when dispersed as an aerosol. The rates range upward from 30% for smallpox to more than 80% for anthrax. Smallpox and anthrax have other advantages in that they can be grown reasonably easily and in large quantities and are sturdy organisms that are resistant to destruction. They are thus especially suited to aerosol dissemination to reach large areas and numbers of people. . . .

LIKELY PERPETRATORS

Some argue that almost anyone with intent can produce and dispense a biological weapon. It is unlikely, however, that more than a few would be successful in obtaining any of the top-rated agents in a form suitable to be dispensed as an aerosol. Naturally occurring cases of plague, anthrax, and botulism do occur on almost every continent and so provide a potential source for strains. However, there is considerable variation in the virulence of different strains, and a high level of expertise, which is much less obtainable than the agents themselves, is needed to identify an especially pathogenic one. Moreover, producing these particular organisms in large quantity and in the ultra-small particle form needed for aerosolization is beyond the average laboratory. . . .

GREATEST THREATS: SMALLPOX AND ANTHRAX

Of the potential biological weapons, smallpox and anthrax pose by far the greatest threats, albeit because of different clinical and epidemiological properties. . . .

Smallpox poses an unusually serious threat; in part, because virtually everyone is now susceptible, vaccination having stopped worldwide 20 or more years ago as a result of the eradication of the disease. Because of waning immunity, it is probable that no more than 20% of the population is protected. Among the unprotected, case fatality rates after infection with smallpox are 30%. There is no treatment. Virus, in aerosol form, can survive for 24 hours or more and is highly infectious even at low dosages.

An outbreak in which as few as 100 people were infected would quickly tax the resources of any community. There would be both actual cases and people with a fever and rash for whom the diagnosis was uncertain. In all, 200 or more patients would probably have to be treated in the first wave of cases. Most of the patients would be extremely ill with severe aching pains and high fever and would normally be hospitalized. . . . [P]atients would have to be confined to rooms under negative pressure that were equipped with special filters to prevent the escape of the virus. Hospitals have few rooms so ventilated; there would, for example, probably be less than 100 in the Washington, D.C., metropolitan area.

A vaccination program would have to be undertaken rapidly to protect as many as possible of those who had been in contact with the patients. Vaccination given within 3 to 4 days after exposure can protect most people against a fatal outcome and may prevent the disease entirely. It is unlikely, however, that smallpox would be diagnosed early enough and vaccination programs launched rapidly enough to prevent infection of many of the people exposed during the first wave. Few physicians have ever seen smallpox and few, if any, have ever received training in its diagnosis. . . .

A second wave of cases would be almost inevitable. From experiences with smallpox imported into Europe over the past 40 years, it is estimated that there would be at least 10 secondary cases for every case in the first wave, or 1000 cases in all, appearing some 14 days after the first wave. Vaccination would initially be needed for health workers, essential service personnel, and contacts of patients at home and at work. With mounting numbers of cases, contacts, and involved areas, mass vaccination would soon be the only practical approach. That would not be possible, however, because present vaccine supplies are too limited, there being approximately 5 to 7 million doses currently available. To put this number in perspective, in New York City in 1947, 6 million people were vaccinated over approximately 1 week in response to a total of eight cases of smallpox. Moreover, there are no longer any manufacturers of smallpox vaccine. Best estimates indicate that substantial additional supplies could not be ensured sooner than 36 months from the initial outbreak. [Ed.–In November 2001, the Bush administration announced a major initiative to increase the vaccine supply; it was followed by the unsuccessful plan, described earlier in this chapter, to vaccinate as many as 500,000 health care workers.]

A scenario for an inhalation anthrax epidemic is of no less concern. Like smallpox, the aerosol would almost certainly be unobtrusively released and would drift throughout a building or even a city without being noticed. After 2 to 3 days, infected individuals would appear in emergency rooms and doctors' offices with a variety of nonspecific symptoms such as fever, cough, and headache. Within a day or two, patients would become critically ill and then die within 24 to 72 hours. It is doubtful that antibiotic therapy given after symptoms develop would be of benefit. The case fatality rate is 80% or greater.

Although anthrax does not spread from person to person, it has another dangerous attribute. Individuals who are exposed to an aerosol may abruptly develop illness up to 8 weeks after the initial exposure. Cases can be prevented by the administration of antibiotics, but such treatment would have to be continued daily for at least 60 days. This period might be shortened by the prompt administration of vaccine. Experimental studies suggest that two doses of vaccine given 15 days apart may provide protection beginning 30 days after the initial inoculation. At this time, however, there is no vaccine available for civilian use; building of stockpiles of antibiotics is still in the planning stage, and no city at present has a plan for distributing antibiotics so as to ensure that drugs are given over a 60-day period. [Ed.–Though not all these problems have been addressed, the Strategic National Stockpile (originally called the National Pharmaceutical Stockpile) was established in 1999.]

A LOOK AT THE FUTURE

... The most effective step now is to strengthen the public health and infectious disease infrastructure. An augmented full-time cadre of professionals at the state and local level would represent, for biological weapons, a counterpart to the National Guard Rapid Assessment and Initial Detection Teams for chemical weapons. Rather than being on a standby basis, however, the biological cadre would also serve to strengthen efforts directed toward dealing with new and emerging infections and food-borne diseases....

National Institutes of Health- and CDC-administered research agendas are needed to attract both university and private sector talents to address a host of constraints and problems. Among the most critical needs now are improved vaccines, available in large supply, for both smallpox and anthrax. Areas for vaccine improvement include increasing overall efficacy; in the case of smallpox, reducing complications and in the case of anthrax, reducing the number of inoculations. Feasibility studies suggest that substantially improved second-generation vaccines can be developed quickly.

Finally, there is a need both now and in the longer term to pursue measures that will prevent acts of terrorism.... The strengthening of our intelligence capabilities so as to anticipate and perhaps interdict terrorists is of the highest priority. The fostering of international cooperative research programs to encourage openness and dialogue as is now being done with Russian laboratories is also important.

B. Securitization of Public Health

Biosecurity refers to the approaches used to protect populations from dangerous microbial agents—both those that occur naturally and those that are deliberately released (Fidler and Gostin 2007). Although it may be common to associate biosecurity only with counterbioterrorism programs, naturally occurring epidemics pose security threats comparable to those presented by biological weapons. In particular, both bioterrorism and infectious disease outbreaks have the potential to cause widespread disruptions in society. As Tara O'Toole (2001, 109), a physician expert in bioterrorism and biodefense, notes:

The forces of globalization offer efficient conduits for the spread of disease. . . . Today a deadly virus or bacteria can traverse the planet in a day. . . . Vast food distribution networks [now] allow widespread dissemination of tainted products and greatly complicate efforts to prevent contamination. Further, the pressures of population growth and commercialization have fueled human intrusion into once remote eco-systems, increasing the chances of contact with previously unknown and potentially dangerous viruses. Finally, the natural evolution and mutation of microbial pathogens . . . have ensured that drug resistance must be factored into strategies to contain infectious disease. All of these factors present a context that demands urgent attention to the perils of biological weapons and epidemic infectious disease.

Historically, a gulf has separated American public health programs and national security imperatives, with their very different policy priorities, ideological underpinnings, and funding sources. Both aim to secure public safety, but the scope of national security is arguably narrower—only acute, large-scale threats are given high priority. Thus national security objectives focus tightly on preventing and mitigating such threats. In contrast, public health aims at securing community health and well-being, a far broader mission that involves norms of justice and equality.

In the wake of the 2001 attacks, it became apparent that public health tools and the public health system in general could further national security interests. Public health approaches to identifying, contain-ing, and treating naturally occurring infectious diseases (e.g., SARS, HIV/AIDS, tuberculosis, and measles) are similar to those required for bioterrorism monitoring and prevention, and a well-functioning public health system would be integral to detecting, monitoring, and respond-ing to biological threats. In 2002, the Office of Homeland Security (the precursor to the Department of Homeland Security) published a national strategy explicitly recognizing the public health system's role in managing and responding to bioweapon threats. The White House's national security reports in 2002 and 2006 characterized specific infectious diseases—HIV/AIDS and pandemic influenza—as national security threats. At the international level, in 2005 the WHO revised its International Health Regulations to address not just infectious dis-eases but also biological, chemical, and radiological attacks (see chap-ter 7). Rapidly, the "concern about bioterrorism . . . transformed public health from unappreciated to a central component of national security" (May 2005, 34).

Since then, a variety of biosecurity measures and securitized health programs have been implemented. In 2003, the National Institutes of Health received $1.5 billion for biodefense research and corresponding labs (Enserink and Kaiser 2005). Research funding also reflected new security interests: from 2001 to 2005, money for grants to study bacterial bioweapon agents increased more than fifteenfold over the amount provided in the previous five years. But at the same time, the change in priorities made it increasingly difficult for scientists to undertake basic research in microbiology and bacteriology, as research grants in those areas declined by 41 percent and 27 percent, respectively (Bettelheim 2006).

The integration of public health and national security measures has been welcomed by many. Not only has the usually strained public health system received needed dollars, but it also has garnered substantially more public attention and support. The securitization of public health programs has also opened new lines of communication, ensuring that epidemiological and medical information can be readily conveyed to security officials. Many politicians and public health practitioners hail biosecuritization as providing the "significant dual benefit" of advancing health and improving security (May 2005, 36).

But critics argue that "partnering with military, national security, and law enforcement agency–led preparedness strategies and programs could ultimately undermine our ability to effectively employ primary prevention against significant health threats" (Sidel, Gould, and Cohen 2002, 82). They point out that the theoretical frameworks of public health and national security are often at odds with each other. The narrower mission of national security—preserving the population against direct and acute threats—excludes much of what concerns public health, particularly its focus on social justice. From a national security standpoint, acquiring intelligence and preventing violence take precedence over the more general well-being of the population and considerations of social justice (e.g., the protection of vulnerable groups). And, on a more practical level, national security is primarily focused on the immediate causes of security breaches. Public health interventions, in contrast, target all factors that compromise the population's health. Some argue that because a narrow national security emphasis fails to take into account the more fundamental causes of the threats—poverty, political instability, and social inequalities—it actually compromises biosecurity (H. Cohen, Gould, and Sidel 2004). Such tensions may damage public trust in health officials: "Given the well documented history of abuses by US military, intelligence, and law enforcement in the name of 'national security,' [public health risks] being tainted by current and future violations of public trust" (Sidel, Gould, and Cohen 2002, 87–88).

C. Health Security, Globalization, and Social Justice

Linked with the threat of infectious disease is the threat of bioterrorism. Many nations and sub-national groups now have the capability to prepare and disseminate pathogenic microbes. . . . The propensity of a group to apply this capability for a malicious purpose will be influenced by a variety of factors, one of which will be the group's perception of social injustice. While it would be foolish to attribute the entire threat of bioterrorism to social injustice, it would be equally foolish to ignore the potential for poverty, insecurity, and injustice to motivate terrorists or provide rationale for their actions. (Gutlove and Thompson 2003, 19)

Public health and related security issues are no longer strictly domestic matters. In a global era, the problems of one country can quickly affect the world's economic, political, and social stability. This was exemplified in the April 2009 outbreak of influenza A (H1N1): in the span of only nine weeks, the WHO raised the pandemic alert to Phase 6, with all regions reporting confirmed cases of the disease (WHO 2009b). As Donald A. Henderson (1999, 179) observes, "If smallpox were to appear anywhere in the world today, the way airplane travel is now, about six weeks would be enough time to seed cases around the world. Dropping an atomic bomb would cause casualties in a specific area, but dropping smallpox would engulf the world."

Although few corners of the world would be untouched by a smallpox epidemic or the intentional release of an infectious bioagent, illness and death would affect each area to different degrees. As figure 10 demonstrates, preexistent social inequities, inadequate health care services, and economic stratification may predispose certain populations to higher rates of illness and death. Such outcomes would inevitably strain already weakened health and political systems, thereby contributing to the troubled social conditions thought to underlie bioviolence (H. Cohen, Gould, and Sidel 2004).

If poverty and political unrest are some of the major factors that may fuel bioterrorist activities and exacerbate casualties, how do they fit into plans to enhance biosecurity? Are biosecurity and social justice conceptually irreconcilable, or are they simply incompatible as currently approached? In the following excerpt, David Heymann, the assistant director-general for health security and environment at the WHO,

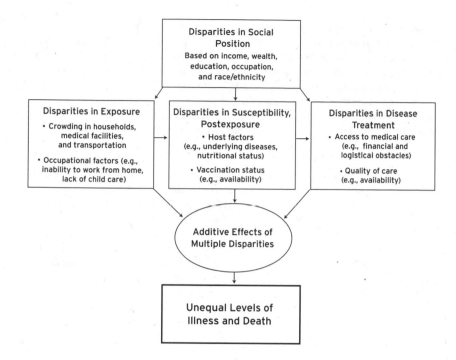

Figure 10. Biosecurity and disparities. Possible sources of disparities in the event of a bioterrorist attack or release of biological weapons that may lead to heightened morbidity and mortality for disadvantaged populations. *Source:* Adapted from Blumenshine et al. 2008, 710.

considers how national and international health security protocols can ensure the public's health and help ameliorate health disparities.

THE EVOLVING INFECTIOUS DISEASE THREAT: IMPLICATIONS FOR NATIONAL AND GLOBAL SECURITY*

David L. Heymann

The deliberate use of anthrax to incite terror . . . changed the profile of the infectious disease threat in a dramatic and definitive way. Prior to these events, the emergence of new diseases . . . had sharpened concern about the infectious disease threat as a disruptive and destabilizing force . . . [to] national security. . . . The reality of bioterrorism immediately raised the infectious disease threat to the level of a high-priority security imperative . . . worthy of attention in defense and intelligence circles. . . . As

*Reprinted from *Journal of Human Development* 4 (2003): 191–207. Reprinted by permission of the publisher Taylor & Francis Ltd., www.informaworld.com.

smallpox again became a disease of greatest concern, both politicians and the public began to comprehend problems long familiar to public health professionals. These have ranged from silent incubation periods that allow pathogens to cross borders undetected and undeterred ... to the simple fact that outbreaks have a potential for international spread that transcends the defenses of any single country. ... This heightened concern has clearly identified a central principle of global public health security: strengthened capacity to detect and contain naturally caused outbreaks is the only rational way to defend the world against the threat of a bioterrorist attack. ...

THE RESURGENCE OF THE INFECTIOUS DISEASE THREAT

During the past 30 years, the infectious disease threat has diverged considerably from previous patterns of epidemiology, drug susceptibility, geographical distribution, and severity. ... Infectious disease agents readily and rapidly multiply, mutate, adapt to new hosts and environments, and evolve to resist drugs. This natural propensity to change has been greatly augmented by the pressures of a crowded, closely interconnected, and highly mobile world. ... As adversaries, microbial pathogens have particular advantages in terms of invisibility, mobility, adaptability, and silent incubation periods that render national borders meaningless. Infectious agents, incubating in symptomless air travelers, can move between any two cities in the world within 36 hours and slip undetected past any border. ... The threat posed by drug resistance is particularly ominous and universal. Health care in all countries is now compromised by the shrinking number of effective first-line antimicrobials and the need to resort to more costly, and often more hazardous, alternative drugs, when available. Fuelled by co-infection with HIV, the return of tuberculosis as a global menace has been accompanied by the emergence of multidrug-resistant forms costing up to 100 times more to treat. ... Drug resistance to common bacterial infections is now so pervasive that ... many life-saving treatments and routine surgical procedures could become too risky to perform

These developments [have] restored the historical significance of infectious diseases as a disruptive force—this time cast in a modern setting characterized by close interdependence of nations and instantaneous communications. Within affected countries, the disruptive potential of outbreaks and epidemics [ranges] from public panic and population displacement to the interruption of routine functions that occurs when containment requires the emergency immunization of populations. ... Affected countries [also] can experience heavy additional burdens in ... lost trade and tourism. At the global level, some of the most telling efforts to measure economic consequences ... have centered on determining what the AIDS epidemic in sub-Saharan Africa means for the economies of wealthy nations. At one extreme, the high mortality caused by this disease [has] been interpreted as the cost to industrialized countries of lost export markets. At the other extreme, the economic costs of AIDS to the international community have been expressed in terms of the price of drugs and services needed to rescue a continent. ...

AIDS: A CLEAR THREAT TO NATIONAL SECURITY

Of all diseases, AIDS provides the most dramatic and disturbing example of the capacity of a previously unknown pathogen to rapidly spread throughout the world ... and cause social and economic upheaval. ... Prior to the events of September and October 2001, AIDS already provided a strong case for considering infectious diseases as a security issue. At the most obvious level, any agent with such high rates of mortality . . . that directly threatens to kill a significant proportion of a state's population constitutes a direct threat to state security. . . . In Africa, AIDS poses an immediate threat to the organization of many different societies as well as to the security of political institutions. . . . Other immediate effects on state capacity include the loss of high-level government officials, an overwhelming of the health care system, and an erosion of traditional systems of social support. . . . More, not less, state failure and insecurity is projected, and this is expected to translate into new forms of transnational security threats. . . .

CHANGING PERCEPTIONS OF SECURITY

In its traditional meaning, "security" has long been a strictly national pursuit aimed at defending territorial integrity and ensuring state survival. . . . Traditional approaches to the defense of national security are military functions: protecting borders, fighting wars, and deterring aggressors. Two events have challenged these . . . views. First, the end of the Cold War meant an end to security issues polarized by the ideological conflict and geopolitical interests of the superpowers. . . . As old threats subsided, more attention focused on threats arising from civil unrest, internal conflicts, mass migration of refugees, and localized wars between neighboring countries. . . . Security issues became broader and more complex, and attention began to focus on . . . the root causes of unrest, conflict, and mass population movement. . . . In the wake of these changes . . . environmental conditions[,] . . . income, education, and health . . . were put forward as determinants of internal state stability. . . . In a second event, the forces of globalization demonstrated the porous nature of national borders and eroded traditional notions of state sovereignty. In a closely interconnected and interdependent world, the repercussions of adverse events abroad easily cross borders to intrude on state affairs in ways that cannot be averted through traditional military defenses. . . . Emerging and epidemic-prone diseases qualified as a transnational threat for obvious reasons: they easily cross borders in ways that defy traditional defenses and cannot be deterred by any state acting alone. . . . In industrialized countries, global pandemics such as influenza, where supplies of vaccines and antivirals are clearly insufficient, have the capacity to destabilize populations, and . . . cause great social disruption. In developing countries, where economies are fragile and infrastructures weak, outbreaks and epidemics are far more directly disruptive. In these countries, the destabilizing effect of high-mortality endemic diseases . . . is amplified by emerging and epidemic-prone diseases, as they disrupt routine control programs and health services. . . . Outbreaks of new or unusual diseases can cause public panic to a degree that calls into question government's capacity to protect its population. In addition, the dramatic interruption of trade, travel, and tourism that can follow news of an outbreak places a further economic burden on impoverished countries with little capacity to absorb such shocks.

HIGH PRIORITY ON THE SECURITY AGENDA?

Several recent events suggest that emerging and epidemic-prone diseases are being taken seriously as a threat to national and global security. . . . The [security] threat posed by microbial agents . . . was . . . acknowledged in 2000 by [a] report from the

US Central Intelligence Agency's National Intelligence Council. Citing the "stagger-ing" and "destabilizing" number of deaths caused by AIDS in sub-Saharan Africa, the report documented specific consequences in the form of diminished gross domestic product, reduced life expectancy, weakened military capacity, social fragmentation, and political destabilization. The report also addressed the growing threat posed by infectious diseases in general, and drew attention to the contributing roles of rapid urban growth, environmental degradation, and cross-border population move-ments. . . . The events of September and October 2001 changed this situation dra-matically, as the prospect of bioterrorism brought infectious disease agents into direct intersection with national security imperatives. It has also brought into sharp focus many of the difficult problems faced by public health on a daily basis. For example, the anthrax incident demonstrated the difficulty of quickly identifying an unfamiliar disease. . . . The rapid determination of whether a disease might be deliberately caused is likewise notoriously difficult. Plague in India, dengue in Cuba, hantavirus in New Mexico, and West Nile virus in New York are just some examples of diseases initially considered to have a deliberate origin in the recent past. . . .

'DUAL USE' DEFENSE

Efforts to prevent the international spread of infectious diseases . . . are currently being revised . . . to serve as an up-to-date framework for global surveillance and response. . . . The WHO has long argued that the most important defense against the infectious disease threat . . . is good intelligence and a rapid response. Intelligence is gleaned through highly sensitive global surveillance systems that keep the world alert to changes in the infectious disease situation. Routine surveillance systems for naturally occurring outbreaks enhance the capacity to detect and investigate those that may be deliberately caused. . . . Adequate background data on the natural behavior of known pathogens provide the epidemiological intelligence needed to recognize an unusual event and to determine whether suspicions of a deliberate cause should be investigated. A global surveillance system, operating in real time, facilitates rapid and rational responses. . . . The performance of routine systems in detecting and containing naturally occurring outbreaks provides an indication of how well they would perform when coping with a deliberately caused outbreak. . . . Strong public health systems are vital, as public health plays the initial and leading role in the response to a deliberately caused outbreak.

The mechanisms for global surveillance and response are in place and opera-tional, on a daily basis, in the Global Outbreak Alert and Response Network. . . . This overarching network interlinks electronically . . . 110 existing laboratory and disease reporting networks [that] together . . . possess much of the data, expertise, and skills needed to keep the international community constantly alert and ready to respond. The network . . . is supported by several new mechanisms and a custom-ized artificial intelligence engine for real-time gathering of disease information. This tool, the Global Public Health Intelligence Network . . . , . . . heightens vigilance by continuously and systematically crawling websites, news wires, local online news-papers, public health e-mail services, and electronic discussion groups for rumors of outbreaks. In this way, the network is able to scan the world for informal news that gives cause for suspecting an unusual event. . . . The network currently picks up—in real time—more than 40% of the outbreaks subsequently verified by the WHO.

However, outbreaks of some diseases ... frequently occur in very remote rural areas that fall outside the reach of electronic communications, thus necessitating contin-ued reliance on other sources, including reports from countries. ...

Once international assistance is needed, ... electronic communications are used to coordinate prompt assistance. ... Surge capacity, insufficient vaccine supplies, and expensive drugs are issues that must be dealt with on a regular basis in order to keep the world ready to respond—issues similar to those needed for preparedness for bio-terrorism. ... The work of coordinating large-scale international assistance ... is facilitated by operational protocols that set out standardized procedures for the alert and verification process, communications, co-ordination of the response, emergency evacuation, research, monitoring, ownership of data and samples, and relations with the media. By setting out a chain of command and bringing order to the containment response, such protocols help protect against the very real risk that samples of a lethal pathogen might be collected for later provision to a terrorist group. ...

A RATIONAL RESPONSE TO A SHARED THREAT

The possibility that biological agents might be deliberately used to cause harm is ... another divergence of the infectious disease threat. ... Its significance as a secu-rity threat is readily appreciated in light of the well-documented ability of naturally caused infectious diseases to invade, surprise, and disrupt. The issues that require attention and resources—vaccine production, stockpiling of antibiotics, and protec-tive clothing—are vital. ... The challenge is to manage this new threat in ways that do not compromise the response to natural outbreaks and epidemics, but rather strengthen the public health infrastructure, locally and globally, for managing both threats. ...

In the US, the initial response to the anthrax incident concentrated almost exclu-sively on the strengthening of domestic public health capacity, with very little atten-tion given to the international dimensions. ... More recent developments indicate a growing awareness of the inadequacy of a strictly national response. They also indi-cate a growing willingness to view improved global capacity to detect and contain naturally caused outbreaks as the most rational ... way to defend nations, individu-ally and collectively, against the threat of a bioterrorist attack. In November 2001, a meeting of G7 + Mexico health ministers culminated in [a] plan acknowledg[ing] bio-terrorism as an international issue requiring international collaboration, and launched a series of collective efforts aimed at improving international prepared-ness and capacity to respond. ... The meeting also launched a global collaborative network of high-security laboratories as a strategy for improving global capacity to rapidly and accurately diagnose diseases "whether naturally or intentionally occurring." In another significant development, the proposed US *Global Pathogen Surveillance Act 2002* acknowledged the universal nature of the infectious disease threat and frankly admitted that "domestic surveillance and monitoring, while abso-lutely essential, are not sufficient" to combat bio-terrorism or ensure adequate domestic preparedness. ... The Act treated natural and intentionally caused out-breaks as closely related threats and recognized that strengthened capacity to mon-itor, detect, and respond to infectious disease outbreaks would offer dual dividends in the form of better protection against both threats. ...

Recent developments provide encouraging evidence that political leaders have

a better understanding of the issues facing public health and ... appreciate both
the need to strengthen public health infrastructures and the universal benefits of
doing so. Equally important is the understanding that strong national and international public health must be considered as elements of national security, and that
increased funding for strengthening national and international public health must
come from government sectors that go beyond health to include national security,
defense, and international development aid. Only then can the world begin to move
towards a degree of security that sees the volatile infectious disease threat matched
by a stable, alert, and universal system of defense. The lasting benefits for the daily
work of outbreak detection and control could be enormous for both industrialized
and developing countries.

II. FROM GENES TO PUBLIC HEALTH

On April 14, 2003, the international scientific community passed a
major milestone: the human genome had been sequenced. Thus began
the genomic era, and with it the complex and arduous task of understanding the relationships among genes, genomics, and human health.
Scientists have long known about hereditary diseases such as cystic
fibrosis, Huntington's chorea, sickle-cell anemia, and Tay-Sachs disease. The Human Genome Project now promises to help us understand
multifactorial illnesses such as cancer, diabetes, heart disease, and
schizophrenia. Scientists today can examine information about a person's general landscape of genes (i.e., his or her genomic information)
as well as information about a particular gene or genes carried by a
person (i.e., genetic information).

Genetic scientists hope to provide many benefits, such as supplying
patients with predictive information about their health status that can
inform their choices, aiding the identification of the origin and physiol-
ogy of diseases, advancing clinical knowledge to better prevent and
treat genetic diseases, and generally enhancing medical research. At the
same time, the increased use of genetic testing, diagnosis, and clinical
intervention raises social concerns. Worries about privacy and the specter of genetic discrimination in employment and health insurance loom
large. Some fear that the benefits and burdens of genetic information
and medicine might be inequitably distributed, favoring the rich and
powerful over society's most vulnerable. And, on a more fundamental
level, some are concerned that genetic technologies—genetic enhance-
ments, artificial reproduction, cloning, and the like—might eventually
alter the "natural" order of life.

This section examines the potential benefits of applying genetic
knowledge to population health. Moreover, it considers how to use

genetic research and biotechnology to reduce health disparities and improve living conditions in developing countries.

A. Public Health Genetics and Genomics

Genomics is the study of the entire human genome, which explores not only the actions of single genes but also the interactions of multiple genes with each other and with the environment (IOM 2005b). Public health genomics is an exciting field that brings all the public health sciences to bear on the emerging challenge of interpreting the significance of genetic and genomic variation within populations. Increasing knowledge of the human genome, gene-gene interactions, and gene-environment interactions has the potential to revolutionize public health interventions and approaches toward health policy.

The very concept of "public health genomics" may at first appear contradictory. As the expert in law and genetics Ellen Wright Clayton (2000, 489) notes,

> For many people, it is difficult to imagine how genetics and public health intersect. We repeatedly hear that genetic information is individual, intensely private, indeed more private than almost any other kind of information, and in today's environment potentially hazardous to one's access to employment and insurance. One person's genetic makeup rarely presents a risk to the health of others; a woman who has a mutation in $BRCA_1$ [breast cancer 1, early onset] and so is more susceptible to breast cancer cannot transmit the disease or even the mutation to her best friend. At the same time, most people think of public health in terms of the interventions that public health agencies impose on large groups of people to improve health, ranging from fluoridation of water to immunization or, in extreme cases, quarantine. Thinking about the conjunction of private concerns and public actions makes it hard even to consider genetics and public health at the same time.

Yet genetic information is already contributing to many areas of study in public health. For example, marked genetic heterogeneity exists in susceptibility to specific infectious agents (e.g., malaria, TB, HIV/ AIDS), sensitivity to environmental toxins or contaminants, and metabolism of nutrients and prescription medications. In short, exposure to certain pathogens, pollutants, diets, and drugs can affect people quite differently depending on individual genetic traits. In addition, genetics may have a role in influencing risk behaviors such as smoking, alcoholic beverage consumption, and illicit drug use, though the relationships are deeply complex.

Genomics offers unprecedented promise to change our understanding of how the health of populations is determined and to provide new tools for improving health and reducing the burden of disease. For example, the notion of personalized medicine—the use of genomic information to classify a disease, select a medication, provide a therapy, or initiate a preventive measure that is particularly suited to a given patient—has been heralded by physicians and researchers as the best way to maximize health care and treatment benefits in the future. Francis Collins (1999, 34–35), the former director of the National Human Genome Research Institute, envisions the long-promised day when personalized medicine has become a reality:

> John, a 23-year-old-man, consults with his doctor in selecting from a battery of genetic tests that will provide information about his personal relative and lifetime risks for a number of common diseases. . . . Confronted with the reality of his own genetic data, [John] arrives at that crucial "teachable moment" when a lifelong change in health-related behavior, focused on reducing specific risks, is possible. And there is so much to offer. By 2010, the field of pharmacogenomics has blossomed, and a prophylactic drug regimen based on the knowledge of John's personal genetic data can be precisely prescribed to reduce his cholesterol level and the risk of coronary artery disease to normal levels. His risk of colon cancer can be addressed by beginning a program of annual colonoscopy at the age of 45, which in his situation is a very cost-effective way to avoid colon cancer. His substantial risk of contracting lung cancer provides the key motivation for him to join a support group of persons at genetically high risk for serious complications of smoking and he successfully kicks the habit.

Although this vision may be overly rosy and remains a distant prospect at best, researchers have made progress in identifying genetic variances that correspond with an increased chance of an adverse reaction to medication or of an enhanced response (e.g., individuals with certain genetic polymorphisms associated with the neurotransmitter serotonin have demonstrated better responses to antidepressants).

As scientists learn how genes and the environment ("nature" and "nurture") interact at the cellular level, policy makers will have important decisions to make about how we regulate environmental exposures, how we determine the risk/reward ratios of different activities, and even when to alter the genome. In a preface to a collection of papers from a major symposium on public health genetics, Jonathan E. Fielding, Lester B. Lave, and Barbara Starfield (2000, vi) explain the complex policy issues raised:

We will need to rethink how standards for environmental and occupational exposures are set, because we will know much more about the variation in human susceptibility to different effects of environmental influences. As one example, will we permit new chemical compounds that cause neurotoxicity in one child per million or the continued manufacture and sale of an existing compound that has this result? Will new laws permit employers to require genetic testing and legally exclude from certain types of jobs those individuals whose genetic predispositions place them at greatly increased risk for adverse health effects? Could an individual who is found to be 10-fold more likely than average to sustain a back injury by lifting heavy objects be legally excluded by a prospective employer from a job that requires these activities? Will prospective employees be required to submit to genetic screening to determine whether they are particularly susceptible to adverse effects of chemicals to which they would be exposed occupationally? Will the FDA change its approach to food labeling based on greater understanding of polymorphism in biotransformational enzymes, which can predispose to cancer, cardiovascular disease, or cerebral degeneration? Although these generic questions of ascertaining risk, workers vs. employer rights, assignment of legal liabilities, and the setting of standards are not new, we will have much better and more quantifiable data to consider in making individual and societal decisions. The looming question is how to translate better data into better decisions.

B. Genetic Knowledge and Health Disparities

In March 2008, the National Institutes of Health established the Center for Genomics and Health Disparities to explore how genetic and socioeconomic factors contribute to differences between races in disease rates and medical responses among races. Though it hoped that such initiatives in public health genomics would improve population health, it is also feared that public health genomics might in fact exacerbate existing health disparities. Even those who undertake health initiatives with the best intentions are not immune to shifting political agendas and socially ingrained prejudices. As genetic knowledge continues to increase, public health and political figures must determine how this knowledge can be used in ways to avoid further marginalization and, ideally, to alleviate ongoing health inequities.

Consider the case of BiDil, a drug used to treat heart failure, and its marketing campaigns that primarily targeted African Americans. On the surface, NitroMed, Inc., the manufacturer of BiDil, seemed to have the worthy objective of addressing the disproportionately high rates of heart failure among African Americans. The company suggested that the disparity might be due to biological or physiological differences between races, which BiDil addressed. At a time when public health and medicine had begun to emphasize the ameliorattion of racial disparities in health, NitroMed's promotion of BiDil as a racially specific drug was viewed by many as progressive, if not laudable. But others criticized the company for reifying race as a biological construct and for its research and marketing strategies. Pamela Sankar and Jonathan. Kahn (2005) argued that treating BiDil as a new drug—when it was in fact a combination of two known and effective generic drugs—cheated African American consumers of a cost-effective therapy. More fundamentally and damagingly, by creating "the impression that the best way to address health disparities is through commercial drug development," BiDil may have drawn attention away from the social determinants of health and "distort[ed] public understanding of health disparities and of efforts to address them" (Sankar and Kahn 2005, 462). At the same time, racial self-identification cannot effectively substitute for genetic classification, since many people self-identify incorrectly.

In addition, some worry that public health genomics may exacerbate health disparities not just within a country but also between countries. If the required technologies are expensive, the genomic era might improve the fate only of the world's most privileged. Worse still, the burden of genomic research might fall disproportionately on the world's poor. Craig Venter, the former president of Celera Genomics, stresses the need to develop cost-effective genomic initiatives:

> The key question for public health, however, is whether [genomic information] will improve the health of all of the world's people, or whether it will just widen the technology gap between rich and poor. Ask people what they understand of the potential of genomics for human health, and many will talk about an unprecedented opportunity to develop new drugs and vaccines. Others are concerned that the poor will gain nothing, while the rich will gain a kind of "boutique medicine": the opportunity to buy a full analysis of their personal genetic makeup, and then purchase designer therapies. If genomics is to make a major impact on global health, it will have to help provide affordable population-wide tools for combating common diseases. (quoted in Brand 2005, 114)

In the following selection, Halla Thorsteinsdóttir and colleagues examine the threat that genomics might become a "club good" instead of a global public good and propose ways to use genomic knowledge to improve the fates of those living in developed and developing countries alike.

GENOMICS—A GLOBAL PUBLIC GOOD?*

Halla Thorsteinsdóttir, Abdallah S. Daar, Richard D. Smith, and Peter A. Singer

In October, 2002, scientists published the sequence of the parasites responsible for most of the world's human malaria, *Plasmodium falciparum* and *P yoelii,* as well as the mosquito that carries it, *Anopheles gambiae.* The knowledge of these genomes and of the human genome, will lead to new drug and vaccine targets against malaria. But how fully will new genomics knowledge be used to the benefit of developing countries?

The WHO Advisory Committee for Health Research recently emphasized the relevance of genomic knowledge for health improvement in developing countries. However, as evidenced by the enormous inequities in global health and global health-research, knowledge—including genomics knowledge—is not developed to the optimum or used for improving the health of people in developing countries. In a closely interconnected world, this growing "genomics divide" will have global repercussions, including increased illnesses and instability. Genomics has significant characteristics as a global public "good," but these are not fully developed in developing countries. . . .

Goods can be defined along a spectrum from pure "private" goods to pure "public" ones. Most goods are private in nature, having clear property rights associated with them. For example, an apple is a private good and its consumption can be withheld until a price is paid (i.e., it is excludable). Eaten by one person, an apple cannot then be eaten by someone else (i.e., it is rivalrous in consumption). By contrast, the benefits of public goods are enjoyed by all (non-excludable) and consumption by one individual does not deplete the good and thus does not restrict its consumption by others (non-rivalrous). For instance, the internet is typically open to all (non-excludable) and downloading information does not deplete the information (non-rivalrous). Global public goods are simply public goods that possess such properties of publicness across national boundaries.

Genomics is principally about knowledge, which is commonly conceived to be the archetypal public good. Genomics knowledge is non-rivalrous in consumption (not depleted by use), and is usually made public by genomics databases on the internet and journal publication, as was the case with the malaria and mosquito genome. It is a global public good in the sense of the knowledge not being bound by national borders, in discovery, transmission, or use. Further, the global public-good nature of genomics is reflected in the way in which the Human Genome Project was funded and undertaken.

Although the development of genomics knowledge has significant global public-good characteristics, its application, especially at the individual level, may have private-good characteristics (excludable and rivalrous in consumption). For example, consumed by one individual, an antimalarial drug cannot also be consumed by

*Reprinted from *The Lancet* 361 (2003): 891–92, with permission from Elsevier. © 2003 by The Lancet, Ltd.

another. However, the application of genomics at the population level—such as by genetically altering mosquitoes to block the cycle of parasite transmission—retains significant public-goods characteristics. The incidence of malaria infection will be reduced both in the region where the modification is done as well as in other regions to which the modified mosquitoes spread. The effects of these interventions are therefore non-excludable and non-rivalrous in consumption.

This analysis shows that genomics knowledge and its application have, in principle, considerable global public-good characteristics. However, in practice, genomics knowledge and its application do not always express these characteristics. Although knowledge is theoretically free to be disseminated, in practice constraints are often put on its use. To absorb and make use of scientific knowledge, considerable investment is required. For example, education and training, physical access to journals or the internet, research infrastructure, and the ability to establish the necessary production processes to turn genomic knowledge into a useful product, all challenge the ability to make practical use of genomics knowledge. The international patent system can accentuate this problem for developing countries. Genomics is only a public good to those countries that have the capacity to exploit genomics knowledge and to conduct genomics research. Because of the need for these "access goods," genomics becomes a "club good," accessible mainly to industrialized countries.

The global public-good concept, applied to genomics, highlights three important issues. First, as with knowledge, the free-market does not have an incentive to produce a nonexcludable good since a price cannot be charged, and thus different mechanisms for finance or production are required. Second, in developing countries, because of the lack of access to goods, genomics becomes a club good. Finally, to achieve the best global production and use of genomics, collective action is required.

Collective action will be required in many areas, including efforts to improve research infrastructure, education, and training to provide developing countries with the access goods they need. These steps will require a financial commitment on the part of industrialized country governments ... [and] the sharing of relevant intellectual property by multinational corporations, for example through public-private partnerships such as the Malaria Vaccine Initiative and the Medicines for Malaria Venture. A global genomics initiative—in partnership with developing countries— would provide a suitable forum to discuss and develop these steps, ... strengthen global genomics governance[,] ... [and] harness genomics to improve global health-equity.

.   .   .   .   .

Although the use of genomic information faces many challenges in developing countries, innovative researchers are employing biotechnology to develop creative solutions. For example, scientists are working on an HIV vaccine based on the cellular immune responses observed in HIV-resistant prostitutes from Nairobi. Researchers are also testing a hepatitis B vaccine for which antigens are bred in transgenic plants and consumed orally; similar immunization techniques are being used for cholera, measles, and human papillomavirus (HPV). These plant-based edible vaccines are ideal for the immunization needs of developing countries because they do not require refrigeration, they can be harvested or freeze-dried and then shipped anywhere, and they are significantly cheaper than other vaccines to produce and transport (Singer and Daar 2001). Resourceful health programs and collaborations with external organizations must be established and maintained in order to include the developing world in the public health genomics movement.

Public health genomics holds great promise to improve the health of populations and to reduce disparities experienced throughout the world. However, this potential can be fully realized only if scientists and policy makers create well-planned and equity-based health initiatives and programs. Personalized medicine is still only a vision, but preparations for managing and disseminating such treatments need to be made far in advance. As the case of BiDil shows, the best-intentioned medical therapies cannot be extricated from their sociopolitical environments. Public health and political officials should work toward creating an environment in which public health genomics can maximize access to premium health care and minimize discrimination between populations.

III. THE OBESITY PANDEMIC: OBESITY-PROMOTING ENVIRONMENTS AND GLOBAL JUSTICE

Traditionally, obesity has been viewed as a condition caused—and ameliorated—by personal choices and behaviors: choosing potato chips over vegetables, preferring sedentary activities to those demanding bodily exertion, and so on. Public health programs have focused on education efforts and media campaigns (such as the CDC's "5 A Day") to promote increased consumption of healthier foods. Even as funding for such dietary instruction grows, waistlines continue to expand (see figure 11). According to the WHO's most recent data, approximately two-thirds of American adults are overweight; of these, half are obese. (For updated data and information on other countries, see the WHO's Global Database on Body Mass Index at www.who.int/bmi—the source of the figures in the following paragraph.) The rise in childhood obesity is a particularly troubling trend; recent studies estimate that 17 percent of children and adolescents are overweight (Ogden et al. 2006). Beyond predisposing children for co-morbid diseases and psychosocial problems, physicians "predict that pediatric obesity may shorten life

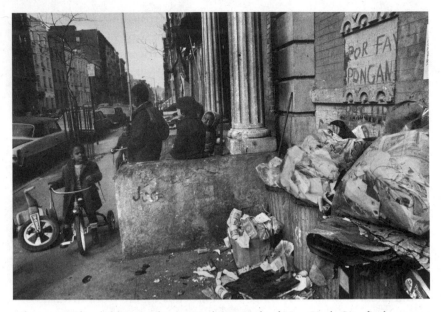

Photo 31. The children in this 1970 photograph of New York City find room to play amid piles of garbage and cement blocks. The built environment—that is, the altered and constructed physical environment in which people live—is a strong determinant of community health. The absence of clean, safe places for exercise and play helps fuel the obesity epidemic in urban areas. Reproduced by permission, © Bettman/Corbis, February 16, 1970.

expectancy in the United States by two to five years by midcentury—an effect equal to that of all cancers combined" (Ludwig 2007, 2325).

The United States is not alone in facing this epidemic. Obesity rates are high in other developed countries as well (e.g., one in four Britons are obese), and they have surged dramatically in developing countries. The island nations of the Micronesian South Pacific have been particularly devastated by the obesity epidemic: according to the WHO, 79 percent of adults are obese in Naura, 56 percent in Tonga, and 41 percent in French Polynesia.

The startling domestic and global numbers on obesity show that obesity does not result solely from the behavior of autonomous agents or from genetic predispositions. The population trends indicate that environmental and cultural factors are also at work. Accordingly, obesity researchers, public health practitioners, and policy makers are all beginning to consider "a broad set of social and environmental explanations"

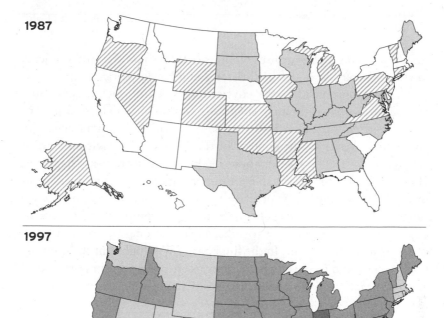

1987

1997

2007

No data | <10% | 10-14% | 15-19% | 20-24% | 25-29% | ≥ 30%

Figure 11. Obesity trends in the United States (1987, 1997, 2007). *Source:* Centers for Disease Control and Prevention, "U.S. Obesity Trends 1985– 2007," www.cdc.gov/nccdphp/dnpa/obesity/trend/maps/

for obesity rates and to devise solutions that focus on the environments in which people live and eat (Christakis and Fowler 2007, 371).

This section considers the environments (built, social, economic, and cultural) that ultimately shape the worlds in which food is consumed and physical activity is conducted. Earlier chapters generally considered obesity in the context of the information environment. In chapter 9, compelled speech about health was featured; in chapter 6, efforts to hold companies liable for distorting the information environment (deceptive marketing practices) were discussed. Here, I describe a range of other environments (e.g., the built environment and the socioeconomic environment) that together create an obesity-promoting, or obesogenic, environment. In the final part, I will highlight the growing obesity epidemic in developing countries, stressing the importance of addressing inequities to tackle the obesity pandemic.

A. *The Obesogenic Environment*

> With rising trends reported in most parts of the world, childhood obesity has reached the stage of pandemic. Essentially, obesity has become rampant because we now tend to eat more and move less, and we are increasingly encouraged to do so by our environments. Obesity, in other words, is a sign of mismatch between our genes—still lingering at the hunter-gatherer epoch—and our current techno-commercial and comfort-oriented lifestyles. (Maziak, Ward, and Stockton 2007, 39)

An ethos of personal responsibility pervades American legal, cultural, and political life, reflecting the society's larger emphasis on individual autonomy. Not surprisingly, law and economics scholars often see ill health in general and obesity in particular in terms of individuals' rational choices. Public health scholars and practitioners have a different explanation, however. They note that behavior is largely determined by the environment in which people live. The principal environmental determinants of health are the *physical or built environment*—for example, transportation, buildings, green spaces, and roads; the *economic environment*—for example, complex interactions among socioeconomic status–related, psychosocial, behavioral, and health care–related factors; the *social environment*—for example, social networks, social support, and loneliness; the *informational environment*—for example, comprehensible information on healthy behaviors and lifestyles; the *natural environment*—for example, clean air, water, and other natural resources; and the *work environment*—for example,

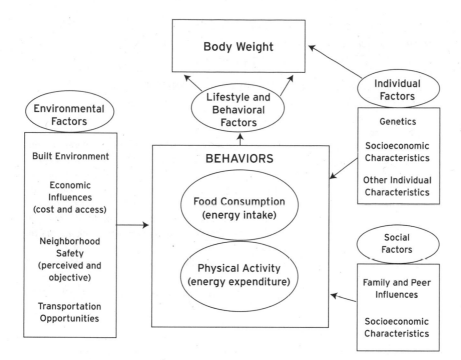

Figure 12. Ecological model: The influence on body weight of factors derived from physical and socioeconomic environments. *Source:* Adapted from Papas et al. 2007.

pay, job demands, control, and job insecurity. In the context of obesity, the built, economic, social, and informational environments exert the greatest influence on weight. (See chapter 9 for a discussion of the informational environment and childhood obesity.)

While personal responsibility has been a prominent theme in popular discussions of obesity—consider the popularity of so-called common-sense consumption laws (discussed in chapter 6)—the media coverage of obesity increasingly reflects the importance of the physical, social, and economic environments (see figure 12). In a June 2008 issue of *Time* magazine, Brian Walsh examined the "skyrocketing increase in childhood obesity," concluding that "who you are, where you are and how much your family has in the bank have a lot to do with whether your child will be claimed by the crisis or emerge unharmed."

In the following excerpt, Wendy C. Perdue, a professor of law and former member of a major county planning council, describes ways in

which the built and socioeconomic environments interact to fuel the
obesity epidemic in the United States.

OBESITY, POVERTY, AND THE BUILT ENVIRONMENT: CHALLENGES AND OPPORTUNITY*

Wendy C. Perdue

Obesity and its associated chronic diseases have become a major health concern in
the United States. . . . Approximately two thirds of adults in the United States are
either overweight or obese, and the condition is linked to diabetes, high blood pressure and other chronic conditions requiring ongoing medical supervision. Obesity is
a particular health concern for the poor. Not only are obesity rates generally higher
among those with lower socioeconomic status, but the chronic conditions caused
by obesity may present a particular challenge for the poor who often lack access to
necessary ongoing medical supervision.

   Obesity is linked to behaviors related to food consumption and physical activity.
Although the factors affecting [these] behaviors are complex, there is growing evidence that the physical characteristics of many of our communities, and particularly
poorer communities, encourage obesity-generating behaviors. . . .

OBESITY AND THE BUILT ENVIRONMENT

Even before researchers began to focus on obesity, the connection between human
behavior and physical surroundings was observed and documented. Jane Jacobs'
pioneering work on public spaces observed that some parks and public spaces feel
welcoming and safe and draw people in, while other spaces, because of their design,
have the opposite effect. . . . Except for people inhabiting highly rural and undevel-
oped areas, the primary features of people's physical environment are man-made,
and encompass everything from land use patterns and urban planning, to the design,
location, uses and interrelations among buildings, to transportation systems. All
of these man-made physical features are known collectively as the "built environment." Increasingly, evidence suggests that the features of the built environment
affect behaviors related to obesity. . . .

   . . . Studies suggest that proximity to stores stocking healthier food choices has
measurable effects on health. Unfortunately, access to healthy foods can be particularly problematic for the poor. . . .

   In the United States, small grocery stores and convenience stores tend not to
stock much selection of healthier foods, and supermarkets are the primary source of
[healthy] foods. However, as supermarkets have moved to larger size store formats,
the total number of grocery stores in the U.S. has actually declined. . . . Fewer stores
that are larger and further apart may not be a problem for affluent residents with
cars, but it can be a challenge for poorer residents. . . .

   While healthy food may be relatively hard to find in poorer neighborhoods, less

*Reprinted from *Georgetown Journal on Poverty Law & Policy* 15 (2008):
821–32.

healthy food may be more plentiful. Studies have found that the concentration of fast food restaurants is greater in poorer neighborhoods than wealthier ones—sometimes 2 to 3 times the density. . . . Empirical evidence shows a correlation between higher calorie consumption and obesity rates on the one hand and, on the other hand, proximity to fast food restaurants. Thus, whatever the merits of individual moderation as a response to weight gain, many poorer communities have limited access to healthy foods and abundant access to unhealthy foods.

In addition to impacting food consumption, characteristics of the built environment may impact levels of physical activity. Studies showed that less dense, automobile-dependent patterns of development correlate with lower levels of physical activity and an increased risk of being overweight. This research has significant implications in light of changing demographic patterns—notably the "suburbanization of poverty." As one study notes, "by 2005, the suburban poor out-numbered their central-city counterparts by at least 1 million" (Berube and Kneebone 2006, 12). Thus, the poor are increasingly located in communities that are spread out and unwalkable. The poor located in urban communities also confront neighborhood characteristics that discourage physical activity. Crime and perceptions of crime are affected by features such as abandoned buildings, vacant lots and poor lighting and may be significant deterrents to outdoor activity such as walking or using parks or playgrounds. . . .

Another factor which may impact levels of physical activity is access to recreation facilities. Although . . . empirical studies do not show consistent results among all populations in all locations, some studies show a clear association between greater proximity to recreation facilities and frequency of exercise or lower weight. . . . One study of over 20,000 adolescents found that not only were private facilities more plentiful in wealthier communities, public and quasi-public facilities including schools, parks, YMCAs and youth organizations were as well.

This brief summary highlights that the behaviors associated with obesity do not occur in a vacuum. The choices that people make concerning food and physical activity are significantly influenced by the environment in which those choices are made. . . .

CHALLENGES TO CHANGING THE BUILT ENVIRONMENT

In light of the studies on food and physical activity, a growing chorus of researchers has begun to argue that changing our built environment may be an important component to our public health strategy. [However,] there are some practical, political, and empirical challenges to such a strategy. . . .

First, the empirical data on the correlations between health, healthy behavior, and particular aspects of the built environment are sometimes inconsistent and, among some populations in some locations, these correlations are weak. Even where there is reasonably strong correlation evidence, we lack data that would allow one to draw general conclusions concerning priorities with respect to changes in the built environment. . . . As one study observes, the data on diet and exercise are "disappointingly ambiguous about the contribution of eating vs. that of a lack of physical activity to the obesity epidemic, much less the contribution of specific behaviors" (Jeffery and Utter 2003, 13S). . . . .

Second, changing our physical environment can be slow and expensive. For example, bringing a supermarket to a community requires finding a site, securing financing and [a] permit, and then designing and constructing the facility. It is a process that can easily take five years or more. Efforts to improve public facilities can be similarly slow and, even with the best of intentions, small design defects can doom the effectiveness of the changes....

Third, the complex web of land use and other laws that impact the built environment may be far outside the expertise of public officials. At the same time, improvements in the built environment will require the collaboration of a variety of professionals for whom public health is outside their training.... Most issues concerning land use, transportation and development are allocated to urban planners, architects, engineers and offices of economic development. Although there is a growing academic literature on the connection between public health and the built environment, this literature has not necessarily penetrated into the day-to-day focus of those who make land use decisions....

Fourth, to the extent land use and transportation decisions turn on input from surrounding neighbors, poor communities may be at a disadvantage. Language barriers, lower education levels, lack of information, and the inability to get child care or time off from work negatively affect the ability of poorer communities to organize effectively. In addition, poorer citizens may have come to expect less and therefore demand less. For all these reasons, land use processes that are dependent on neighborhood-initiated requests or complaints may be less effective in addressing the needs of poorer communities. For example, some have advocated that fast food restaurants be subject to a special use permit process that would require a showing of need or a demonstration that there is not already an undue concentration. Yet, if this process is structured as a quasi-adversarial proceeding that requires communities to come forward in opposition, such a process may not be particularly effective in slowing the expansion of fast food restaurants into poorer communities.... The point is not that planning decisions should be disconnected from the community, but rather that attention must be paid to the procedures used to assure both that the community's voice can be effectively heard and that needed change is not *dependent* on communities becoming politically engaged....

Finally, it is important to appreciate that efforts to change the built environment may encounter some resistance from entrenched interests that have a stake in the status quo. The built environment as it currently exists has been structured by a complex web of laws, regulations, and incentives, and private property and investment decisions may have been made in reliance on these rules. Changes in these rules can create a complex "politics of 'place making'" (Corburn 2004, 543)....
Moreover, efforts to alter the built environment are sometime understood as an inappropriate government intrusion into the private sphere. Thus, some public officials have questioned whether encouraging supermarket development in underserved communities is properly within their mission.... .

OPPORTUNITIES TO CHANGE THE BUILT ENVIRONMENT

Notwithstanding these challenges, there are several reasons why attention to the built environment should continue as a component of our public health agenda. First, small changes in behavior may yield significant long-term benefits to obesity and other such chronic diseases and conditions.... Noting that a pound of body weight typically represents 3500 calories, one research study has estimated that "most of the weight gain seen in the population could be eliminated by some combination of increasing energy expenditure and reducing energy intake by 100 kcal/day" (Hill et al. 2003, 854–55). . . . One hundred calories is equivalent to walking a mile . . . or drinking a 12 ounce serving of Coca-Cola. Thus, environmental changes that cause people to be even a little more active or to eat a little more healthy diet, can produce over-all public health benefits. . . .

Second, while some changes to the built environment can be slow and expensive, changes are constantly occurring and will continue to occur, regardless of the engagement of the public health community. . . . Roads are constructed or repaired, government facilities, private homes and business are all being sited and constructed. To the extent that these changes are happening anyway, there may be an opportunity to locate and build in ways that are more likely . . . to be health promoting. Some improvements may not require new money but may be accomplished by spending old money more wisely. [Thus, where] projects are likely to occur anyway, we can locate, design and construct them so that they are more likely to contribute to a healthy environment. Moreover . . . focusing on the potential health benefits of such investments may bring renewed urgency and funding priority to the infrastructure needs of neglected communities. If parks, sidewalks and recreation facilities are understood as an important part of a broader agenda to improve public health, maybe that can provide a justification for further necessary fiscal resources. Finally, not all useful changes are necessarily large and expensive. Small improvements, such as adding lights to pathways, may increase safety and therefore increase usage.

In addition to public projects, private owners are also constantly building and changing their properties. What and where owners build is influenced by a complex web of zoning, land use, and environmental laws, building codes, and tax laws. Changes in the legal framework that shape these incentives can change what gets built. Indeed, some of our current zoning and land use laws may have the effect of discouraging a healthy environment. . . . Building codes written for new construction that are applied to existing buildings may have the effect of discouraging the rehabilitation of old properties and thereby contribute to neighborhood deterioration. Thoughtful reexamination of these laws can encourage a redirection of private investment without necessarily requiring an infusion of public money. . . .

Third, the challenge of gaining institutional expertise of other critical players is beginning to be addressed. . . . City and state planning departments have begun to try systematically to integrate planning and public health. For example, San Francisco convened a multi-stakeholder process that brought together community representatives as well as professionals from multiple fields. The group developed the Healthy Development Measurement Tool which identifies a number of health related data such as neighborhood proximity to grocery stores and recreation facilities along with basic health data. . . . The Tool is not intended to be regulatory but nonetheless applies "a community health 'lens' to planning" (San Francisco Department of Public Health 2006). The San Francisco experience is noteworthy not only for the tool that was ultimately developed but also for the inclusive process that was used. As one commentary by a public health official observed, "Public health, by definition, is a group activity."

Finally, although most of the physical components of the built environment are

privately owned, those components are profoundly affected by government investments, incentives, and laws. Zoning and building codes, the home mortgage deduc-
tion and other tax provisions, how and where roads, highways and transportation
systems have been built, environmental laws, and urban renewal projects all have
changed the parameters of private decisions and private investments with respect
to the built environment. Government laws and policies help shape a world that
encourages unhealthful behaviors. Those same laws and policies can be restruc-
tured to shape a different, more healthful physical environment. . . .

CONCLUSION

A hundred years ago, progressive reformers concerned about the health of the poor
understood that they needed to focus considerable attention on the built environment. In an age of infectious disease, frequent epidemics, and squalid tenements,
it became apparent that improving health of the urban poor required improving the
physical environment in which they lived and worked. For the poor in the United
States today, the health crisis is more likely to be chronic rather than infectious
diseases, but attention to the physical environment should remain as an important
public health tool.

.   .   .   .   .

Beyond the built, economic, and informational environments, the social
environment appears to play a significant role in determining obesity
levels. Social connectedness and the social capital that such networks
yield are correlated with obesity rates—those with greater social capital
are less likely to be obese than those who are socially isolated. In a
further complication, being overweight or obese seems to contribute to
social isolation, thereby promoting a vicious cycle in which weight gain
and its psychosocial correlates fuel one another.

Some researchers have begun to examine the nature of social networks and their impact on obesity more closely. In 2007, Nicholas
Christakis and James Fowler, two well-regarded social scientists, published a study tracking the weight patterns of participants and of persons within their social networks. The results indicated that obesity is
"socially contagious." The likelihood of an individual becoming obese
jumped by 57 percent if a friend within his or her social network was
obese. Christakis and Fowler's work suggests that overweight and obesity are closely linked to social norms and interpersonal relationships.
If so, social networks might also be useful for spreading "good" behaviors, such as a healthful diet and active lifestyle. Although Christakis
and Fowler's study remains controversial, it "highlights the necessity of
approaching obesity not only as a clinical problem but also as a public
health problem" (2007, 378).

B. The Obesity Pandemic

In the developing world, an obesity time bomb
awaits[:] . . . *overnourishment will soon outpace*
malnutrition in the poorer half of the world.

Brian Vastag, 2004

Internationally, as well as domestically, obesity is no longer a disease
of affluence. Instead, obesity most severely plagues the global poor.
Rapid globalization and urbanization have prompted abrupt and problematic changes in diet and lifestyle, and resource-poor countries that
have traditionally struggled to feed their citizens are suddenly straining to cope with the growing burden of obesity-related diseases. These
countries continue to bear the brunt of the world's infectious disease
burden (e.g., malaria, yellow fever, TB), and, in many, HIV/AIDS
already overwhelms the health system. Within resource-poor countries,
obesity disproportionately burdens the urban poor, widening existing
socioeconomic health disparities. The WHO Commission on the Social
Determinants of Health (2008, 1) found that

> The poor health of the poor, the social gradient in health within coun-
> tries, and the marked health inequities between countries are caused by
> the unequal distribution of power, income, goods, and services, glob-
> ally and nationally, the consequent unfairness in the immediate, visible
> circumstances of people's lives—their access to health care, schools, and
> education, their conditions of work and leisure, their homes, communi-
> ties, towns, or cities—and their chances of leading a flourishing life. This
> unequal distribution of health-damaging experiences is not in any sense
> a "natural" phenomenon but is the result of a toxic combination of poor
> social policies and programmes, unfair economic arrangements, and bad
> politics. Together, the structural determinants and conditions of daily
> life constitute the social determinants of health and are responsible for a
> major part of health inequities between and within countries.

Sharon Friel, Mickey Chopra, and David Satcher argue that social
and economic inequities such as those highlighted by the WHO Commission on the Social Determinants of Health underlie rising obesity
rates. They suggest that policies and interventions to reduce obesity
rates must focus on ameliorating health disparities.

> Obesity and its unequal distribution is a consequence of the complex
> system operating at global, national, and local levels, shaping how we
> trade, live, learn, and work. Focusing only on direct action to make people
> eat more healthily and be more physically active misses the heart of the

> problem: the underlying unequal distribution of factors that support the
> opportunity to be a healthy weight. Unless this oversight is addressed the
> obesity epidemic and its inequities will persist and possibly increase. . . .
> Dealing with inequalities in obesity requires a different policy agenda from
> the one currently being promoted. Action is needed that is grounded in
> principles of health equity. (Friel, Chopra, and Satcher 2007, 1241)

The obesity-causing "energy imbalance between and among societies" (Friel, Chopra, and Satcher 2007, 1241) results from a number of
interlocking factors. In addition to the state of the built environment,
discussed in the article by Perdue in the previous section, living and
working conditions, place in the social hierarchy, and the increased
availability of energy-dense foods can all contribute to a person's intake
of energy exceeding his or her output of energy. The liberalization of
trade has brought new types of energy-rich foods to many countries.
Many foods that are produced with government subsidies and that
are being exported most cheaply around the world are high in energy
but low in nutritional value. Unfortunately, many of the foods that
are most beneficial are more expensive than less healthy food options.
Food advertising also seeks to turn people—particularly children and
teenagers—toward foods that are less conducive to their good health.
Consumers' material and psychosocial resources, which are affected
significantly by the precariousness of their employment, can support or
undermine their capacity to make sound decisions about their health.
Individual position in the social hierarchy is an exacerbating factor, as
social inequality contributes to the unequal impact of obesity.

In looking for solutions, Friel and her colleagues focus on policies
and programs that are aimed at changing the underlying determinants
of health and achieving "an equitable distribution of ample and nutri-
tious global and national food supplies; built environments that lend
themselves to easy access and uptake of healthier options by all; and
living and working conditions that produce more equal material and
psychosocial resources between and within social groups" (Friel,
Chopra, and Satcher 2007, 1241). Domestic and international cooperation is of paramount importance in addressing the global obesity
epidemic. Much can be achieved through successful international
collaborations, such as those that resulted in the WHO Framework
Convention on Tobacco Control. However, it is also worth considering ways in which agreements between states, which are implemented
and take effect at the country level, may also undermine health. Many
analysts have expressed concern about the role that certain provisos of
trade agreements may play in creating conditions that foster obesity.

Constructive national interventions to address obesity are also essential. For example, efforts can be made at the national level—through subsidies, price regulation, labeling, consumer education, and the like—to make energy-dense foods less readily available and to create greater local access to affordable healthier foods. At the national level, a "whole of government" approach must also be achieved, in which all departments or ministries coordinate their policies to advance health goals. A government's labor, education, trade, and economic policies can have as great an impact on the health of its citizens as the decisions of its department of health. Furthermore, unless public health practitioners, physicians, political figures, urban planners, and community members collaborate, the environmental factors that contribute to obesity and overweight will remain entrenched, because the underlying physical, social, and economic frameworks will not change. For international and domestic efforts to succeed, adequate financial and other resources must be dedicated to the long-term task of reducing obesity.

Fortunately, addressing the obesity epidemic, especially through equity-based programs and policies, may improve overall living conditions for some of the most disadvantaged people and regions of the world. But until socioeconomic and health disparities are reduced, as the physician Ben Caballero (2005, 1516) warns, "we will continue to find malnourished children in the arms of overweight mothers."

IV. CONCLUSION

This chapter, like the *Reader* as a whole, demonstrates the complexity of public health theory and practice. As a society, we want to achieve health and well-being in the community and distribute benefits fairly among all members. At the same time, we want to respect the inviolability of each individual. The values of population health, social justice, and strong personal autonomy are not always in harmony. Society's only sensible course is to search for answers based on rigorous ethical principles, respect for democratic institutions, and adherence to legal doctrine and human rights.

RECOMMENDED READINGS

"Public Health in Reverse": Bioterrorism and Biosecurity

Ban, Jonathan. 2003. Health as a global security challenge. *Seton Hall Journal of Diplomacy and International Relations* 4: 19–28. (Advocates for the inclusion of public health initiatives in security measures, suggesting that the threat posed by individual health issues should be ranked on a predetermined scale)

Blumenshine, Philip, Arthur Reingold, Susan Egerter, Robin Mockenhaupt, Paula Braveman, and James Marks. 2008. Pandemic influenza planning in the United States from a health disparities perspective. *Emerging Infectious Diseases* 14: 709–15. (Considers how populations of lower socioeconomic status and minority ethnic groups may fare in the event of pandemic influenza and makes suggestions for improving health care access and delivery)

Fidler, David P., and Lawrence O. Gostin. 2007. *Biosecurity in the Global Age: Biological Weapons, Public Health, and the Rule of Law,* 121–45. Stanford, CA: Stanford Univ. Press. (Provides a comprehensive overview of domestic and international biosecurity measures, highlighting the implications of public health's intersection with security imperatives)

Goldsmith, Jeff. 2002. Facing reality in preparing for biological warfare: A conversation with George Poste. *Health Affairs* (June 2002 Web Exclusive): W219–W228. http://content.healthaffairs.org/cgi/reprint/hlthaff.w2.219v1. (Discusses what public health and government priorities should be in the event of a bioterrorist attack, suggesting that collaborations between public health and legislative authorities, national and local governments, and domestic and international agencies are crucial for preparation)

Institute of Medicine. 2005. *The Smallpox Vaccination Program: Public Health in an Age of Terrorism.* Washington, DC: National Academies Press. (Provides a concluding report on the smallpox vaccination program and notes the need for greater interaction between public health scientists and national defense officials)

Koplow, David A. 2004. *Smallpox: The Fight to Eradicate a Global Source.* Berkley: Univ. of California Press. (Examines the case for and against eradicating the last remaining sources of the smallpox virus)

From Genes to Public Health

Halliday, Jane L., Veronica R. Collins, Mary Anne Aitkan, Martin P. M. Richards, and Craig A. Olsson. 2004. Genetics and public health—evolution or revolution? *Journal of Epidemiology and Community Health* 58: 894–99. (Outlines valid concerns, as well as misconceptions, about public health genetics and suggests that using genomic information for public health purposes will encourage more interdisciplinary approaches to public health initiatives and policy)

Khoury, Muin J., Marta Gwinn, Wylie Burke, Scott Bowen, and Ron Zimmern. 2007. Will genomics widen or help heal the schism between medicine and public health? *American Journal of Preventive Medicine* 33: 310–17. (Provides an informative and historical overview of the underlying tensions between public health and primary care medicine, suggesting that well-implemented genomic programs may improve cooperation between the fields as well as overall health outcomes)

Smith, Richard D., Halla Thorsteinsdóttir, Abdallah S. Daar, E. Richard Gold, and Peter A. Singer. 2004. Genomics knowledge and equity: A global public goods perspective of the patent system. *Bulletin of the World Health Organization* 82: 385–89. (Suggests reconsidering national patent systems and international collaborations to improve access to and the application of public health genomics information in developing countries)

The Obesity Pandemic: Obesity-Promoting Environments and Global Justice

Caballero, Benjamin. 2005. A nutrition paradox—underweight and obesity in developing countries. *New England Journal of Medicine* 352: 1514–16. (Suggests that the "dual burden" of obese and malnourished persons within communities and families in developing countries may arise from metabolic disturbances during pregnancy and the urbanization of middle-income countries)

Friel, Sharon, Mickey Chopra, and David Satcher. 2007. Unequal weight: Equity oriented policy responses to the global obesity epidemic. *British Medical Journal* 335: 1241–43. (Examines global problems and global solutions to the obesity epidemic with a particular focus on equity)

Perdue, Wendy Collins, Lesley A. Stone, and Lawrence O. Gostin. 2003. The built environment and its relationship to the public's health: The legal framework. *American Journal of Public Health* 93: 1390–94. (Provides an overview of how physical spaces shape health conditions and what legal interventions, such as zoning ordinances and tax incentives, may best address issues of the built environment)

Prentice, Andrew M. 2006. The emerging epidemic of obesity in developing countries. *International Journal of Epidemiology* 35: 93–99. (Expounds on the multiple factors contributing to the obesity pandemic in developing countries, pointing to demographic changes, nutritional transitions, globalization, and urbanization efforts as the main influences)

Story, Mary, Karen M. Kaphingst, Ramona Robinson-O'Brien, and Karen Glanz. 2008. Creating healthy food and eating environments: Policy and environmental approaches. *Annual Review of Public Health* 29: 253–72. (Delves into environmental factors and macro-level influences, such as social structures and agricultural policy, that contribute to overweight and obesity of communities, especially those who are of lower socioeconomic status or are otherwise marginalized)

Selected Bibliography

Ackerman, Frank, and Lisa Heinzerling. 2004. *Priceless: On Knowing the Price of Everything and the Value of Nothing.* New York: New Press.

Advisory Committee on Human Radiation Experiments. 1996. *Final Report.* Washington, DC: Department of Energy.

Advisory Council for the Elimination of Tuberculosis. 1993. Initial therapy for tuberculosis in the era of multidrug resistance: Recommendations of the Advisory Council for the Elimination of Tuberculosis. *Morbidity and Mortality Weekly Report Recommendations and Reports* 42 (RR15): 1–28.

Alaska Dental Society. 2007. Judge rules—DHATS beyond state law. *Alaska Update,* July: 1.

Albert, Michael, Kristen Ostheimer, and Joel Breman. 2001. The last smallpox epidemic in Boston and the vaccination controversy, 1901–1903. *New England Journal of Medicine* 344: 375–79.

Alderman, Jess, and Richard A. Daynard. 2006. Applying lessons from tobacco litigation to obesity lawsuits. *American Journal of Preventive Medicine* 30: 82–88.

American Medical Association. 2008. AMA apologizes for history of racial inequality and works to include and promote minority physicians. American Medical Association website. Press release, July 10. www.ama-assn.org/ama/no-index/news-events/18773.shtml.

Annas, George J. 2002. Bioterrorism, public health, and human rights. *Health Affairs* 21 (6): 94–97.

Arras, John D. 2005. Rationing vaccine during an avian influenza pandemic: Why it won't be easy. *Yale Journal of Biology and Medicine* 78: 283–96.

Arrow, Kenneth J., Maureen L. Cropper, George C. Eads, Robert W. Hahn, Lester B. Lave, Roger G. Noll, Paul R. Portney, et al. 1996. Is there a role for benefit-cost analysis in environmental, health, and safety regulation? *Science* 272: 221–22.

Bailey, Tracey M., Timothy Caulfield, and Nola M. Ries, eds. 2005. *Public Health Law and Policy in Canada*. Markham, ON: Butterworths.

Baker, Robert B., Harriet A. Washington, Ololade Olakanmi, Todd L. Savitt, Elizabeth A. Jacobs, Eddie Hoover, and Matthew K. Wynia. 2008. African American physicians and organized medicine, 1846–1968: Origins of a racial divide. *JAMA* 300: 306–13.

Baker, Susan P. 1980. On lobbies, liberty, and the public good. *American Journal of Public Health* 70: 573.

Baker, Susan P., and Stephen P. Teret. 1981. Freedom and protection: A balancing of interests. *American Journal of Public Health* 71: 295–96.

Ban, Jonathan. 2003. Health as a global security challenge. *Seton Hall Journal of Diplomacy and International Relations* 4: 19–28.

Barbera, Joseph, Anthony Macintyre, Larry Gostin, Tom Inglesby, Tara O'Toole, Craig DeAtley, Kevin Tonat, and Marci Layton. 2001. Large-scale quarantine following biological terrorism in the United States: Scientific examination, logistic and legal limits, and possible consequences. *JAMA* 286: 2711–17.

Bayer, Ronald. 1994. Ethical challenges posed by zidovudine treatment to reduce vertical transmission of HIV. *New England Journal of Medicine* 331: 1223–25.

———. 2002. Tobacco, commercial speech, and libertarian values: The end of the line for restrictions on advertising? *American Journal of Public Health* 92: 356–59.

Bayer, Ronald, and Laurence Dupuis. 1995. Tuberculosis, public health, and civil liberties. *Annual Review of Public Health* 16: 307–26.

Bayer, Ronald, and Amy L. Fairchild. 2000. Public health: Surveillance and privacy. *Science* 290: 1898–99.

———. 2004. The genesis of public health ethics. *Bioethics* 18: 473–92.

———. 2006. Changing the paradigm for HIV testing—The end of exceptionalism. *New England Journal of Medicine* 355: 647–49.

Bayer, Ronald, Lawrence O. Gostin, Bruce Jennings, and Bonnie Steinbock, eds. 2007. *Public Health Ethics: Theory, Policy and Practice*. New York: Oxford Univ. Press.

Bayer, Ronald, Catherine Stayton, Moise Desvarieus, Cheryl Healton, Sheldon Landesman, and Wei-Yann Tsai. 1998. Directly observed therapy and treatment completion for tuberculosis in the United States: Is universal supervised therapy necessary? *American Journal of Public Health* 88: 1052–58.

Bayer, Ronald, and Kathleen E. Toomey. 1992. HIV prevention and the two faces of partner notification. *American Journal of Public Health* 82: 1158–64.

Bayer, Ronald, and David Wilkinson. 1995. Directly observed therapy for tuberculosis: History of an idea. *Lancet* 345: 1545–48.

Beaglehole, Robert, and Ruth Bonita. 1997. *Public Health at the Crossroads: Achievements and Prospects*. Cambridge: Cambridge Univ. Press.

Beauchamp, Dan. 1985. Community: The neglected tradition of public health. *Hastings Center Report* 15 (6): 28–36.

———. 1988. *The Health of the Republic: Epidemics, Medicine, and Moralism as Challenges to Democracy.* Philadelphia: Temple Univ. Press.

———. 1999. Public health as social justice. In *New Ethics for the Public's Health,* ed. Dan Beauchamp and Bonnie Steinbock, 105–14. New York: Oxford Univ. Press.

Berube, Alan, and Elizabeth Kneebone. 2006. Two steps back: City and suburban poverty trend 1999–2005. Washington, DC: Brookings Institution. www.brookings.edu/reports/2006/12poverty_berube.aspx.

Bettelheim, Adriel. 2006. Public health, political priorities of bioterrorism research. *CQ Weekly,* January 23.

Biber, Eric. 2007. Two sides of the same coin: Judicial review under APA sections 706(1) and 706(2). *Virginia Environmental Law Journal* 26: 461–503.

Bloche, M. Gregg, and Elizabeth R. Jungman. 2003. Health policy and the WTO. *Journal of Law, Medicine & Ethics* 31: 529–45.

Blumenshine, Philip, Arthur Reingold, Susan Egerter, Robin Mockenhaupt, Paula Braveman, and James Marks. 2008. Pandemic influenza planning in the United States from a health disparities perspective. *Emerging Infectious Diseases* 14: 709–15.

Bohmer, Richard. 2007. The rise of in-store clinics—threat or opportunity? *New England Journal of Medicine* 356: 765–68.

Bradley, Peter, and Amanda Burls, eds. 2000. *Ethics in Public and Community Health.* New York: Routledge.

Brand, Angela. 2005. Public health and genetics—a dangerous combination? *European Journal of Public Health* 15 (2): 114–16.

Brandt, Allan M. 1978. Racism and research: The case of the Tuskegee Syphilis Study. *Hastings Center Report* 8 (6): 21–29.

———. 1987. *No Magic Bullet: A Social History of Venereal Disease in the United States since 1880.* New York: Oxford Univ. Press.

———. 2007. *The Cigarette Century: The Rise, Fall, and Deadly Persistence of the Product That Defined America.* New York: Basic Books.

Breyer, Stephen. 1993. *Breaking the Vicious Circle: Toward Effective Risk Regulation.* Cambridge, MA: Harvard Univ. Press.

Bryans, Nathaniel. 2007. *New Hampshire Motor Transport Association v. Rowe:* Federal preemption of Maine's attempt to regulate Internet sales of tobacco to minors. *Maine Law Review* 59: 481–510.

Buchanan, Allen, Dan W. Brock, Norman Daniels, and Daniel Winkler. 2000. Introduction to *From Chance to Choice: Genetics and Justice,* 1–24. Cambridge: Cambridge Univ. Press.

Buchanan, David R. 2000. Disquietudes. In *An Ethic for Health Promotion: Rethinking the Sources of Human Well-Being,* 1–22. Oxford: Oxford Univ. Press.

———. 2008. Autonomy, paternalism, and justice: Ethical priorities in public health. *American Journal of Public Health* 98: 15–20.

Buchanan, David R., and Franklin G. Miller. 2006. Justice and fairness in the Kennedy Krieger Institute lead paint study: The ethics of public health research on less expensive, less effective interventions. *American Journal of Public Health* 96: 781–87.

Bureau of National Affairs. 2008. Second amendment shields individual rights, is violated by D.C.'s prohibition of handguns. *United States Law Week* 77: 1011–13.

Burris, Scott. 1997. The invisibility of public health: Population-level measures in a politics of market individualism. *American Journal of Public Health* 87: 1607–10.

———. 2003. Legal aspects of regulating bathhouses. In *Gay Bathhouses and Public Health Policy,* ed. William J. Woods and Diane Binson, 131–49. New York: Harrington Park Press.

Burton, Scot, Elizabeth Creyer, Jeremy Kees, and Kyle Huggins. 2006. Attacking the obesity epidemic: The potential health benefits of providing nutrition information in restaurants. *American Journal of Public Health* 96: 1669–75.

Caballero, Benjamin. 2005. A nutrition paradox—underweight and obesity in developing countries. *New England Journal of Medicine* 352: 1514–16.

Calandrillo, Steve. 2004. Vanishing vaccinations: Why are so many Americans opting out of vaccinating their children? *University of Michigan Journal of Law Reform* 37: 353–440.

Callahan, Daniel, and Bruce Jennings. 2002. Ethics and public health: Forging a strong relationship. *American Journal of Public Health* 92: 169–76.

Caruso, David. 2005. City proposes tracking diabetes, raising privacy questions. *New York Sun,* July 26.

Carver, Krista Hessler. 2008. A global view of the First Amendment constraints on the FDA. *Food and Drug Law Journal* 63: 151–215.

Centers for Disease Control and Prevention (CDC). 1999. CDC guidelines for national human immunodeficiency virus case surveillance. *Morbidity and Mortality Weekly Report Recommendations and Reports* 48 (RR13): 1–23.

———. 2000a. Recommendations for human immunodeficiency virus screening of pregnant women. *Morbidity and Mortality Weekly Report Recommendations and Reports* 50 (RR19): 59–86.

———. 2000b. Surveillance for adverse events associated with anthrax vaccination—U.S. Department of Defense, 1998–2000. *Morbidity and Mortality Weekly Report* 49 (16): 341–45.

———. 2003. Use of quarantine to prevent severe acute respiratory syndrome—Taiwan. *Morbidity and Mortality Weekly Report* 52 (29): 680–83.

———. 2006. *Expedited Partner Therapy in the Management of Sexually Transmitted Diseases.* Atlanta: Department of Health and Human Services.

———. 2008. Measles—United States, January 1–April 25, 2008. *Morbidity and Mortality Weekly Report* 57: 494–98.

Centers for Disease Control and Prevention and Department of Health and Human Services. 2003. HIPAA Privacy Rule and public health: Guidance from CDC and the U.S. Department for Health and Human Services. *Morbidity and Mortality Weekly* 52: S1–S17.

Charo, R. Alta. 2007. The partial death of abortion rights. *New England Journal of Medicine* 356: 2125–28.

Childress, James F., Ruth R. Faden, Ruth D. Gaare, Lawrence O. Gostin, Jeffrey Kahn, Richard J. Bonnie, Nancy E. Kass, Anna C. Mastroianni, Jonathan D. Moreno, and Phillip Nieburg. 2002. Public health ethics: Mapping the terrain. *Journal of Law, Medicine & Ethics* 30: 170–78.

Christakis, Nicholas A., and James H. Fowler. 2007. The spread of obesity in a large social network over 32 years. *New England Journal of Medicine* 357: 370–79.

Christoffel, Tom, and Stephen P. Teret. 1991. Epidemiology and the law: Courts and confidence intervals. *American Journal of Public Health* 81: 1661–66.

Clayton, Ellen Wright. 2000. Genetics, public health, and the law. In *Genetics and Public Health in the 21st Century: Using Genetic Information to Improve Health and Prevent Disease,* ed. Muin J. Khoury, Wylie Burke, and Elizabeth J. Thomson, 489–503. New York: Oxford Univ. Press.

Cleary, Paul, Michael Barry, Kenneth Mayer, Allan M. Brandt, Lawrence O. Gostin, and Harvey V. Fineberg. 1987. Compulsory premarital screening for the human immunodeficiency virus: Technical and public health considerations. *JAMA* 258: 1757–62.

Clemow, F. G. 1929. The origin of "quarantine." *British Medical Journal* 1: 122–23.

Clifford, Stephanie. 2008. Tug of war in food marketing to children. *New York Times,* July 30.

Cohen, Hillel W., Robert M. Gould, and Victor M. Sidel. 1999. Bioterrorism initiatives: Public health in reverse? *American Journal of Public Health* 89: 1629–31.

———. 2004. The pitfalls of bioterrorism preparedness: The anthrax and smallpox experiences. *American Journal of Public Health* 94: 1667–71.

Cohen, Jon. 2006. The new world of global health. *Science* 311: 162–67.

Cole, Philip. 1995. The moral bases for public health interventions. *Epidemiology* 6: 78–83.

Colgrove, James. 2006. Expansion and backlash: Vaccination at the turn of the twenty-first century. In *State of Immunity: The Politics of Vaccination in Twentieth-Century America,* 218–51. Berkeley: Univ. of California Press.

Colgrove, James, and Ronald Bayer. 2005. Manifold restraints: Liberty, public health, and the legacy of *Jacobson v. Massachusetts. American Journal of Public Health* 95: 571–76.

Collins, Francis S. 1999. Shattuck lecture—medical and societal consequences of the Human Genome Project. *New England Journal of Medicine* 341: 28–37.

Commission on Social Determinants of Health. 2008. *Closing the Gap in a Generation: Health Equity through Action on the Social Determinants of Health.* Geneva: World Health Organization.

Corburn, Jason. 2004. Confronting the challenges in reconnecting urban planning and public health. *American Journal of Public Health* 94: 541–46.

Coughlin, Steven S., and Thomas L. Beauchamp, eds. 1996. *Ethics and Epidemiology*. New York: Oxford Univ. Press.

Croley, Stephen P. 2007. *Regulation and Public Interest*. Princeton, NJ: Princeton Univ. Press.

Cross, Frank B. 1994. The public role in risk control. *Environmental Law* 24: 887–969.

Csete, Joanne. 2006. Scaling up HIV testing: Human rights and hidden cost. *HIV/AIDS Policy and Law Review* 11: 1–10.

Curtis, Valerie A., Nana Garbrah-Aidoo, and Beth Scott. 2007. Masters of marketing: Bringing private sector skills to public health partnerships. *American Journal of Public Health* 97: 634–41.

Daar, Abdallah S., Peter A. Singer, Deepa Leah Persad, Stig K. Pramming, David R. Matthews, Robert Beaglehole, et al. 2007. Grand challenges in chronic non-communicable diseases. *Nature* 450: 494–96.

Dahlgren, Goran, and Margaret Whitehead. 1991. *Policies and Strategies to Promote Social Equality in Health*. Stockholm: Institute of Future Studies.

Daniels, Norman. 2000. Accountability for reasonableness. *British Medical Journal* 321: 1300–1301.

———. 2006. Equity and population health: Toward a broader bioethics agenda. *Hastings Center Report* 36 (4): 22–35.

Daniels, Norman, Bruce Kennedy, and Ichiro Kawachi. 2000. Justice is good for our health. *Boston Review*, February/March: 6–15.

Dawson, Angus. 2007. Vaccination ethics. In *Principles of Health Care Ethics*, ed. Richard E. Ashcroft, Angus Dawson, Heather Draper, and John McMillan, 617–22. 2d ed. Chichester: Wiley.

Dawson, Angus, and Marcel Verweij, eds. 2007. *Ethics, Prevention, and Public Health*. Oxford: Clarendon Press.

Deaton, Angus. 2002. Policy implications of the gradient of health and wealth. *Health Affairs* 21 (2): 13–30.

Dowdle, Walter. 1997. The 1976 experience. *Journal of Infectious Diseases* 176: 69S–72S.

Drazen, Jeffrey M. 2007. Government in medicine. *New England Journal of Medicine* 356: 2195.

Drazen, Jeffrey M., Stephen Morrissey, and Gregory D. Curfman. 2008. Guns and health. *New England Journal of Medicine* 359: 517–18.

Dresser, Rebecca. 2007. Protecting women from their abortion choices. *Hastings Center Report* 37 (6): 13–14.

Dubois, René, and Jean Dubois. 1987. *The White Plague: Tuberculosis, Man and Society*. New Brunswick, NJ: Rutgers Univ. Press.

Dugger, Celia W. 2008. South Africa confines the ill to fight severe TB. *New York Times*, March 25.

Dworkin, Gerald. 2008. Paternalism. In *Philosophy of Law*, ed. Joel Feinberg and Jules Coleman, 281–91. 8th ed. Belmont, CA: Wadsworth Publishing.

Eager, J.M. 1903. *The Early History of Quarantine: Origin of Sanitary Measures Directed against Yellow Fever*. Washington, DC: Government Printing Office.

Editor's Choice. 1996. *British Medical Journal* 312: 985.

Emanuel, Ezekiel J., and Alan Wertheimer. 2006. Who should get influenza vaccine when not all can? *Science* 312: 854–55.

Enserink, Martin, and Jocelyn Kaiser. 2005. Has biodefense gone overboard? *Science* 307: 1396–98.

Epstein, Richard A. 2003. Let the shoemaker stick to his last: A defense of the "old" public health. *Perspectives in Biology and Medicine* 46: 138–59.

Ewald, P. W. 2000. Biobombs. In *Plague Time: How Stealth Infections Cause Cancers, Heart Disease, and Other Deadly Ailments*, 177–95. New York: Free Press.

Ezzati, Majid, Stephen Vander Hoorn, Carlene M. M. Lawes, Rachel Leach, W. Phillip T. James, Alan D. Lopez, Anthony Rodgers, and Christopher J. L. Murray. 2005. Rethinking the "diseases of affluence" paradigm: Global patterns of nutritional risks in relation to economic development. *Public Library of Science Medicine* 2: 404–11. Available at www.plosmedicine.org.

Faden, Ruth R. 1987. Ethical issues in government-sponsored public health campaigns. *Health Education Quarterly* 14: 27–37.

Faden, Ruth R., Nancy Kass, and Madison Powers. 1991. Warrants for screening programs: Public health, legal and ethical frameworks. In *AIDS, Women and the Next Generation: Towards a Morally Acceptable Public Policy for HIV Testing of Pregnant Women and Newborns*, ed. Ruth R. Faden, Gail Geller, and Madison Powers, 3–24. New York: Oxford Univ. Press.

Fairchild, Amy L., and Ava Alkon. 2007. Back to the future? Diabetes, HIV, and the boundaries of public health. *Journal of Health Politics, Policy, and Law* 32: 561–93.

Fairchild, Amy L., and Ronald Bayer. 2004. Ethics and the conduct of public health surveillance. *Science* 303: 631–32.

Fairchild, Amy L., Ronald Bayer, and James Colgrove. 2007. *Searching Eyes: Privacy, the State, and Disease Surveillance in America*. Berkeley: Univ. of California Press.

Farmer, Paul, Fernet Leandre, Joia Mukherjee, Rajesh Gupta, Laura Tarter, and Jim Yong Kim. 2001. Community-based treatment of advanced HIV disease: Introducing DOT-HAART (directly observed therapy with highly active antiretroviral therapy). *Bulletin of the World Health Organization* 79: 1145–51.

Federal Trade Commission. 2008. *Marketing Food to Children and Adolescents: A Review of Industry Expenditures, Activities, and Self-Regulation*. Washington, DC: Federal Trade Commission.

Feldman, Eric A., and Ronald Bayer. 2004. *Unfiltered: Conflicts over Tobacco Policy and Public Health*. Cambridge, MA: Harvard Univ. Press.

Fidler, David P. 2003. SARS: Political pathology of the first post-Westphalian pathogen. *Journal of Law, Medicine & Ethics* 31: 485–505.

———. 2004. *SARS: Governance and the Globalization of Disease*. New York: Palgrave Macmillan.

Fidler, David P., and Lawrence O. Gostin. 2006. The new International Health Regulations: An historic development for international law and public health. *Journal of Law, Medicine & Ethics* 33: 85–94.

———. 2007. *Biosecurity in the Global Age: Biological Weapons, Public Health, and the Rule of Law.* Stanford, CA: Stanford Univ. Press.

Fielding, Jonathan E., Lester B. Lave, and Barbara Starfield. 2000. Preface. *Annual Review of Public Health* 21: 1–13.

Fox, Daniel M. 1986. From TB to AIDS: Value conflicts in reporting disease. *Hastings Center Report* 16 (6): 11–16.

Freeman, Jody. 2003. Public values in an era of privatization: Extending public law norms through privatization. *Harvard Law Review* 116: 1285–1352.

Freeman, Jody, and Adrian Vermeule. 2007. *Massachusetts v. EPA*: From politics to expertise. *Supreme Court Review* 2007: 51–110.

Fried, Charles. 1991. *Order and Law: Arguing the Reagan Revolution: A Firsthand Account.* New York: Simon & Schuster.

Frieden, Thomas R. 2004. Asleep at the switch: Local public health and chronic diseases. *American Journal of Public Health* 94: 2059–61.

———. 2006. Interview by Frank Stasio, *Talk of the Nation*, NPR, January 12.

Frieden, Thomas R., Moupali Das-Douglas, Scott E. Kellerman, and Kelly J. Henning. 2005. Applying public health principles to the HIV epidemic. *New England Journal of Medicine* 353: 2397–2402.

Friel, Sharon, Mickey Chopra, and David Satcher. 2007. Unequal weight: Equity oriented policy responses to the global obesity epidemic. *British Medical Journal* 335: 1241–43.

Garrett, Laurie. 2000. *Betrayal of Trust: The Collapse of Global Public Health.* New York: Hyperion.

———. 2007. The challenge of global health. *Foreign Affairs* 86: 15–38.

Goldsmith, Jeff. 2002. Facing reality in preparing for biological warfare: A conversation with George Poste. *Health Affairs* (June Web Exclusive): W219–W228. http://content.healthaffairs.org/cgi/reprint/hlthaff.w2.219v1.

Goodin, Robert. 1989. *No Smoking: The Ethical Issues.* Chicago: Univ. of Chicago Press.

Goodman, Richard, Richard E. Hoffman, Wilfredo Lopez, Gene W. Matthews, Mark A. Rothstein, and Karen L. Foster, eds. 2007. *Law in Public Health Practice.* 2d ed. Oxford: Oxford Univ. Press.

Gostin, Lawrence O. 2002. Public health law in an age of terrorism: Rethinking individual rights and common goods. *Health Affairs* 21 (6): 79–93.

———. 2005a. *Jacobson v. Massachusetts* at 100 years: Police power and civil liberties in tension. *American Journal of Public Health* 95: 576–81.

———. 2005b. Medical marijuana, American federalism, and the Supreme Court. *JAMA* 294: 824–44.

———. 2005c. The Supreme Court's impact on medicine and health: The Rehnquist Court, 1986–2005. *JAMA* 294: 1685–87.

———. 2006a. HIV screening in health care settings: Public health and civil liberties in conflict? *JAMA* 296: 2023–25.

———. 2006b. The International Health Regulations: A new paradigm for global health governance? In *First Do No Harm: Law, Ethics and Healthcare,* ed. Sheila A.M. McLean, 59–80. Burlington, VT: Ashgate Publishing.

———. 2006c. Medical countermeasures for pandemic influenza: Ethics and the law. *JAMA* 295: 554–56.

———. 2006d. Physician-assisted suicide: A legitimate medical practice? *JAMA* 296: 1941–43.

———. 2006e. Property rights and the common good. *Hastings Center Report* 36 (5): 10–11.

———. 2006f. Public health strategies for pandemic influenza: Ethics and the law. *JAMA* 296: 1700–1704.

———. 2007a. Abortion politics: Clinical freedom, trust in the judiciary, and the autonomy of women. *JAMA* 298: 1562–64.

———. 2007b. Global regulatory strategies for tobacco control. *JAMA* 298: 2057–59.

———. 2007c. Law as a tool to facilitate healthier lifestyles and prevent obesity. *JAMA* 297: 87–90.

———. 2007d. Meeting the survival needs of the world's least healthy people: A proposed model for global health governance. *JAMA* 298: 225–28.

———. 2007e. Police powers and public health paternalism: HIV and diabetes surveillance. *Hastings Center Report* 37 (2): 9–10.

———. 2007f. The "Tobacco Wars": Global litigation strategies. *JAMA* 298: 2537–39.

———. 2007g. Why rich countries should care about the world's least healthy people. *JAMA* 289: 89–92.

———. 2008a. The deregulatory effects of preempting tort litigation. *JAMA* 299: 2313–16.

———. 2008b. The deregulatory state. *Hastings Center Report* 38 (2): 10–11.

———. 2008c. Meeting basic survival needs of the world's least healthy people: Toward a framework convention on global health. *Georgetown Law Journal* 96: 331–92.

———. 2008d. *Public Health Law: Power, Duty, Restraint*. 2d ed. Berkeley: Univ. of California Press; New York: Milbank Memorial Fund.

———. 2008e. The right to bear arms: Constitutional law, politics, and public health. *JAMA* 300: 1575–77.

———. 2009. Influenza A(H1N1) and pandemic preparedness under the rule of international law. *JAMA* 301: 2376–78.

Gostin, Lawrence O., Ronald Bayer, and Amy L. Fairchild. 2003. Ethical and legal challenges posed by severe acute respiratory syndrome: Implications for the control of severe infectious disease threats. *JAMA* 290: 3229–37.

Gostin, Lawrence O., and Benjamin E. Berkman. 2007. Pandemic influenza: Ethics, law, and the public's health. *Administrative Law Review* 59: 121–75.

Gostin, Lawrence O., and M. Gregg Bloche. 2003. The politics of public health: A response to Epstein. *Perspectives in Biology and Medicine* 46: 160–75.

Gostin, Lawrence O., Jo Ivey Boufford, and Rose Marie Martinez. 2004. The future of the public's health: Vision, values, and strategies. *Health Affairs* 23 (4): 96–107.

Gostin, Lawrence O., and Catherine D. DeAngelis. 2007. Mandatory HPV vaccination: Public health vs. private wealth. *JAMA* 297: 1921–23.

Gostin, Lawrence O., and Kieran G. Gostin. 2009. A broader liberty: J.S. Mill, paternalism and the public's health. *Public Health* 123: 214–21.

Gostin, Lawrence O., James G. Hodge Jr., and Ronald O. Valdiserri. 2001. Informational privacy and the public's health: The model state public health privacy act. *American Journal of Public Health* 91: 1388–92.

Gostin, Lawrence O., and Gail H. Javitt. 2001. Health promotion and the First Amendment: Government control of the information environment. *Milbank Quarterly* 79: 547–78.

Gostin, Lawrence O., and Zita Lazzarini. 1995. Childhood immunization registries: A national review of public health information systems and the protection of privacy. *JAMA* 274: 1793–99.

———. 1997. *Human Rights and Public Health in the AIDS Pandemic.* New York: Oxford Univ. Press.

Gostin, Lawrence O., and Madison Powers. 2006. What does social justice require for the public's health? Public health ethics and policy imperatives. *Health Affairs* 25 (4): 1053–60.

Gostin, Lawrence O., and Allyn L. Taylor. 2008. Global health law: A definition and grand challenges. *Public Health Ethics* 1 (1): 53–63.

Government Accounting Office. 1991. *Highway Safety Motorcycle Helmet Laws Save Lives and Reduce Costs to Society.* Washington, DC: Government Accounting Office.

Grad, Frank. 2004. *Public Health Law Manual.* 3d ed. New York: American Public Health Association.

Graham, John D., Phaedra S. Corso, Jill M. Morris, Maria Segui-Gomez, and Milton C. Weinstein. 1998. Evaluating the cost-effectiveness of clinical and public health measures. *Annual Review of Public Health* 19: 125–52.

Grier, Sonya, and Carol A. Bryant. 2005. Social marketing in public health. *Annual Review of Public Health* 26: 319–39.

Griffin, Robert, Kathleen Stratton, and Rosemary Chalk. 2004. Childhood vaccine finance and safety issues. *Health Affairs* 23 (5): 98–111.

Gruskin, Sofia, ed. 2005. *Perspectives on Health and Human Rights.* New York: Routledge.

Gutlove, Paula, and Gordon Thompson. 2003. Human security: Expanding the scope of public health. *Medicine, Conflict, & Survival* 19: 17–34.

Guttman, Nurit, and William Harris Ressler. 2001. On being responsible: Ethical issues in appeals to personal responsibility in health campaigns. *Journal of Health Communication* 6: 117–36.

Halliday, Jane L., Veronica R. Collins, Mary Anne Aitkan, Martin P.M. Richards, and Craig A. Olsson. 2004. Genetics and public health—evolution or revolution? *Journal of Epidemiology and Community Health* 58: 894–99.

Handl, Gunter. 1991. Environmental security and global change: The challenge of international law. In *Environmental Protection and International Law*, 59–87. London: Graham & Trotman/Martinus Nijhoff.

Hardin, Garrett. 1968. The tragedy of the commons. *Science* 162: 1234–48.

Hawkes, Corinna. 2007. Regulating food marketing to young people worldwide: Trends and policy drivers. *American Journal of Public Health* 97: 1962–73.

Heinzerling, Lisa. 1998a. The perils of precision. *Environmental Forum,* September/October: 38–43.

———. 1998b. Regulatory costs of mythic proportions. *Yale Law Journal* 107: 1981–2070.

———. 2006. Doubting *Daubert. Journal of Law and Policy* 14: 65–83.

———. 2008. Climate change, human health, and the post-precautionary principle. *Georgetown Law Journal* 96: 445–60.

Henderson, Donald A. 1999. The looming threat of bioterrorism. *Science* 283: 1279–82.

Henderson, Donald A., Thomas V. Inglesby, John G. Bartlett, Michael S. Ascher, Edward Eitzen Jr., P. B. Jahrling, Jerome Hauer, M. Layton, Joseph McDade, Michael T. Osterholm, Tara O'Toole, Gerald Parker, Trisk M. Perl, Philip K. Russel, and Keven Tonat. 1999. Smallpox as a biological weapon: Medical and public health management. *JAMA* 281: 2127-37.

Heymann, David L. 2003. The evolving infectious disease threat: Implications for national and global security. *Journal of Human Development* 4: 191–207.

Hill, James O., Holly R. Wyatt, George W. Reed, and John C. Peters. 2003. Obesity and the environment: Where do we go from here? *Science* 299: 853–55.

Hodge, James G., Jr. 1997. Implementing modern public health goals through government: An examination of new federalism and public health law. *Journal of Contemporary Health Law and Policy* 14: 93–126.

———. 1998. The role of new federalism and public health law. *Journal of Law and Health* 12: 309–57.

———. 2005. An enhanced approach to distinguishing public health practice from human subjects research. *Journal of Law, Medicine & Ethics* 33: 125–40.

Hodge, James, and Lawrence O. Gostin. 2002. School vaccination requirements: Historical, social, and legal perspectives. *Kentucky Law Journal* 90: 831–90.

Hodge, James, Amy Pulver, Matthew Hogben, Dhrubajyoti Bhattacharya, and Erin Fuse Brown. 2008. Expedited partner therapy for sexually transmitted diseases: Assessing the legal environment. *American Journal of Public Health* 98: 238–43.

Hogben, Matthew. 2007. Partner notification for sexually transmitted diseases. *Clinical Infectious Diseases* 44 (Supp. 3): S160–S174.

Hollis, Aidan, and Thomas Pogge. 2008. *The Health Impact Fund: Making New Medicines Accessible for All.* www.yale.edu/macmillan/igh/hif_book .pdf.

Holmes, O. W., Jr. 1881. *The Common Law.* Boston: Little, Brown.

Houston, David J., and Lilliard E. Richardson Jr. 2007. Motorcycle safety and the repeal of universal helmet laws. *American Journal of Public Health* 97: 2063–69.

Huber, Peter W. 1991. *Galileo's Revenge: Junk Science in the Courtroom.* New York: Basic Books.

Institute of Medicine. 1988. *The Future of Public Health.* Washington, DC: National Academies Press.

———. 1994. *Growing Up Tobacco Free: Preventing Nicotine Addiction in Children and Youths.* Washington, DC: National Academies Press.

———. 1999. *Reducing the Odds: Preventing Perinatal Transmission of HIV in the United States.* Washington, DC: National Academies Press.

———. 2003. *The Future of the Public's Health in the 21st Century.* Washington, DC: National Academies Press.

———. 2004. *Immunization and Safety Review: Vaccines and Autism.* Washington, DC: National Academies Press.

———. 2005a. *Food Marketing to Children: Threat or Opportunity?* Washington, DC: National Academies Press.

———. 2005b. *Implications of Genomics for Public Health. Workshop Summary.* Washington, DC: National Academies Press.

———. 2005c. *The Smallpox Vaccination Program: Public Health in an Age of Terrorism.* Washington, DC: National Academies Press.

International Health Regulations (IHR). 2005. *Revision of the International Health Regulations,* WHO Doc. WHA58.3. May 23. www.who.int/ihr/en.

Jacobson, Peter D., and Wendy E. Parmet. 2007. A new era of unapproved drugs: The case of *Abigail Alliance v. Von Eschenbach. JAMA* 297: 205–8.

Jacobson, Peter D., and Soheil Soliman. 2002. Litigation as public health policy: Theory or reality? *Journal of Law, Medicine & Ethics* 30: 224–38.

Jeffery, Robert W., and Jennifer Utter. 2003. The changing environment and population obesity in the United States. *Obesity* 11 (Supp.): 12S–22S.

Jennings, Bruce. 2009. Public health and liberty: Beyond the Millian paradigm. *Public Health Ethics* 2 (2): 123–34.

Johnson, Niall P. A. S., and Juergen Mueller. 2002. Updating the accounts: Global mortality of the 1918–1920 "Spanish" influenza pandemic. *Bulletin of the History of Medicine* 76: 105–15.

Jones, Marian Moser, and Ronald Bayer. 2007. Paternalism and its discontents: Motorcycle helmet laws, libertarian values, and public health. *American Journal of Public Health* 97: 208–17.

Kass, Nancy E. 2000. A change in approach to prenatal HIV screening. *American Journal of Public Health* 90: 1026–27.

———. 2001. An ethics framework for public health. *American Journal of Public Health* 91: 1776–82.

———. 2004. Public health ethics: From foundations and frameworks to injustice and global public health. *Journal of Law Medicine and Ethics* 32: 232–42.

Kaul, Inge, Isabelle Grunberg, and Marc A. Stern. 1999. Defining global public goods. In *Global Public Goods: International Cooperation in the 21st Century,* ed. Inge Kaul, Isabelle Grunberg, and Marc A. Stern, 2–20. New York: Oxford Univ. Press

Kawachi, Ichiro, and Lisa F. Berkman. 2000. Social cohesion, social capital and health. In *Social Epidemiology,* ed. Lisa F. Berkman and Ichiro Kawachi, 174–90. Oxford: Oxford Univ. Press.

Kessel, Reuben A. 1970. The A.M.A. and the supply of physicians. *Law & Contemporary Problems* 35: 267–83.

Kesselheim, Aaron S., and Jerry Avon. 2006. Biomedical patents and the public's health: Is there a role for eminent domain? *JAMA* 295: 434–37.

Kessler, David A., and David C. Vladeck. 2008. A critical examination of the FDA's efforts to preempt failure-to-warn claims. *Georgetown Law Journal* 96: 461–95.

Khoury, Muin J., Marta Gwinn, Wylie Burke, Scott Bowen, and Ron Zimmern. 2007. Will genomics widen or help heal the schism between medicine and public health? *American Journal of Preventive Medicine* 33: 310–17.

King, Patricia A. 2004. Reflections on race and bioethics in the United States. *Health Matrix* 14: 149–53.

Koplow, David A. 2004. *Smallpox: The Fight to Eradicate a Global Source.* Berkley: Univ. of California Press.

Kotalik, Jaro. 2005. Preparing for an influenza pandemic: Ethical issues. *Bioethics* 19: 422–31.

Lasso, Jose Ayala, and Peter Piot. 1997. Foreword to *Human Rights and Public Health in the AIDS Pandemic,* by Lawrence O. Gostin and Zita Lazzarini, vii–viii. New York: Oxford Univ. Press.

Leavitt, Judith Walzer. 1997. *Typhoid Mary.* Boston: Beacon Press.

Legarre, Santiago. 2007. The historical background of the police power. *University of Pennsylvania Journal of Constitutional Law* 9: 745–96.

Leggiadro, Robert J. 2000. The threat of biological terrorism: A public health and infection control reality. *Infection Control and Hospital Epidemiology* 21: 53–56.

Lewin, Nancy L., Jon S. Vernick, Peter L. Beilenson, Julie S. Mair, Melisa M. Lindamood, Stephen P. Teret, Daniel W. Webster, et al. 2005. The Baltimore Youth Ammunition Initiative: A model application of local public health authority in preventing gun violence. *American Journal of Public Health* 95: 762–65.

Lobel, Orly. 2004. The renew deal: The fall of regulation and the rise of governance in contemporary legal thought. *Minnesota Law Review* 89: 262–390.

Loftin, Colin, David McDowall, Brian Wiersema, and Talbert J. Cottey. 1991. Effects of restrictive licensing of handguns on homicide and suicide in the District of Columbia. *New England Journal of Medicine* 325: 1615–20.

Ludwig, David S. 2007. Childhood obesity—the shape of things to come. *New England Journal of Medicine* 357: 2325–27.

Lynch, John, George Davey Smith, Sam Harper, Marianne Hillemeier, Nancy Ross, George A. Kaplan, and Michael Wolfson. 2004. Is income inequality a determinant of population health? Part 1: A systematic review. *Milbank Quarterly* 82: 5–95.

MacKenzie, Debora. 1998. Bioarmageddon. *New Scientist* 159: 42–46.

Magnusson, Roger S. 2007. Non-communicable diseases and global health governance: Enhancing global processes to improve health development.

Globalization & Health 3 (2). www.globalizationandhealth.com/content/
3/1/2.

Malone, Kevin, and Alan Hinman. 2007. Vaccination mandates: The public
health imperative and individual rights. In *Law in Public Health in Practice,*
ed. Richard A. Goodman, Richard E. Hoffman, Wilfredo Lopez, Gene W.
Matthews, Mark A. Rothstein, and Karen L. Foster, 338–60. 2d ed. Oxford:
Oxford Univ. Press.

Mann, Jonathan M. 1997. Medicine and public health, ethics, and human
rights. *Hastings Center Report* 27 (3): 6–13.

Mann, Jonathan M., Lawrence O. Gostin, Sofia Gruskin, Troyen Brennan,
Zita Lazzarini, and Harvey Fineberg. 1994. Health and human rights. *Journal of Health and Human Rights* 1: 6–23.

Mariner, Wendy K., George J. Annas, and Leonard H. Glantz. 2005. *Jacobson
v. Massachusetts:* It's not your great-great-grandfather's public health law.
American Journal of Public Health 95: 581–90.

Markel, Howard, Lawrence O. Gostin, and David P. Fidler. 2007. Extensively
drug-resistant tuberculosis: An isolation order, public health powers, and a
global crisis. *JAMA* 298: 83–86.

Marmot, Michael. 2004. *The Status Syndrome: How Social Standing Affects
Our Health and Longevity.* New York: Times Books.

———. 2006. Status syndrome: A challenge to medicine. *JAMA* 295: 1304–7.

Marmot, Michael, on Behalf of the Commission on Social Determinants of
Health. 2007. Achieving health equity: From root causes to fair outcomes.
Lancet 370: 1153–63.

Marmot, Michael, and Richard G. Wilkinson, eds. 1999. *Social Determinants
of Health.* Oxford: Oxford Univ. Press.

Martin, Robyn, and Linda Johnson, eds. 2001. *Law and the Public Dimension
of Health.* London: Cavendish Publishing.

Masenior, Nicole Franck, and Chris Beyrer. 2007. The US anti-prostitution
pledge: First Amendment challenges and public health priorities. *Public
Library of Science Medicine* 4: e207. Available at www.plosmedicine.org.

Mastroianni, Anna C., and Jeffrey P. Kahn. 2002. Risk and responsibility:
Ethics, *Grimes v. Kennedy Krieger,* and public health research involving
children. *American Journal of Public Health* 92: 1073–76.

Mather, Lynn. 1998. Theorizing about trial courts: Lawyers, policymaking,
and tobacco litigation. *Law and Social Inquiry* 23: 897–940.

May, Thomas. 2005. Funding agendas: Has bioterror defense been over-prioritized? *American Journal of Bioethics* 5 (4): 34–44.

May, Thomas, and Ross D. Silverman. 2005. Free riding, fairness and the
rights of minority groups in exemption from mandatory childhood vaccination. *Human Vaccines* 1 (1): 12–15.

Maziak, W., K. D. Ward, and M. B. Stockton. 2007. Childhood obesity: Are we
missing the big picture? *Obesity Reviews* 9 (1): 35–42.

McCann, Michael W. 1992. Reform litigation on trial. *Law and Social Inquiry*
17: 715–43.

McGarity, Thomas O. 2007. Frankenfood free: Consumer sovereignty, federal
regulation, and industry control in marketing and choosing foods in the

United States. In *Labeling Genetically Modified Food: The Philosophical and Legal Debate,* ed. Paul Weirich, 128–50. Oxford: Oxford Univ. Press.

McGinnis, J. Michael, and William H. Foege. 1993. Actual causes of death in the United States. *JAMA* 270: 2207–12.

McMichael, Anthony, and Rosalie Woodruff. 2004. Climate change and risk to health: The risk is complex, and more than a sum of risks due to individual climatic factors. *British Medical Journal* 329: 1416–17.

McMichael, Anthony J., Rosalie E. Woodruff, and Simon Hales. 2006. Climate change and human health: Present and future risks. *Lancet* 367: 859–65.

Meacham, Katherine R., and Jo Ann T. Croom. 2004. Tricksters, *The Plague,* and mirrors: Biotechnology, bioterrorism, and justice. In *Cross-Cultural Biotechnology: A Reader,* ed. Michael C. Brannigan, 177–92. Lanham, MD: Rowman & Littlefield.

Mello, Michelle, David Studdert, and Troyen A. Brennan. 2006. Obesity—the new frontier of health law. *New England Journal of Medicine* 354: 2601–10.

Meyer, Ilan H., and Sharon Schwartz. 2000. Social issues as public health: Promise and peril. *American Journal of Public Health* 90: 1189–91.

Mill, John Stuart. 1961. *The Philosophy of John Stuart Mill,* ed. Marshall Cohen. New York: Random House.

Mokdad, Ali H., James S. Marks, Donna F. Stroup, and Julie L. Gerberding. 2004. Actual causes of death in the United States, 2000. *JAMA* 291: 1238–45.

Morrall, John. 1986. A review of the record. *Regulation* 10: 25–34.

Musto, David F. 1986. Quarantine and the problem of AIDS. *Milbank Quarterly* 64 (Supp. I): 97–117.

Narayan, Raj K. 1987. How many deaths will it take? *Texas Medicine* 83: 5–6.

National Commission for the Protection of Human Subjects of Biomedical and Behavioral Research. 1978. *Belmont Report: Ethical Principles and Guidelines for the Protection of Human Subjects of Research.* Washington, DC: Government Printing Office.

National Restaurant Association. 2006. Model commonsense consumption act. www.restaurant.org/government/state/nutrition/resources/nra_200602_modelbilltext.doc.

Nestle, Marion. 2006. Food marketing and childhood obesity—a matter of policy. *New England Journal of Medicine* 354: 2527–29.

New York City Department of Health and Mental Hygiene. 2005. Board of Health, Notice of Intention to Amend Article 13 of the New York City Health Code, Notice of Public Hearing. http://home2.nyc.gov/html/doh/downloads/pdf/public/notice-intention-art-13.pdf.

Novak, William J. 1993. Public economy and the well-ordered market: Law and economic regulation in 19th-century America. *Law and Social Inquiry* 18: 1–32.

———. 1996. Governance, police, and American liberal mythology. In *The*

People's Welfare: Law and Regulation in Nineteenth-Century America, 1–18. Chapel Hill: Univ. of North Carolina Press.

Office of Homeland Security. 2002. *The National Strategy for Homeland Security.* Washington, DC: Office of Homeland Security.

Offit, Paul A. 2007. Fatal exemption. *Wall Street Journal,* January 20.

———. 2008. Vaccines and autism revisited—the Hanna Poling case. *New England Journal of Medicine* 358: 2089–91.

Ogden, Cynthia L., Margaret D. Carroll, Lester R. Curtin, Margaret A. McDowell, Carolyn J. Tabak, and Katherine M. Flegal. 2006. Prevalence of overweight and obesity in the United States, 1999–2004. *JAMA* 295: 1549–55.

Omer, Saad B., William K. Y. Pan, Neal A. Halsey, Shannon Stokley, Lawrence H. Moulton, Ann Marie Navar, Matthew Pierce, and Daniel A. Salmon. 2006. Nonmedical exemptions to school immunization requirements: Secular trends and association of state policies with pertussis incidence. *JAMA* 296: 1757–63.

O'Neill, Onora. 2004. Informed consent and public health. *Philosophical Transactions of the Royal Society of London* 359: 1133–36.

O'Toole, Tara. 2001. The problem with biological weapons: The next steps for the nation. *Public Health Reports* 116: 109.

Oxford Health Alliance. 2008. Sydney Resolution. Available at www.oxha .org/knowledge/publications/.

Ozonoff, David. 2005. Legal causation and responsibility for causing harm. *American Journal of Public Health* 95 (S1): S35–S38.

Paine, Thomas. 1945. Common sense [1776]. In *The Complete Writings of Thomas Paine,* ed. Philip S. Foner, 1–45. New York: Citadel.

Papas, Mia A., Anthony J. Alberg, Reid Ewing, Kathy J. Helzlsouer, Tiffany L. Gary, and Ann. C. Klassen. 2007. The built environment and obesity. *Epidemiologic Reviews* 29: 129–43.

Parmet, Wendy E. 1992. Health care and the Constitution: Public health and the role of the state in the Framing Era. *Hastings Constitutional Law Quarterly* 20: 267–335.

———. 1996. From *Slaughter-House* to *Lochner:* The rise and fall of the constitutionalization of public health. *American Journal of Legal History* 40: 476–503.

———. 2007. Legal power and legal rights—isolation and quarantine in the case of drug-resistant tuberculosis. *New England Journal of Medicine* 357: 433–35.

———. 2009. *Populations, Public Health, and the Law.* Washington, DC: Georgetown Univ. Press.

Parmet, Wendy E., and Richard A. Daynard. 2000. The new public health litigation. *Annual Review of Public Health* 21: 437–54.

Parmet, Wendy E., Richard A. Goodman, and Amy Farber. 2005. Individual rights versus the public's health—100 years after *Jacobson v. Massachusetts. New England Journal of Medicine* 352: 652–54.

Parmet, Wendy E., and Jason A. Smith. 2006. Free speech and public health: A population-based approach to the First Amendment. *Loyola of Los Angeles Law Review* 39: 363–446.

Pearce, Neil, and George Davey Smith. 2003. Is social capital the key to inequalities in health? *American Journal of Public Health* 93: 122–29.

Perdue, Wendy C. 2008. Obesity, poverty, and the built environment: Challenges and opportunity. *Georgetown Journal on Poverty Law & Policy* 15: 821–32.

Perdue, Wendy Collins, Lesley A. Stone, and Lawrence O. Gostin. 2003. The built environment and its relationship to the public's health: The legal framework. *American Journal of Public Health* 93: 1390–94.

Perkins, Richard J. 1981. Perspective on the public good. *American Journal of Public Health* 71: 294–95.

Porter, Margaret J. 1997. The *Lohr* decision: FDA perspective and position. *Food and Drug Law Journal* 52: 7–11.

Powers, Madison, and Ruth Faden. 2000. Inequalities in health, inequalities in health care: Four generations of discussion about justice and cost-effectiveness analysis. *Kennedy Institute of Ethics Journal* 10: 109–27.

————. 2006. *Social Justice: The Moral Foundations of Public Health and Health Policy.* New York: Oxford Univ. Press.

Prentice, Andrew M. 2006. The emerging epidemic of obesity in developing countries. *International Journal of Epidemiology* 35: 93–99.

Putnam, Robert D. 2000. Health and happiness. In *Bowling Alone: The Collapse and Revival of American Community,* 326–35. New York: Simon & Schuster.

Rabin, Robert. 1992. A socio-legal history of the tobacco tort litigation. *Stanford Law Review* 44: 853–78.

Rawls, John. 1999. *A Theory of Justice.* Rev. ed. Cambridge, MA: Belknap Press of Harvard Univ. Press.

Resnick, David B. 2000. Ethical dilemmas in communicating health information to the public. *Health Policy* 55: 129–49.

Reynolds, Christopher, with Genevieve Howse. 2004. *Public Health: Law and Regulation.* Sydney: Federation Press.

Rodricks, Joseph V. 1994. Risk assessment, the environment, and public health. *Environmental Health Perspectives* 102: 258–64.

Roemer, Ruth, Allyn Taylor, and Jean Lariviere. 2005. Origins of the WHO Framework Convention on Tobacco Control. *American Journal of Public Health* 95: 936–38.

Rose, Geoffrey. 1981. Strategy of prevention: Lessons from cardiovascular disease. *British Journal of Medicine* 282: 1847–51.

————. 1985. Sick individuals and sick populations. *International Journal of Epidemiology* 14: 32–38.

Rosenbaum, Sara, and Taylor Burke. 2003. *Lawrence v. Texas:* Implications for public health policy and practice. *Public Health Reports* 118: 559–61.

Rosenberg, Gerald N. 1991. *The Hollow Hope: Can Courts Bring About Social Change?* Chicago: Univ. of Chicago Press.

Rothstein, Mark A. 2002. Rethinking the meaning of public health. *Journal of Law, Medicine & Ethics* 30: 144–49.

Roush, Sandra, Guthrie Birkhead, Denise Koo, Angela Cobb, and David Fleming. 1999. Mandatory reporting of diseases and conditions by health care providers and laboratories. *JAMA* 282: 164–70.

SafeMinds [Sensible Action for Ending Mercury-Induced Neurological Disorders]. 2004. SafeMinds Analysis of IOM Report: The Failures, the Flaws and Conflicts of Interest. Press release, May 19. www.safeminds.org/news/pressroom/press_releases/040519-PR11.pdf.

Sage, William M. 1999. Regulating through information: Disclosure laws and American health care. *Columbia Law Review* 100: 1701–1829.

Salmon, Daniel A., Michael Haber, Eugene J. Gangarosa, Lynelle Phillips, Natalie J. Smith, and Robert T. Chen. 1999. Health consequences of religious and philosophical exemptions from immunization laws: Individual and societal risk of measles. *JAMA* 282: 47–53.

Salmon, Daniel A., and Saad B. Omer. 2006. Individual freedoms versus collective responsibility: Immunization decision-making in the face of occasionally competing values. *Emerging Themes in Epidemiology* 3: 13–15.

Salmon, Daniel A., Jason Sapsin, Stephen Teret, Richard Jacobs, Joseph Thompson, Kevin Ryan, and Neal Halsey. 2005. Public health and the politics of school immunization requirements. *American Journal of Public Health* 95: 778–83.

San Francisco Department of Public Health. 2006. Healthy Development Measurement Tool. www.thehdmt.org/tool.php.

Sankar, Pamela, and Jonathan Kahn. 2005. BiDil: Race medicine or race marketing? *Health Affairs* W5: 455–63.

Santora, Marc. 2006. Overhaul urged for laws on AIDS tests and data. *New York Times*, February 2.

Sapsin, Jason W., Theresa M. Thompson, Lesley Stone, and Katherine E. DeLand. 2003. International trade, law, and public health advocacy. *Journal of Law, Medicine & Ethics* 31: 546–56.

Savitt, Todd L. 1984. The education of black physicians at Shaw University, 1882–1918. In *Black Americans in North Carolina and the South*, ed. Jeffrey J. Crow and Flora J. Hatley, 680–715. Chapel Hill: Univ. of North Carolina Press.

Sciarrino, Alfred J. 2003. The grapes of wrath and the speckled monster (epidemics, biological terrorism, and the early legal history of two major defenses—quarantine and vaccination). *Journal of Medicine and Law* 7: 117–76.

Seidman, Louis M., and Mark V. Tushnet. 1996. *Remnants of Belief: Contemporary Constitutional Issues*. New York: Oxford Univ. Press.

Sekiguchi, Eugene, Albert H. Guay, L. Jackson Brown, and Thomas J. Spangler. 2005. Improving the oral health of Alaska Natives. *American Journal of Public Health* 95: 769–73.

Sen, Amartya. 2002. Why health equity? *Health Economics* 11: 659–66.

Sharkey, Catherine M. 2007. Federalism in action: FDA regulatory preemption in pharmaceutical cases in state versus federal courts. *Brooklyn Journal of Law and Policy* 15: 1013–48.

Sidel, Victor W., Robert M. Gould, and Hillel W. Cohen. 2002. Bioterrorism preparedness: Cooptation of public health? *Medicine & Global Survival* 7 (2): 82–88.

Silberschmidt, Gaudenz, Don Matheson, and Ilona Kickbusch. 2008. Creating a Committee C of the World Health Assembly. *Lancet* 371: 1483–86.

Silverman, Ross D. 2003. No more kidding around: Restructuring non-medical childhood immunization exemptions to ensure public health protection. *Annals of Health Law* 12 (2): 277–94.

Singer, Peter A., and Abdallah S. Daar. 2001. Harnessing genomics and biotechnology to improve global health equity. *Science* 294: 87–89.

Smith, Richard D., Halla Thorsteinsdóttir, Abdallah S. Daar, E. Richard Gold, and Peter A. Singer. 2004. Genomics knowledge and equity: A global public goods perspective of the patent system. *Bulletin of the World Health Organization* 82: 385–89.

Sobel, Richard. 2007. The HIPAA paradox: The privacy rule that's not. *Hastings Center Report* 37 (4): 40–50.

Stephenson, Kathryn. 2004. The quarantine war: The burning of the New York Marine Hospital in 1858. *Public Health Reports* 119: 79–92.

Stoddard, Thomas B., and Walter Rieman. 1990. AIDS and the rights of the individual: Toward a more sophisticated understanding of discrimination. *Milbank Quarterly* 8 (Supp. 1): 143–74.

Story, Mary, Karen M. Kaphingst, Ramona Robinson-O'Brien, and Karen Glanz. 2008. Creating healthy food and eating environments: Policy and environmental approaches. *Annual Review of Public Health* 29: 253–72.

Studdert, David, Michelle Mello, and Troyen Brennan. 2003. Medical monitoring for pharmaceutical injuries. *JAMA* 289: 889–94.

Sugarman, Stephen. 2002. Mixed results from recent United States tobacco litigation. *Tort Law Review* 10: 94–126. Available at www.law.berkeley .edu/faculty/sugarmans/#Tobacco.

Sugarman, Stephen, and Nirit Sandman. 2007. Fighting childhood obesity through performance-based regulation of the food industry. *Duke Law Review* 56: 1403–90.

Sunstein, Cass R. 1996. Health-health tradeoffs. *University of Chicago Law Review* 63: 1533–71.

———. 2006. *Chevron* step zero. *Virginia Law Review* 92: 187–249.

Tandy, Elizabeth C. 1923. Local quarantine and inoculation for smallpox in the American colonies. *American Journal of Public Health* 13: 810–13.

Taylor, Allyn L. 2004. Governing the globalization of public health. *Journal of Law, Medicine & Ethics* 32: 500–508.

Taylor, Allyn L., and Douglas W. Bettcher. 2000. WHO Framework Convention on Tobacco Control: A global "good" for public health. *Bulletin of the World Health Organization* 78: 920–29.

Teret, Stephen P. 1986. Litigating for the public health. *American Journal of Public Health* 76: 1027–29.

Thomas, James C., Michael Sage, Jack Dillenberg, and V. James Guillory. 2002. A code of ethics for public health. *American Journal of Public Health* 92: 1057–59.

Thorsteinsdóttir, Halla, Abdallah S. Daar, Richard D. Smith, and Peter A. Singer. 2003. Genomics—a global public good? *Lancet* 361: 891–92.

Trebilcock, Michael J., and Robert Howse. 2005. *The Regulation of International Trade.* 3d ed. New York: Routledge.

Tribe, Laurence. 1988. *American Constitutional Law.* 2d ed. Los Angeles: Foundation Press.

Tucker, Jonathan B. 2003. Biosecurity: Limiting terrorist access to deadly pathogens. *Peaceworks* 52: 5–49.

Turnock, Bernard J. 2001. *Public Health: What It Is and How It Works.* Gaithersburg, MD: Aspen.

Tussman, Joseph. 1960. *Obligations and the Body Politic.* New York: Oxford Univ. Press.

UNAIDS [Joint United Nations Programme on HIV/AIDS]. 2008. *Report on the Global AIDS Epidemic 2008.* UNAIDS/08.25E / JC1510E. www.unaids.org/en/KnowledgeCentre/HIVData/GlobalReport/2008/2008_Global_report.asp.

Union of Concerned Scientists. 2004a. *Scientific Integrity in Policy Making: Investigation of the Bush Administration's Abuse of Science.* www.ucsusa.org/assets/documents/scientific_integrity/rsi_final_fullreport_1.pdf.

———. 2004b. *Scientific Integrity in Policy Making: Further Investigation of the Bush Administration's Misuse of Science.* www.ucsusa.org/assets/documents/scientific_integrity/scientific_integrity_in_policy_making_july_2004_1.pdf.

United Nations Commission on Human Rights, Economic and Social Council. 2004. *Economic, Social and Cultural Rights: The Right of Everyone to the Highest Attainable Level of Physical and Mental Health. Report of the Special Rapporteur, Paul Hunt. Addendum: Mission to the World Trade Organization.* UN Doc. E/CN.4/2004/49/Add.1. www.unhchr.ch/Huridocda/Huridoca.nsf/e06a5300f90fa023802566870051 8ca4/5860d7d863239d82c1256e660056432a/$FILE/G0411390.pdf.

United Nations Committee on Economic, Social, and Cultural Rights. 2000. *The Right to the Highest Attainable Standard of Health,* General Comment 14. CESCR, E/C. 12/2000/4. Available at www.unhcr.org/refworld/docid/4538838do.html.

United Nations Secretary-General. 2005. *In Larger Freedom: Towards Development, Security, and Human Rights for All.* UN Doc. A/59/2005. www.un.org/largerfreedom.

U.S. Congress. House. Committee on Government Reform. Minority Staff Special Investigations Division. 2006. *Congressional Preemption of State Laws and Regulations* (Prepared for Representative Henry A. Waxman). Available at http://oversight.house.gov/story.asp?ID=1062.

U.S. Department of Health and Human Services. 1994. *Preventing Tobacco Use among Young People: A Report of the Surgeon General.* Atlanta: U.S. Department of Health and Human Services.

———. [2000a]. *Healthy People 2010.* Washington, DC: U.S. Department of Health and Human Services.

———. 2000b. *National Call to Promote Oral Health*. Rockville, MD: U.S. Department of Health and Human Services.

———. 2005a. *HHS Pandemic Influenza Plan*. Part 1, Appendix D: NVAC/ ACIP recommendations for prioritization of pandemic influenza vaccine and NVAC recommendations on pandemic antiviral drug use. www.hhs .gov/pandemicflu/plan/pdf/AppD.pdf.

———. 2005b. *HHS Pandemic Influenza Plan*. Part 2, Supplement 6: Vaccine distribution and use. www.hhs.gov/pandemicflu/plan/pdf/S06.pdf.

Uscher-Pines, Lori, Patrick S. Duggan, Joshua P. Garoon, Ruth A. Karron, and Ruth R. Faden. 2007. Planning for an influenza pandemic: Social justice and disadvantaged groups. *Hastings Center Report* 37 (4): 32–39.

Vastag, Brian. 2004. Obesity is now on everyone's plate. *JAMA* 291: 1186–88.

Vernick, Jon S., Lainie Rutkow, and Stephen P. Teret. 2007. Public health benefits of recent litigation against the tobacco industry. *JAMA* 298: 86–89.

Vernick, Jon S., Jason W. Sapsin, Stephen P. Teret, and Julie Samia Mair. 2004. How litigation can promote product safety. *Journal of Law, Medicine & Ethics* 32: 551–55.

Vladeck, David C. 2005. Preemption and regulatory failure. *Pepperdine Law Review* 33: 95–97.

———. 2006. Unreasonable delay, unreasonable intervention: The battle to force regulation of ethylene oxide. In *Administrative Law Stories*, ed. Peter L. Strauss, 191–226. New York: Foundation Press.

———. 2008. The FDA and deference lost: A self-inflicted wound or the product of a wounded agency? A response to Professor O'Reilly. *Cornell Law Review* 93: 981–1002.

Vladeck, David C., Gerald Weber, and Lawrence O. Gostin. 2004. Commercial speech and the public's health: Regulating advertisements of tobacco, alcohol, high fat foods and other potentially hazardous products. *Journal of Law, Medicine & Ethics* 32: S32–S34.

Walsh, Bryan. 2008. It's not just genetics. *Time*, June 23.

Walzer, Michael. 1983. *Spheres of Justice: A Defense of Pluralism and Equality*. New York: Basic Books.

Warner, Kenneth E. 2005. The role of research in international tobacco control. *American Journal of Public Health* 95: 976–84.

Watt, Holly. 2008. Doctors' group plans apology for racism. *Washington Post*, July 10.

Webster's Third New International Dictionary. 1986. Springfield, MA: Merriam-Webster.

Weeks, Elizabeth. 2006. After the catastrophe: Disaster relief for hospitals. *North Carolina Law Review* 85: 223–300.

———. 2007. Beyond compensation: Using torts to promote public health. *Journal of Health Care Law and Policy* 10: 27–59.

Weiss, Martin Meyer, Peter D. Weiss, and Joseph B. Weiss. 2007. Anthrax vaccine and public health policy. *American Journal of Public Health* 97: 1945–51.

Wendel, O.T., and Michael Glick. 2008. Lessons learned: Implications for workforce change. *Journal of the American Dental Association* 139: 232–34.

White House. 2002. *The National Security Strategy of the United States of America*. Washington, DC: The White House.

———. 2006. *The National Security Strategy of the United States of America*. Washington, DC: The White House.

Wilson, J. M. G., and F. Jungner. 1968. *Principles and Practice of Screening for Disease*. Public Health Papers 34. Geneva: World Health Organization.

Wilson, Richard, and E. A. C. Crouch. 1987. Risk assessment and comparisons: An introduction. *Science* 236: 267–70.

Wing, Kenneth R. 2003. *The Law and the Public's Health*. 6th ed. Chicago: Health Administration Press.

Winslow, Charles-Edward A. 1920. The untilled fields of public health. *Science* 51: 20–30.

Wintemute, Garen J. 2008. Guns, fear, the Constitution, and the public's health. *New England Journal of Medicine* 358: 1421–24.

Wintour, Patrick, and Colin Blackstock. 2004. Let the poor smoke, says health secretary. *Guardian,* June 9.

World Bank. 1999. *Curbing the Epidemic: Governments and the Economics of Tobacco Control*. Washington, DC: World Bank.

World Health Organization. 1946. Constitution of the World Health Organization. 14 U.N.T.S. 185. www.who.int/governance/eb/who_constitution_en.pdf.

———. 2003a. *Climate Change and Human Health—Risks and Responses: Summary*. Geneva: World Health Organization.

———. 2003b. *World Health Report*. Geneva: World Health Organization.

———. 2009a. Global alert and response. Current WHO phase of pandemic alert. www.who.int/csr/disease/avian_influenza/phase/en/index.html.

———. 2009b. Global alert and response. Situation updates—pandemic (H1N1) 2009. www.who.int/csr/disease/swineflu/updates/en/index.html.

———. 2009c. Swine influenza. Statement by WHO director-general, Dr Margaret Chan, April 25. www.who.int/mediacentre/news/statements/2009/h1n1_20090425/en/index.html.

World Health Organization, Commission on Macroeconomics and Health. 2001, 2003. *Macroeconomics and Health: Investing in Health for Development*. Geneva: World Health Organization.

World Health Organization, Commission on the Social Determinants of Health. 2008. *Closing the Gap in a Generation: Health Equity through Action on the Social Determinants of Health*. Geneva: World Health Organization.

World Health Organization and World Trade Organization. 2002. *WTO Agreements & Public Health: A Joint Study by the WHO and WTO Secretariat*. Geneva: World Trade Organization/World Health Organization.

World Health Organization Global Task Force on XDR-TB. 2007. Control of XDR-TB: Update on progress since the Global XDR-TB Task Force Meeting, 9–10 October 2006. www.who.int/tb/xdr/globaltaskforce_update_feb07.pdf.

World Trade Organization. 2001. *European Communities—Measures Affecting Asbestos and Asbestos-Containing Products.* WT/DS135/AB/R. www.wto.org/english/tratop_E/dispu_e/cases_e/ds135_e.htm.

——— . 2007. *Brazil—Measures Affecting Imports of Retreaded Tyres.* T/DS332/AB/R. www.wto.org/english/tratop_E/dispu_e/cases_e/ds332_e.htm. http://docsonline.wto.org/DDFDocuments/t/WT/DS/332ABR.doc.

Yach, Derek. 1999. The tobacco-free initiative (TFI) responding to the globalization of tobacco consumption. Paper presented at Conference on Globalization: Perspectives, Trends and Impacts on Human Welfare. London School of Hygiene and Tropical Medicine (April 19).

Yach, Derek, Corinna Hawkes, C. Linn Gould, and Karen J. Hofman. 2004. The global burden of chronic diseases: Overcoming impediments to prevention and control. *JAMA* 291: 2616–22.

Yardley, William. 2005. After eminent domain victory, disputed project goes nowhere. *New York Times,* November 21.

Younger, Steve. 1987. Alcoholic beverage advertising on the airwaves: Alternatives to a ban on counteradvertising. *University of California Los Angeles Law Review* 34: 1139–93.

Table of Cases

Index

Italicized page numbers refer to an illustration.

About the Author

Lawrence O. Gostin, an internationally acclaimed scholar, is the Linda D. and Timothy J. O'Neill Professor of Global Health Law at the Georgetown University Law Center, where he directs the O'Neill Institute for National and Global Health Law. He is a professor at the Johns Hopkins Bloomberg School of Public Health and director of the Center for Law & the Public's Health—a Collaborating Center of the World Health Organization and the Centers for Disease Control and Prevention. In addition, he is Visiting Professor of Public Health (Faculty of Medical Sciences) and a research fellow (Centre for Socio-Legal Studies) at Oxford University. He is the health law and ethics editor of the *Journal of the American Medical Association* and also serves as a contributing writer and columnist.

Professor Gostin has led major law reform initiatives in the United States, including the drafting of the Model Emergency Health Powers Act (MEHPA), intended to combat bioterrorism in the wake of the anthrax attacks in 2001, and the "Turning Point" Model State Public Health Act.

Professor Gostin, an elected lifetime member of the Institute of Medicine (IOM)/National Academy of Sciences, serves on the Board on Health Sciences Policy and the Committee on Science, Technology, and Law. He has also served as the chair of four IOM committees.

The IOM awarded Professor Gostin the Adam Yarmolinsky Medal for distinguished service in furthering its mission of science and health. The Public Health Law Association awarded him the Distinguished

Lifetime Achievement Award "in recognition of a career devoted to using law to improve the public's health." In the United Kingdom, the Royal Society of Public Health designated Professor Gostin an honorary fellow; and for his work on human rights, he received the Rosemary Delbridge Memorial Award from the National Consumer Council, given to the person "who has most influenced Parliament and government to act for the welfare of society." He also received the Key to Tohoko University (Japan) for distinguished contributions to human rights in mental health. He holds honorary degrees from Cardiff University (Wales) and the State University of New York.

Text:	10/13 Sabon
Display:	Sabon
Compositor:	BookMatters, Berkeley
Printer:	Sheridan Books, Inc.